Radiology of Iatrogenic Disorders

Series Editor:
Morton A. Meyers, M.D.

Also in this series

Iatrogenic Gastrointestinal Complications

Morton A. Meyers, M.D.
Professor and Chairman
Department of Radiology
School of Medicine
State University of New York at Stony Brook

Gary G. Ghahremani, M.D.
Professor and Chairman
Department of Diagnostic Radiology
Evanston Hospital-Northwestern University

With 587 Illustrations

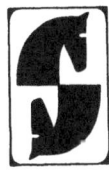

Springer-Verlag
New York Heidelberg Berlin

Series Editor

Morton A. Meyers, M.D.
Professor and Chairman
Department of Radiology
School of Medicine
State University of New York at Stony Brook
Long Island, New York 11794 U.S.A.

Volume Editors

Morton A. Meyers, M.D.

Gary G. Ghahremani, M.D.
Professor and Chairman
Department of Diagnostic Radiology
Evanston Hospital-Northwestern University
Evanston, Illinois 60611 U.S.A.

Library of Congress Cataloging in Publication Data
Main entry under title:
Iatrogenic gastrointestinal complications.
    (Radiology of iatrogenic disorders)
    Bibliography: p.
    Includes index.
    1. Gastrointestinal system—Diseases.
2. Iatrogenic diseases. I. Meyers, Morton A.
II. Ghahremani, Gary G. III. Series. [DNLM:
1. Gastrointestinal system—Radiography. 2. Gastro-
intestinal diseases—Complications. 3. Iatrogenic
disease. 4. Postoperative complications. W1
RA354M v. 1 / WI 100 I12]
RC802.I18   617′.4301   80-27150

© 1981 by Springer-Verlag New York Inc.
Softcover reprint of the hardcover 1st edition 1981

9 8 7 6 5 4 3 2 1

ISBN-13: 978-1-4612-5855-1   e-ISBN-13: 978-1-4612-5853-7
DOI: 10.1007/978-1-4612-5853-7

Contents

Dedicated to our wives
Bea and Zohreh
for their love, patience, and encouragement,
and to our children
Richard and Amy Meyers
Lilly and Susan Ghahremani

Series Editor's Foreword

The purpose of this series of volumes is to present a comprehensive view of the complications that result from the use of acceptable diagnostic and therapeutic procedures. Individual volumes will deal with iatrogenic complications involving (1) the alimentary system, (2) the urinary system, (3) the respiratory and cardiac systems, (4) the skeletal system and (5) the pediatric patient.

The term *iatrogenic*, derived from two Greek words, means physician-induced. Originally, it applied only to psychiatric disorders generated in the patient by autosuggestion, based on misinterpretation of the doctor's attitude and comments. As clinically used, it now pertains to the inadvertent side-effects and complications created in the course of diagnosis and treatment. The classic categories of disease have included: (1) congenital and developmental, (2) traumatic, (3) infectious and inflammatory, (4) metabolic, (5) neoplastic, and (6) degenerative. To these must be added, however, iatrogenic disorders—a major, although generally unacknowledged, source of illness. While great advances in medical care in both diagnosis and therapy have been accomplished in the past few decades, many are at times associated with certain side-effects and risks which may result in distress equal to or greater than the basic condition. Iatrogenic complications, which may be referred to as "diseases of medical progress," have become a new dimension in the causation of human disease.

A highly accurate index of the overall incidence of iatrogenic illnesses is difficult to establish, but there is little doubt that it approaches epidemic proportions in certain instances. The literature indicates that paramount causes include drugs and hospital-associated risks:

• Every year in the United States, up to one and a half million people—between 3 and 5 percent of all hospital admissions—are admitted primarily because of drug reactions. Once in the hospital, between 18 and 30 percent of all patients have a drug reaction. The length of their stay is about doubled as a result[1-3].

• In one study of a general medical unit over a twelve-month period, one-quarter of the 67 deaths in the unit were due to adverse drug reactions[3]. In acutely ill hospitalized patients, the drug-related death rate has been recently reported to be nearly one per thousand[4].

• Hospital-acquired infections occur in about one in 20 patients and there is approximately 25 percent excess mortality among patients with nosocomial bloodstream infections. About one-third of all infections seen in hospital practice are nosocomial in origin[5]. The incidence of postoperative wound infections is about 7.4 percent[6].

• It has been reported that one out of every five patients admitted to the medical service of a typical university teaching hospital suffers an iatrogenic episode, which is classified as moderate or severe in 40 percent. Over one-fourth of the episodes result from diagnostic and therapeutic procedures[7].

• Of all patients admitted to a multidisciplinary intensive care unit in one recent study[8], over 12 percent were admitted because of iatrogenic disease. Potentially avoidable therapeutic and technical errors accounted for half of these; the remaining adverse reactions that were determined to be unpreventable represent the risk-benefit ratio of a treatment compared with the natural history of the illness. Furthermore, once in a medical-surgical intensive care unit, patients are subject to often harmful adverse occurrences[9].

• Ten percent of hospital deaths are associated with a diagnostic or therapeutic procedure which is considered a contributing, precipitating or primary cause of obitus[10].

This series is not intended to support or encourage any concept of diagnostic or therapeutic nihilism. Rather, it is intended to assess and detail the broad spectrum of the mechanisms and effects of complications experienced in order to further refine clinical practice. Undue conservatism would effectively prohibit the meaningful application of any diagnostic or therapeutic method, virtually any of which carries a potential risk to the patient. Many inherent complications of medical and surgical techniques can be controlled only to an irreducible minimum, despite the exercise of utmost care and skill. In this series, areas of practical clinical concern are addressed rather than topics of pure academic interest. Radiologic documentation is often critical to uncover or confirm the presence and to evaluate the extent of many iatrogenic complications. The large number of illustrations used in each volume attest to the aim of fully employing the power of visual instruction.

Oscar Wilde's wry statement that "experience is the name men give to their mistakes" is beneficial only if physicians continue to be open-minded and to learn from each other. It is a medical axiom that advances introduce new problems which, in turn, generate solutions and further advances. Lewis Thomas[11] affirms that "Mistakes are at the very base of human thought . . . What is needed, for progress to be made, is the move based on the error." This series is designed in the hope that iatrogenic illnesses may be minimized, or appropriately anticipated and promptly recognized and managed, so that the prime injunction of clinical medicine can be further fulfilled: "Physician, do no harm."

Morton A. Meyers, M.D.

References

1. Wade N: Drug regulation: FDA replies to charges by economists and industry. Science 179:775–777, 1973
2. Seidl LG, Thornton GF, Smith JW, et al: Studies on the epidemiology of adverse drug reactions. III. Reaction in patients on a general medical service. Bull Johns Hopk Hosp 119:299–315, 1966
3. Ogilvie RI, Reudy J: Adverse drug reactions during hospitalization. Canad Med Assn J 97:1450–1457, 1967
4. Porter J, Jick H: Drug-related deaths among medical inpatients. JAMA 237 No 9:879–881, 1977
5. Hospital Infections. Bennett John V., Brachman Philip S. (eds). Little, Brown and Company, Boston, 1979
6. Altemeier WA: Postsurgical infections. Antibiotics Chemother 21:11–21, 1976
7. McLamb JT, Huntley RR: The hazards of hospitalization. Southern Med J 60:469–472, 1967
8. Trunet P, LeGall J-P, Lhoste F, et al: The role of iatrogenic disease in admissions to intensive care. JAMA 244:2617–2620, 1980
9. Abramson N, Ward K, Grenvik A, et al: Adverse occurrences in intensive care units. JAMA 244:1582–1584, 1980
10. Schimmel EM: The hazards of hospitalization. Ann Intern Med 60:100–116, 1964
11. Thomas L: The Medusa and the Snail. The Viking Press, New York, 1979

Preface

Nearly four thousand years ago Hammurabi's code of practice not only made the payment for medical care dependent upon successful recovery of the patient, but worse yet, it imposed harsh reprisals for operative mishaps. This law of retribution for failure to cure fortunately was not enforced beyond a brief period in Babylonian history. Advancements in medicine have been based upon triumphs and oversights, both of which have contributed toward strengthening the foundation of our current knowledge. Just as D. H. Lawrence stated that the greatest secret of Victorian England was sex—in the sense that many more people were participating in it than openly discussing it—so it might be said that the understated effects of many advances in the diagnosis and treatment of digestive disorders are iatrogenic complications.

In this context, the present volume is aimed to review the broad spectrum of clinical gastrointestinal disorders caused by application of modern diagnostic and therapeutic methods. The purpose is not to emphasize dangers but rather to provide a perspective of the underlying mechanisms and clinical presentations of iatrogenic gastrointestinal complications. Guidelines and characteristic features are established which help in their anticipation, prompt recognition, and management. Every physician will do well by looking ahead for such often inevitable problems, and using the past experiences for guidance in their solution.

The first chapter includes a comprehensive review of drug-induced gastrointestinal disorders, probably the most common iatrogenic problem in medicine today. Voltaire had once stated that "A physician is one who pours drugs of which he knows little into a body of which he knows less." The text and references listed in the first chapter challenge that widely quoted opinion, clearly reflecting the depth of current medical knowledge on this subject.

Gastrointestinal endoscopy and intubation have become particularly valuable methods in the diagnosis and management of digestive disorders. Their widespread use has led to an increasing frequency of the complications described in Chapters 2 and 3. The iatrogenic problems associated with the performance of radiologic procedures are reviewed in detail in Chapter 4.

By far the largest portion of this book, Chapters 5 through 11, is devoted to the complications of surgery. The coverage of this subject, which carries significant morbidity and mortality, has been made relatively extensive for two reasons: to permit a review of postoperative anatomy which is a prerequisite for accurate diagnosis of abnormalities superimposed on the distorted gastrointestinal landmarks; and to detail a wide range of surgical complications even though some perhaps elude a clear definition in terms of being iatrogenic versus inherent risk of operation.

The final section in this volume, Chapter 12, deals with gastrointestinal sequelae of radiation therapy. Awareness of their pathophysiology and manifestations should become even more important in the future considering the apparent increase in the incidence of cancer and the number of patients treated with this modality.

Both the text and the accompanying illustrations emphasize the critical role of diagnostic imaging in the evaluation of iatrogenic gastrointestinal disorders. Their correct diagnosis and management depend upon close consultation between the clinician and radiologist.

Morton A. Meyers, M.D.
Gary G. Ghahremani, M.D.

Contributors

Morton A. Meyers, M.D., F.A.C.R.
Professor and Chairman, Department of Radiology, State University
of New York School of Medicine, Stony Brook, New York, U.S.A.
Chapters 2, 9, 10, 11

Gary G. Ghahremani, M.D., F.A.C.R.
Professor and Chairman, Department of Diagnostic Radiology,
Evanston Hospital—Northwestern University, Evanston, Illinois,
U.S.A.
Chapters 2, 3, 9, 10, 11

William H. Brewer, M.D.
Assistant Professor, Department of Radiology, Medical College of
Virginia, Richmond, Virginia, U.S.A.
Chapter 9

H. Joachim Burhenne, M.D., F.R.C.P. (C)
Professor and Head, Department of Diagnostic Radiology, Univer-
sity of British Columbia, Vancouver, British Columbia, Canada
Chapter 7

Morton Burrell, M.D.
Professor, Department of Diagnostic Radiology, Yale University
School of Medicine, New Haven, Connecticut, U.S.A.
Chapters 1, 6

Leonid Calenoff, M.D.
Professor, Department of Radiology, Northwestern University Med-
ical School, Chicago, Illinois, U.S.A.
Chapter 5

James L. Clements, Jr., M.D.
Professor, Department of Radiology, Emory University School of
Medicine, Atlanta, Georgia, U.S.A.
Chapter 8

Peter Cooperberg, M.D., F.R.C.P. (C)
Associate Professor, Department of Radiology, University of British Columbia, Vancouver, British Columbia, Canada
Chapter 7

David W. Gelfand, M.D.
Professor, Department of Radiology, Bowman Gray School of Medicine, Wake Forest University, Winston-Salem, North Carolina, U.S.A.
Chapter 4

Burton M. Gold, M.D.
Assistant Professor, Department of Radiology, School of Medicine, State University of New York at Stony Brook, Long Island, New York, U.S.A.
Chapter 10

Sven-Ola Hietala, M.D.
Assistant Professor, Department of Radiology, Medical College of Virginia, Richmond, Virginia, U.S.A.
Chapter 9

Thomas H. Hunt, M.D.
Assistant Professor, Department of Radiology, Bowman Gray School of Medicine, Wake Forest University, Winston-Salem, North Carolina, U.S.A.
Chapter 4

Eric A. Hyson, M.D.
Attending Radiologist, Waterbury Hospital, Waterbury, Connecticut, U.S.A.
Chapter 1

Bernard S. Jay, M.D.
Department of Diagnostic Radiology, Yale University School of Medicine, New Haven, Connecticut, U.S.A.
Chapter 6

David J. Ott, M.D.
Assistant Professor, Department of Radiology, Bowman Gray School of Medicine, Wake Forest University, Winston-Salem, North Carolina, U.S.A.
Chapter 4

James V. Rogers, Jr., M.D.
Professor, Department of Radiology, Emory University School of
Medicine, Atlanta, Georgia, U.S.A.
Chapter 8

Lee F. Rogers, M.D.
Professor and Chairman, Department of Radiology, Northwestern
University Medical School, Chicago, Illinois, U.S.A.
Chapters 5, 12

Robert Toffler, M.D.
Clinical Associate Professor, Department of Diagnostic Radiology,
Yale University School of Medicine, New Haven, Connecticut,
U.S.A.
Chapter 1

William E. Torres, M.D.
Assistant Professor, Department of Radiology, Emory University
School of Medicine, Atlanta, Georgia, U.S.A.
Chapter 8

1 Drug-Induced Gastrointestinal Disorders

Eric A. Hyson, Morton Burrell, and Robert Toffler

Gastrointestinal disorder related to drug administration is a common phenomenon (1–6). In one study, drug reactions occurred in 16% of all hospital inpatients, with gastrointestinal reactions accounting for 26.9% of the total (1). Although frequently the reaction may be minor, such as mild nausea, vomiting, or diarrhea, serious drug-induced disease is often encountered as well. Outpatient illness serious enough to warrant medical service admission included 2.9% drug-induced cases in one series, excluding suicide attempts and drug abuse (5). Gastrointestinal reactions, usually hemorrhage, were the second most common manifestation (18.5%) after cardiovascular (22.2%).

The radiologist is often in a unique position to assist in making the diagnosis of drug-induced gastrointestinal disease. Radiographic changes may result from ulceration, vascular disease, motility disturbances, alteration of gastrointestinal tract flora, allergic phenomena, and other drug effects (7,8). Although the diagnosis may be suggested by radiographic studies, the clinical history of drug administration is usually essential.

Following is a list of drugs and their associated gastrointestinal complications.

Gastrointestinal Erosions and Ulcerations
Salicylates
Corticosteroids
Other antiarthritics (indomethacin, phenylbutazone, oxyphenbutazone, ibuprofen, naproxen, tolmetin, fenoprofen)
Miscellaneous (reserpine, spironolactone, iron)
Potassium supplements (enteric-coated, potassium gluconate, slow-release)

Hypomotility disorders
Ganglionic blockers (hexamethonium, mecamylamine, pentolinium)
Psychoactive drugs (antiparkinsonian anticholinergics, phenothiazines, tricyclic antidepressants)
Narcotics
Miscellaneous (clonidine, vincristine, dantrolene, ^{131}I-induced myxedema)

Bleeding disorders
Heparin
Oral anticoagulants

Ischemic-thrombotic disease
Oral contraceptives
Digitalis
Ergot derivatives

Cathartic colon
Castor oil
Phenolphthalein
Bisacodyl
Senna
Danthron
Cascara sagrada

Retroperitoneal fibrosis
Methysergide
Miscellaneous (ergotamine, dihydroergotamine, LSD, ? others)

Liver tumors
Estrogens
Androgens

Esophageal moniliasis
Corticosteroids
Immunosuppressives
Antibiotics

Enterocolitis
  Pseudomembranous enterocolitis
  Antibiotics (tetracycline, chloramphenicol, penicillin, ampicillin, cephalexin, neomycin, erythromycin, sulfamethoxazole-trimethoprim, lincomycin, clindamycin)
  Acute, transient antibiotic colitis (penicillin, ampicillin, amoxicillin)
  Gold enterocolitis
  Gastrointestinal urticaria (penicillin)
Miscellaneous
  Obstruction (Drug masses: aluminum hydroxide, cholestyramine, bulk laxative, tablets)
  Pancreatitis (corticosteroids, estrogens, diuretics, salicylazosulfapyridine, antineoplastic agents, indomethacin, anticoagulants, phenformin)
  Gallstones (estrogens, clofibrate)
  Fibrotic peritonitis (practolol)
  Enzyme esophagitis (papain)

Ulceration

Salicylates

Many drugs have been reported as possibly related to gastric ulceration, but the most convincing evidence relates to aspirin (9,10). Superficial gastric erosions following aspirin ingestion have been well documented by endoscopy (11–13), and even the cellular mechanism of gastric mucosal injury by aspirin has been established (11). In the acid environment of the gastric lumen, aspirin remains in its nonionized form and hence readily crosses into the cells of the gastric mucosa. However, once inside the mucosal cell in a more alkaline medium, aspirin (acetylsalicylic acid, a weak acid) ionizes, leading to cellular injury, sloughing of gastric mucosa, and superficial erosion. Other salicylates may be less damaging to the stomach, but the evidence is less clear (13,14).

In the past, radiographic demonstration of gastritis and superficial erosions, such as those caused by aspirin, was difficult with the conventional upper gastrointestinal barium contrast studies. Even with erosions documented by endoscopy, the upper gastrointestinal tract series might show merely slightly enlarged gastric mucosal folds in only a minority of cases (14). However, with the newer double-contrast methods for examination of the stomach, superficial gastric erosions are more readily seen (15,-16) (Fig. 1-1) although endoscopy is still more sensitive (12). Patients with "aspirin gastritis"

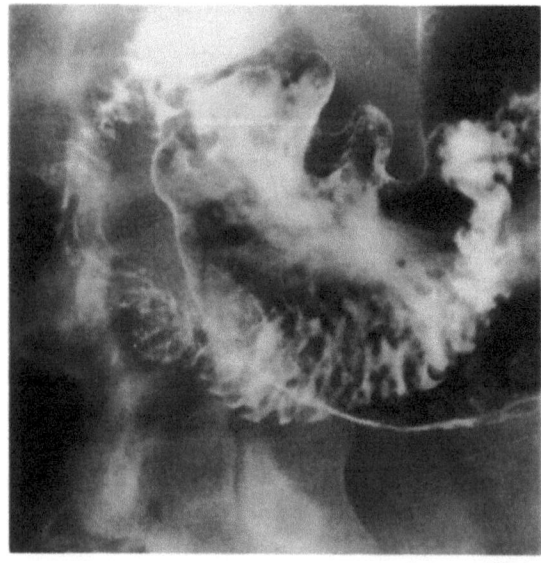

a

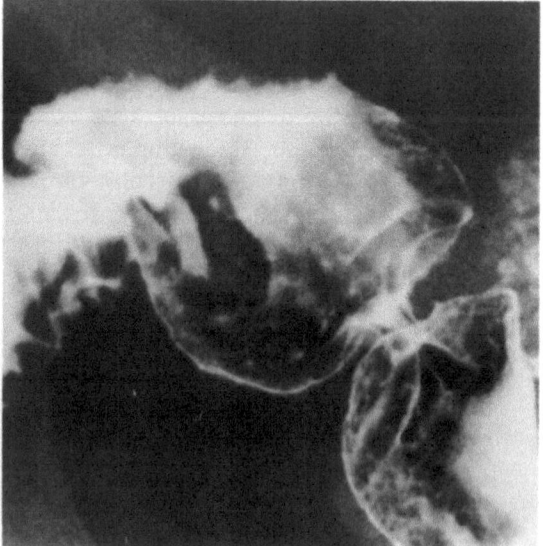

b

Fig. 1-1, a and b. Multiple superficial gastric erosions. Evident in the antrum (**a**) and duodenum (**b**), these probably do not extend below the muscularis mucosae and thus are too superficial to be called ulcers. They are shown to best advantage in double-contrast examinations. This patient had epigastric pain, guaiac-positive stools, and a history of repeated aspirin ingestion.

typically have gastrointestinal bleeding, either gross or occult (11).

Evidence has accumulated that use of aspirin is also related to chronic gastric ulcer. The earliest evidence came from Australia where a high incidence of gastric ulcer was discovered in middle-aged females who regularly ingested analgesics (17–20). More recent studies in the United States have also shown significant association between heavy aspirin intake and chronic gastric ulcer; considering the widespread use of aspirin in this country, the risk of gastric ulcer in any one individual aspirin user is probably small (21,22). No significant relationship between salicylates and duodenal ulcer or gastric carcinoma has been demonstrated (17,18,20,21).

Aspirin-associated gastric ulcer usually has no radiologic features to distinguish it from idiopathic ulcer. However, some evidence indicates that "aspirin ulcer" is relatively more common in the gastric antrum (22). One report noted a high frequency of hourglass stomach in gastric ulcer patients with a history of prolonged aspirin use (23).

Corticosteroids

While early reports stressed that corticosteroids are associated with peptic ulcer disease, particularly gastric ulcer (24–27), others have found no significant relationship (28–30). The controversy has been rekindled by Conn and Blitzer who, on the basis of a statistical review of the literature, concluded that there is an insignificant difference in the incidence of peptic ulcer disease in patients treated with steroids and in those not treated with steroids (31). The arguments continue (32,33), but the ulcerogenic properties of corticosteroids have been neither completely established nor refuted (10). Much of the controversy centers around patients with rheumatoid arthritis who seem to have a higher incidence of peptic ulcer disease even without steroid therapy (28–30).

The radiographic description of "steroid ulcers" varies. Peptic ulcers in corticosteroid-treated patients tend to be predominantly gastric (usually antral) rather than duodenal, the reverse of the control population (25,34). Descriptions of the individual ulcers, however, range from large and deep (34), to shallow (25), to indistinguishable from idiopathic ulcers (35). There has been

general agreement that peptic ulcers in patients taking steroids show less surrounding edema, spasm, and scarring, a situation that is perhaps related to the anti-inflammatory effect of the corticosteroids (25,36,37). Some reports have emphasized the relatively silent nature of peptic ulcer disease in patients receiving corticosteroids and an associated high complication rate from bleeding and perforation (25,34,36).

The possibility of a relation between colonic perforation and corticosteroid use has also been raised, both in a diseased colon involved with diverticulitis or ulcerative colitis and in an otherwise normal colon with punched-out ulcerations (29,38,39). A causal relationship has not been established, but steroid therapy does tend to make clinical recognition of perforation more difficult since the patient's symptoms and physical findings are often of mild degree.

Other Antiarthritics

Gastritis and chronic gastric ulcer have also been associated with some of the newer antiinflammatory medications (40). The association has been strongest for indomethacin, phenylbutazone, and oxyphenbutazone (41–47). Preliminary reports suggest that there is less gastric mucosal injury with the most recently introduced antiarthritics, ibuprofen, naproxen, tolmetin, and fenoprofen (11,48–52). Occasionally more distal gastrointestinal tract ulcerations and perforations in the small bowel and colon have been linked to ingestion of certain of these new "super aspirins" (53–56).

Miscellaneous

Reserpine and other Rauwolfia alkaloids, now used principally for treatment of hypertension, increase gastric acid secretion when given in large oral doses, and there is some evidence for association with peptic ulcer disease (57–60). However, in routine oral doses, the increase in acid secretion is probably insignificant and ulcerogenic potential minimal (59). Sporadic cases of gastric ulceration associated with spironolactone have been reported (61). In children ingestion of toxic amounts of iron preparations has resulted in several cases of ulcerative gastric stricture and one case of mesenteric infarction due to caustic effects (62–67). Esophageal ulceration has been noted in three patients who took tetracycline just before going to bed, raising the possibility of stasis of the pills in the esophageal lumen as a contributing factor (68).

Potassium Supplements

As potassium-wasting diuretics have come into widespread use for hypertension and cardiac failure in recent years, a need for a simple means of potassium replacement has arisen. To avoid gastric irritation from orally ingested potassium chloride, an enteric-coated form was developed to dissolve in the more alkaline environment of the small bowel. However, as use of enteric-coated potassium chloride tablets increased in the early 1960s, it became clear that they were occasionally ulcerogenic in the small intestinal mucosa (69–73). Most affected patients had increasing postprandial crampy abdominal pain of days' to months' duration, suggesting partial small bowel obstruction. Barium contrast studies typically show a transition in small bowel caliber due to the partial obstruction (Fig. 1-2a) and occasionally define the cause, a short segmental ulcerated stricture with proximal bowel dilatation (70,74) (Fig. 1-2b). Although the short circumferential ulceration is seen grossly in the

resected small bowel specimen (Figs 1-3, 1-4) the lesion usually appears radiographically as a short stricture without an ulcer niche (Fig. 1-5). The ulcer-strictures occur usually in the midjejunum and are uncommonly multiple. Surgical resection of the involved segment of bowel has been the treatment of choice (72). Less common manifestations of enteric-coated potassium chloride ulcerations include free small intestinal perforation and hemorrhage (69,72) (Fig. 1-6).

Potassium chloride injury to the small bowel probably results when accumulation of a locally high concentration of ionized potassium bathes the mucosa in the immediate vicinity of a tablet (71). It has been suggested that the high potassium level causes local vascular damage followed by circumferential hemorrhagic infarction and mucosal slough (75). At this point the lesion may perforate or bleed, but usually healing simply leads to a stricture.

Enteric-coated potassium chloride tablets have been withdrawn from the market in the United States but are still in use in other countries. Other forms of oral potassium supplements still in use in this country, however, have occasionally been associated with gastrointestinal tract ulceration. Potassium gluconate liquid and the new slow-release potassium chloride tablets

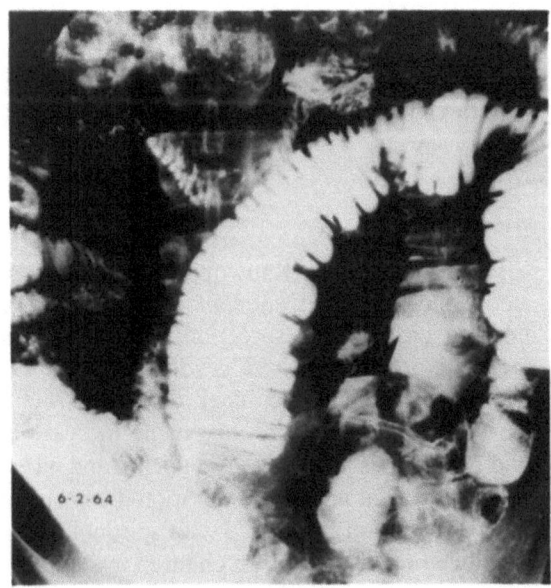 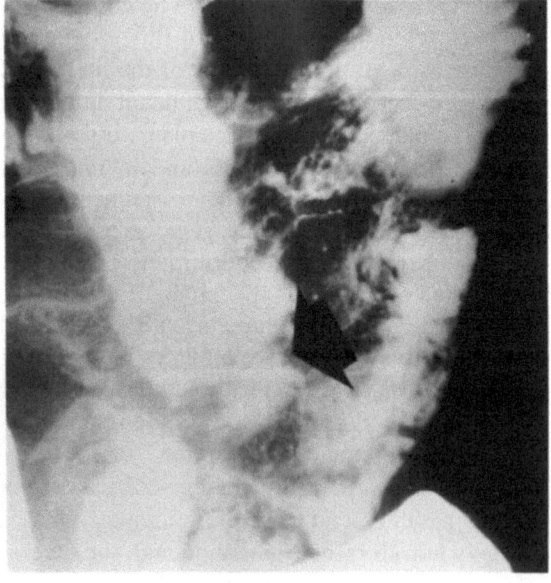

a   b

Fig. 1-2, a and b. Partial small bowel obstruction associated with ingestion of enteric-coated potassium chloride tablets. a Arrow indicates level of obstruction. **b** Close-up of area of obstruction demonstrates short, segmental ulcerated stricture. (Courtesy of S. Schwartz, MD, New Haven, Connecticut)

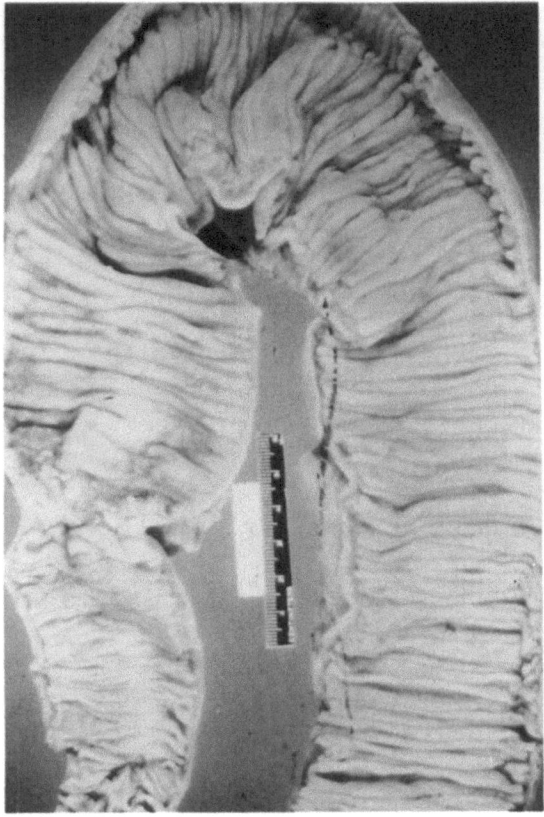 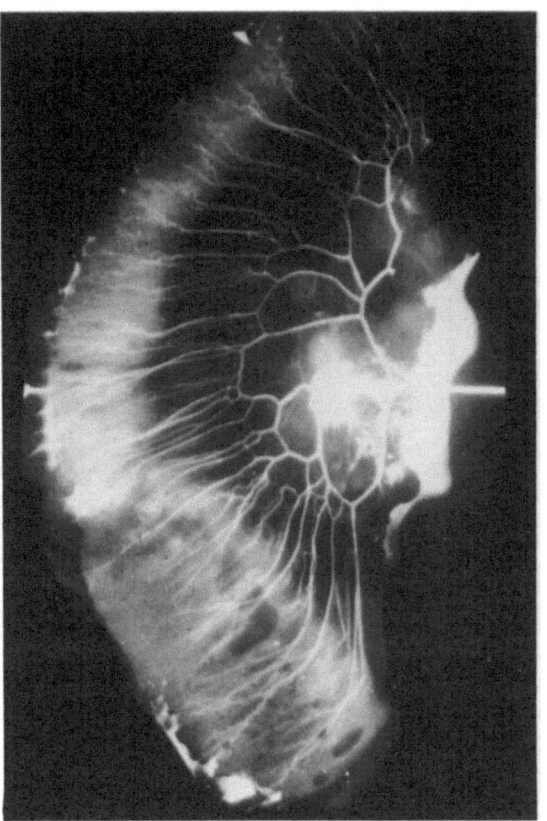

Fig. 1-3. Potassium chloride–induced ulceration. Secondary segmental annular narrowing and dilation of proximal bowel are present. (Courtesy of S. Schwartz, MD, New Haven, Connecticut)

Fig. 1-4. Potassium chloride–induced ulceration. Marked peripheral tapering of vessels in area of ulceration is evident on injected specimen. (Courtesy of S. Schwartz, MD, New Haven, Connecticut)

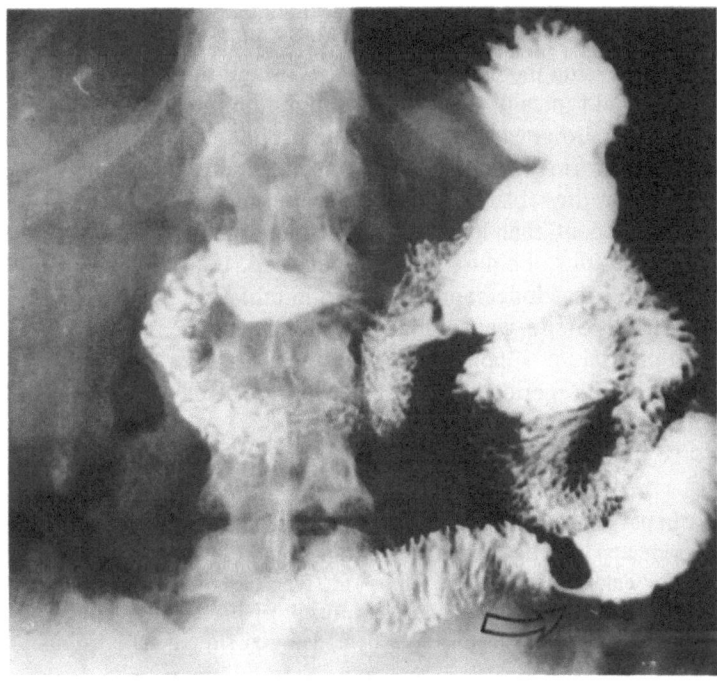

Fig. 1-5. Ischemic ulceration due to potassium chloride ingestion. The short, smooth stricture (*arrow*) without visible ulceration is characteristic.

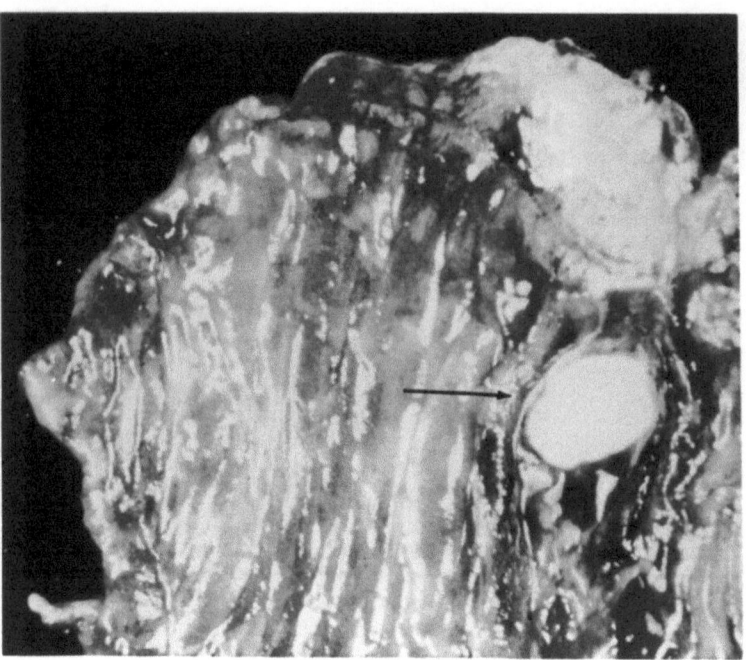

in a wax matrix (Slow-K) have rarely been associated with the same short ulcerated small-bowel strictures seen with use of enteric-coated tablets (70,76–79). In a few instances, enteric-coated and slow-release potassium tablets have been associated with gastric ulceration (80,81).

In the British literature there have been numerous reports of association of slow-release potassium chloride tablets with ulcerative strictures of the esophagus (82–86). In almost all of the cases the left cardiac atrium was enlarged and impressing the esophagus (Fig. 1-7), and the patient had typically received the potassium tablets after cardiac surgery. Since the esophageal strictures formed at the level of the left atrial impression the tablets may have been temporarily arrested at that level, allowing ulcerogenic concentrations of potassium to be released. In at least two cases lodgment of potassium tablets at the stricture site was demonstrated (83,85). If oral potassium supplements are given in the postoperative period to a patient with left atrial enlargement, the liquid form is preferred.

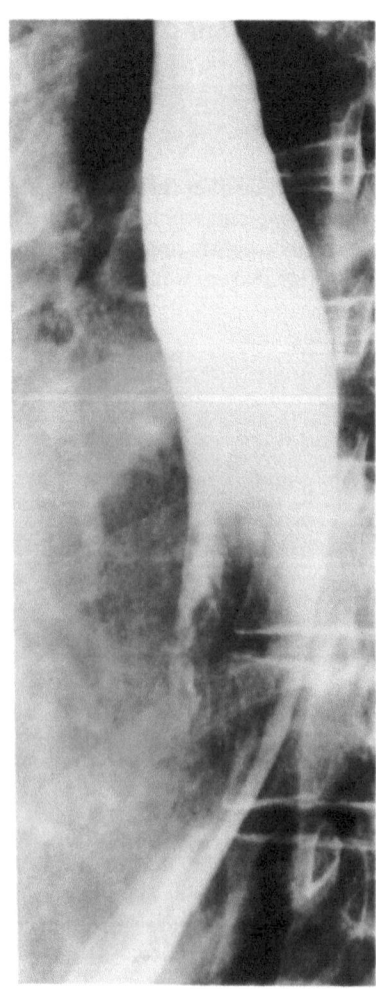

Fig. 1-7. Esophagitis due to potassium chloride ingestion. Barium swallow in patient with mitral insufficiency, who had been taking potassium chloride and diuretics, reveals significant compression upon the esophagus by enlarged left atrium. This is the type of patient in whom strictures of the esophagus develop as a result of ingestion of potassium chloride. Endoscopy at this time demonstrated superficial erosions in the area of stasis.

Hypomotility Disorders

Ganglionic Blockers

In the differential diagnosis of mechanical bowel obstruction, the possibility of drug-induced paralytic ileus or pseudo-obstruction should always be kept in mind. The long-acting ganglionic blocking agents formerly used in the treatment of hypertension provide a classic example of drugs capable of inducing ileus, although these medications are now mostly of historical interest since they have been replaced by more effective antihypertensive agents (87). Patients taking the ganglionic blockers hexamethonium, mecamylamine, or pentolinium occasionally have apparent small bowel obstruction (88–96). Plain abdominal radiographs usually show dilated gas-filled loops of small bowel, occasionally associated with gastric dilatation. Peristaltic rushes on abdominal auscultation have been described, in spite of the term "paralytic" ileus (96). There was no mechanically obstructing lesion of the bowel in patients who underwent laparotomy, but there was atonic dilatation. In patients in whom an appropriate drug history was obtained, nonoperative therapy, including withdrawal of the ganglionic blocker, nasogastric or long-tube suction, and parenteral administration of fluids, has often been successful. However, several fatalities have been recorded, probably related to bowel infarction and fluid-electrolyte abnormalities from prolonged ileus.

Psychoactive Drugs

Currently psychoactive medications, because of their anticholingeric effects, form the largest group of drugs producing pseudo-obstruction of the bowel (Fig. 1-8). They differ from the ganglionic blockers in that they cause principally large bowel dilatation, simulating mechanical colonic obstruction. Drug effect is thus part of a large

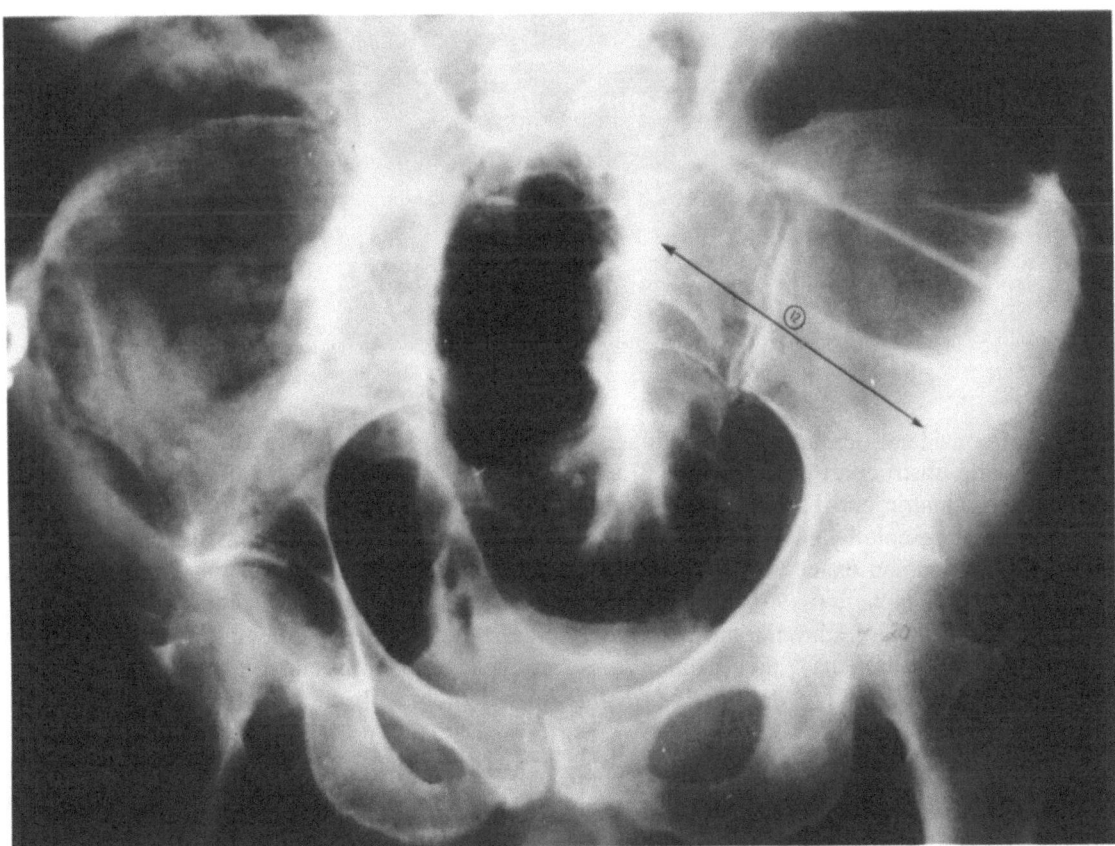

Fig. 1-8. Pseudo-obstruction of the colon associated with ingestion of a phenothiazine derivative (Stelazine). The plain film demonstrates marked distention of the entire colon. The width of the transverse colon is 12 cm. Barium enema study revealed no evidence of mechanical obstruction.

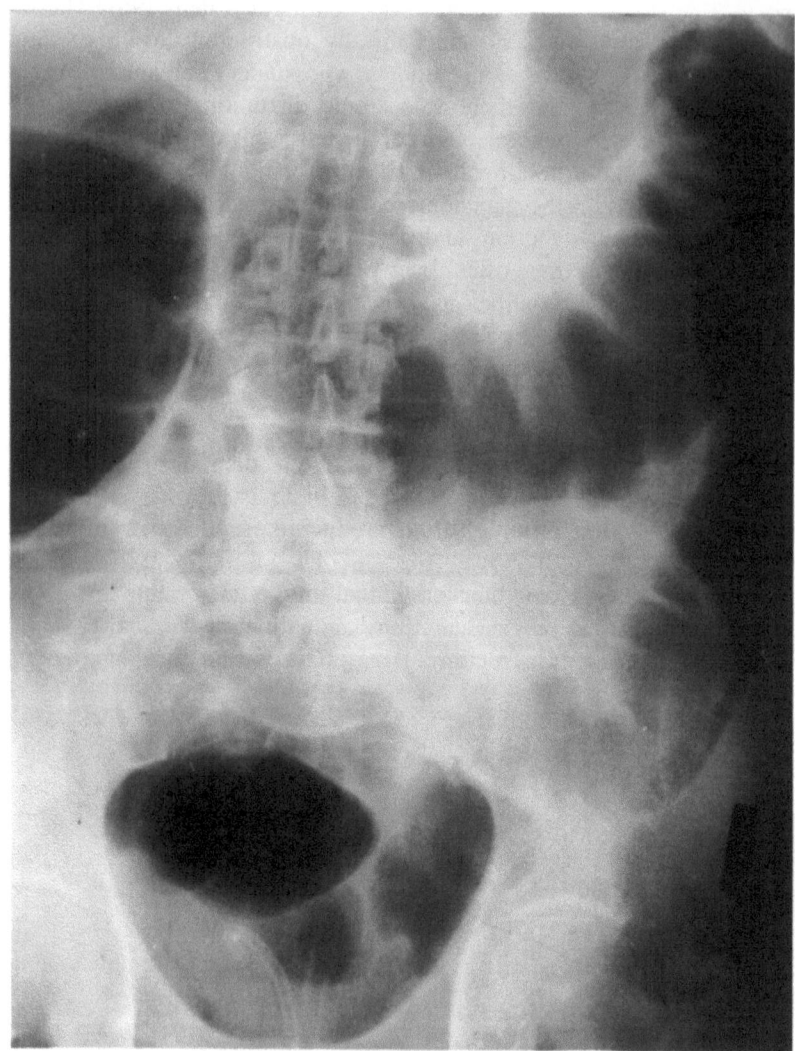

Fig. 1-9. Megacolon. This is present in a patient with Parkinson's disease who was taking procyclidine hydrochloride (Kemadrin).

number of considerations in differential diagnosis for pseudo-obstruction of the colon (97,98). Although psychiatric and Parkinsonian patients often have megacolon independent of drug effect, medication can exacerbate the situation, leading to fecal impaction (99). Patients may have no symptoms of chronic megacolon or pseudo-obstruction but may have acute symptoms of mechanical obstruction in the distal colon due to fecaliths.

Patients with Parkinson's disease are frequently treated with anticholinergic drugs, including trihexyphenidyl and benzotropine, further impairing already poor colonic motility (Fig. 1-9). Acute worsening of the patient's longstanding constipation may signify obstruction by fecal impaction, but these patients are also more liable to sigmoid volvulus since the colon has become chronically dilated and elongated (100–102). (Fig. 1-10). Phenothiazines have a similar anticholinergic influence, leading to fecal impaction; morbidity and mortality in psychiatric patients may be due to its delayed recognition (99,103, 104). Anticholinergic effects are also seen with tricyclic antidepressants; gastrointestinal complications have been reported with amitriptyline (Fig. 1-11) and nortriptyline. In addition to fecal impaction (105,106), marked paralytic ileus, leading to surgery in a few cases, has also been described (107–110). In some instances, psychoactive drugs and anticholinergic medications are combined in a single preparation. Such a combination can cause changes in small and large bowel (Fig. 1-12).

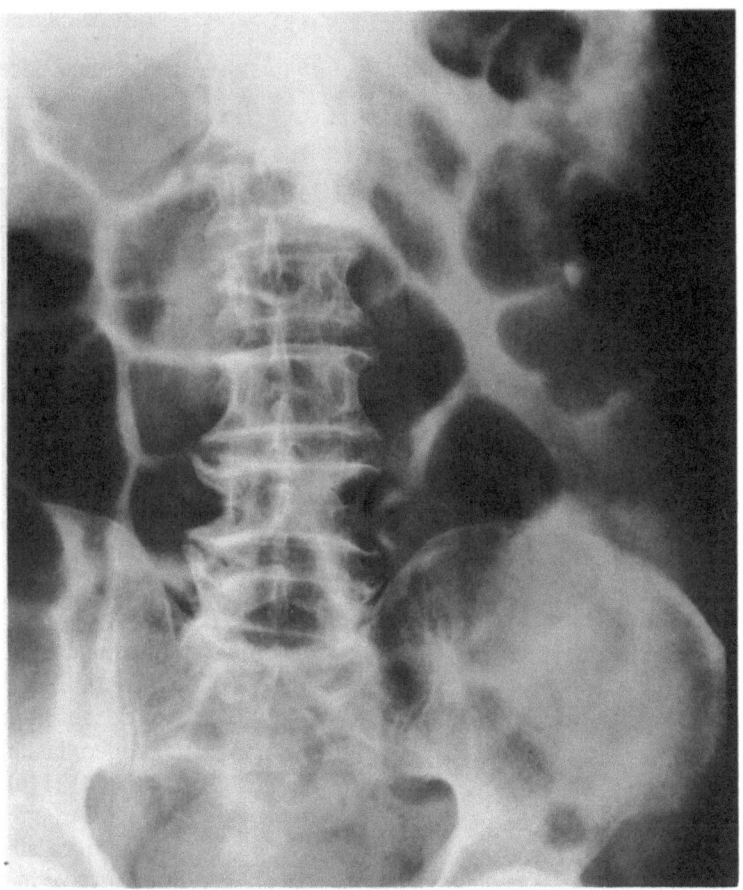

Fig. 1-10. Marked colonic dilatation. A patient with Parkinson's disease had been receiving long-term therapy with trihexyphenidyl (Artane). Although no mechanical obstruction was found on barium examination, marked redundancy was noted.

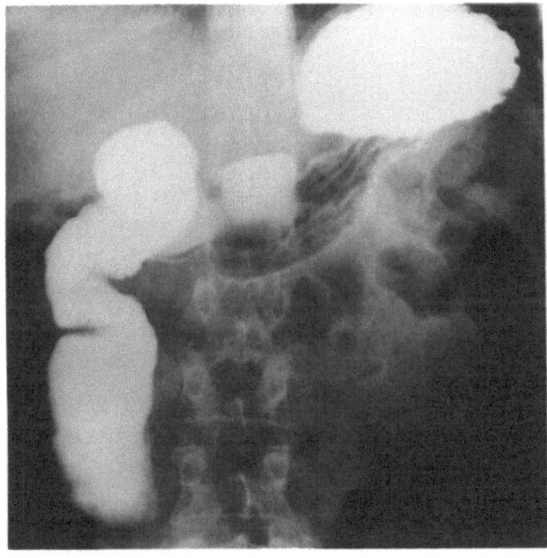

a

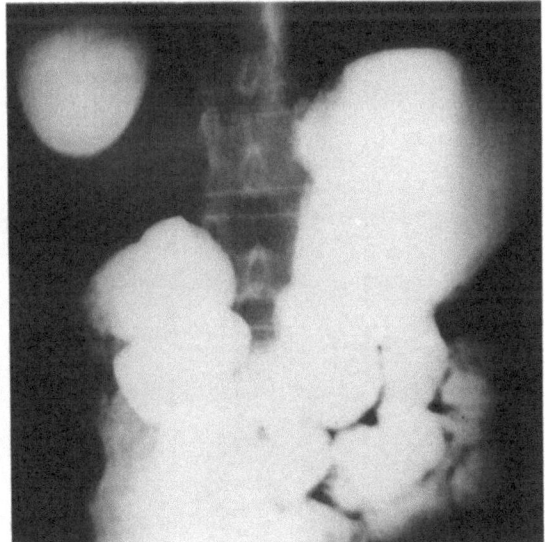

b

Fig. 1-11, a and b. Obstruction of the third portion of the duodenum due to compression by the superior mesenteric artery. The patient was receiving amitriptyline (Elavil) therapy. a Perhaps the dilatation of the bowel produced the superior mesenteric artery syndrome in this patient with a predisposition for obstruction. b With the patient in the knee-chest position the film reveals passage of contrast material beyond this area into remaining small bowel. (Density in the right upper quadrant is the patient's breast outlined by air.)

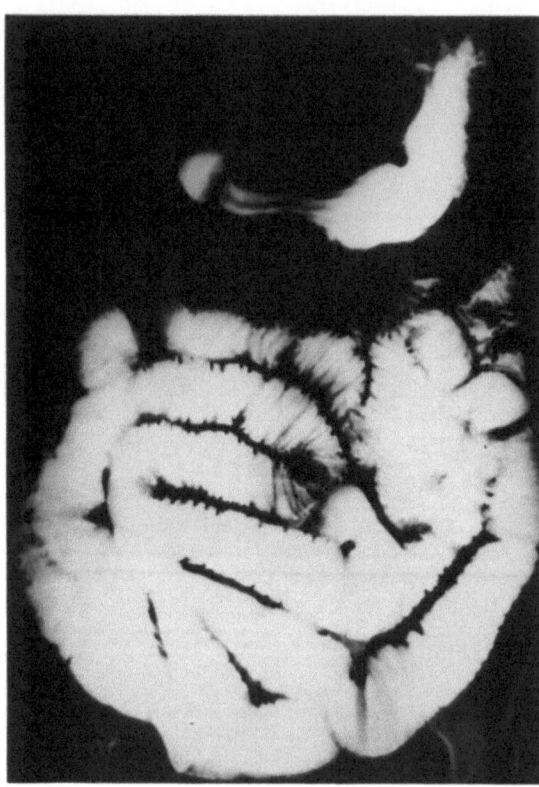
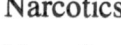

Fig. 1-12. Small bowel dilatation induced by a drug combination. A 62-year-old woman was taking Milpath, a combination of meprobomate, a tranquilizing agent, and tridihexethyl chloride, an anticholinergic agent.

Narcotics

Narcotics decrease intestinal motility, allowing increased water absorption from the colonic fecal contents but occasionally resulting in impaction of a serious nature. Long-term treatment with methadone in particular has at times led to a presentation clinically and radiographically similar to mechanical obstruction (111) (Fig. 1-13). The key findings are a stool-laden colon supporting the appropriate drug history. Nasogastric or long-tube suction, high enemas, and rectal bisacodyl suppositories may be adequate treatment, as with impactions due to other medication, although a fatality due to delay in seeking medical attention has been reported (112).

Miscellaneous

Intestinal hypomotility, paralytic ileus, or fecal impaction has also been associated with clonidine (antihypertensive) (113,114), vincristine (antineoplastic) (115), and dantrolene (muscle relaxant) (116). Myxedema, a known complication of treatment of hyperthyroidism with ^{131}I (117), has also been associated with pseudo-obstructive megacolon (118,119) (Fig. 1-14).

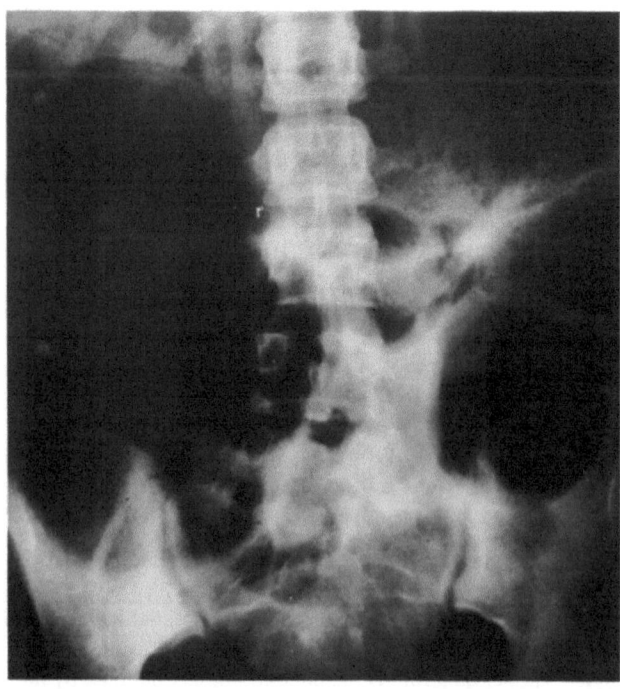

Fig. 1-13. Marked ileus associated with methadone treatment. The patient subsequently died from bowel necrosis. (Courtesy of J. Farman, MD, Brooklyn, New York)

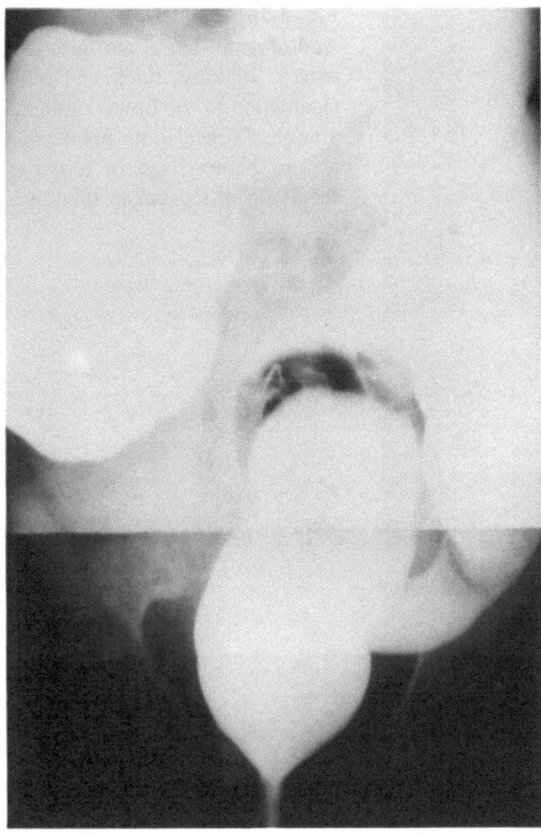

Fig. 1-14. Myxedema megacolon. Barium enema study confirms a dilated atonic large intestine.

fever, abdominal distention and tenderness, hypoactive bowel sounds, rebound tenderness, and sometimes a vague mass caused by hematoma in the bowel wall and mesentery. Laboratory studies may show anemia and coagulation time indicating anticoagulation beyond the therapeutic range. Plain abdominal radiographs often demonstrate a pattern of obstruction or paralytic ileus with distended bowel loops containing air-fluid levels (122–126). If present, thickening of the bowel wall and mucosal folds (Fig. 1-15) must be differentiated from a similar appearance seen in infarction (since patients receiving anticoagulants usually have preexisting vascular disease) and other entities such as tuberculosis, lymphoma, and regional enteritis. A pseudotumor from hematoma in the mesentery may be seen, or there may be evidence of free fluid since more than half of patients with intramural hemorrhage have intraperitoneal blood as well (120).

If small bowel intramural hemorrhage due to anticoagulants is suspected, contrast studies are indicated. The barium column demonstrates segmental involvement of the intestine with rigidity and thickened mucosal folds such that the barium contrast between the folds forms spiked projections or a picket-fence appearance (122,123) (Figs. 1-16, 1-17). As on the plain films, bowel-

Bleeding Disorders

Anticoagulants

The major complication of widely used heparin and oral anticoagulants is certainly hemorrhage. Bleeding has been reported in 5–48% of nonhospitalized patients receiving anticoagulants; it was major in 0.8–12% (120). Gastrointestinal bleeding can be intraluminal (spontaneous or secondary to a preexisting lesion), intramural, retroperitoneal, into solid abdominal organs (ovary, pancreas, liver, adrenals), or into the rectus abdominis muscle (120,121).

Spontaneous intramural small bowel hemorrhage is the most common type of bleeding, other than radiographically undetectable intraluminal bleeding. Clinical presentation includes crampy abdominal pain, nausea and vomiting, and bleeding, frequently from other sites (120, 121). Physical examination typically reveals mild

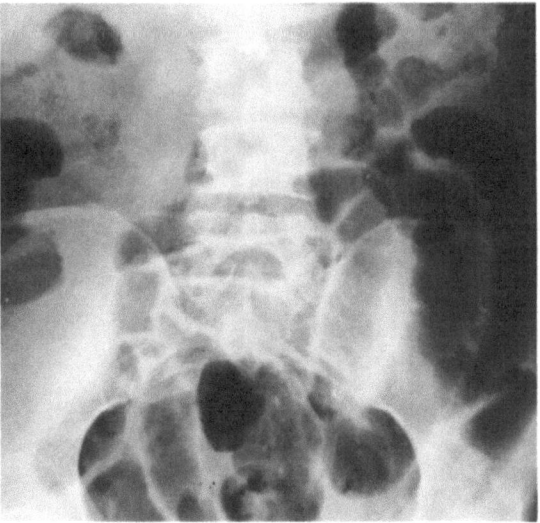

Fig. 1-15. Nodular indentations in the right colon secondary to hemorrhage. The patient had been receiving warfarin sodium (Coumadin). The indentations are well seen on the plain film.

E. A. Hyson, M. Burrell, and R. Toffler

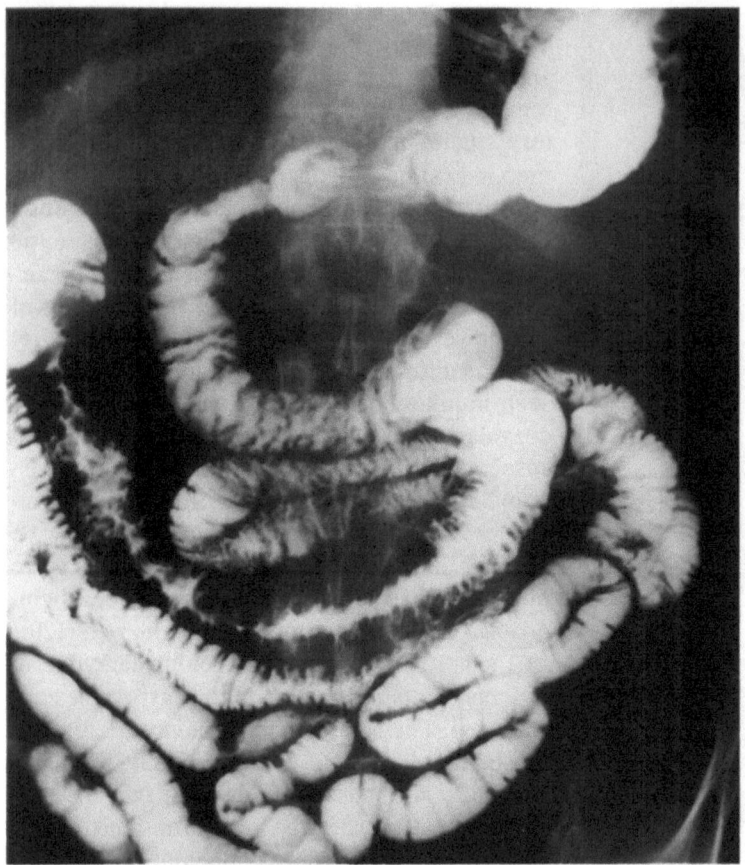

a

Fig. 1-16, a and **b. Bleeding into wall of small bowel and into mesentery.** Rigidity, thickened folds, spiculation of the bowel, and separation of bowel loops are secondary to hemorrhage in a patient receiving anticoagulant therapy.

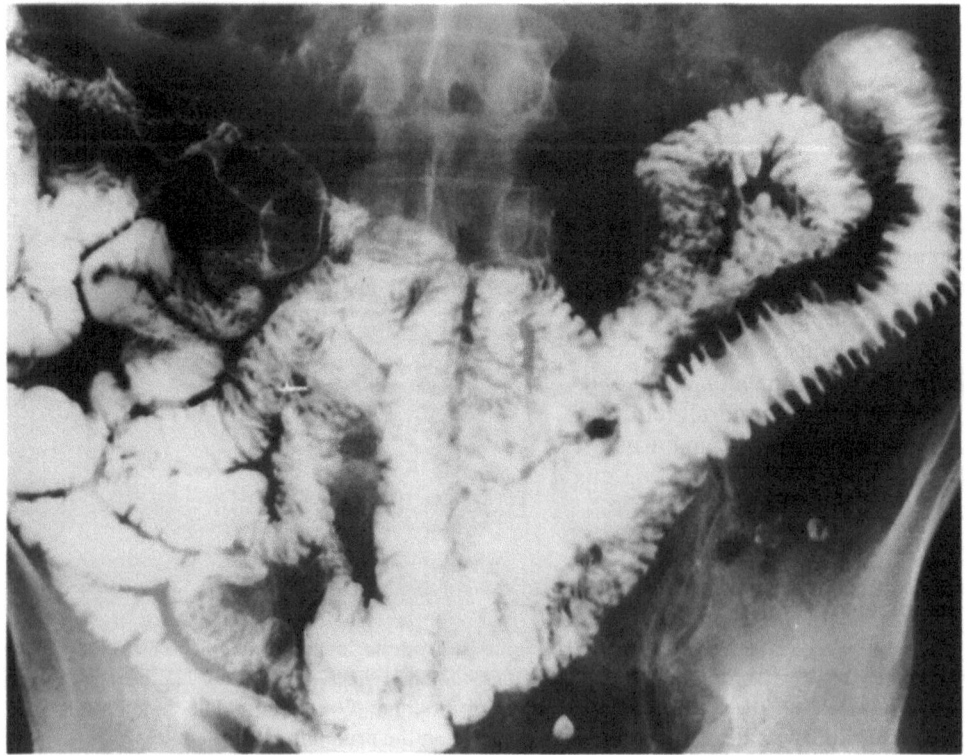

b

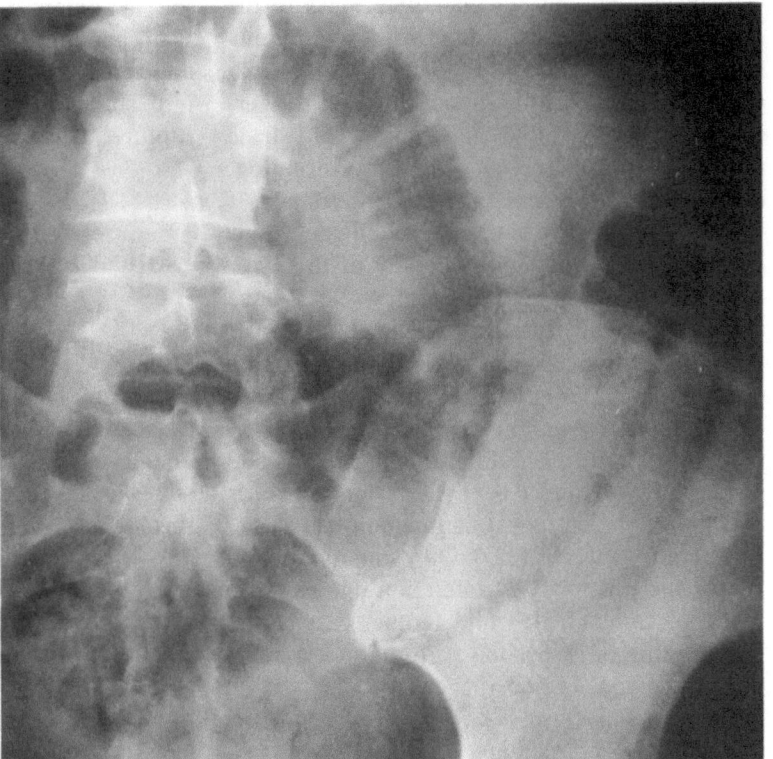

a

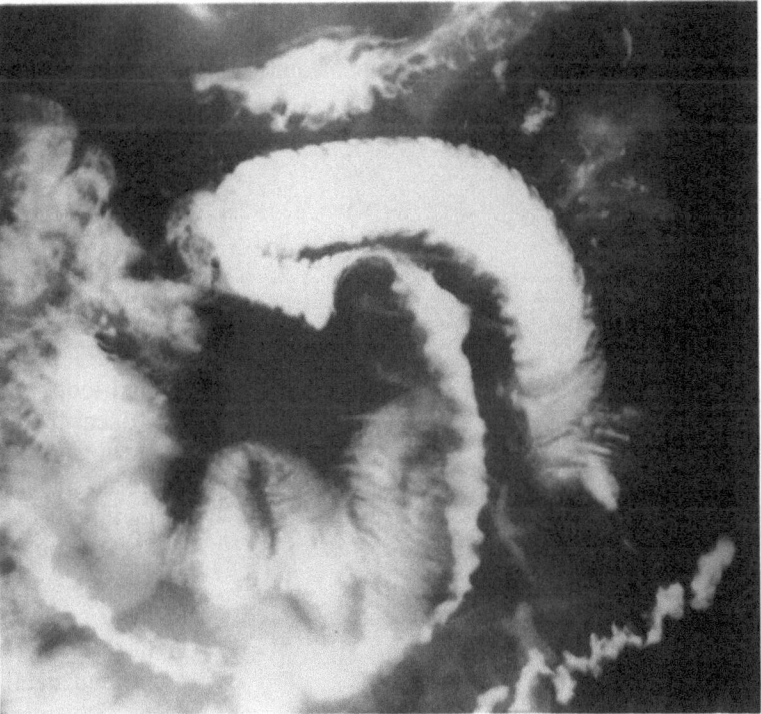

b

Fig. 1-17, a and **b. Marked hemorrhage into bowel and mesentery producing separation of loops and partial obstruction.** This is seen on plain film (**a**) and barium contrast study (**b**). The patient had been receiving Coumadin therapy. At follow-up examination the appearance was completely normal.

wall thickening and evidence of a mass in the mesentery may be seen. Most commonly involved is the jejunum, followed by the proximal ileum, and then the duodenum and the terminal ileum (125,127). The intramural hemorrhage may be extensive enough to cause obstruction, even involving the duodenum (128,129).

Intramural hemorrhage due to anticoagulants has been reported less commonly in the large bowel (129–131) (Fig. 1-18). A few cases have also been noted in the upper alimentary tract, involving the esophagus (132,133) and retropharyngeal region (134).

Treatment for intramural bleeding is conservative with correction of coagulation values and nasogastric suction if necessary. The bowel is usually normal on repeat barium contrast examination in 2–3 weeks (125). Only one report suggested the possibility of infarction due to intramural bleeding (135), while another case raised the question of associated perforation 2 months after small bowel hemorrhage (136).

Spontaneous retroperitoneal bleeding occurs uncommonly in patients receiving anticoagulants; usually they have abdominal or flank pain, bleeding from other sites, and shock (121). Findings include abdominal tenderness, hypoactive bowel sounds, and sometimes a palpable mass in

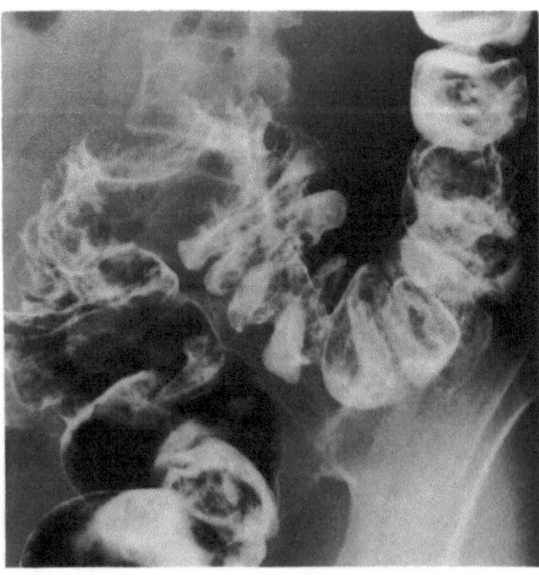

Fig. 1-18. Intramural hemorrhage, seen as a mass defect in the sigmoid. The patient was taking anticoagulants.

the abdomen or flank and neuropathy (137). Plain abdominal films may show adynamic ileus and a mass effect due to hematoma. Hemorrhage into solid abdominal organs, including hepatic rupture, has been noted (120, 138).

Ischemic-Thrombotic Disease

Oral Contraceptives

Oral contraceptives and estrogens have been associated with an increased incidence of thromboembolic complications, including deep and superficial thrombophlebitis, cerebral vein thrombosis, and mesenteric vein thrombosis (139–144), perhaps related to induced coagulation abnormalities (145). Mesenteric vein thrombosis may lead to hemorrhagic infarction of the small bowel virtually throughout or segmentally (Fig. 1-19). The onset of symptoms is usually more gradual than with mesenteric artery occlusion, typically with crampy abdominal pain, nausea, vomiting, and diarrhea (often with blood) developing over hours to several weeks. Mild premonitory symptoms may occur many weeks before (139). The duration of treatment with oral contraceptives is not significant since cases have been reported after 10 days and after 10 years of use; a previous history of thrombophlebitis is unusual (143). Abdominal findings may vary from mild to acute distention with peritoneal signs and absence of bowel sounds, depending on the stage of evolution. Similarly, plain abdominal radiographs may be normal early in the course, but later often demonstrate distended loops of bowel with air-fluid levels and peritoneal fluid. Evidence of infarction is often seen: bowel segments with thickened walls and mucosal folds, unchanged in configuration on serial films.

The treatment of choice has been considered to be early surgical resection of the involved segment of small bowel, which results in high survival rates (Fig. 1-20). Otherwise intestinal gangrene and death can be expected in advanced cases. Several cases of ischemic changes in the small bowel, however, have resolved spontaneously after cessation of oral contraceptive use (146,147). "Second-look" laparotomy 24–48

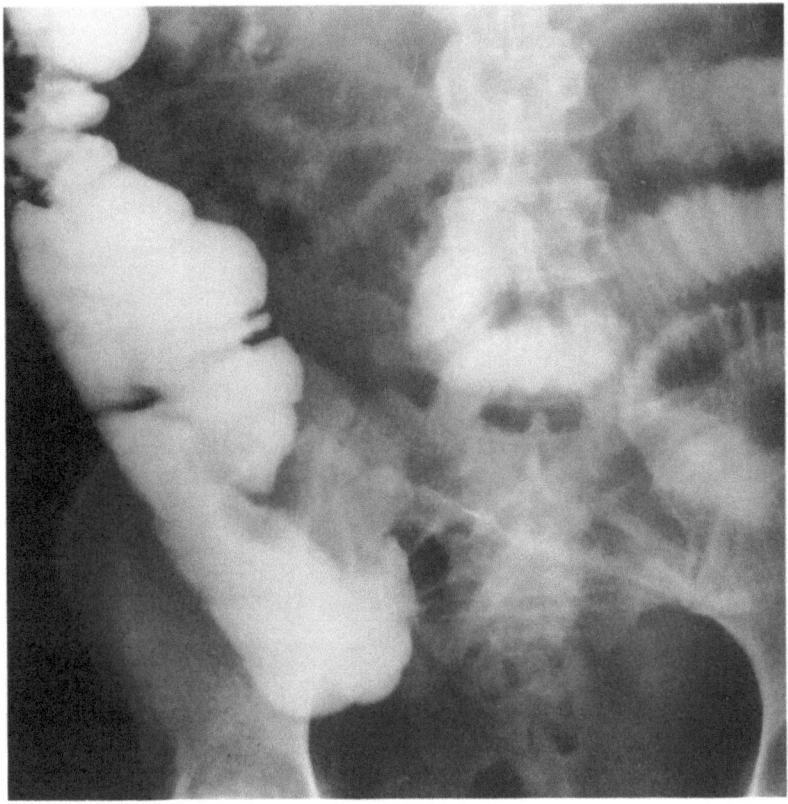

a

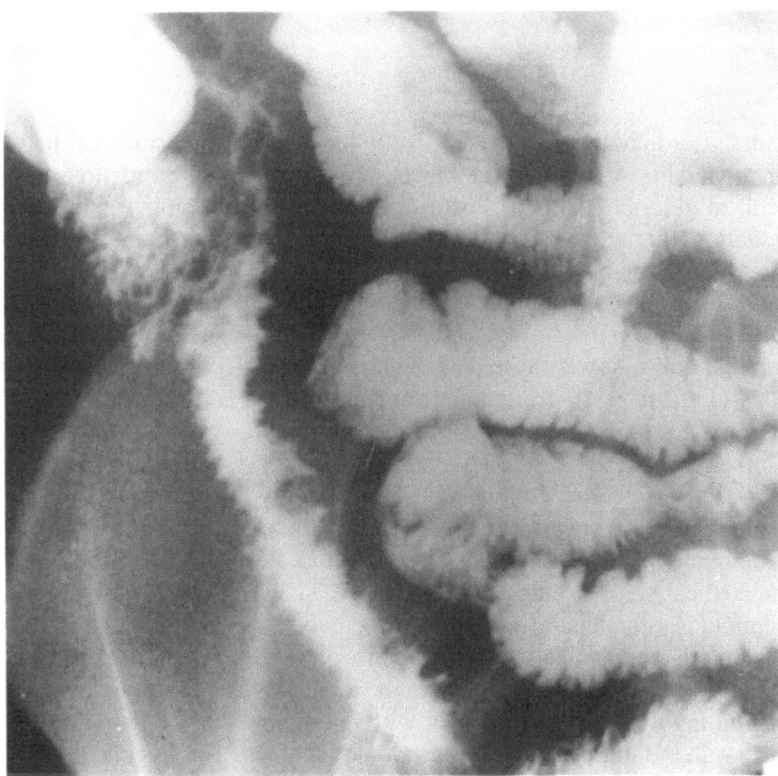

Fig. 1-19, a and b. Ischemic changes in distal ileum associated with use of oral contraceptives. a Initial small bowel series demonstrates irregular narrowing of the distal ileum with mucosal edema, "thumbprints," and separation of the loops. b On follow-up examination 7 days later there is partial resolution with increased patency of the lumen. This eventually went on to complete resolution.

b

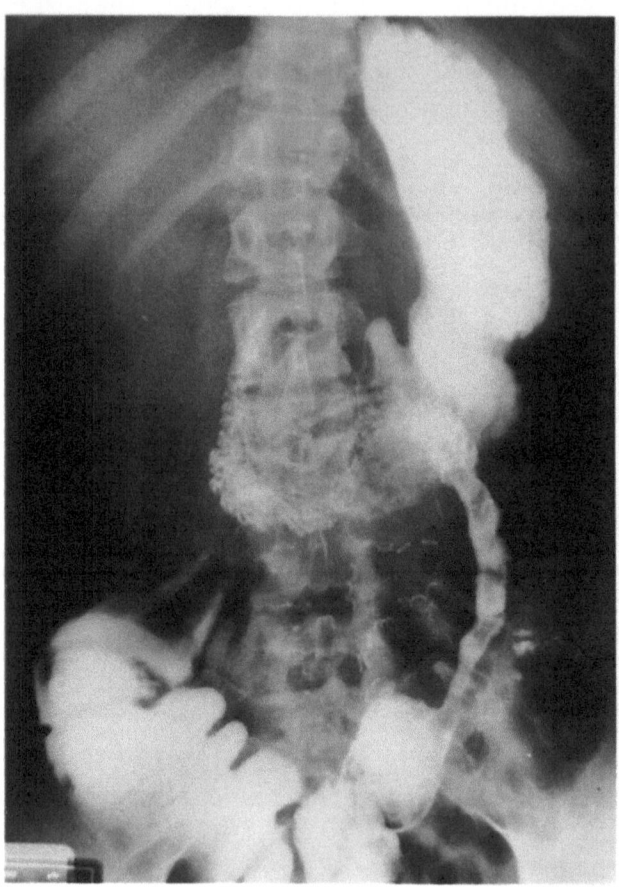

Fig. 1-20. Ischemic stricture of small bowel associated with use of oral contraceptives. Upper gastrointestinal series in a 22-year-old female several weeks after resection of 22 ft of small bowel for massive infarction demonstrates narrowing and mucosal effacement of the remaining small bowel.

hours after initial resection is probably indicated since viability of some of the bowel may be difficult to determine at first. Postoperative anticoagulation therapy is recommended because of the recurrent nature of the disease.

Oral contraceptives tend to cause reversible ischemic colitis, in contrast to the generally irreversible small bowel mesenteric venous infarctions (140,148–151). In addition to oral contraceptives, conjugated estrogens and depot synthetic progestogens have also been associated with ischemic colitis (152,153). Patients usually have a day or two of crampy lower abdominal pain and bloody diarrhea before seeking medical help; bleeding may be massive (151). Sigmoidoscopy demonstrates that the mucosa is edematous and friable with ulcerations. Typical findings on barium enema study are long segmental involvement of the colon with edema of the wall, "thumbprinting," narrowing of the lumen, and mucosal ulceration (Figs. 1-21, 1-22) and involvement of the terminal ileum with

thickening of the wall and mucosal folds if there are contiguous changes in the right colon. The etiology of the findings is unclear. In one case arteriographic findings suggested infarction via the microvasculature or intramural hemorrhage, since the large vessels were normal (154). Treatment of contraceptive-related ischemic colitis is conservative. The contraceptive is discontinued, and in a repeat barium enema study in a few weeks to months the findings return to normal.

The thrombotic complications of oral contraceptives have also included occasional cases of the Budd-Chiari syndrome (155,156). This possibility should be considered in a young female who is taking contraceptives and who develops abdominal pain, hepatomegaly, and ascites (Fig. 1-23). Recovery is possible after taking of the medication is stopped, although death from bleeding varices or even spontaneous rupture of the liver has been reported (157). Radiographically the diagnosis can be substantiated by hepatic venography (158).

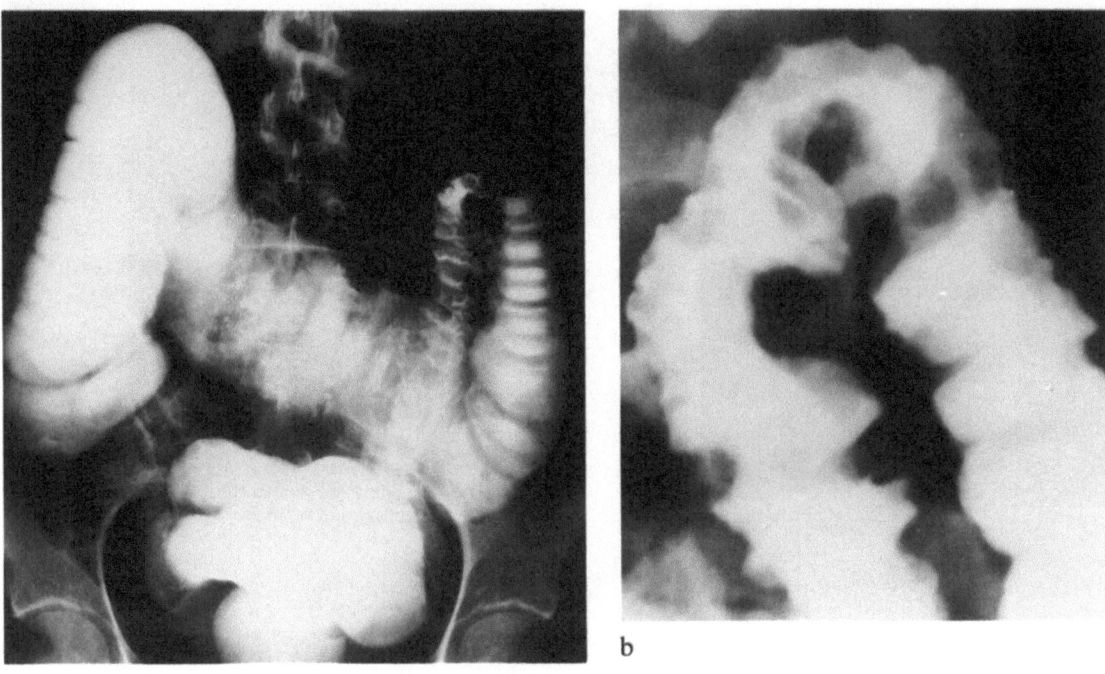

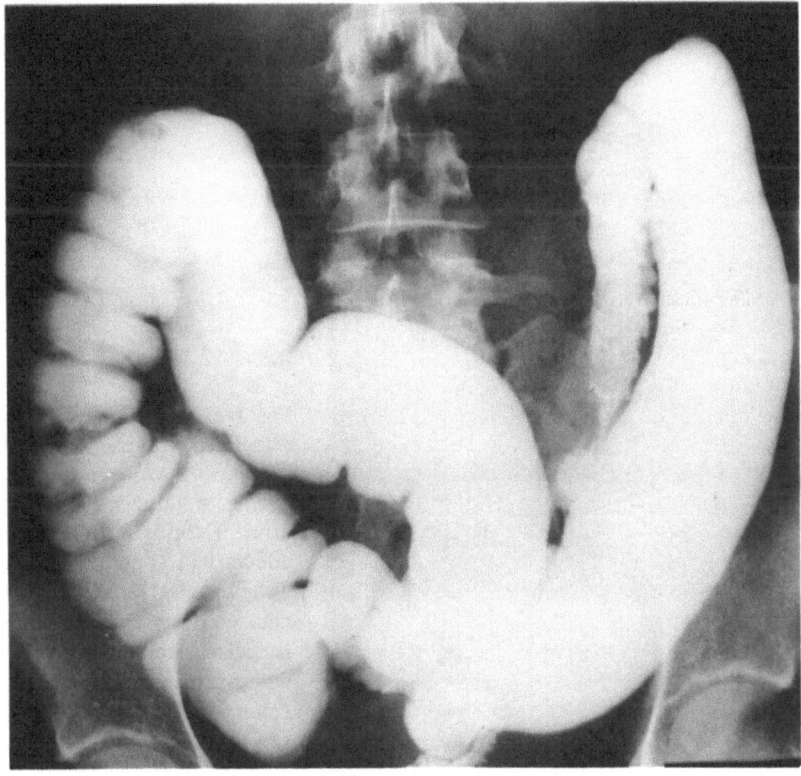

Fig. 1-21, a–c. Ischemic changes of the left colon secondary to use of oral contraceptives. a Long segmental involvement, submucosal ridging, and luminal narrowing are evident in this study from a 28-year-old female. b Close-up of hepatic flexure demonstrates the ridging and thumbprinting. c Two weeks later the abnormalities are resolving.

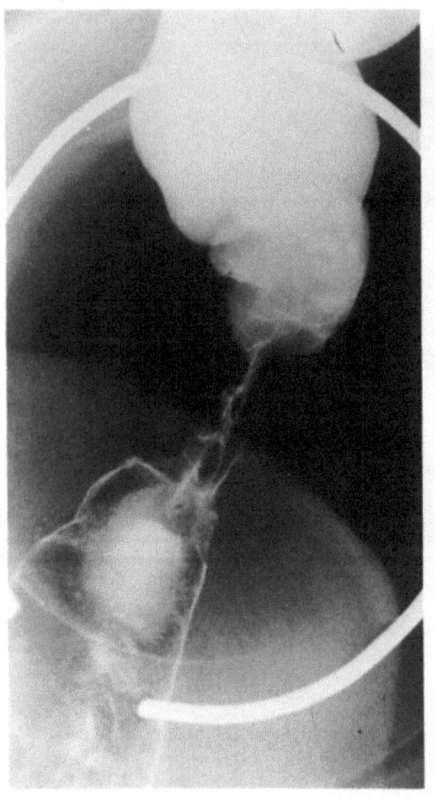

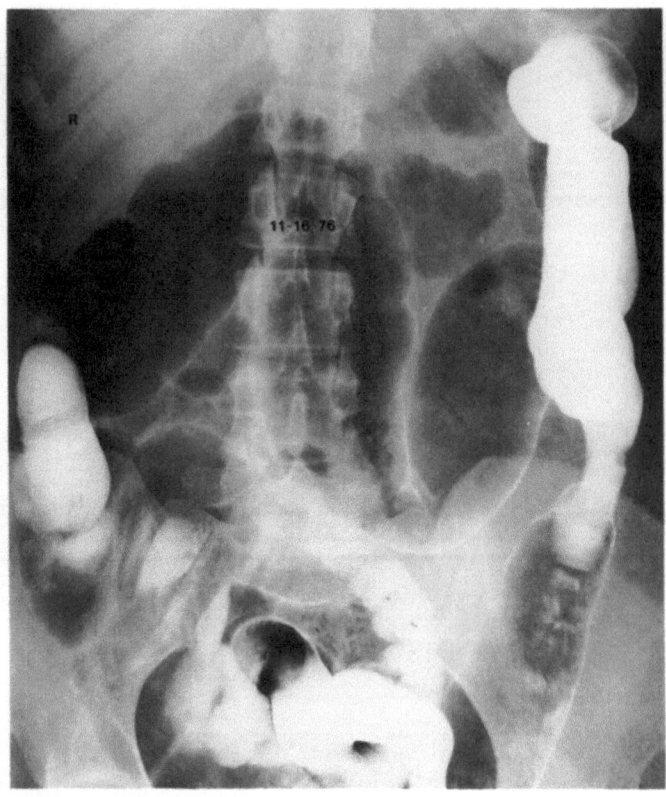

a   b

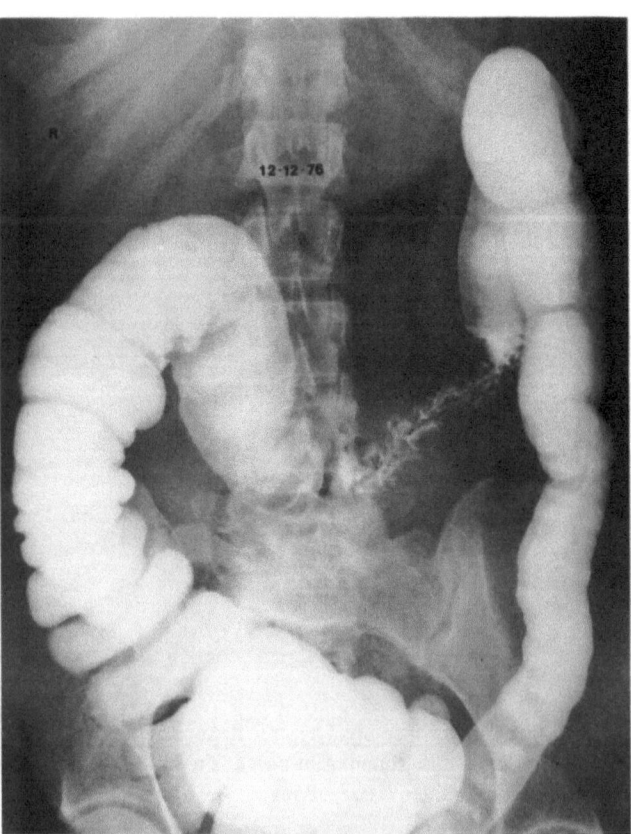

Fig. 1-22, a–c. Ischemic changes of the colon associated with use of oral contraceptives. A 22-year-old woman who had been taking cyclical contraceptive medication, norethindrone (Norinyl), for 2 years without side effects had symptoms of cerebral transient ischemic attacks as well as lower abdominal pain and one episode of rectal bleeding. **a** Localized colonic narrowing with nodular mucosa is seen on spot film of descending colon. **b** Following injection of glucagon, spasm is relieved but luminal narrowing persists. **c** Barium enema study 25 days later demonstrates complete disappearance of segmental ischemic colitis. (Ghahremani GG, et al: Ischemic disease of the small bowel and colon associated with oral contraceptives. Gastrointest Radiol 2:221–228, 1977)

c

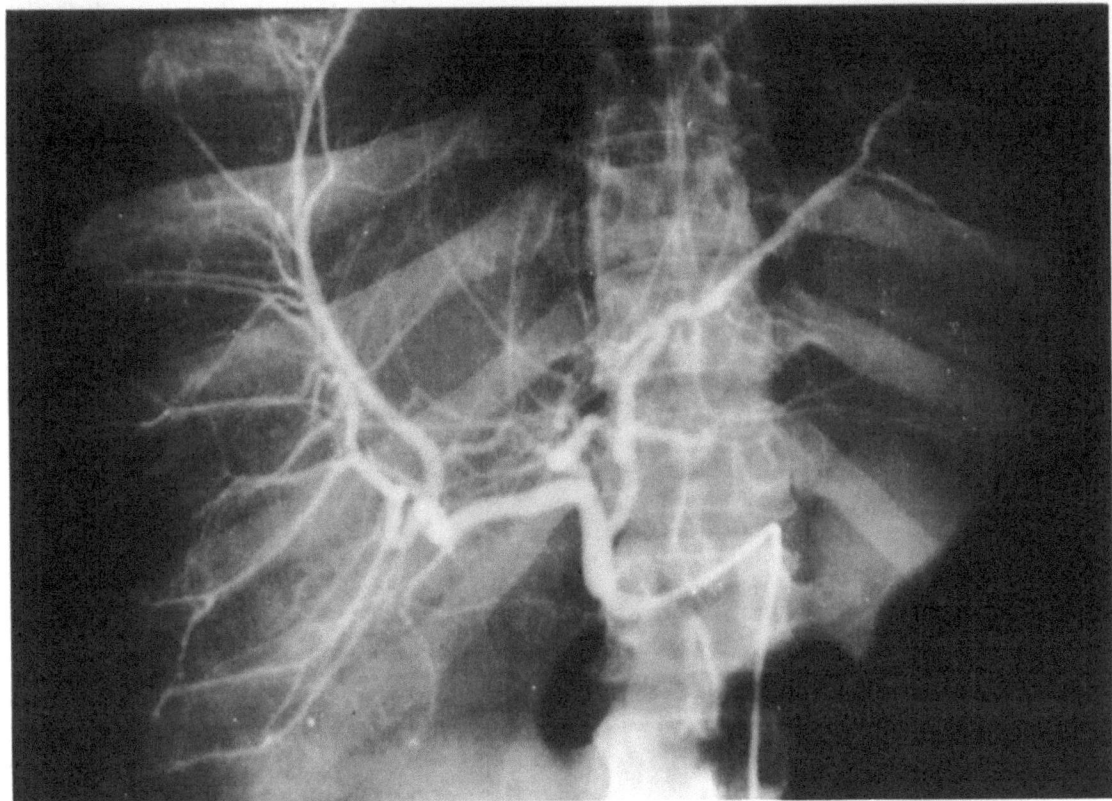

a

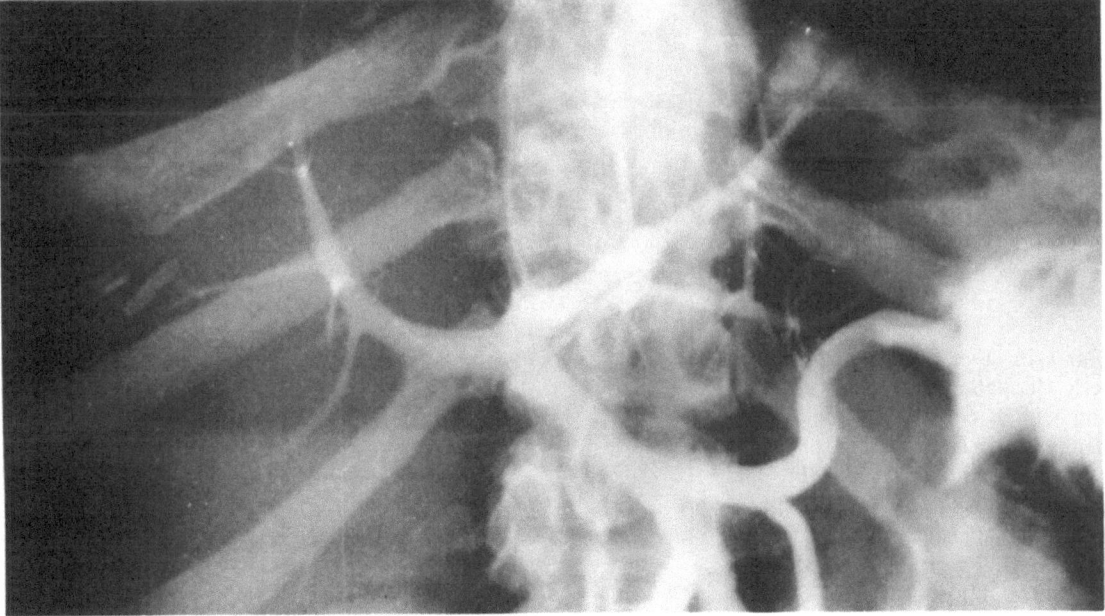

b

Fig. 1-23, a and **b. Budd-Chiari syndrome.** In a 47-year-old woman who had been taking birth control pills for the previous 8 years there was sudden onset of ascites 6 weeks prior to admission. **a** Hepatic arteriogram shows increase in size of the liver, particularly the left lobe. A mesenteric arteriogram obtained after administration of tolazoline (Priscoline) revealed no filling of the portal vein. **b** Splenoportogram shows lit-tle blood flow to the liver, which demonstrates small intrahepatic radicals. There is retrograde flow down the superior and inferior mesenteric veins secondary to increased portal pressure. The absence of large esophageal varices suggests that the process is acute. Hepatic venography demonstrated only tapered stumps.

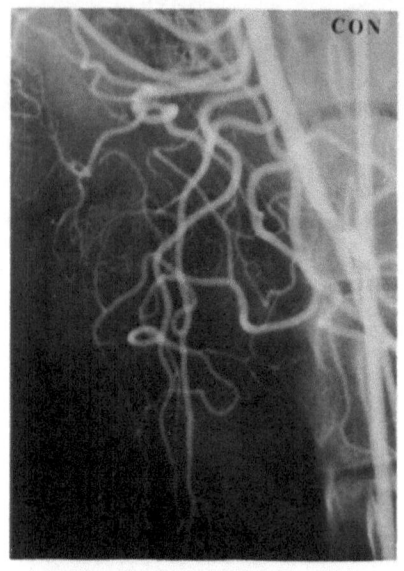

a

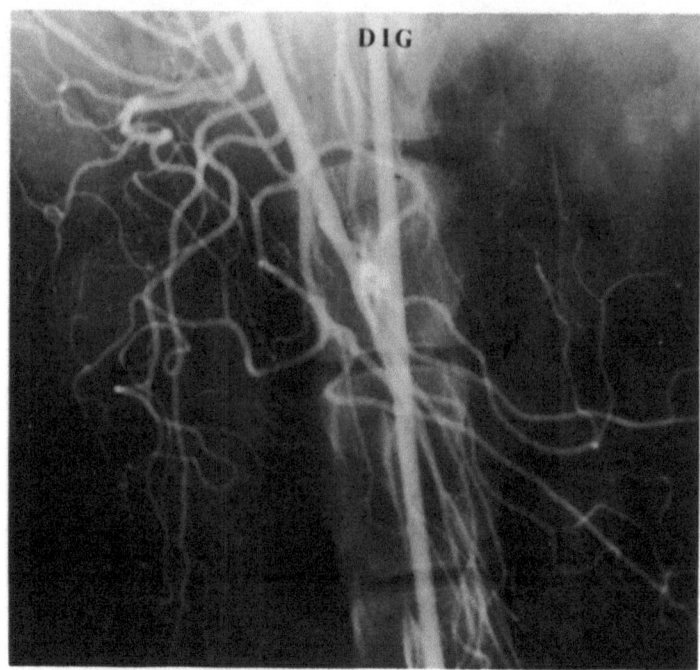

b

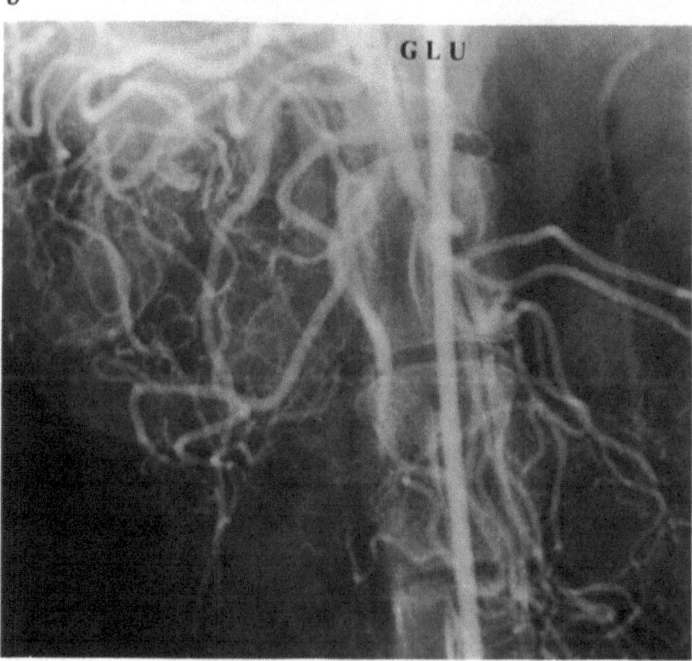

c

Fig. 1-24, a–c. Evaluation of mesenteric circulation in dogs. In comparison with a control (**a**), angiography demonstrates a decrease in splanchnic perfusion with digitalis (**b**) and increase with glucagon (**c**). *CON*, control; DIG, digitalis; GLU, glucagon. (Courtesy of R. Danford, MD, Worcester, Massachusetts)

Digitalis

Nonocclusive intestinal infarction has been noted in patients being treated with digitalis derivatives (159–162). Although these patients usually have cardiac disease with splanchnic vasoconstriction and poor perfusion in the first place, digitalis has been shown to increase vaso-constriction further (163,164) (Fig. 1-24). Mesenteric arterial spasm has been demonstrated by arteriography (165). A large percentage of patients with possible digitalis-precipitated intestinal infarction were receiving high doses or in fact had digitalis toxicity (Fig. 1-25). Therefore it is suggested that digitalis preparations be used with caution in patients in shock.

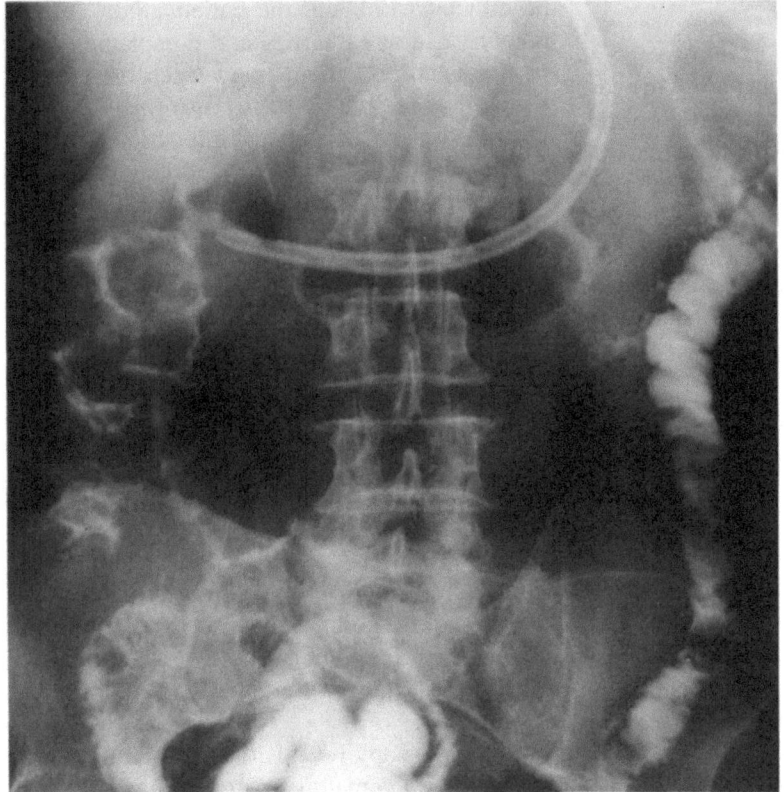

a

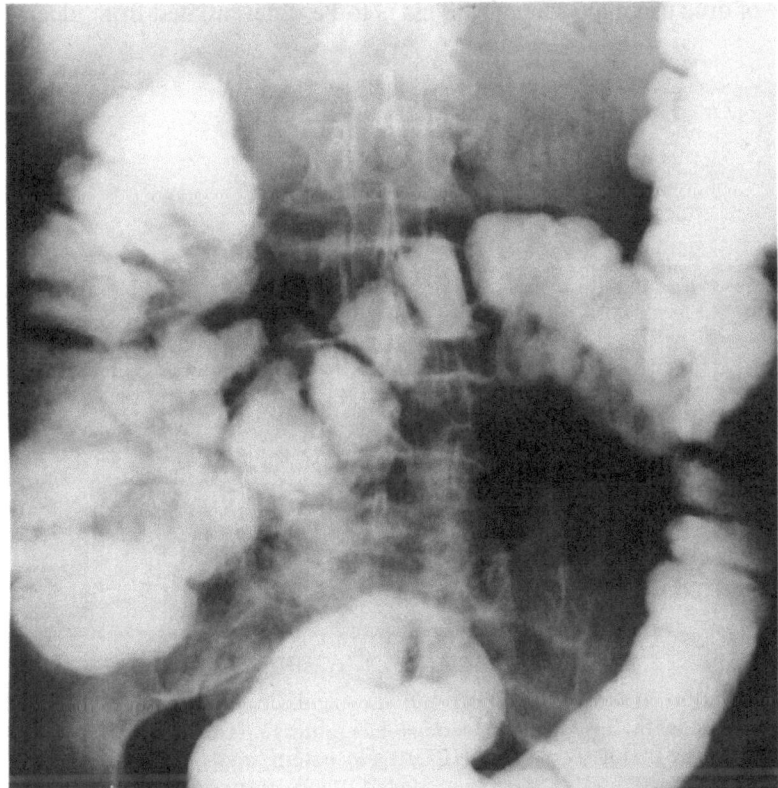

b

Fig. 1-25, a and b. Ischemic changes associated with use of digitalis. a Radiographic changes of infarct at hepatic flexure are seen in a 60-year-old man with lower gastrointestinal bleeding. He was taking digitalis at the time and had clinical and ECG evidence of digitalis toxicity. b Resolution of radiographic findings 1 week later.

In this age group and in most cardiac patients it is clinically impossible to determine whether the ischemic changes are secondary to the effects of digitalis or to underlying vascular disease.

Ergot Derivatives

High doses of the ergot alkaloids are capable of causing intense vasoconstriction (166); however, clinical reports involving the mesenteric arterial tree are unusual (Fig. 1-26). Two cases, one due to ergotamine and the other due to methysergide, have been noted; vasospasm was observed by arteriography (167, 168). Intestinal infarction did not occur, and after cessation of the medication, follow-up arteriography was normal in both cases.

"Cathartic Colon"

The entity of so-called cathartic colon due to prolonged use of stimulant-irritant cathartics has been described principally in the radiologic literature (169–173). Currently the most frequently used stimulant-irritant cathartics include castor oil, phenolphthalein, bisacodyl, senna, danthron, and cascara sagrada derivatives (174). The typical patient with cathartic colon is female and has habitually used irritant cathartics for more than 15 years. The history of drug use may

be difficult to obtain, the patient often initially denying use of cathartics and complaining only of constipation. Patients may reach the point at which they feel that a bowel movement without laxative assistance is almost impossible.

The diagnosis of cathartic colon is usually based on the barium enema study in the setting of an appropriate history. Although the entire colon can be involved, right-sided changes alone are very common. The findings of the barium enema study closely simulate those of "burned-out" ulcerative colitis—dilated, atonic, ahaustral colon, patulous ileocecal valve, and dilated terminal ileum suggestive of "backwash ileitis" (Figs. 1-27, 1-28). Longstanding ulcerative colitis, however, tends to display more colonic shortening, true strictures, and a more ragged mucosal surface. Cathartic colon, on the other hand, may show transient pseudostrictures due to spasm of the colon (Fig. 1-29), but it maintains its pliability. Predominantly right-sided involvement necessitates differentiation from amebic colitis.

Sigmoidoscopy reveals the colonic mucosa to be pale and edematous, or occasionally melanosis coli is observed when cascara has been used heavily. This is to be differentiated from ulcera-

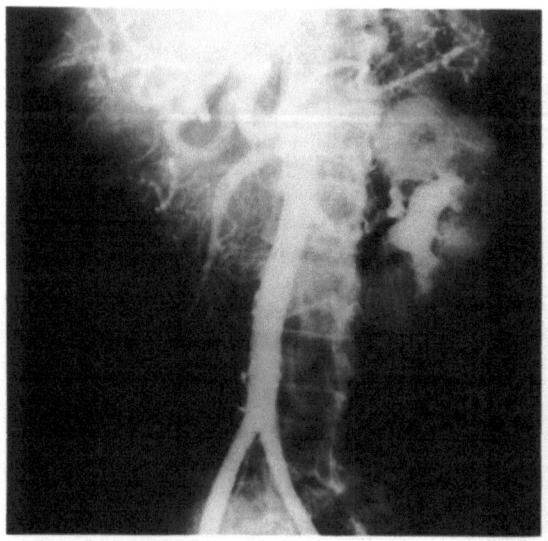

a

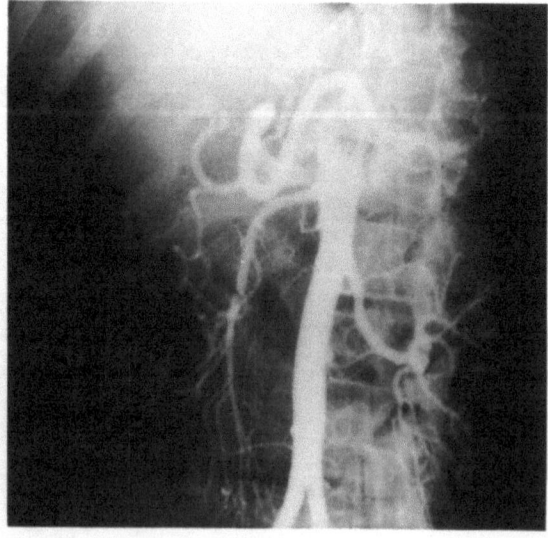

b

Fig. 1-26, a and b. Prominent changes in the mesenteric circulation associated with ergotism. a In this patient with history of ergotamine abuse there is slight dilatation of the proximal mesenteric artery and marked vasoconstriction of the peripheral branches to

the bowel. **b** Following discontinuation of ergot, normal appearance has returned. (Greene FL, Ariyan S, Stansel HC Jr.: Mesenteric and peripheral vascular ischemia secondary to ergotism. Surgery 81:176–179, 1977)

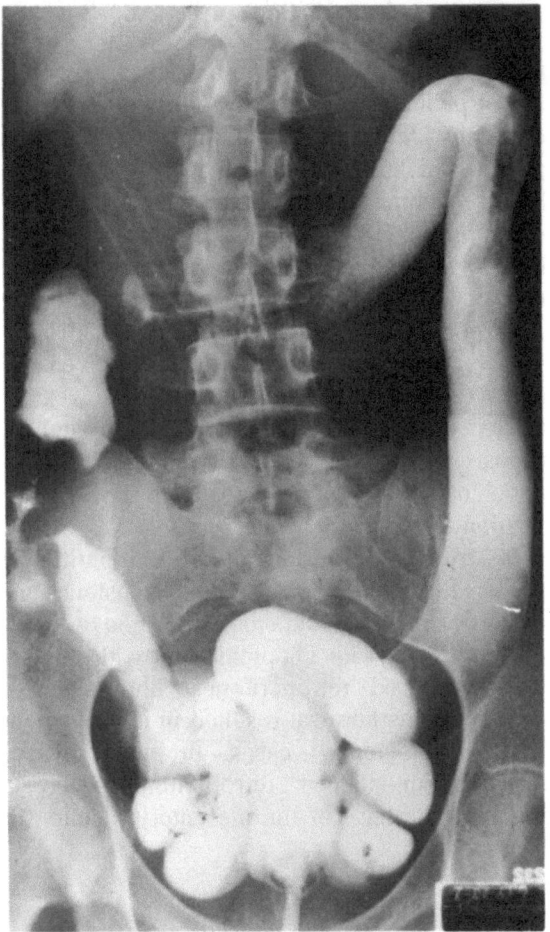

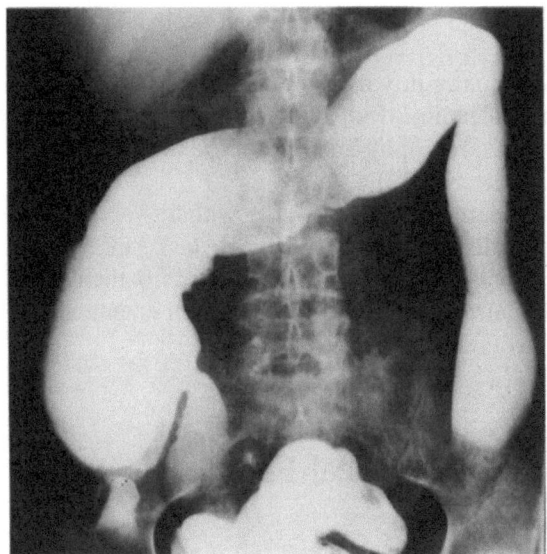

Fig. 1-28. Cathartic colon. Present are dilatation of most of the colon, loss of haustral definition, and changes in the ileocecal region simulating backwash ileitis. The patient complained of constipation and had used cascara sagrada cathartics for many years.

Fig. 1-27. Cathartic colon. Tubular ahaustral colon, patulous ileocecal valve, and dilated terminal ileum with effaced mucosal pattern are all present in this patient with history of long-standing cathartic ingestion.

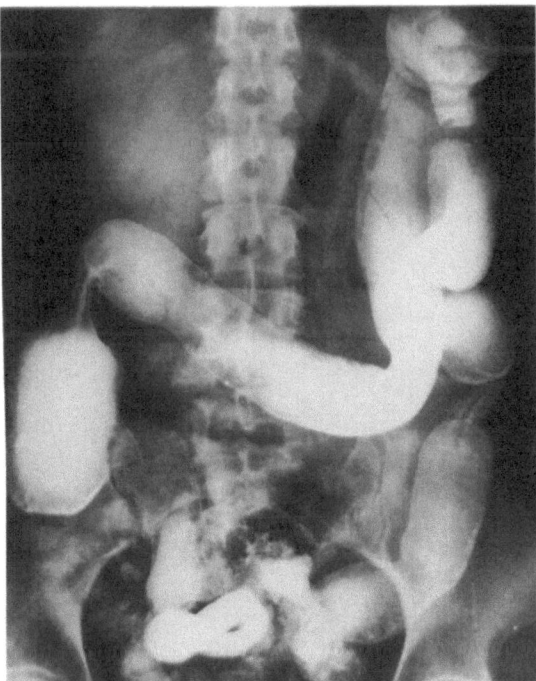

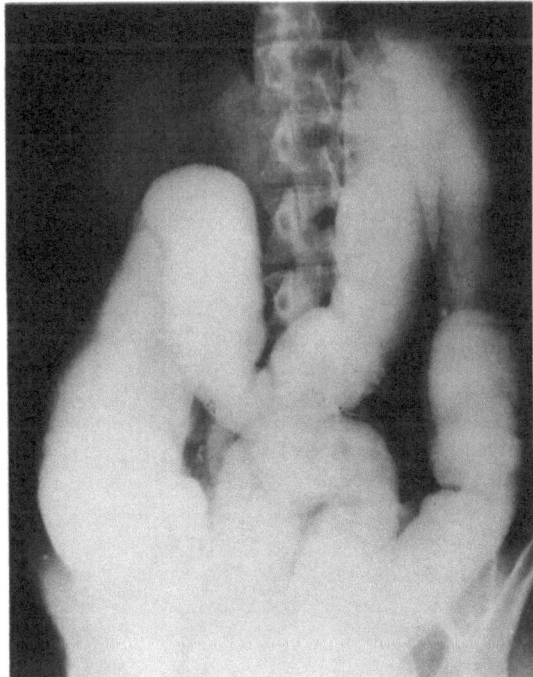

Fig. 1-29. Cathartic colon. a (left) Apparent strictures are secondary to spasm and are transient. b (right) Subsequent film demonstrates distensibility of entire colon. Despite loss of haustral pattern there is no shortening of colon in this patient, a feature that helps to distinguish cathartic colon from ulcerative colitis.

tive colitis in which the mucosa is red, friable, and bleeding. Biopsy of cathartic colon shows mucosal atrophy and loss of the normal glandular pattern (173).

Treatment consists of withdrawal of the offending laxatives, a difficult task since these patients have become habituated to their use. Abnormalities noted in the barium enema study may then improve (170).

Retroperitoneal Fibrosis

Methysergide

Although retroperitoneal fibrosis is usually idiopathic, there are many known causes such as surgery, trauma, abdominal aneurysm leakage, inflammatory disorders, thrombophlebitis, urine leakage, extravasation of contrast material, and tumors (175). In the 1960s methysergide, an ergot derivative used for migraine headache, became a conspicuous cause (176,177). Retro-

peritoneal fibrosis occurs in approximately 1%–2% of patients taking methysergide and is pathologically identical to the idiopathic variety, displaying a nonspecific inflammatory infiltrate followed by fibrosis, even though the mechanism is otherwise unclear (176,177). A fibrous plaque usually forms over the region of the sacral promontory and as a result, ureteral involvement is most common. Other fibrotic lesions associated with methysergide ingestion have involved the heart valves, lungs, pleurae, and great vessels (178). Methysergide-induced retroperitoneal fibrosis is potentially reversible after discontinuation of the drug, at times making surgical intervention unnecessary (176,177).

Gastrointestinal lesions due to retroperitoneal fibrosis are rare (Fig. 1-30). Several instances of extrinsic rectosigmoid narrowing have been reported both with idiopathic and with methysergide-induced retroperitoneal fibrosis (179–182). Drug withdrawal resulted in improvement in the drug-induced cases. In another case, methysergide-induced retroperitoneal fibrosis involved the base of the mesentery, leading to

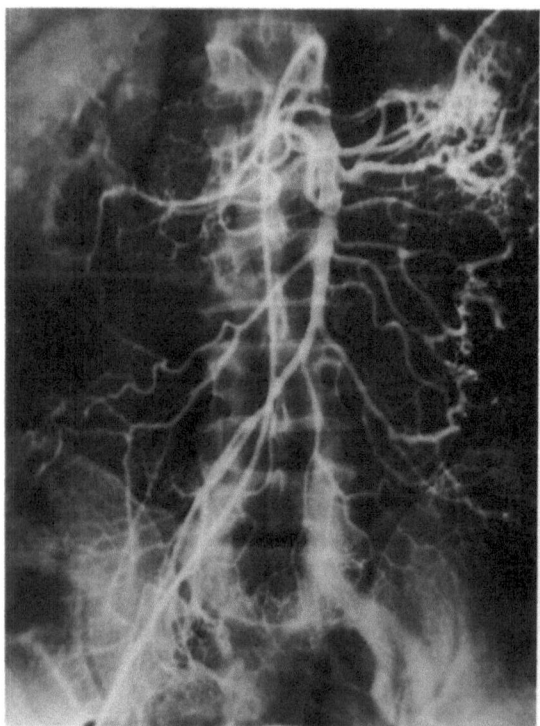 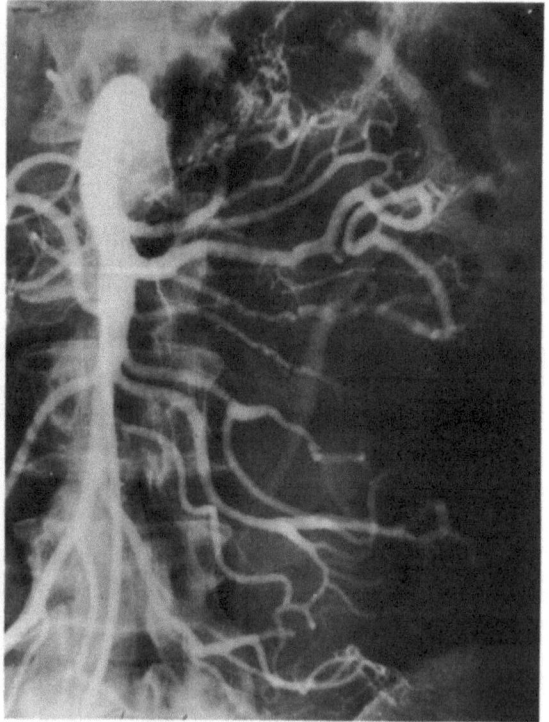

a   b

Fig. 1-30, a and **b. Mesenteric fibrosis.** Angiography demonstrates kinking and beading of mesenteric vasculature in a patient who had been treated with methysergide (Sansert). (Courtesy of D. Bloom, MD, Morristown, New Jersey)

intestinal angina (183). Angiography demonstrated high-grade superior mesenteric artery stenosis that was thought to be due to the extrinsic constricting fibrosis found at surgery. After release of the fibrosis the patient improved, but later mesenteric infarction occurred, probably secondary to recurrent fibrosis which was seen at autopsy. In a second patient taking methysergide, in whom segmental ileal infarction occurred, adventitial fibrosis was demonstrated in vessels of the resected specimen (184).

Many variant fibrotic syndromes are known to involve the gastrointestinal tract directly or indirectly, although they have not yet been associated with methysergide or other medications. Fibrotic masses have obstructed the duodenum (180,185,186), common bile duct (185,187), portal vein (188), and hepatic artery (189). It has been suggested that idiopathic mediastinal fibrosis and sclerosing cholangitis may also be related to retroperitoneal fibrosis (189–191).

Miscellaneous

Several other medications have been associated with retroperitoneal fibrosis in a few cases and potentially could cause gastrointestinal manifestations, although none has been reported. Ergotamine, dihydroergotamine, and LSD are all ergot derivatives (as is methysergide) that have been implicated as causes of retroperitoneal fibrosis (176,192,193); and analgesics (194), hydralazine (175), methyldopa (195), and antibiotics (196,197) have been circumstantially associated.

Liver Tumors

Estrogens

In 1973 possible association between use of oral contraceptives and occurrence of benign liver tumors was first reported (198). Since then numerous other reports have appeared (199–205). Although one report suggests no statistically significant association between use of contraceptives and occurrence of hepatic adenoma, the data were unclear in the case of focal nodular hyperplasia of the liver (206). The contraceptives incriminated most often contained mestranol as

the estrogenic component (202). Benign hepatic tumors—the incidence of which has apparently increased in recent years, coinciding with widespread use of oral contraceptives—are usually classified as adenoma or focal nodular hyperplasia. Both contain hepatocytes, but adenomas classically have capsules and no nodularity, bile ducts, ductules, or sinusoidal vascularity (201).

Clinically there are several modes of presentation (199). The duration of contraceptive use varies, from 6 months to many years; prior liver disease is unusual. Approximately one-third of patients are asymptomatic, and hepatomegaly is discovered on routine physical examination. Another third are first seen because of right upper quadrant pain of days' to months' duration, probably due to hemorrhage into the tumor. The final third also have right upper quadrant pain, but this is then accompanied by "acute abdomen" and shock from intraperitoneal rupture of the tumor. This final group is the main source of concern in these otherwise benign tumors. In review of 35 reported cases of benign hepatic tumors associated with use of oral contraceptives there were 12 cases of massive hemoperitoneum, resulting in 5 deaths (201).

Radiographic evaluation of these tumors is useful in diagnosis and follow-up. Plain abdominal films and barium contrast studies are not useful other than to demonstrate a mass effect in the liver; no calcifications have been seen (199).

Liver scanning with technetium ^{99m}Tc sulfur colloid can be helpful in following the size of hepatic adenomas since these lesions usually show no uptake of the radiopharmaceutical; scanning is of little differential value because malignant hepatomas present a similar appearance (207–209). In some cases, though, even a large hepatic adenoma may not be apparent on liver scan if it is of a pendunculated nature (199). In focal nodular hyperplasia the lesion tends to take up the isotope similar to normal liver since it contains reticuloendothelial cells, but hemorrhage in the tumor may make it "cold" (208,209).

Selective hepatic arteriography is the most useful diagnostic radiographic examination (Figs. 1-31 to 1-34). Preoperative differentiation of a benign tumor from a hepatoma is usually possible (208,210). Both are very vascular with an intense tumor blush and may be quite large (e.g., 15 cm in diameter), but the benign lesions

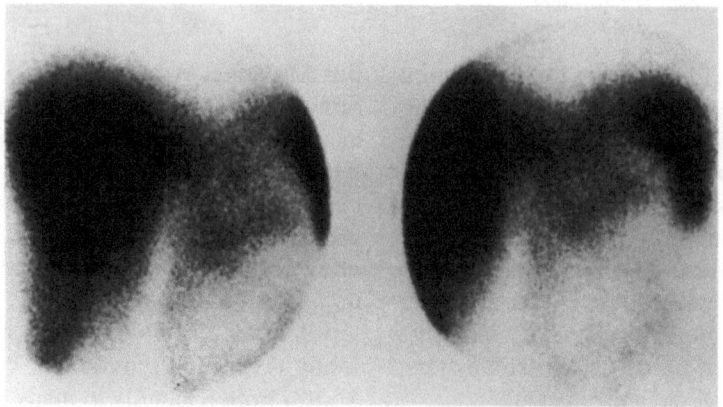

a

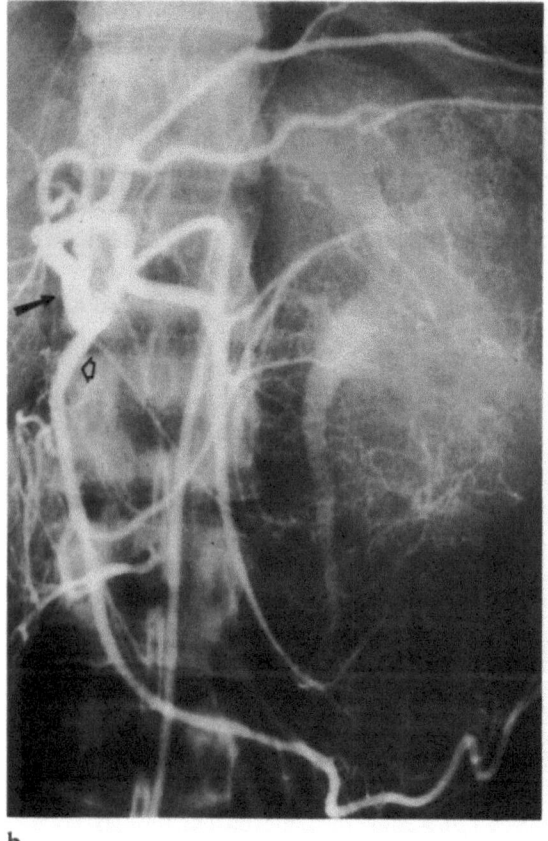

b

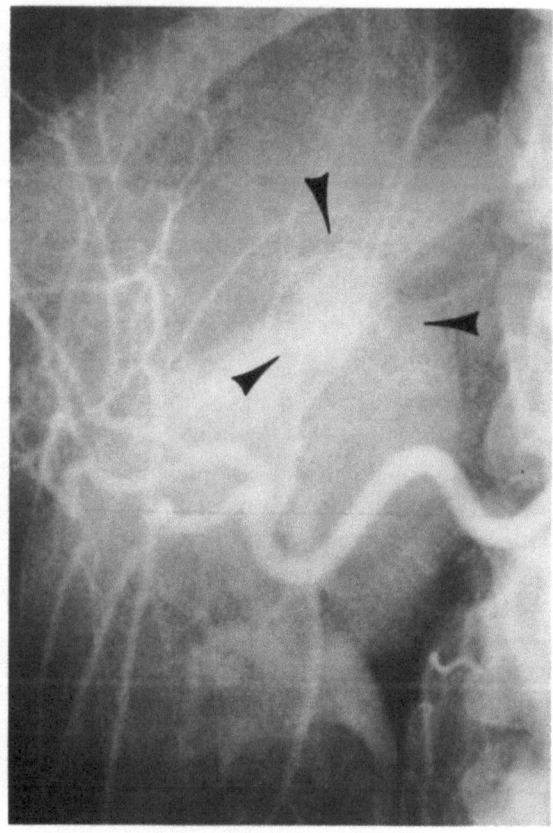

c

Fig. 1-31, a–c. Focal nodular hyperplasia of the liver associated with use of oral contraceptives. A palpable midepigastric mass was noted on routine physical examination in a 26-year-old woman who had been taking the combined contraceptive norethindrone-mestranol (Ortho-Novum 1/80) for 7 years. She had no history of liver disease. **a** Technetium Tc 99-m sulfur colloid scan reveals a large defect in the inferior aspect of the left hepatic lobe with lack of nuclide uptake centrally.

b Left hepatic arteriogram demonstrates a vascular mass with peripheral circumferential arterial supply and multiple parallel branches coursing centrally. *Solid arrow* is the left hepatic artery. There was minimal vascular stain in the parenchymal phase compared to the normal contiguous liver. *Open arrow* is the gastroduodenal–right gastroepipoploic arterial complex, which does not supply blood to the hepatic mass.

The left lobe was surgically resected and histologic section revealed focal nodular hyperplasia with cords of well-differentiated hepatocytes containing thin strands of fibrous tissue with occasional ductal proliferation. The right lobe appeared normal although right hepatic artery injection (c) demonstrated a 1.5-cm vascular lesion *(arrowheads)* in the medial aspect of the right lobe, presumably another area of focal nodular hyperplasia. (Davis TJ, Berk N: Benign hepatic lesions in women taking oral contraceptives. Gastrointest Radiol 2:213–219, 1977)

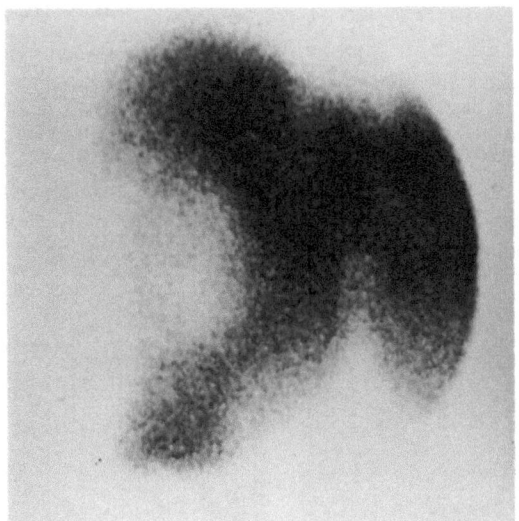

a

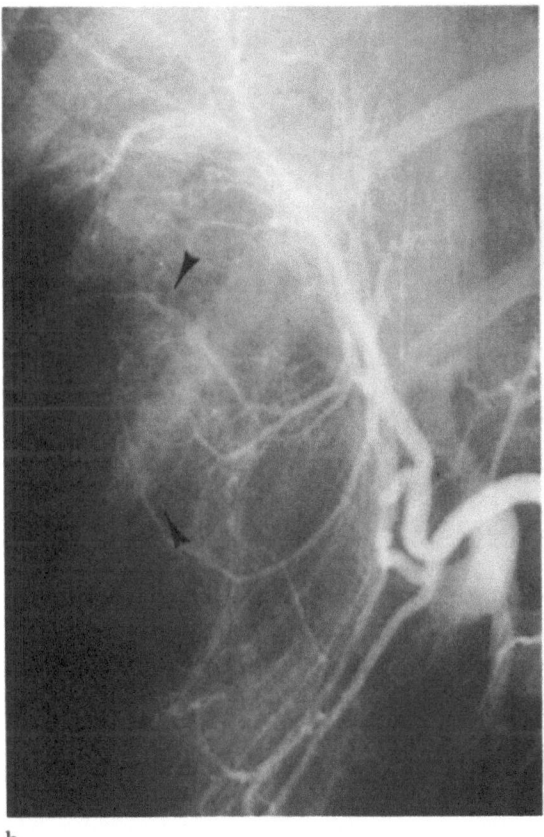

b

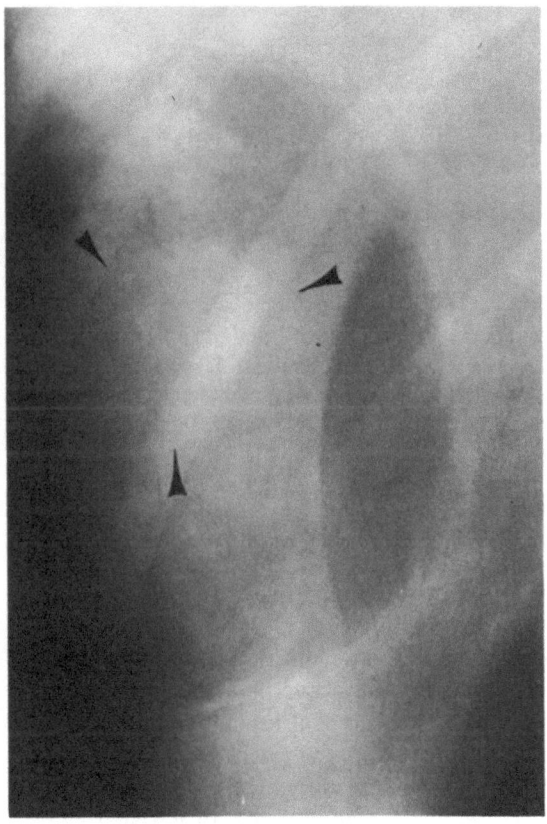

c

Fig. 1-32, a–c. Hepatic adenoma associated with use of oral contraceptives. This 23-year-old woman, who had been taking birth control pills continuously for 7 years, had acute onset of midepigastric pain. The hematocrit fell from 40% to 34% over 24 hours. **a** Radionuclide liver scan (technetium Tc 99-m sulfur colloid) reveals a large defect in the lateral aspect of the right lobe. **b** Arteriography demonstrates a moderately vascular lesion *(arrowheads)* with peripheral circumferential arterial supply, a few branches coursing centrally, and a surrounding avascular zone representing hematoma. **c** The parenchymal phase demonstrates the tumor stain and surrounding hematoma *(arrowheads),* which in turn is surrounded by a rim of compressed hepatic parenchyma.

The patient underwent right hepatic lobectomy at which time a 6-cm mass with surrounding hematoma was found. No extrahepatic extension or bleeding was noted. Histologic sections revealed cords of normal liver cells without portal tracts or visible bile ducts. The diagnosis was hepatic adenoma. (Davis TJ, Berk RN: Benign hepatic lesions in women taking oral contraceptives. Gastrointest Radiol 2:213–219, 1977)

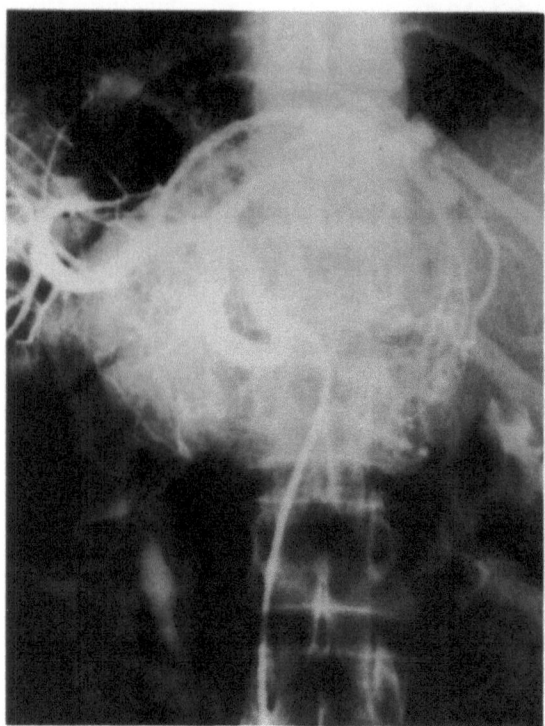

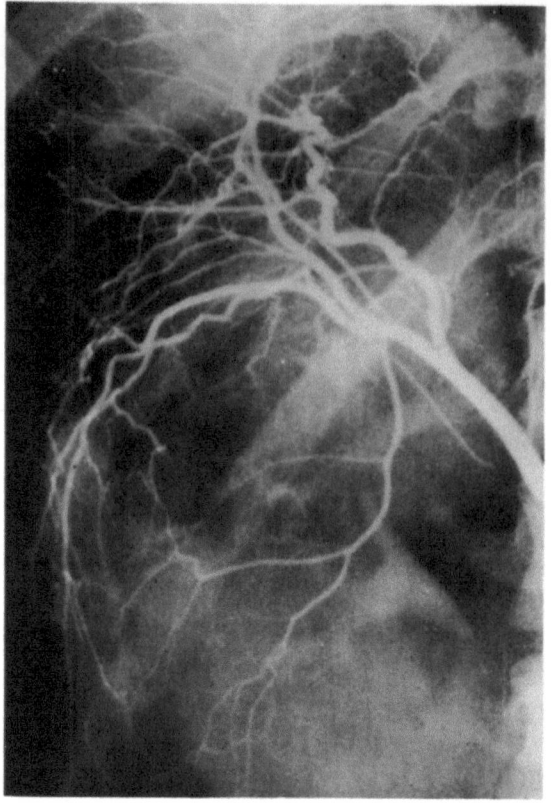

Fig. 1-33. Hepatic adenoma associated with the use of birth control pills. This young woman had umbilical pain, decreasing hematocrit, and a palpable epigastric mass; a liver scan was abnormal. Hepatic arteriogram demonstrates a large tumor mass, characterized by wild tumor vessels and the main vessels entering from the periphery. The parenchymal phase demonstrated a sharp margin without infiltration.

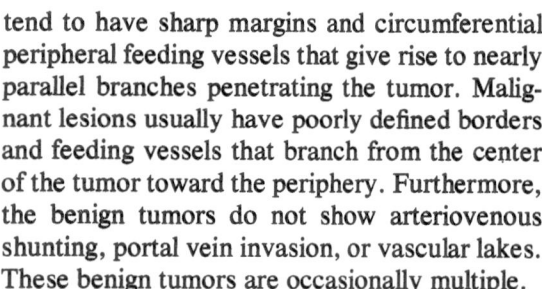

Fig. 1-34. Hepatic lesion associated with use of oral contraceptives. The poorly vascularized mass in the right lobe of the liver in a young woman is a variety of hepatic tumor midway between benign and malignant. (Courtesy of S. Galloway, MD, New Haven, Connecticut)

tend to have sharp margins and circumferential peripheral feeding vessels that give rise to nearly parallel branches penetrating the tumor. Malignant lesions usually have poorly defined borders and feeding vessels that branch from the center of the tumor toward the periphery. Furthermore, the benign tumors do not show arteriovenous shunting, portal vein invasion, or vascular lakes. These benign tumors are occasionally multiple.

Treatment usually consists of discontinuation of use of oral contraceptives and resection of the tumor if possible because of the propensity for rupture and any uncertainty in absolutely differentiating it from a malignant hepatoma. Reports of regression of these benign tumors after cessation of use of contraceptives raise the possibility of nonoperative management (211,212). Some

recommend needle biopsy of the tumor after the diagnosis is suspected on the basis of history and angiography, but this may carry some risk because of the vascular nature of the tumors (211).

The possibility of estrogen-induced cancer arising in these otherwise benign liver tumors, or independent of the benign lesions, has been raised (203,213–215).

Androgens

A possible connection between androgenic-anabolic steroid therapy and malignant hepatoma has been made. Reports have usually involved patients being treated for aplastic anemias. (216–218).

Esophageal Moniliasis

Corticosteroids, Immunosuppressives, Antibiotics, Chemotherapeutic Agents

Candida albicans is a common inhabitant of the normal healthy alimentary tract, primarily in the mouth and large bowel, where the fungus lives as a saprophyte. However, the organism can be a low-grade pathogen when host immunity and normal gastrointestinal tract flora are altered by debilitating disease (usually in patients with transplants, myeloproliferative disorders, or diabetes mellitus) or drug therapy (corticosteroids, immunosuppressives, or antibiotics) (219–221). Antibiotic therapy usually has been prolonged, or broad-spectrum agents have been used. Odynophagia, dysphagia, and persistent chest pain are the most common presenting complaints, although the patient may be asymptomatic (221). The chest pain may initially suggest cardiac or pericardial pain. Examination usually reveals oral thrush.

Endoscopy, to demonstrate typical pseudomembranes containing *Candida* and debris, is diagnostically more sensitive than the barium swallow. Radiographically the esophagus may appear entirely normal or display no more than hypomotility in mild cases (221). In cases of moderate to severe involvement, barium swallow usually shows significant abnormality (219, 222–227) (Figs. 1-35 to 1-37). Findings are typically most marked in the lower and middle areas of the esophagus. Decreased peristaltic activity (Fig. 1-38) and thickened folds, which may simulate varices, are seen as early changes. Submucosal edema then leads to a nodular or cobblestone appearance, followed by ulceration, with a shaggy esophageal border (Fig. 1-37), and spasm in the more advanced cases. Normal distensibility of the esophageal lumen usually remains, but localized narrowing may occur in severe cases when inflammation and fibrosis extend deeply. Pseudodiverticulosis of the esophagus has been thought to be secondary to deep ulceration or undermining of the pseudomembrane. However, there have been examples in which this appearance is explained by widened submucosal glands (228,229) (Figs. 1-39, 1-40). One report describes an unusual radio-graphic presentation as a single polypoid lesion (230).

Treatment for candida esophagitis usually consists of oral administration of nystatin, to which patients respond quickly (219,221).

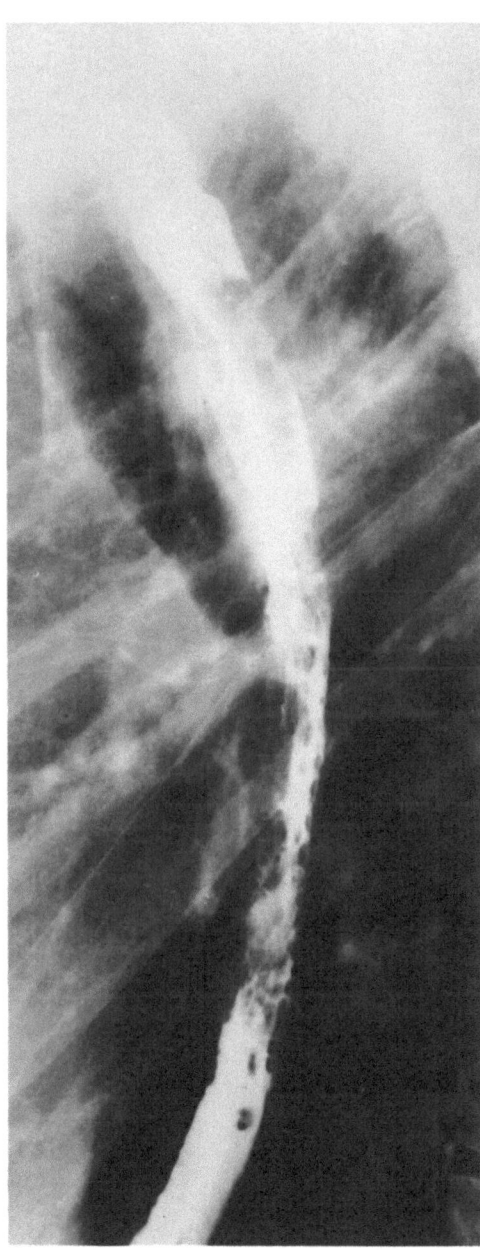

Fig. 1-35. Esophageal moniliasis. Marked irregularity of the midesophagus, thickened folds, ulcerations, and plaque-like defects are secondary to moniliasis in this patient receiving immunosuppressive therapy.

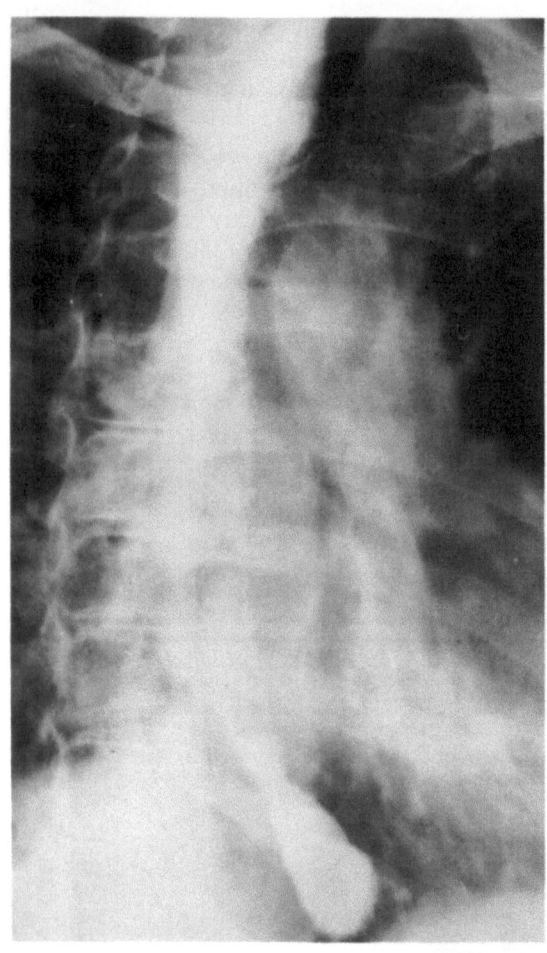

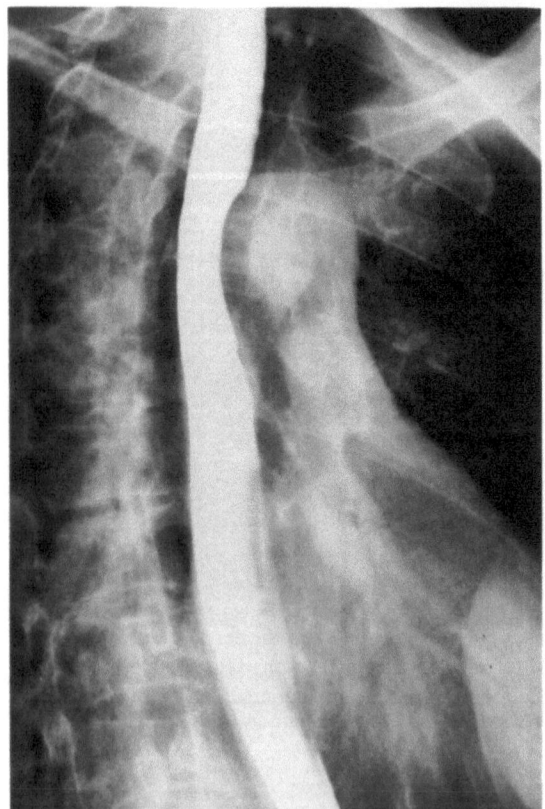

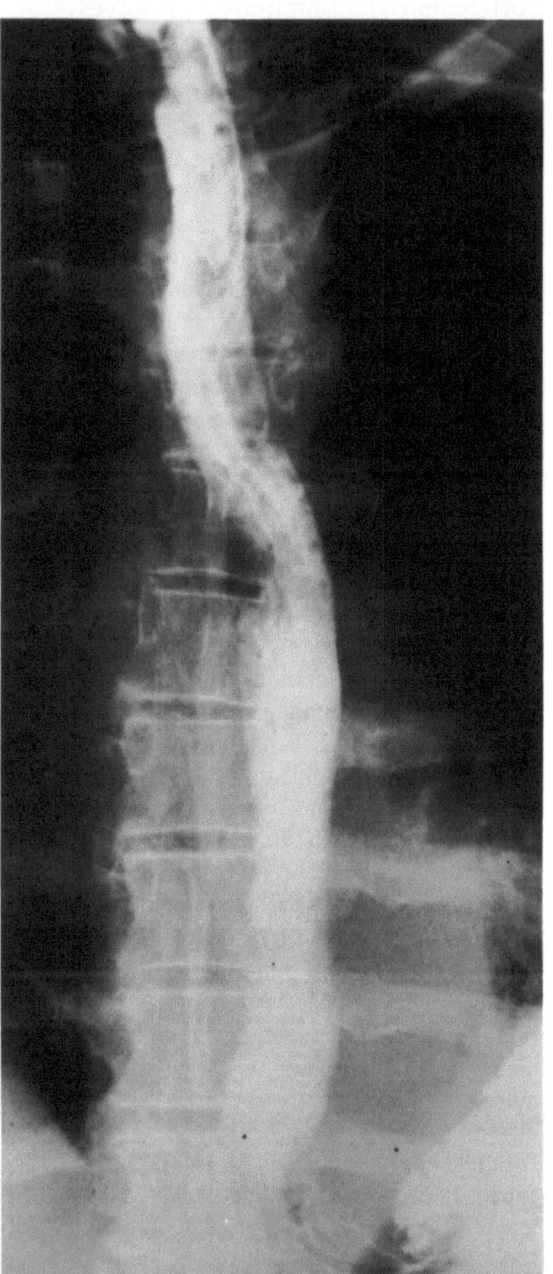

Fig. 1-36. (Top, left) **Monilial esophagitis.** The patient, who had leukemia and was receiving combined chemotherapy, developed monilial esophagitis and diffuse pulmonary infiltrates secondary to candida pneumonitis.

▲
Fig. 1-37. **Marked irregularity of esophageal border associated with moniliasis.** The patient had been receiving long-term steroid therapy for ulcerative colitis.

◀ Fig. 1-38. **Candida esophagitis.** The patient has total aperistalsis of the esophagus. Despite the apparent regularity of the esophageal margin, the absence of peristalsis is a significant sign of extensive involvement.

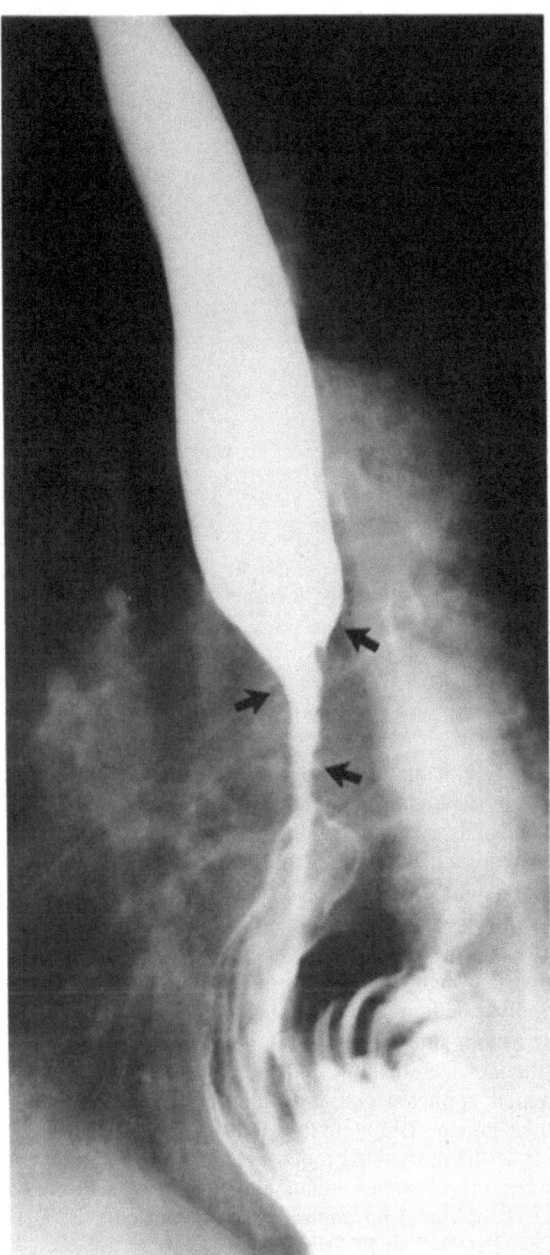

a

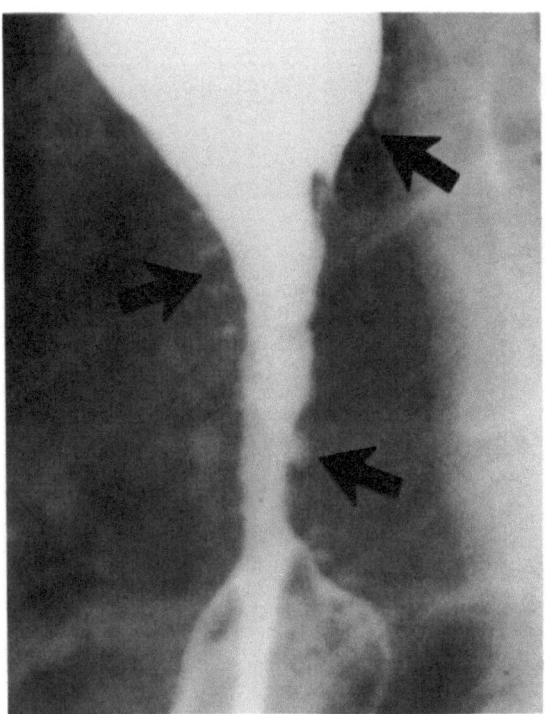

b

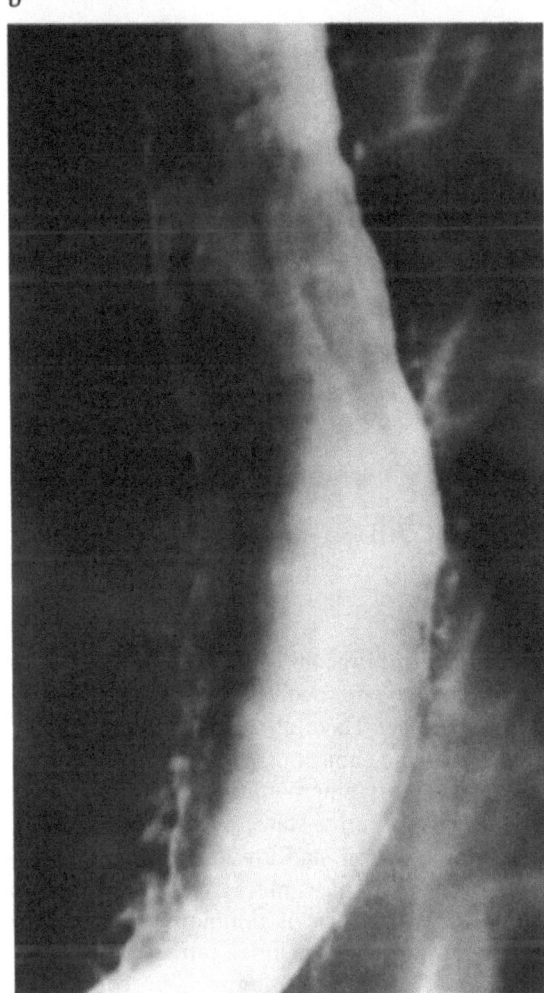

c

Fig. 1-39, a–c. Esophageal moniliasis. Multiple sac-like outpouchings filled with barium represent dilated intramural glands in these two patients. **a** and **b** Narrowing of distal esophagus with tiny barium collections *(arrows)* perpendicular to axis of esophagus is seen in a 55-year-old woman being treated with antibiotics for gram-negative sepsis. (These collections are seen better on the spot film.) **c** In a different patient, multiple pseudodiverticular outpouchings are demonstrated throughout the length of the esophagus. (Fromkes JJ et al: Esophageal intramural pseudo-diverticulosis. Dig Dis 22:690–700, 1977)

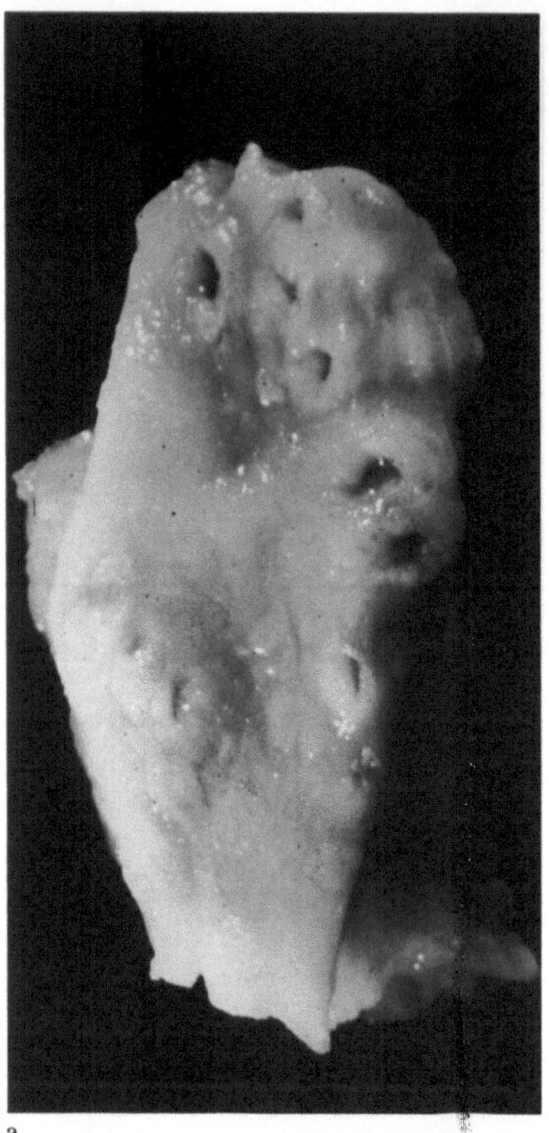

a

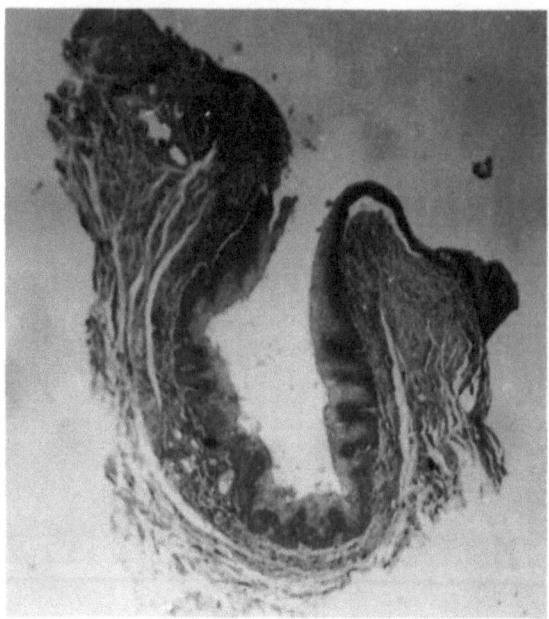

b

Fig. 1-40, a and b. Pseudodiverticulosis of the esophagus associated with moniliasis. a Gross specimen of esophagus in patient with moniliasis and pseudodiverticulosis demonstrates multiple ostia measuring 1–2 mm opening onto mucosal surface. These correspond to the openings of the main excretory ducts of the esophageal submucosal glands. b Microscopic sections through the ostium, neck, and complete pseudodiverticulum shows cavitary dilatation of the main excretory duct. These ducts are lined with stratified squamous epithelium and generally contain desquamated epithelial cells and amorphous debris within their lumen. These cavities indented but did not penetrate the muscularis mucosae, and surrounding them were rims of intense inflammatory infiltrate. (Fromkes JJ: Esophageal intramural pseudodiverticulosis. Dig. Dis. 22:690–700, 1977)

Enterocolitis

Antibiotics

In this era of burgeoning antibiotic use, pseudomembranous enterocolitis has become a well-defined entity. There are two excellent detailed reviews of the subject (231,232). Forms of pseudomembranous enterocolitis have been related to the postoperative state, hypotension, staphylococcal infection, and low birth weight in neonates. Of particular interest here is the form associated with use of antibiotics. The list of probable offenders includes tetracycline, chloramphenicol, penicillin, ampicillin, cephalexin, neomycin, erythromycin, sulfamethoxazole-trimethoprim, lincomycin, and, most commonly in recent years, clindamycin (232–234). The incidence of clindamycin-associated pseudomembranous enterocolitis has been reported to be as high as 10% when proctoscopy was utilized in all patients taking the drug and having diarrhea (235).

Clinically the patient with pseudomembranous enterocolitis complains of crampy abdominal pain, fever, and diarrhea, usually without blood. A history of concurrent antibiotic use is typically obtained, although cases appearing 2 to 3 weeks following cessation of antibiotic therapy are not rare. Early diagnosis is important because an acute abdominal condition may develop with severe involvement, leading to colonic perforation and death. The diagnostic mode of choice is sigmoidoscopy; the characteristic pseudomembranous plaques are seen with intervening edematous nonulcerated mucosa (Figs. 1-41, 1-42). The plaques are composed of fibrin, mucin, white cells, and sloughed mucosal cells. The mechanism of antibiotic induction of the disease has recently been shown to be through overgrowth of a toxin-producing bacterium, *Clostridium difficile* (236).

Until recently the radiographic findings in pseudomembranous enterocolitis were considered to be nonspecific, indistinguishable from those in other forms of colitis (237). However, on detailed study, the diagnosis can be made if the pseudomembranous plaques can be demonstrated (231,238,239) (Figs. 1-43, 1-44). Involvement is generally restricted to the colon. Plain abdominal radiographs may show moderate gaseous distention and distorted haustra with thumbprinting and thickening of the colonic

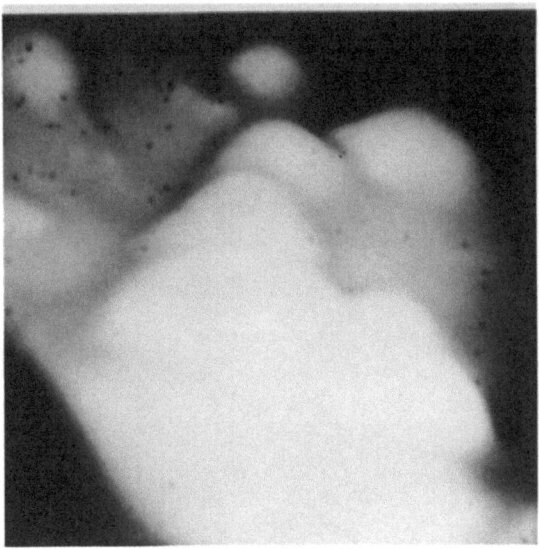

Fig. 1-41. Pseudomembranous colitis associated with use of clindamycin. Endoscopically the characteristic plaques are seen on a background of edematous nonulcerated mucosa. (Courtesy of The Upjohn Company)

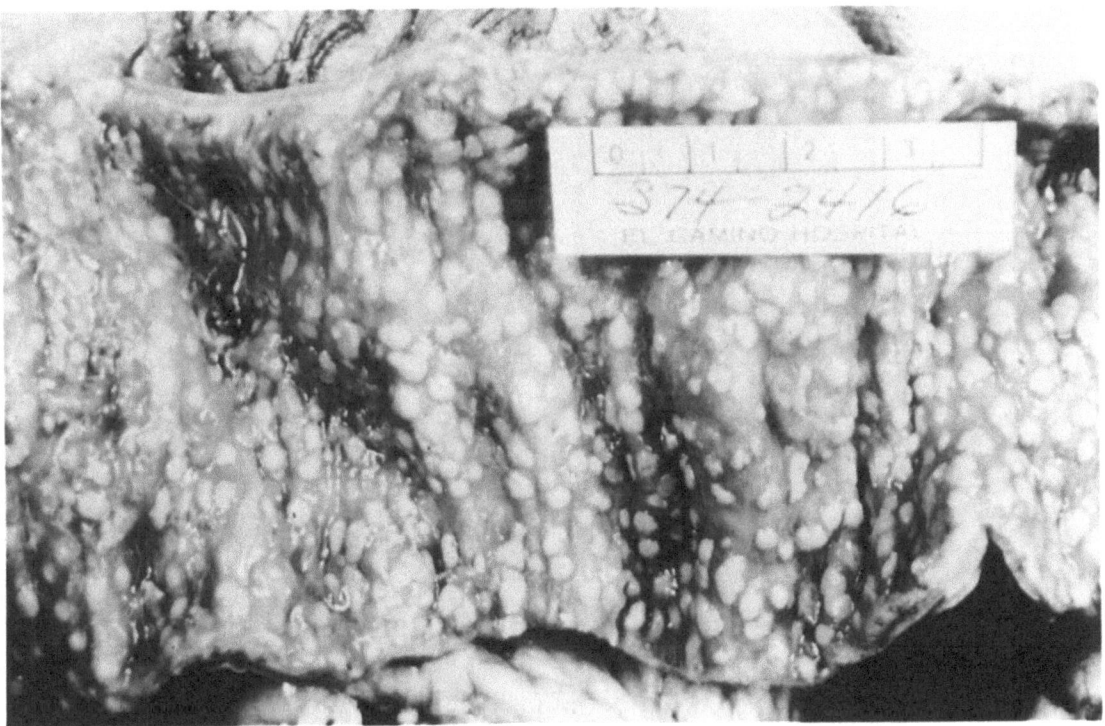

Fig. 1-42. Pseudomembranous colitis associated with use of clindamycin. The pathologic specimen demonstrates multiple plaques that form the pseudomembrane and the intervening edematous nonulcerating mucosa. (Courtesy of The Upjohn Company)

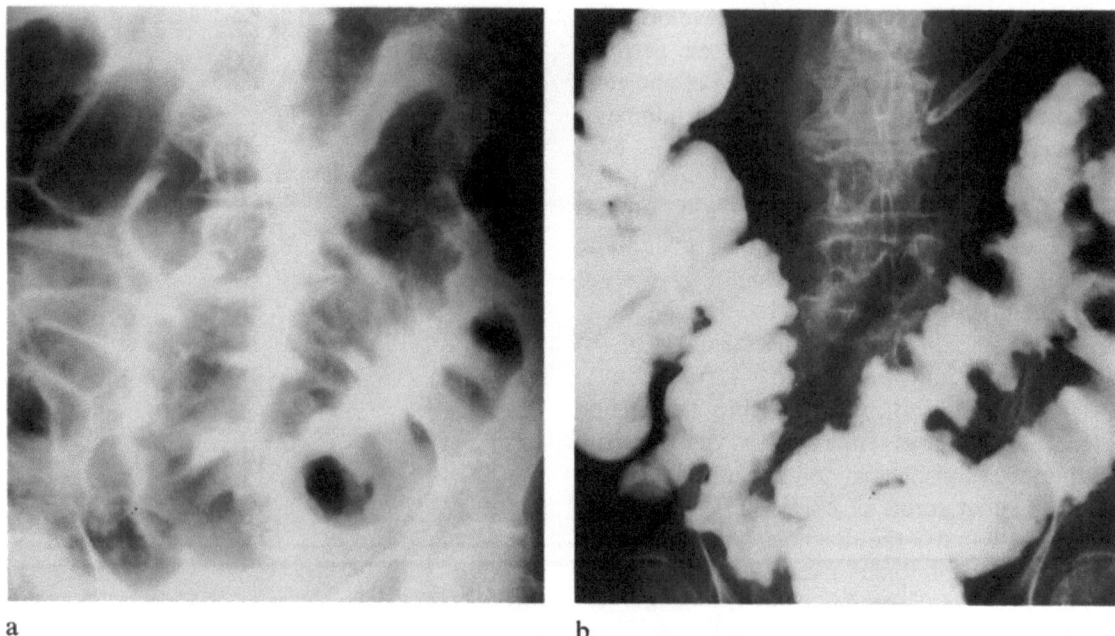

a   b

Fig. 1-43, a and b. Pseudomembranous colitis. a Plain film demonstrates ridging of left colon and irregularity of transverse colon. **b** These findings are confirmed on barium enema study, which shows the shaggy irregular margin of the bowel with several localized defects suggesting plaque formation.

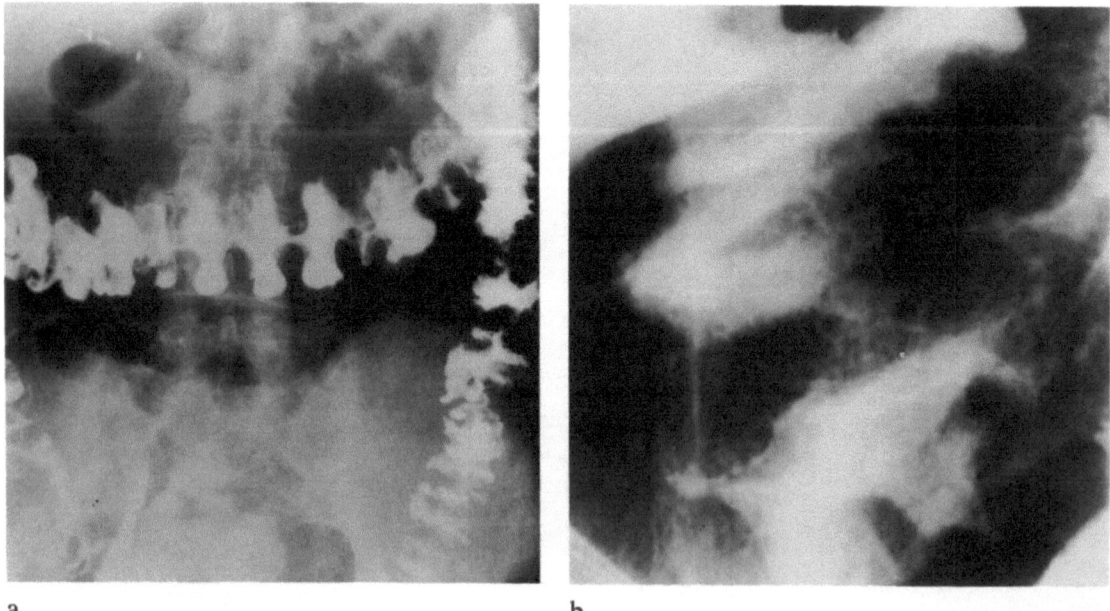

a   b

Fig. 1-44, a and b. Pseudomembranous colitis associated with use of clindamycin. a Generalized colonic involvement is evident. **b** Close-up of right colon demonstrates multiple plaque-like defects.

wall. Small mucosal irregularities on the plain film may indicate the presence of pseudomembranous plaques. Barium enema study should not be performed in severe toxic cases, which can simply be followed with plain films, but it is otherwise a safe procedure if done without excessive colonic distention. Colonic involvement is usually generalized (Fig. 1-44). Unless the plaques are demonstrated clearly, a shaggy appearance (Fig. 1-43) to the mucosa, suggesting nonspecific ulceration, may be noted. An air contrast technique may be of aid.

Treatment of antibiotic-induced pseudomembranous enterocolitis is usually supportive following cessation of the drug (231,240). However, discovery of the place of *Clostridium difficile* in the disease has led to a therapeutic role for vancomycin, to which the organism is sensitive (236). Severe cases in the past were sometimes treated with subtotal colectomy and temporary diverting ileostomy, but ileostomy alone may be sufficient (231,241).

Several cases of acute transient antibiotic colitis related to penicillin, ampicillin, and amoxicillin, but differing from the usual picture of pseudomembranous enterocolitis, have been described (242). (Fig. 1-45). In these cases, bloody diarrhea initiated an illness that resolved rapidly within a few days. Sigmoidoscopy showed no evidence of pseudomembranous plaque formation. Colonic involvement as demonstrated on barium enema study was predominantly right-sided, with submucosal edema and ulceration but no plaques. The etiology for this acute, transient form of antibiotic colitis is unclear, but the condition may be an allergic manifestation (242).

Actual urticarial lesions have, very rarely, been seen in the colon during barium enema examination of a patient undergoing a severe hypersensitivity reaction to penicillin (243,244). A mosaic pattern to the mucosa is produced by focal raised plaques of submucosal edema (Figs. 1-46, 1-47). The pattern is much more regular than the plaques of pseudomembranous enterocolitis (Fig. 1-48). One case of probable gastric urticaria due to penicillin has also been noted, with an appearance of submucosal infiltration on barium contrast examination of the stomach (245).

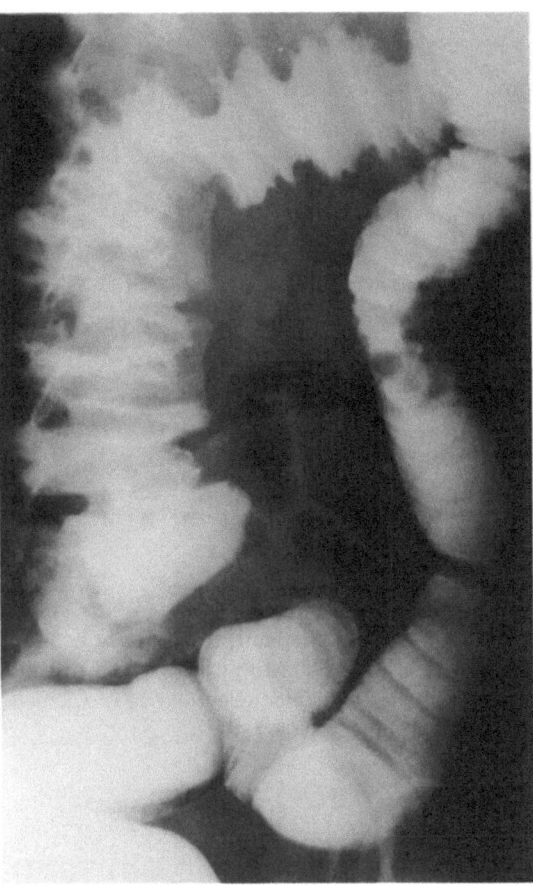

Fig. 1-45. Acute transient antibiotic colitis. The patient had lower gastrointestinal bleeding following ampicillin therapy. Barium enema findings consist of submucosal ridging involving predominantly the right colon. Sigmoidoscopy was normal, and on follow-up barium enema study several days later the appearance of the colon had returned to normal.

Gold

During gold therapy for rheumatoid arthritis, enterocolitis may rarely develop with fever, nausea, vomiting, abdominal cramps, and diarrhea (sometimes bloody) (246). Ulcerative changes with edematous mucosa have been described in the colon and small bowel on barium contrast study (247,248) (Fig. 1-49). Gold enterocolitis may be fatal and has been found at autopsy to be capable of involving the entire gastrointestinal tract from esophagus to rectum. The mechanism of mucosal damage is unknown. After gold therapy is stopped, treatment is supportive; steroids may possibly have a role.

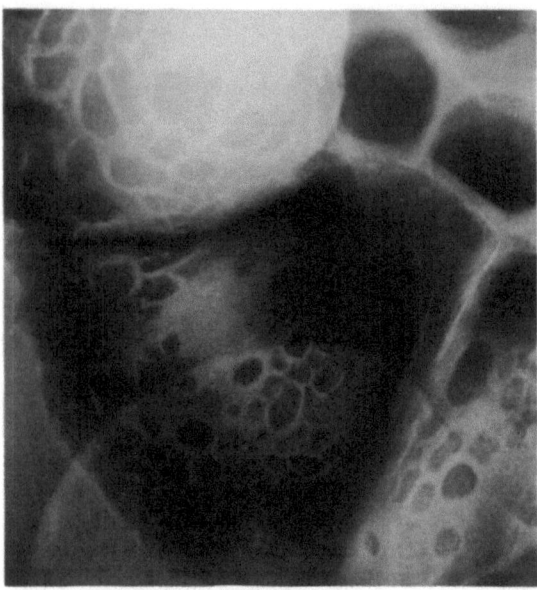

Fig. 1-46. Gastrointestinal urticaria. Localized allergic urticarial reaction to penicillin produces this mosaic pattern in the colon. (Courtesy of A. Clemett, MD, New York, New York)

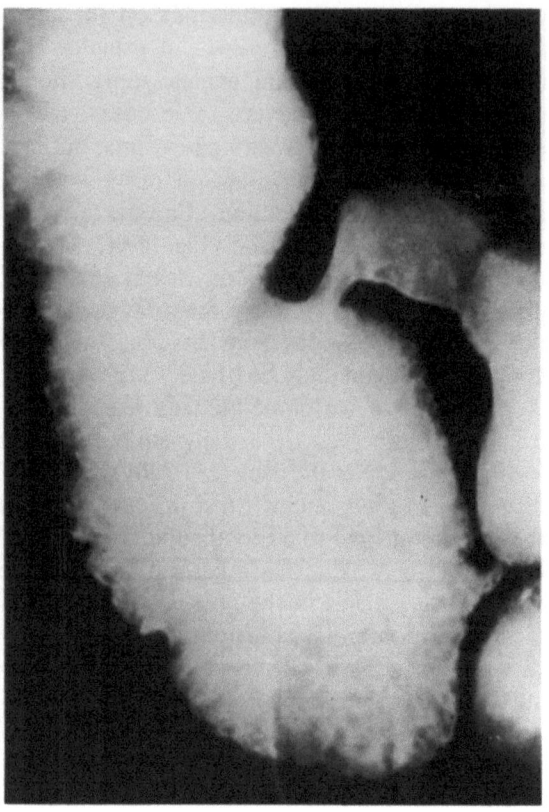

Fig. 1-47. Gastrointestinal urticaria. Multiple, small, very regular plaque-like defects in the right colon are manifestations of urticaria. (Courtesy of A. Clemett, MD, New York, New York)

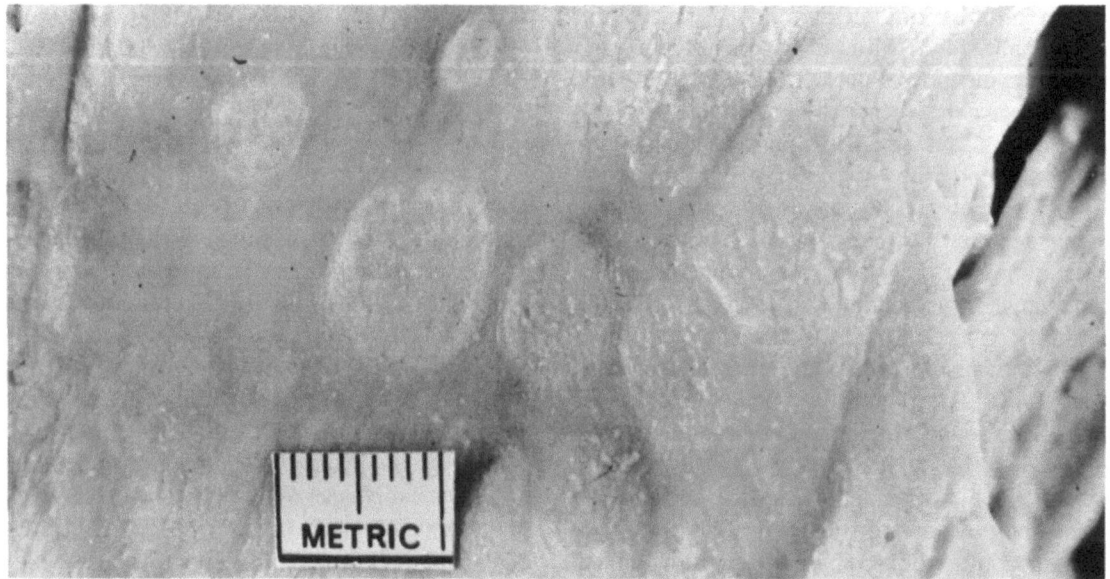

Fig. 1-48. Gastrointestinal urticaria. Gross specimen of colon in patient with generalized urticarial reaction of bowel reveals multiple lesions. (Courtesy of R. Berk, MD, San Diego, California)

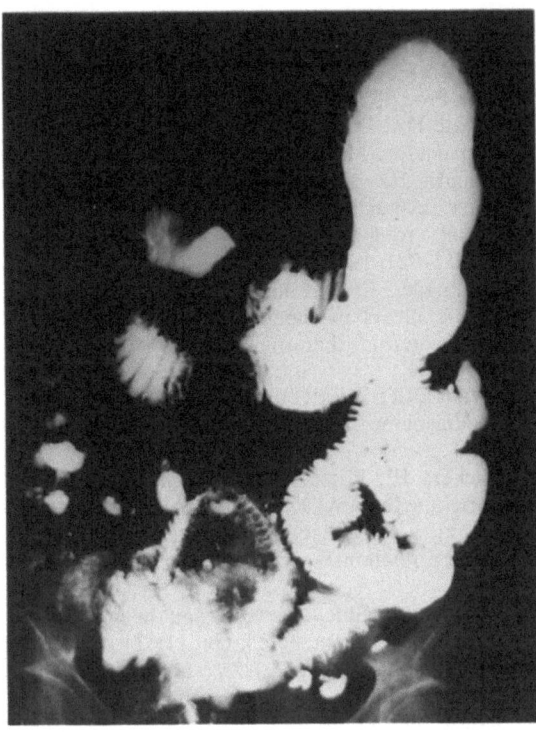

Fig. 1-49. Gold enteritis. A 61-year-old woman with severe rheumatoid arthritis had abdominal pain and guaiac-positive stools after repeated gold injections. Marked edema is present in the distal small bowel. (Courtesy of G. Ghahremani, MD, Evanston, Illinois)

Miscellaneous

Obstruction

Drugs can occasionally obstruct the gastrointestinal tract simply by virtue of their physical mass. Insoluble antacids such as aluminum hydroxide have become impacted in both large and small bowel (249–251). Cholestyramine, an insoluble exchange resin used to decrease bile salt reabsorption, has also caused impaction in several cases (252,253). A hygroscopic bulk laxative taken with insufficient water can form an obstructing rubbery mass in the esophagus (254). Even vitamin C tablets when swallowed whole have obstructed the ileocecal valve (255).

Pancreatitis

Many medications have shown a possible role in the induction of pancreatitis. Drugs incriminated include corticosteroids, estrogens, diuretics, salicylazosulfapyridine, antineoplastic agents, indomethacin, anticoagulants, and phenformin (256–266).

Gallstones

Several reports have indicated a relationship between estrogens, i.e., oral contraceptives and conjugated estrogens, and an increased incidence of gallstones (267–270). Similar findings have appeared for clofibrate, a drug used in the treatment of hyperlipidemia (271–273). Both drugs share an ability to increase the concentration of cholesterol in the bile.

Fibrotic Peritonitis

Practolol is a new β-adrenergic blocking agent not marketed in the United States but used extensively in Great Britain for the treatment of angina, hypertension, arrhythmias, and thyrotoxicosis. A unique fibrotic reaction of the visceral and parietal peritoneum has been described after long-term use of practolol (274). Patients have obstructive symptoms of abdominal pain, distention, nausea, vomiting, and often an apparent lower abdominal mass. The fibrotic peritoneal process encases the bowel like a cocoon, causing shortening and constriction. Small-bowel barium studies often demonstrate obstruction, prolonged transit time, bowel dilatation, loop separation by the "cocooning" process, fixation and rigidity of bowel loops, and an abnormal mucosal pattern (274). When obstructive symptoms arise an abdominal surgical procedure is necessary to strip off the encasing fibrous sheath (275).

Enzyme Esophagitis

A bolus of meat often becomes impacted in the distal esophagus at a prominent Schatzki's ring. Swallowing of papain (Adolph's meat tenderizer) to effect enzymatic digestion of the meat has been recommended as an alternative to endoscopic removal (276). However, there is a hazard of esophageal mucosal digestion and resulting esophagitis. Esophageal perforation has been reported.

References

1. Stewart RB, Cluff LE: Gastrointestinal manifestations of adverse drug reactions. Am J Dig Dis 19:1–7, 1974
2. Das KM: Iatrogenic alimentary disorders. J Indian Med Assoc 63:125–129, 1974
3. Rowe WS: Some of the clinically more important side effects of drug therapy. Part 2. Med J Aust 1:506–508, 1975
4. Shun DCH: Iatrogenic gastrointestinal diseases in the aged. Geriatrics 27:89–95 (Sept), 1972
5. Caranasos GJ, Stewart RB, Cluff LE: Drug-induced illness leading to hospitalization. JAMA 228:713–717, 1974
6. Berman PM, Kirsner JB: Recognizing and avoiding adverse gastrointestinal effects of drugs. Geriatrics 29:59–62, June, 1974
7. Ferrucci JT, Eaton AB: Complications of drug therapy. In Margulis AR, Burhenne HJ (eds): Alimentary Tract Roentgenology, 2nd ed. St. Louis: Mosby 1973, pp 281–293
8. Ansell G: Radiological manifestations of drug-induced disease. Clin Radiol 20:133–148, 1969
9. Roth JLA: Ulcerogenic drugs. Bockus HL (ed): Gastroenterology, 3rd ed., vol 1. Philadelphia: Saunders 1974, pp 491–514
10. Cooke AR: Drugs and gastric damage. Drugs 11:36–44, 1976
11. Loebl DH, Craig RM, Culie DD, et al: Gastrointestinal blood loss. Effect of aspirin, fenoprofen, and acetaminophen in rheumatoid arthritis as determined by sequential gastroscopy and radioactive fecal markers. JAMA 237:976–981, 1977
12. Laufer I, Hamilton J, Mullen JE: Demonstration of superficial gastric erosions by double contrast radiography. Gastroenterology 68:387–391, 1975
13. Mills JA: Nonsteroidal anti-inflammatory drugs. N Engl J Med 290:781–784, 1002–1005, 1974
14. Edmar D: Effects of salicylates on the gastric mucosa as revealed by roentgen examination and the gastrocamera. Acta Radiol 11:57–64, 1971
15. Poplack W, Paul RE, Goldsmith M, et al: Demonstration of erosive gastritis by the double-contrast technique. Radiology 117:519–521, 1975
16. Laufer I: A simple method for routine double-contrast study of the upper gastrointestinal tract. Radiology 117:513–518, 1975
17. Duggan JM, Chapman BL: The incidence of aspirin ingestion in patients with peptic ulcer. Med J Aust 1:797–800, 1970
18. Duggan JM: Aspirin in chronic gastric ulcer: An Australian experience. Gut 17:378–384, 1976
19. Douglas RA, Johnston ED: Aspirin and chronic gastric ulcer. Med J Aust 2:893–897, 1961
20. Gillies MA, Skyring A: Gastric and duodenal ulcer: The association between aspirin ingestion, smoking and family history of ulcer. Med J Aust 2:280–285, 1969
21. Levy M: Aspirin use in patients with major upper gastrointestinal bleeding and peptic-ulcer disease. N Engl J Med 290:1158–1162, 1974
22. Cameron AJ: Aspirin and gastric ulcer. Mayo Clin Proc 50:565–570, 1975
23. Floate DA, Duggan JM: Hour-glass stomach, an explanation. Med J Aust 2:674–676, 1976
24. Bulgrin JG, Dubois EL, Jacobson G: Peptic ulcer associated with corticosteroid therapy: Serial roentgenographic studies. Radiology 75:712–721, 1960
25. Freiberger RH, Kammerer WH, Rivelis AL: Peptic ulcers in rheumatoid patients receiving corticosteroid therapy. Radiology 71:542–547, 1958
26. Evans KT: Peptic ulceration associated with prednisolone therapy. Br J Radiol 31:307–312, 1958
27. Vickers JE: Recurrent gastric ulcer incident to cortisone therapy. Radiology 69:412–414, 1957
28. Cooke AR: Corticosteroids and peptic ulcer: Is there a relationship? Am J Dig Dis 12:323–329, 1967
29. Cushman P: Glucocorticoids and the gastrointestinal tract: Current status. Gut 11:534–539, 1970
30. Meltzer LE, Bockman AA, Kanenson W, et al: The incidence of peptic ulcer among patients on long term prednisone therapy. Gastroenterology 35:351–356, 1958
31. Conn HO, Blitzer BL: Nonassociation of adrenocorticosteroid therapy and peptic ulcer. N Engl J Med 294:473–479, 1976
32. Green SB, Gail MH, Byar DP: Steroids and peptic ulcer (letter). N Engl J Med 294:1291, 1976
33. Conn HO, Blitzer BL: Steroids and peptic ulcer (letter). N Engl J Med 294:1293, 1976
34. Laitinen H, Meurman K, Virkkunen M: Roentgenological appearance of corticosteroid-produced peptic ulcers. Acta Rheumatol Scand 4:205–217, 1958
35. Garb AE, Soule EH, Bartholomew LG, et al: Steroid-induced gastric ulcer. Arch Intern Med 116:899–906, 1965
36. Fenster LF: The ulcerogenic potential of glucocorticoids and possible prophylactic measures. Med Clin North Am 57:1289–1294, 1973
37. Hilbish TF, Black RL: X-ray manifestations of peptic ulceration during corticosteroid therapy of rheumatoid arthritis. Arch Intern Med 101:932–942, 1958
38. Weiner JJ, Sala AM: Perforation of the cecum due to hypercortisonism. Am J Proctol 12:387–391, 1961
39. Warshaw AL, Welch JP, Ottinger LW: Acute perforation of the colon associated with chronic corticosteroid therapy. Am J Surg 131:442–446, 1976
40. Emmanuel JH, Montgomery RD: Gastric ulcer and the anti-arthritic drugs. Postgrad Med J 47:227–232, 1971
41. Mauer EF: The toxic effects of phenylbutazone (butazolidin). N Engl J Med 253:404–410, 1955

42. Taylor RT, Huskisson EC, Whitehouse GH, et al: Gastric ulceration occurring during indomethacin therapy. Br Med J 4:734–737, 1968

43. Rothermich NO: An extended study of indomethacin. JAMA 195:531–536, 1966

44. Lovgren O, Allander E: Side-effects of indomethacin. Br Med J 1:118, 1964

45. Shields WE, Adamson NE: Peptic ulcer perforation following administration of phenylbutazone. JAMA 152:28–30, 1953

46. Raffensperger EC: Multiple gastric ulcers occurring during phenylbutazone therapy. JAMA 152:30–31, 1953

47. Krainin P: Gastric ulcer with massive hemorrhage following use of phenylbutazone. JAMA 152:31–32, 1953

48. Lewis JR: Evaluation of ibuprofen (motrin), a new antirheumatic agent. JAMA 233:364–365, 1975

49. Halvorsen L, Dotevall G, Sevelius H: Comparative effects of aspirin and naproxen on gastric mucosa. Scand J Rheumatol 2 (suppl 2):43–47, 1973

50. Roth SH, Boost G: An open trial of naproxen in rheumatoid arthritis patients with significant esophageal, gastric, and duodenal lesions. J Clin Pharmacol 51:378–384, 1975

51. Brogden RN, Pinder RM, Sawyer PR, et al: Naproxen: A review of its pharmacological properties and therapeutic efficacy and use. Drugs 9:326–363, 1975

52. Lewis JR: New antirheumatic agents: Fenoprofen calcium (nalfon), naproxen (naprosyn), and tolmetin sodium (tolectin). JAMA 237:1260–1261, 1977

53. Sturges HF, Krone CL: Ulceration and stricture of the jejunum in a patient on long term indomethacin therapy. Am J Gastroenterol 59:162–169, 1973

54. Shack ME: Drug induced ulceration and perforation of the small intestine. Ariz Med 23:517–523, 1966

55. Bravo AJ, Lowman RM: Benign ulcer of the sigmoid colon. Radiology 90:113–115, 1968

56. Debenham GP: Ulcer of the cecum during oxyphenbutazone (tandearil) therapy. Can Med Assoc J 94:1182–1184, 1966

57. Wofford JD, Cummins AJ: Hemorrhage from duodenal ulcer during the administration of reserpine. N Engl J Med 255:1193–1194, 1956

58. Hussar AE, Bruno E: Acute duodenal ulcer associated with reserpine therapy. Gastroenterology 31:500–504, 1956

59. Bachrach WH: Reserpine, gastric secretion, and peptic ulcer. Am J Dig Dis 4:117–124, 1959

60. Hollister LE: Hematemesis and melena complicating treatment with rauwolfia alkaloids. Arch Intern Med 99:218–221, 1957

61. Mackay A, Stevenson RD: Gastric ulceration induced by spironolactone (letter). Lancet 1:481, 1977

62. Wilmers MJ, Heriot AJ: Pyloric stenosis complicating acute poisoning by ferrous sulphate. Lancet 2:68–69, 1954

63. Warden MR, Munro GA, Lanier RR: Fibrous stricture of the stomach due to iron (feosol) poisoning. Radiology 71:732–734, 1958

64. Gandhi RK, Robarts FH: Hour-glass stricture of the stomach and pyloric stenosis due to ferrous sulphate poisoning. Br J Surg 49:613–617, 1962

65. Vuthibhagdee A, Harris NF: Antral stricture as a delayed complication of iron intoxication. Radiology 103:163–164, 1972

66. Filpi RG, Majd M, LoPresti JM: Reversible gastric stricture following iron ingestion. South Med J 66:845–846, 1973

67. Roberts RJ, Nayfield S, Soper R, et al: Acute iron intoxication with intestinal infarction managed in part by small bowel resection. Clin Toxicol 8:3–12, 1975

68. Crowson TD, Head LH, Ferrante WA: Esophageal ulcers associated with tetracycline therapy. JAMA 235:2747–2748, 1976

69. Baker DR, Schrader WH, Hitchcock CR: Small-bowel ulceration apparently associated with thiazide and potassium therapy. JAMA 190:586–590, 1964

70. Morgenstern L, Freilich M, Parish JF: The circumferential small-bowel ulcer. JAMA 191:637–640, 1965

71. Lawrason FD, Alpert E, Mohr FL, et al: Ulcerative-obstructive lesions of the small intestine. JAMA 191:641–644, 1965

72. Boley SJ, Allen AC, Schultz L, et al: Potassium-induced lesions of the small bowel. I. Clinical aspects. JAMA 193:997–1000, 1965

73. Raf LE: Enteric-coated potassium chloride tablets and ulcer of the small intestine. Acta Chir Scand, suppl 374, 1967

74. Dietz MW: Iatrogenic jejunal ulcer. Am J Roentgenol 99:136–138, 1967

75. Allen AC, Boley SJ, Schultz L, et al: Potassium-induced lesions of the small bowel. II. Pathology and pathogenesis. JAMA 193:1001–1006, 1965

76. Warr OS, Nash JP: Jejunal ulceration: Report of a case apparently associated with potassium gluconate. JAMA 199:317–318, 1967

77. Weiss SM, Rutenberg HL, Paskin DL, et al: Gut lesions due to slow-release KCl tablets (letter). N Engl J Med 296:111–112, 1977

78. Farquharson-Roberts MA, Giddings AEB, Nunn AJ: Perforation of small bowel due to slow release potassium chloride (slow-K). Br Med J 3:206, 1975

79. Heffernan SJ, Murphy JJ: Ulceration of small intestine and slow-release potassium tablets (letter). Br Med J 2:746, 1975

80. Jacobs E, Pringot J: Gastric ulcers due to the intake of potassium chloride. Am J Dig Dis 18:289–294, 1973

81. McMahon FG, Akdamer K: Gastric ulceration

after "slow-K" (letter). N Engl J Med 295:733–734, 1976

82. Pemberton J: Oesophageal obstruction and ulceration caused by oral potassium therapy. Br Heart J 32:267–268, 1970

83. Whitney B, Croxon R: Dysphagia caused by cardiac enlargement. Clin Radiol 23:147–152, 1972

84. Peters JL: Benign oesophageal stricture following oral potassium chloride therapy. Br J Surg 63:698–699, 1976

85. Howie AD, Strachan RW: Slow release potassium chloride treatment. Br Med J 2:176, 1975

86. McCall AJ: Slow-K ulceration of oesophagus with aneurysmal left atrium. Br Med J 3:230–231, 1975

87. Volle RL, Koelle GB: Ganglionic blocking drugs. Goodman LS, Gilman A (eds) In The Pharmacological Basis of Therapeutics, 5th ed. New York:MacMillan, 1975, pp 570–573

88. Bourne G, Hosford J: Methonium compounds in hypertension (letter). Lancet 1:527, 1951

89. Mackey WA, Shaw GB: Paralytic ileus after hexamethonium (letter). Br Med J 1:1205, 1951

90. Ettman IK, Bouchillon CD, Halford HH: Gastrointestinal roentgen findings due to untoward effects of hexamethonium. Radiology 68:673–678, 1957

91. Melamed M, Kubian E: Relationship of the autonomic nervous system to "functional" obstruction of the intestinal tract. Radiology 80:22–29, 1963

92. Goldsmith HJ: Death from hexamethonium ileus. Br Med J 1:522–523, 1955

93. Furste W, Phelps D, Taylor PL: Antihypertensive drugs as a cause of the acute abdomen. JAMA 166:2111–2114, 1958

94. Munster A, Milton GW: Paralytic ileus due to ganglion-blocking agents. Med J Aust 2:210–213, 1961

95. Gibson DS: A case of intestinal obstruction following the administration of pentapyrrolidinium bitartrate ("ansolysen"). Med J Aust 2:860–861, 1957

96. Becker KL, Sutnick AI: Paralytic ileus simulating acute intestinal obstruction due to pentolinium tartrate (ansolysen). Ann Intern Med 54:313–319, 1961

97. Bryk D, Soong KY: Colonic ileus and its differential roentgen diagnosis. Am J Roentgenol 101:329–337, 1967

98. Spira IA, Rodrigues R, Wolff WI: Pseudo-obstruction of the colon. Am J Gastroenterol 65:397–408, 1976

99. Warnes H, Lehmann HE, Ban TA: Adynamic ileus during psychoactive medication. Can Med Assoc J 96:1112–1113, 1967

100. Lewitan A, Nathanson L, Slade WR: Megacolon and dilatation of the small bowel in Parkinsonism. Gastroenterology 17:367–374, 1951

101. Caplan LH, Jacobson HG, Rubinstein BM, et al: Megacolon and volvulus in Parkinson's disease. Radiology 85:73–79, 1965

102. Daggett P, Ibrahim SZ: Intestinal obstruction complicating orphenadrine treatment. Br Med J 1:21–22, 1976

103. Davis JT, Nusbaum M: Chlorpromazine therapy and functional large bowel obstruction. Am J Gastroenterol 60:635–639, 1973

104. Giordano J, Huang A, Canter JW: Fatal paralytic ileus complicating phenothiazine therapy. South Med J 68:351–353, 1975

105. Gander DR, Devlin HB: Ileus after amitriptyline (letter). Br Med J 1:1160, 1963

106. Milner G, Buckler EG: Adynamic ileus and amitriptyline. Med J Aust 1:921–922, 1964

107. Burkitt EA, Sutcliffe CK: Paralytic ileus after amitriptyline ("tryptizol") (letter). Br Med J 2:1648–1649, 1961

108. Milner G, Hills NF: Adynamic ileus and nortriptyline. Br Med J 1:841–842, 1966

109. McNeill DC: Adynamic ileus and nortriptyline (letter). Br Med J 1:1360, 1966

110. McClarke I: Adynamic ileus and amitriptyline (letter). Br Med J 2:531, 1971

111. Spira IA, Rubenstein R, Wolff D, et al: Fecal impaction following methadone ingestion simulating acute intestinal obstruction. Ann Surg 181:15–19, 1975

112. Rubenstein RB, Wolff WI: Methadone ileus syndrome: Report of a fatal case. Dis Colon Rectum 19:357–359, 1976

113. Bear R, Steer K: Pseudo-obstruction due to clonidine. Br Med J 1:197, 1976

114. Bauer GE, Hellestrand KJ: Pseudo-obstruction due to clonidine (letter). Br Med J 1:769, 1976

115. Toghill PJ, Burke JD: Death from paralytic ileus following vincristine therapy. Postgrad Med J 46:330–331, 1970

116. Shaivitz SA: Dantrolene (letter). JAMA 229:1282–1283, 1974

117. Segal RL, Silver S, Yohalem SB, et al: Myxedema following radioactive iodine therapy of hyperthyroidism. Am J Med 31:354–364, 1961

118. Bacharach T, Evans JR: Enlargement of the colon secondary to hypothyroidism. Ann Intern Med 47:121–124, 1957

119. Haley HB, Leigh C, Bronsky D, et al: Ascites and intestinal obstruction in myxedema. Arch Surg 85:328–333, 1962

120. Babb RR, Spittell JA, Bartholomew LG: Gastroenterologic complications of anticoagulant therapy. Mayo Clin Proc 43:738–751, 1968

121. Stanton PE, Wilson JP, Lamis PA, et al: Acute abdominal conditions induced by anticoagulant therapy. Am Surg 40:1–14, 1974

122. Senturia HR, Susman N, Shyken H: The roentgen appearance of spontaneous intramural hemorrhage of the small intestine associated with anticoagulant therapy. Am J Roentgenol 86:62–69, 1961

123. Wiot JF, Weinstein AS, Felson B: Duodenal hematoma induced by coumarin. Am J Roentgenol 86:70–75, 1961

124. Sears AD, Hawkins J, Kilgore BB, et al: Plain roentgenographic findings in drug induced intramural hematoma of the small bowel. Am J Roentgenol 91:808–813, 1964

125. Lloyd DA, Immelman EJ, Wright MGE: Anticoagulant-induced intramural haematoma of the bowel. S Afr Med J 47:734–738, 1973

126. Wiot JF: Intramural small intestinal hemorrhage—A differential diagnosis. Semin Roengenol 1:219–233, 1966

127. Herbert DC: Anticoagulant therapy and the acute abdomen. Br J Surg 55:353–357, 1968

128. Cocks JR: Anticoagulants and the acute abdomen. Med J Aust 1:1138–1141, 1970

129. Goldfarb WB: Coumadin-induced intestinal obstruction. Ann Surg 161:27–34, 1965

130. Gabriele OF, Conte M: Spontaneous intramural hemorrhage of the colon. Arch Surg 89:522–526, 1964

131. Patel DR, Shrivastav R, Hand G: Intestinal obstruction due to intramural hematoma of the colon, a complication of sodium warfarin therapy. Dis Colon Rectum 16:416–418, 1973

132. Andress M: Submucosal haematoma of the esophagus due to anticoagulant therapy. Acta Radiol 11:216–219, 1971

133. Snyder N, Patterson M, Hughes WS: Esophageal hematoma. South Med J 66:1079–1080, 1973

134. Owens DE, Calcaterra TC, Aarstad RA: Retropharyngeal hematoma: A complication of therapy with anticoagulants. Arch Otolaryngol 101:565–568, 1975

135. Levine S, Whelan TJ: Small-bowel infarction due to intramural hematoma during anticoagulant therapy. Arch Surg 95:245–248, 1967

136. Raine JWE: Abdominal complications of anticoagulant therapy. NZ Med J 62:85–87, 1963

137. Curry PVL, Bacon PA: Retroperitoneal haemorrhage and neuropathy complicating anticoagulant therapy. Postgrad Med J 50:37–40, 1974

138. Roberts MH, Johnston FR: Hepatic rupture from anticoagulant therapy. Arch Surg 110:1152, 1975

139. Brennan MF, Clarke AM, MacBeth WAAG: Infarction of the midgut associated with oral contraceptives. N Engl Med 279:1213–1214, 1968

140. Hurwitz RL, Martin AJ, Grossman BE, et al: Oral contraceptives and gastrointestinal disorders. Ann Surg 172:892–896, 1970

141. Rose MB: Superior mesenteric vein thrombosis and oral contraceptives. Postgrad Med J 48:430–433, 1972

142. Ellis DL, Heifetz CJ: Mesenteric venous thrombosis in two women taking oral contraceptives. Am J Surg 125:641–644, 1973

143. Nesbit RR Jr, Deweese JA: Mesenteric venous thrombosis and oral contraceptives. South Med J 70:360–362, 1977

144. Appleberg M: Mesenteric venous thrombosis and suppression of lactation using stilboestrol. S Afr J Surg 9:105–109, 1971

145. Carvalho ACA, Vaillancourt RA, Cabral RB, et al: Coagulation abnormalities in women taking oral contraceptives. JAMA 237:875–878, 1977

146. Nothmann BJ, Chittinand S, Schuster MM: Reversible mesenteric vascular occlusion associated with oral contraceptives. Am J Dig Dis 18:361–368, 1973

147. Ghahremani GG, Meyers MA, Farman J, et al: Ischemic disease of the small bowel and colon associated with oral contraceptives. Gastrointest Radiol 2:221–228, 1977

148. Kilpatrick ZM, Silverman JF, Betancourt E, et al: Vascular occlusion of the colon and oral contraceptives. N Engl J Med 278:438–440, 1968

149. Egger G, Mangold R: Ischaemic colitis and oral contraceptives: Case report and brief review of the literature. Acta Hepatogastroenterol 21:221–224, 1974

150. Prust FW, Kumar GK: Massive colonic bleeding and oral contraceptive "pills." Am J Obstet Gynecol 125:695–698, 1976

151. Bernardino ME, Lawson TL: Discrete colonic ulcers associated with oral contraceptives. Am J Dig Dis 21:503–506, 1976

152. McClennan BL: Ischemic colitis secondary to premarin: Report of a case. Dis Colon Rectum 19:618–620, 1976

153. Gelfand MD: Ischemic colitis associated with a depot synthetic progestogen. Am J Dig Dis 17:275–277, 1972

154. Morowitz DA, Epstein BH: Spectrum of bowel disease associated with use of contraceptives. Med Ann DC 42:6–10, 1973

155. Hoyumpa AM, Schiff L, Helfman EL: Budd-Chiari syndrome in women taking oral contraceptives. Am J Med 50:137–140, 1971

156. Alpert LI: Veno-occlusive disease of the liver associated with oral contraceptives: Case report and review of literature. Hum Pathol 7:709–718, 1976

157. Frederick WC, Howard RG, Spatola S: Spontaneous rupture of the liver in patient using contraceptive pills. Arch Surg 108:93–95, 1974

158. Clain D, Freston J, Kreel L, et al: Clinical diagnosis of the Budd-Chiari syndrome. Am J Med 43:544–554, 1967

159. Gazes PC, Holmes CR, Moseley V, et al: Acute hemorrhage and necrosis of the intestines associated with digitalization. Circulation 23:358–364, 1961

160. Polansky BJ, Berger RL, Byrne JJ: Massive nonocclusive intestinal infarction associated with digitalis toxicity (abstract). Circulation 30:(suppl 3) 141, 1964

161. Muggia FM: Hemorrhagic necrosis of the intestine: Its occurrence with digitalis intoxication. Am J Med Sci 253:263–271, 1967

162. Pierce GE, Brockenbrough EC: The spectrum of mesenteric infarction. Am J Surg 119:233–239, 1970

163. Ferrer MI, Bradley SE, Wheeler HO, et al: The effect of digoxin in the splanchnic circulation in ventricular failure. Circulation 32:524–537, 1965

164. Shanbour LL, Jacobson ED: Digitalis and the mesenteric circulation. Am J Dig Dis 17:826–828, 1972

165. Hess T, Stucki P: Mesenterialinfarkt bei digitalis intoxication. Schweiz Med Wochenschr 105:1237–1240, 1975

166. Brazeau P: Ergot and the ergot alkaloids. Goodman LS, Gilman A (eds): In The Pharmacological Basis of Therapeutics, 5th ed. New York: MacMillan 1975, pp 872–878

167. Greene FL, Ariyan S, Stansel HC Jr: Mesenteric and peripheral vascular ischemia secondary to ergotism. Surgery 81:176–179, 1977

168. Buenger RE, Hunter JA; Reversible mesenteric artery stenoses due to methysergide maleate. JAMA 198:558–560, 1966

169. Heilbrun N: Roentgen evidence suggesting enterocolitis associated with prolonged cathartic abuse. Radiology 44:486–491, 1943

170. Heilbrun N, Bernstein C: Roentgen abnormalities of the large and small intestine associated with prolonged cathartic ingestion. Radiology 65:549–556, 1955

171. Plum GE, Weber HM, Sauer WG: Prolonged cathartic abuse resulting in roentgen evidence suggestive of enterocolitis. Am J Roentgenol 83:919–925, 1960

172. Rawson MD: Cathartic colon. Lancet 1:1121–1124, 1966

173. Urso FP, Urso MJ, Lee CH: The cathartic colon: Pathological findings and radiological/pathological correlation. Radiology 116:557–559, 1975

174. Fingl E: Contact (stimulant) cathartics. Goodman LS, Gilman A (eds): In The Pharmacological Basis of Therapeutics, 5th ed. New York: MacMillan 1975, pp 981–984

175. Case Records of the Massachusetts General Hospital (Case 13–1976). N Engl J Med 294:712–720, 1976

176. Graham JF, Suby HI, LeCompte PR, et al: Fibrotic disorders associated with methysergide therapy for headache. N Engl J Med 274:359–368, 1966

177. Elkind AH, Friedman AP, Bachman A, et al: Silent retroperitoneal fibrosis associated with methysergide therapy. JAMA 206:1041–1044, 1968

178. Kunkel RS: Fibrotic syndromes with chronic use of methysergide. Headache 11:1–5, 1971

179. Leffall LD, White JE, Mann M: Retroperitoneal fibrosis—Two unusual cases. Arch Surg 89:1070–1076, 1964

180. Hissong SL, Freimanis AK: Retroperitoneal fibrosis: Extraretroperitoneal lesions. Am J Roentgenol 107:776–786, 1969

181. Corriere JN, Mackie JA, Murphy JJ: Retroperitoneal fibrosis presenting with large bowel symptoms: Report of two cases. J Urol 96:161–166, 1966

182. Gelford GJ, Cromwell DK: Methysergide, retroperitoneal fibrosis and rectosigmoid stricture. Am J Roentgenol 104:566–570, 1968

183. Crummy AB, Whittaker WB, Morrissey JF, et al: Intestinal infarction secondary to retroperitoneal fibrosis. N Engl J Med 285:28–29, 1971

184. Regan JF, Poletti BJ: Vascular adventitial fibrosis in a patient taking methysergide maleate. JAMA 203:1069–1071, 1968

185. Schneider CF: Idiopathic retroperitoneal fibrosis producing vena caval, biliary, ureteral and duodenal obstructions. Ann Surg 159:316–320, 1964

186. Chew CK, Jarzylo SV, Valberg LS: Idiopathic retroperitoneal fibrosis with protein-losing enteropathy and duodenal obstruction successfully treated with corticosteroids. Can Med Assoc J 95:1183–1188, 1966

187. Raper FP: Idiopathic retroperitoneal fibrosis involving the ureters. Br J Urol 28:436–446, 1956

188. Dalinka MK, McGee JW: The variable manifestations of sclerosing fibrosis. J Can Assoc Radiol 21:280–286, 1971

189. Romanucci D, Stapleton LA: Hepatic artery insufficiency secondary to retroperitoneal fibrosis. Angiology 19:435, 1968

190. Inkley SR, Abbott GR: Unilateral pulmonary arteriosclerosis. Arch Intern Med 108:903–915, 1961

191. Hellstrom HR, Perez-Stable EC: Retroperitoneal fibrosis with disseminated vasculitis and intrahepatic sclerosing cholangitis. Am J Med 40:184–187, 1966

192. Aptekar RG, Mitchinson MJ: Retroperitoneal fibrosis in two patients previously exposed to LSD. Calif Med 113:77–79, 1970

193. Stecker JF, Rawls HP, Devine CJ, et al: Retroperitoneal fibrosis and ergot derivatives. J Urol 112:30–32, 1974

194. Lewis CT, Molland EA, Marshall VR, et al: Analgesic abuse, ureteric obstruction, and retroperitoneal fibrosis. Br Med J 2:76–78, 1975

195. Iversen BM, Johannesen JW, Nordahl E, et al: Retroperitoneal fibrosis during treatment with methyldopa. Lancet 2:302–304, 1975

196. Viskoper JR, Chwat S, Ullmann TD: Recurrent hydronephrosis, retroperitoneal fibrosis and eosinophilia in a patient with previous evidence of Loeffler's infiltrate in the lungs. Isr J Med Sci 5:1071–1076, 1969

197. Schainuck LI, Hano JE: Bilateral ureteral obstruction following sulfamethoxazole. J Urol 98:466–469, 1967

198. Baum JK, Bookstein JJ, Holtz F, et al: Possible association between benign hepatomas and oral contraceptives. Lancet 2:926–929, 1973

199. Ameriks JA, Thompson NW, Frey CF, et al: Hepatic cell adenomas, spontaneous liver rupture, and oral contraceptives. Arch Surg 110:548–557, 1975

200. Stauffer JQ, Lapinski MW, Honold DJ, et al: Focal nodular hyperplasia of the liver and intrahepatic hemorrhage in young women on oral contraceptives. Ann Inter Med 83:301–306, 1975

201. McAvoy JM, Tompkins RK, Longmire WP: Benign hepatic tumors and their association with

oral contraceptives. Arch Surg 111:761–767, 1976

202. Edmondson HA, Henderson B, Benton B: Liver-cell adenomas associated with use of oral contraceptives. N Engl J Med 294:470–472, 1976

203. Mays ET, Christopherson WM, Mahr MM, et al: Hepatic changes in young women ingesting contraceptive steroids. JAMA 235:730–732, 1976

204. Lansing PB, McQuitty JT, Bradburn DM: Benign liver tumors: What is their relationship to oral contraceptives. Am Surg 42:744–760, 1976

205. Kalra TMS, Mangla JC, DePapp EW: Benign hepatic tumors and oral contraceptive pills. Am J Med 61:871–877, 1976

206. Grabowski M, Stenram U, Bergqvist A: Focal nodular hyperplasia of the liver, benign hepatomas, oral contraceptives and other drugs affecting the liver. Acta Pathol Microbiol Scand 83:615–622, 1975

207. Sackett JF, Mosenthal WT, House RK, et al: Scintillation scanning of liver cell adenoma. Am J Roentgenol 113:56–60, 1971

208. McLoughlin MJ, Gilday DL: Angiography and colloid scanning of benign mass lesions of the liver. Clin Radiol 23:377–381, 1972

209. Jhingran SG, Mukhopadhyay AK, Ajmani SK, et al: Hepatic adenomas and focal nodular hyperplasia of the liver in young women on oral contraceptives: Case Reports. J Nucl Med 18:263–266, 1977

210. Goldstein HM, Neiman HL, Mena E, et al: Angiographic findings in benign liver cell tumors. Radiology 110:339–343, 1974

211. Edmondson HA, Reynolds TB, Henderson B, et al: Regression of liver cell adenomas associated with oral contraceptives. Ann Intern Med 86:180–182, 1977

212. Ross D, Pina J, Mirza M, et al: Regression of focal nodular hyperplasia after discontinuation of oral contraceptives (letter). Ann Intern Med 85:203–204, 1976

213. Thalassinos NC, Lymberatos C, Hadjioannou J, et al: Liver-cell carcinoma after long-term oestrogen-like drugs. Lancet 1:270, 1974

214. Meyer P, LiVolsi VA, Cornog JL: Hepatoblastoma associated with an oral contraceptive (letter). Lancet 2:1387, 1974

215. Davis M, Portmann B, Searle M, et al: Histological evidence of carcinoma in a hepatic tumour associated with oral contraceptives. Br Med J 4:496–498, 1975

216. Johnson FL, Feagler JR, Lerner KG, et al: Association of androgenic-anabolic steroid therapy with development of hepatocellular carcinoma. Lancet 2:1273–1276, 1972

217. Farrell GC, Joshua DE, Uren RF, et al: Androgen-induced hepatoma. Lancet 1:430–432, 1975

218. Holder LE, Gnarra DJ, Lampkin BC, et al: Hepatoma associated with anabolic steroid therapy. Am J Roentgenol 124:638–642, 1975

219. Sheft DJ, Shrago G: Esophageal moniliasis. JAMA 213:1859–1862, 1970

220. vHolt JM: Candida infection of the oesophagus. Gut 9:227–231, 1968

221. Kodsi BE, Wickremesinghe PC, Kozinn PJ, et al: Candida esophagitis. Gastroenterology 71:715–719, 1976

222. Marsh AP: Esophageal moniliasis. Am J Roentgenol 82:1063–1066, 1959

223. Kaufman SA, Scheff S, Levene G: Esophageal moniliasis. Radiology 75:726–732, 1960

224. Weiss J, Epstein BS: Esophageal moniliasis. Am J Roentgenol 88:718–720, 1962

225. Goldberg HI, Dodds WJ: Cobblestone esophagus due to monilial infection. Am J Roentgenol 104:608–612, 1968

226. Guyer PB, Brunton FJ, Rooke HWP: Candidiasis of the oesophagus. Br J Radiol 44:131–136, 1971

227. Gonzalez G: Esophageal moniliasis. Am J Roentgenol 113:233–236, 1971

228. Troupin RH: Intramural esophageal diverticulosis and moniliasis. Am J Roentgenol 104:613–616, 1968

229. Simulewicz JJ, Dorfman J: Esophageal intramural diverticulosis: A re-evaluation. Radiology 101:527–529, 1971

230. Ho C, Cullen JB, Gray RR: An unusual manifestation of esophageal moniliasis. Radiology 123:287–288, 1977

231. Stanley RJ, Tedesco FJ: Antibiotic-associated pseudomembranous colitis. CRC Crit Rev Clin Radiol Nucl Med 8:255–277, 1976

232. Bartlett JG, Gorbach SL: Pseudomembranous enterocolitis (antibiotic-related colitis). Adv Intern Med 22:455–476, 1977

233. Ecker JA, Williams RG, McKittick JE, et al: Pseudomembranous enterocolitis—an unwelcome gastrointestinal complication of antibiotic therapy. Am J Gastroenterol 54:214–228, 1970

234. Slagle GW, Boggs HW: Drug-induced pseudomembranous enterocolitis: A new etiologic agent. Dis Colon Rectum 19:253–255, 1976

235. Tedesco FJ, Barton RW, Alpers DH: Clindamycin-associated colitis: A prospective study. Ann Intern Med 81:429–433, 1974

236. Larson HE, Price AB, Honour P, et al: *Clostridium difficile* and the aetiology of pseudomembranous colitis. Lancet 1:1063–1066, 1978

237. Schapiro RL, Newman A: Acute enterocolitis: A complication of antibiotic therapy. Radiology 108:263–268, 1973

238. Stanley RJ, Melson GL, Tedesco FJ: The spectrum of radiographic findings in antibiotic-related pseudomembranous colitis. Radiology 111:519–524, 1974

239. Stanley FJ, Melson GL, Tedesco FJ, et al: Plain film findings in severe pseudomembranous colitis. Radiology 118:7–11, 1976

240. Burbige EJ, Milligan FD: Pseudomembranous colitis: Association with antibiotics and therapy with cholestyramine. JAMA 231:1157–1158, 1975

241. Levine B, Peskin GW, Saik RP: Drug-induced

colitis as a surgical disease. Arch Surg 111:987–989, 1976

242. Toffler RB, Pingoud EG, Burrell MI: Acute, transient antibiotic colitis: Ischemic colitis and bloody diarrhea related to penicillin and penicillin derivatives. Presented at the annual meeting of the Society of Gastrointestinal Radiologists, September 1976

243. Clemett AR, Fishbone G, Gevine RJ, et al: Gastrointestinal lesions in mastocytosis. Am J Roentgenol 103:405–412, 1968

244. Berk RN, Millman SJ: Urticaria of the colon. Radiology 99:539–540, 1971

245. Bralow SP, Girsh LS: Urticaria of the gastric mucosa with massive hemorrhage following oral penicillin anaphylaxis. Ann Intern Med 51:384–390, 1959

246. Stein HB, Urowitz MB: Gold-induced enterocolitis: Case report and literature review. J Rheumatol 3:21–26, 1976

247. Roe M, Sears AD, Arndt JH: Gold reaction panenteritis. Radiology 104:59–60, 1972

248. Kaplinsky N, Pras M, Frankl O: Severe enterocolitis complicating chrysotherapy. Ann Rheum Dis 32:574–577, 1973

249. Levinsky L, Urca I: Intestinal obstruction due to antacid treatment for duodenal ulcer. Dis Colon Rectum 15:55–56, 1972

250. Townsend CM, Remmers AR, Sarles HE, et al: Intestinal obstruction from medication bezoar in patients with renal failure. N Engl J Med 288:1058–1059, 1973

251. Potyk D: Intestinal obstruction from impacted antacid tablets. N Engl J Med 283:134–135, 1970

252. Cohen MI, Winslow PR, Boley SJ: Intestinal obstruction associated with cholestyramine therapy. N Engl J Med 280:1285–1286, 1969

253. Lloyd-Still JD: Cholestyramine therapy and intestinal obstruction in infants. Pediatrics 59:626–627, 1977

254. Melamed A, Marck A: Esophageal obstruction due to serutan. JAMA 152:318–319, 1953

255. Vickery RE: Unusual complication of excessive ingestion of vitamin C tablets. Int Surg 58:422–423, 1973

256. Schmidt H, Creutzfeldt W: Etiology and pathogenesis of pancreatitis, drugs, hormones. Bockus HL (ed): Gastroenterology, 3rd ed, vol 3. Philadelphia: Saunders 1976, p 1010

257. Carone FA, Liebow AA: Acute pancreatic lesions in patients treated with ACTH and adrenal corticoids. N Engl J Med 257:690–697, 1957

258. Nelp WB: Acute pancreatitis associated with steroid therapy. Arch Intern Med 108:702–710, 1961

259. Davidoff F, Tishler S, Rosoff C: Marked hyperlipidemia and pancreatitis associated with oral contraceptive therapy. N Engl J Med 289:552–555, 1973

260. Cornish AL, McClellan JT, Johnston DH: Effects of chlorothiazide on the pancreas. N Engl J Med 265:673–675, 1961

261. Stein D, Sharma OP: Acute pancreatitis and thiazides (letter). Gastroenterology 62:695, 1972

262. Jones PE, Oelbaum MH: Frusemide-induced pancreatitis. Br Med J 1:133–134, 1975

263. Land VJ, Sutow WW, Fernback DJ, et al: Toxicity of L-asparaginase in children with advanced leukemia. Cancer 30:339–347, 1972

264. Weetman RM, Bachner RL: Latent onset of clinical pancreatitis in children receiving L-asparaginase therapy. Cancer 34:780–785, 1974

265. Wilde H: Pancreatitis and phenformin (letter). Ann Intern Med 77:324, 1972

266. Graeber GM, Marmor BM, Hendel RC, et al: Pancreatitis and severe metabolic abnormalities due to phenformin therapy. Arch Surg 111:1014–1016, 1976

267. Boston Collaborative Drug Surveillance Program: Surgically confirmed gallbladder disease, venous thromboembolism, and breast tumors in relation to postmenopausal estrogen therapy. N Engl J Med 290:15–19, 1974

268. Weiss GN, Weiss EB: Hormonal therapy and cholelithiasis. Int Surg 61:472–474, 1976

269. Bennion LJ, Ginsberg RL, Garnick MB, et al: Effects of oral contraceptives on the gallbladder bile of normal women. N Engl J Med 294:189–192, 1976

270. Editorial: Iatrogenic gallstones. Lancet 1:859–860, 1976

271. Coronary Drug Project Research Group: Colfibrate and niacin in coronary heart disease. JAMA 231:360–381, 1975

272. Cooper J, Geizerova H, Oliver MF: Clofibrate and gallstones (letter). Lancet 1:1083, 1975

273. Case Records of the Massachusetts General Hospital (Case 12–1973). N Engl J Med 288:620–629, 1973

274. Lee REJ, Baddeldy H, Marshall AJ, et al: Practolol peritonitis. Clin Radiol 28:119–128, 1977

275. Eltringham WK, Espiner HJ, Windsor CWO, et al: Sclerosing peritonitis due to proctolol: A report on 9 cases and their surgical management. Br J Surg 64:229–235, 1977

276. Hargrove MD Jr, Boyce HW Jr: Meat impaction of the esophagus. Arch Intern Med 125:277–281, 1970

2 Complications of Gastrointestinal Endoscopy

Morton A. Meyers and Gary G. Ghahremani

The technical refinements and widespread application of modern flexible fiberoptic endoscopes have significantly improved the diagnosis of gastrointestinal disorders. Advances in the last several years permit panendoscopy of the esophagus, stomach, and duodenum and endoscopy of the entire large intestine, each in a single examination with minimal patient distress and added optical resolution and visibility. Nevertheless, some of the resultant iatrogenic trauma may not be readily apparent to the endoscopist during the procedure, or its clinical manifestation may be delayed. Radiologic evaluation may document many of the major gastrointestinal complications of fiberoptic endoscopy and their extent.

Upper Gastrointestinal Endoscopy

A survey of the members of the American Society for Gastrointestinal Endoscopy has shown an overall complication rate of 1.32 per 1000 peroral endoscopic examinations (1). The complication rates for esophageal dilatation ranged from 4.25 to 18.4 per 1000. Major complications included perforation, hemorrhage from biopsy, aspiration, myocardial infarction, cardiac arrest and arrhythmia, and respiratory arrest.

It appears that the more frequent use of upper gastrointestinal fiberendoscopes instead of the previously standard semirigid instruments has led to a definite increase in the actual number of perforations and that mortality secondary to iatrogenic perforations has increased (2).

The original fibergastroscope was marketed with the claim that it was 100% flexible and therefore completely safe (3). Complete confidence in the safety of the fibergastroscope is unjustified, however, because its rather large, rigid, bullet-shaped head tends to produce a true transmural rupture, whereas the standard gastroscope occasionally produced a mucosal tear that resulted in benign escape of air (4). Radiologic examination is the most valuable diagnostic test in suspected esophageal or gastric perforation (2,5–7).

Esophageal Perforation

The most common cause of esophageal perforation continues to be instrumentation during esophagoscopy, gastroscopy, or esophageal dilation (5,7). Fiberesophagoscopy alone has a perforation rate of nearly 0.1%, representing no significant improvement in safety over older semirigid esophagoscopes (4).

Anselm et al. have reported five cases of fiberscope-induced perforation of an anatomically normal esophagus (8). The risk is even greater if the esophageal wall is involved by an inflammatory or neoplastic process, particularly when endoscopy is combined with biopsy or dilatation of a stricture (7). Davis emphasized that "in final perspective . . . every such perforation must be considered an error in technique no matter how unusual the anatomy, how poorly the patient cooperates, or how skillful the endoscopist" (9).

Perforation of the esophagus is the most serious and most rapidly fatal type of perforation of the gastrointestinal tract (10). Early diagnosis is essential since successful management requires prompt and vigorous treatment. The mortality is 9%–31% (5,7,11). The prognosis is even less favorable if mediastinitis is complicated by involvement of the pleural spaces. Treatment generally requires antibiotics and surgical drainage and, if possible, primary closure (12,13).

Early and careful radiologic evaluation following fiberendoscopy is important because perforation may not be recognized by the endoscopist (6,11).

Perforation of the cervical esophagus may be due to the tip of the instrument becoming engaged in the pyriform sinus laterally or causing the posterior pharyngeal wall to bulge above the cricopharyngeal muscle (Fig. 2-1). Contributory factors include faulty positioning of the head, lack of control of the tongue, or gagging. When perforation has occurred in this region the operator has usually been astonished at the lack of any sensation of rupture (Fig. 2-2). Lateral radiographs of the neck almost invariably demonstrate evidence of air in the prevertebral space, followed, perhaps, by signs of retropharyngeal abscess formation. Esophagography with water-soluble contrast material may reveal the site of

perforation in only 50% of cases (7). It is more valuable in perforations of the thoracic esophagus, showing extravasation at the site in 75%–86% (5–7). Chest radiographs are also important since they can facilitate evaluation of the extent of spread and possible development of further complications. Plain films may show mediastinal or subcutaneous air, pneumothorax, widening of the mediastinum, and pleural fluid.

Perforation of the cervical esophagus sometimes extends down the mediastinum for a considerable length (2,14) (Figs. 2-2, 2-3). Treatment usually requires cervical mediastinotomy with drainage of the prevertebral space (7), but occasionally prompt conservative management may be successful (2).

Another anatomic point of narrowing of the esophagus that may present some difficulty to instrumental passage is at the level of a tortuous aortic arch and the left main bronchus (2) (Fig. 2-4). Acquired friable strictures may develop at these same points of narrowing, further increasing the possibility of perforation from endoscopy, biopsy, or dilatation (Fig. 2-5).

Perforation commonly occurs in the lower third of the esophagus, being found primarily at

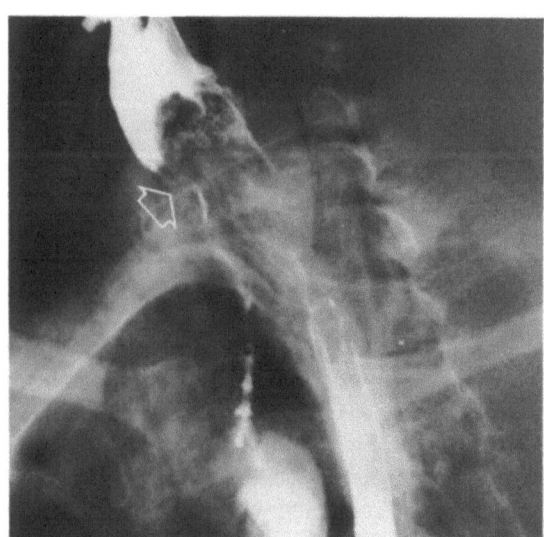
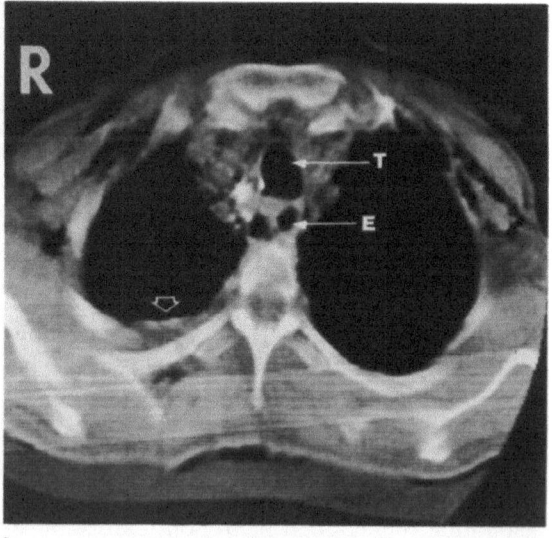

a   b

Fig. 2-1, a and b. Perforation of right pyriform sinus during esophagoscopy. a Spot film shows extravasation of contrast material from the apex of the right pyriform sinus *(arrow)*. The extraluminal passage of the fiberscope has created a longitudinal tract that ends in a cavity caused by insufflated air. **b** Computed chest tomogram at the level of the manubrium demonstrates pneumomediastinum, soft-tissue emphysema of the anterior chest wall, and a right pleural effusion *(arrow)*. There is some retained contrast material in the mediastinum just to the right of the trachea (*T*) and esophagus (*E*).

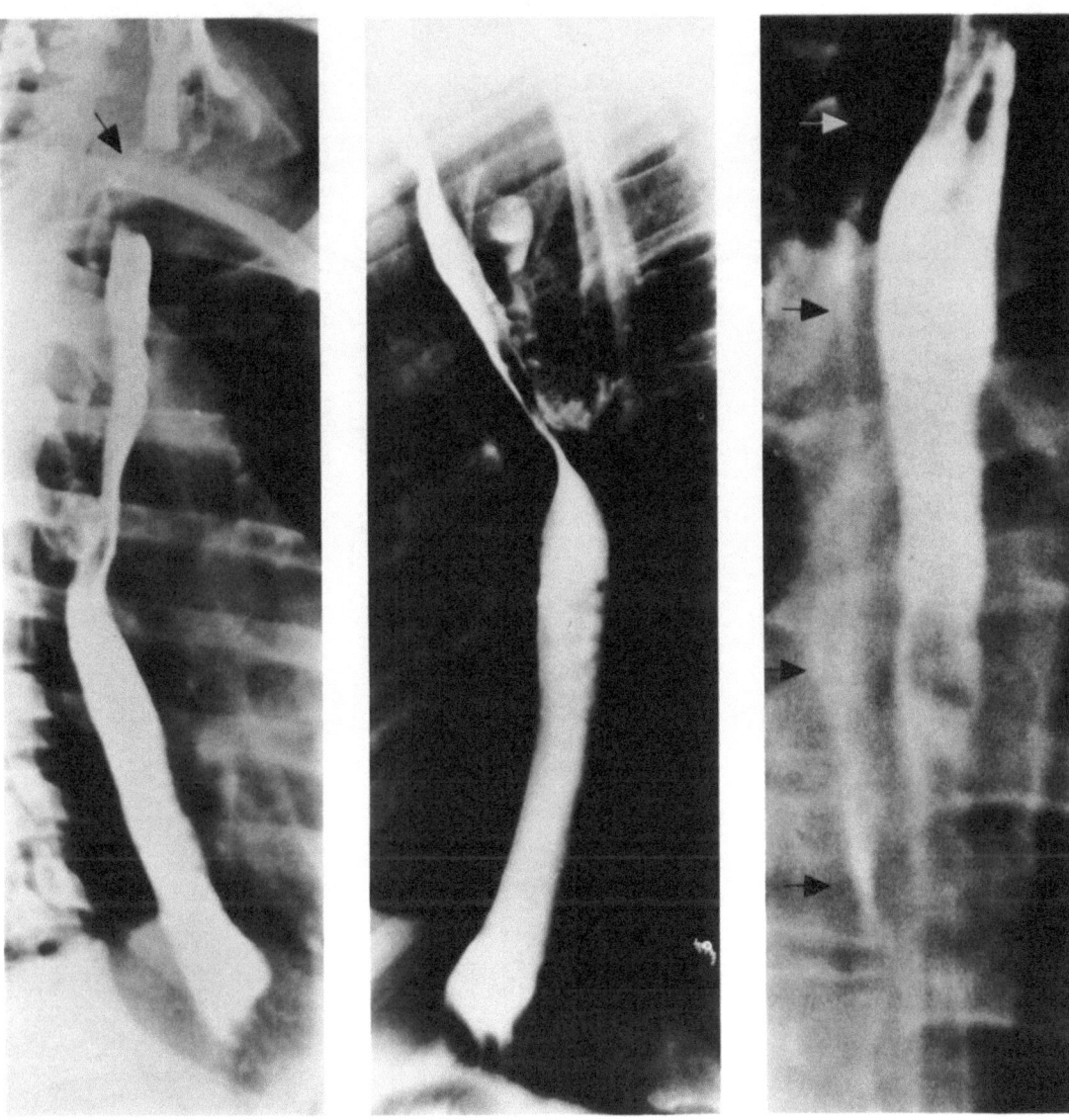

a   b

Fig. 2-2. a and **b. Perforation of cervical esophagus.** There were no unusual findings during fibergastroscopy in a 41-year-old woman. Following development of cervical subcutaneous emphysema shortly after the procedure, a chest radiograph showed pneumomediastinum. Examination with water-soluble contrast material documented extravasation through a 6-mm perforation of the cervical esophagus at the level of C-7. The patient appeared to improve with antibiotic therapy and parenteral feeding. Ten days later, however, this barium contrast study not only again showed the posterior perforation of the lower cervical esophagus *(arrow)* but also revealed its extension into a loculated abscess cavity extending below the level of the aortic arch in the retro-esophageal mediastinal tissues. This was subsequently drained, and follow-up study showed no further communication. (Meyers MA, Ghahremani GG: Complications of fiberoptic endoscopy. I. Esophagoscopy and gastroscopy. Radiology 115:293–300, 1975)

Fig. 2-3. Perforation of cervical esophagus. The patient had cervical subcutaneous emphysema and dysphagia following fiberesophagoscopy. A deep mediastinal sinus tract *(arrows)* extending to the level of T-8 is due to perforation of the pharynx. (Meyers MA, Ghahremani GG: Complications of fiberoptic endoscopy. I. Esophagoscopy and gastroscopy. Radiology 115:293–300, 1975)

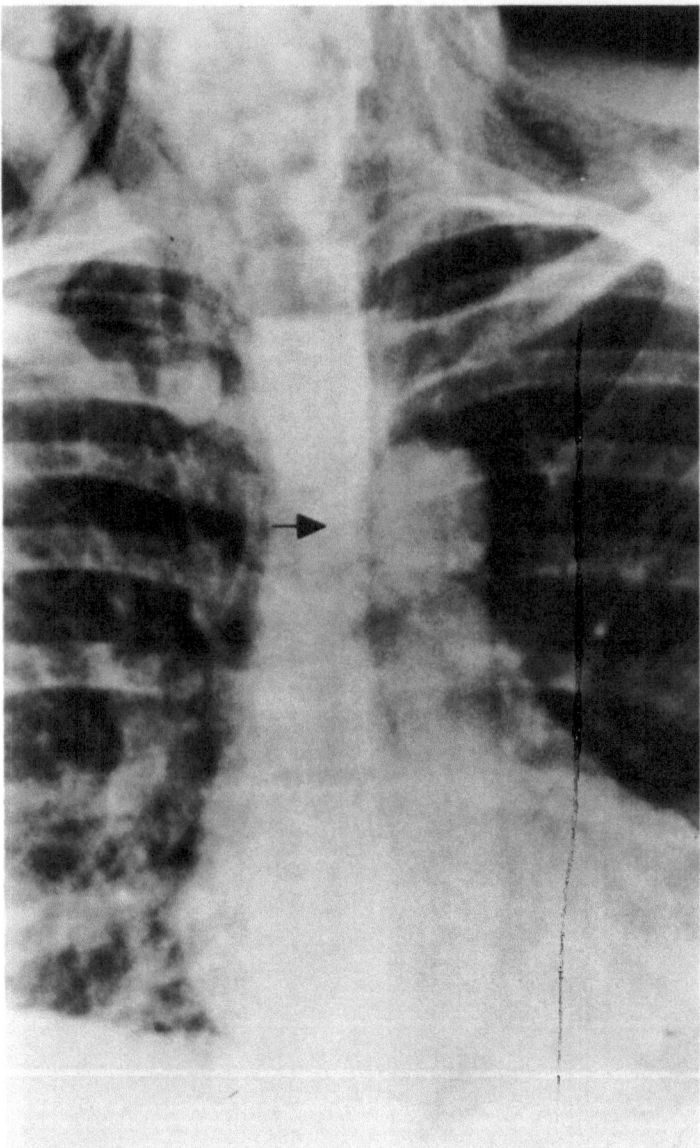

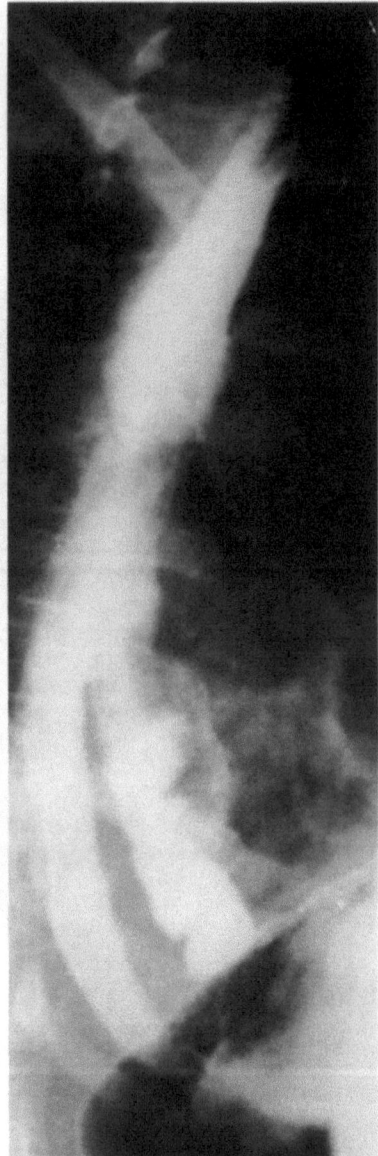

Fig. 2-4. Perforations of cervical and mid-thoracic esophagus. Fibergastroscopy was discontinued in a patient with linitis plastica because of excessive resistance in the lower esophagus and rapid development of massive subcutaneous emphysema.

On this posteroanterior chest film obtained with water-soluble contrast material in the esophagus, note partial esophageal obstruction at the level of anatomic narrowing at the aortic arch and left main bronchus *(arrow).* Considerable pneumomediastinum and subcutaneous emphysema are evident.

Immediate exploratory mediastinotomy showed perforation of the cervical esophagus with a false passage into the thoracic mediastinum, accompanied by localized perforation and hematoma in the midthoracic esophagus. The patient responded well to drainage and chest intubation. (Meyers MA, Ghahremani GG: Complications of fiberoptic endoscopy. I. Esophagoscopy and gastroscopy. Radiology 115:293–300, 1975)

Fig. 2-5. Corrosive esophagitis with large mediastinal sinus tract following fiberesophagoscopy. Perforation occurred at the site of a lye stricture that developed at the anatomic narrowing at the level of the left main bronchus. The tract extends to the level of the diaphragm, presenting the appearance of a double esophagus. (Meyers MA, Ghahremani GG: Complications of fiberoptic endoscopy. I. Esophagoscopy and gastroscopy. Radiology 115:293–300, 1975)

this site in several series (5,6,13) (Fig. 2-6). This may be due to thinning and segmental defects in the circular layer of the muscle at the lower end of the esophagus (15), the segment most frequently involved by inflammation or neoplasm. Endoscopic perforation through an inflammatory stricture or carcinoma (Fig. 2-7) can occur with surprising ease and yet remain clinically silent (5,16) rather than resulting in acute, dramatic mediastinitis. Conservative medical treatment may suffice in some patients with small perforations with minimal signs of leakage (5). Cohen and Katz reported 29 patients with esophageal carcinoma who had radiologic evaluation

with contrast material following esophagoscopy (16). A total of 45% had esophageal perforation. In 3 patients the trauma could be directly attributed to esophagoscopy, since chest films and esophagograms were obtained both before and after the procedure. Of the 13 patients with esophageal perforation, only 1 had symptoms of mediastinitis or pneumonitis. Abrams pointed out that acquired tracheoesophageal fistulas, which are sometimes secondary to instrumentation, may exist for years before symptoms are noted, possibly because of a ball-valve mechanism or muscular closure of the tract during deglutition (17). If postesophagoscopic radio-

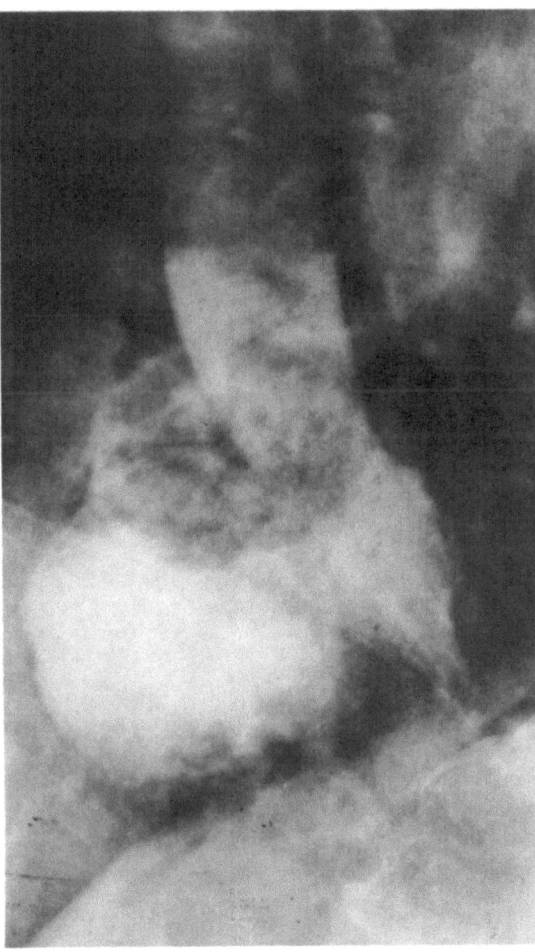

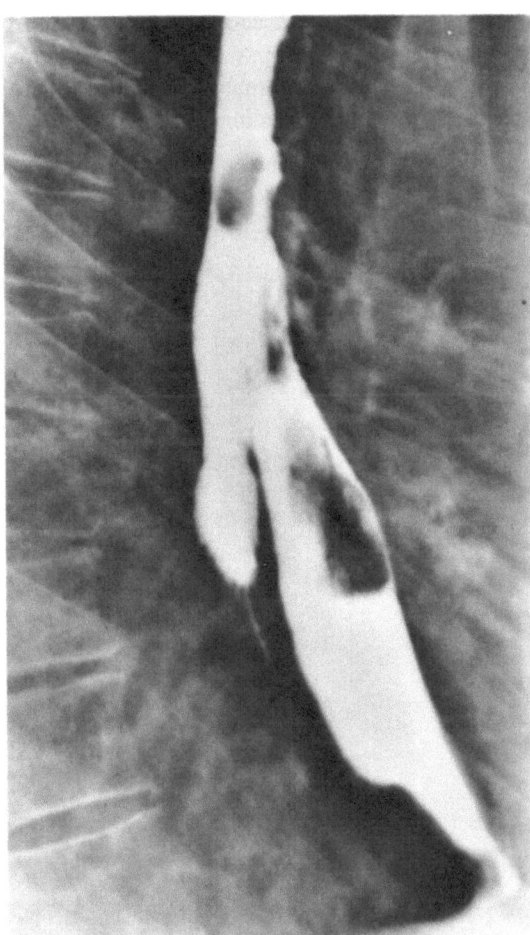

Fig. 2-6. Perforation of distal esophagus. Loculated mediastinal collection can be seen following fiberscopic perforation after removal of impacted piece of meat. (Meyers MA, Ghahremani GG: Complications of gastrointestinal fiberoptic endoscopy. Gastrointest Radiol 2:273–280, 1977)

Fig. 2-7. Perforation of esophagus through carcinoma. Carcinoma of the esophagus is shown with a large mediastinal sinus tract secondary to fiberesophagoscopy. (Meyers MA, Ghahremani GG: Complications of gastrointestinal fiberoptic endoscopy. Gastrointest Radiol 2:273–280, 1977)

graphic examinations are performed routinely, the reported frequency of perforation due to instrumentation may be much higher, particularly if a contrast study is performed with the patient in the Trendelenburg position (16).

Endoscopic biopsy of a friable lesion may also result in perforation. Although biopsy is usually superficial and produces no complication, mural transgression can result if an area of ulceration, weakening of the wall, or relative ischemia is entered (2) (Fig. 2-8). Leigh and Achord studied two cases of esophageal perforation secondary to endoscopic biopsy (11). In one case, which was complicated by an esophagopleural fistula and a tension pneumothorax, the biopsy was later reported as showing normal lung tissue. Wychulis et al. reported esophageal perforation following endoscopic biopsy in two cases of carcinoma and one of inflammatory stricture (7). In each case the biopsy specimen contained mediastinal fat.

Impaction of the Fiberscope

Despite its flexibility, and sometimes because of it, the instrument may curve back upon itself and become impacted within the esophagus (2,18, 19). The reason for the difficulty in further passage and the occasionally unexpected field of visualization is readily confirmed radiologically (Fig. 2-9). In various methods of management the impacted endoscope has been withdrawn in its looped position (18), straightened with a Jackson esophagoscope (20), and advanced into the stomach, straightened, and then withdrawn (19).

Within the stomach, inversion gastroscopy or retroflexion of the distal tip of the instrument to visualize the fundus has also resulted in impaction (21,22). This complication occurs within a small gastric pouch, in the fundus of a cascade stomach, or within a hiatus hernia. Considerable manipulation under fluroscopic control may be helpful in reducing the impaction, but an emer-

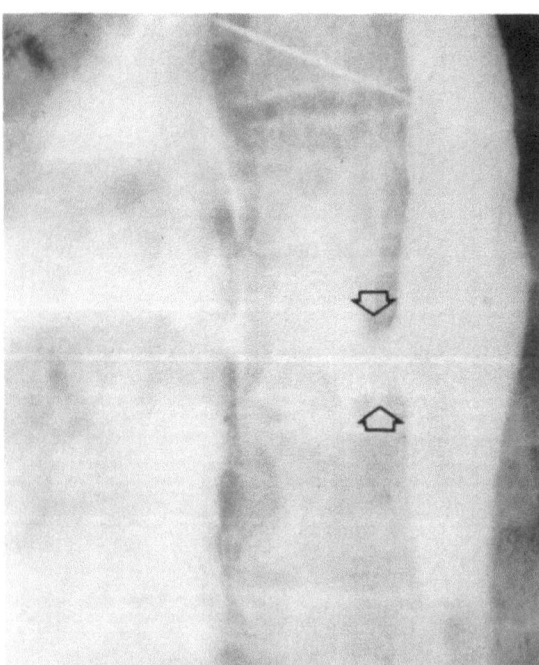

Fig. 2-8. Esophageal perforation due to endoscopic biopsy. Following fiberesophagoscopy and multiple biopsies of an ulcerated esophageal carcinoma the site of an esophagopleural fistula *(arrows)* is documented with water-soluble contrast material. The patient died following a complicated postoperative course. (Meyers MA, Ghahremani GG: Complications of fiberoptic endoscopy. I. Esophagoscopy and gastroscopy. Radiology 115:293–300, 1975)

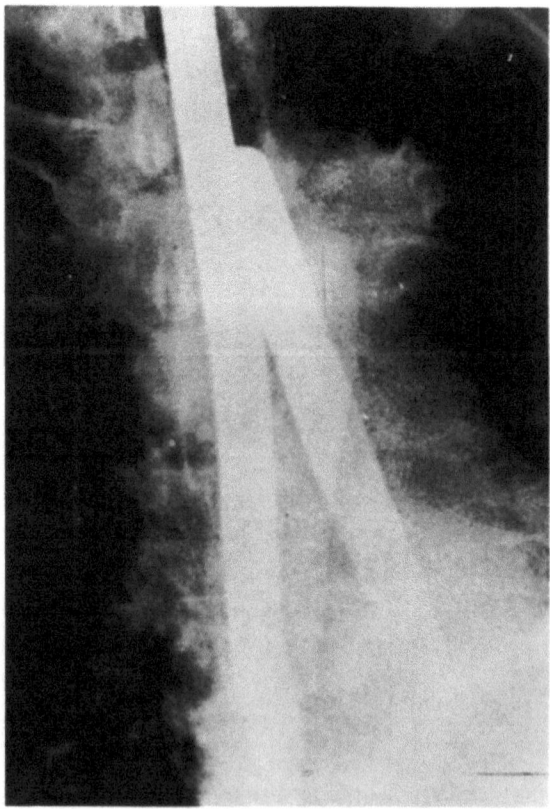

Fig. 2-9. Impaction of fiberscope in esophagus. This was due to looping, which can be seen on this film. (Parker LS: Impacted fibrescope in the oesophagus. J Laryngol Otol 83:1123–1125, 1969)

gency laparotomy may be unavoidable (23). Burke and Roling provided radiologic evidence suggesting that impaction is less likely to occur when the fundus is examined in the supine rather than the standard left lateral position, as the tip then tends to stay farther from the esophagogastric junction (24).

Gastric Perforation

Within the stomach, perforation usually occurs posteriorly into the lesser sac at or just beyond the esophagogastric junction (25). This can be explained on an anatomic basis. Just beyond the cardia the posterior wall is angulated anteriorly by the bulk of the retroperitoneal organs. Trauma, ranging from intramural hematoma

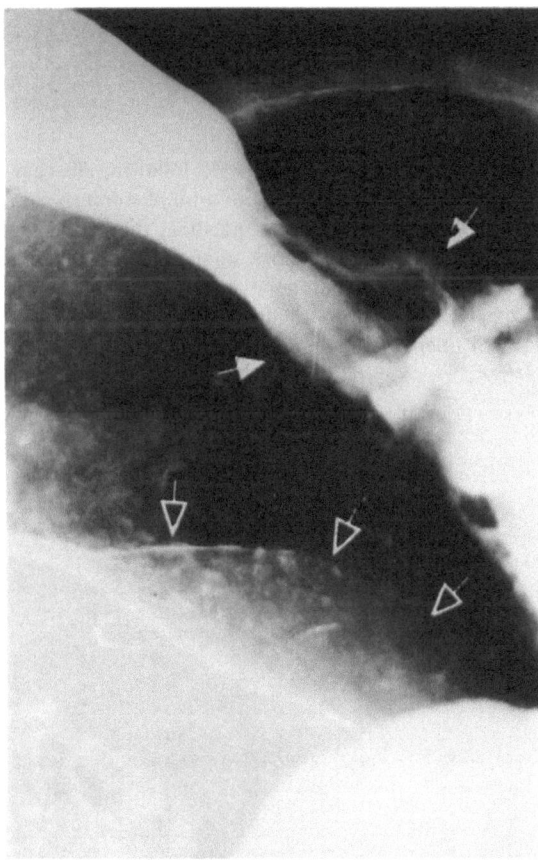

Fig. 2-10. Gastric hematomas induced by fibergastroscopic trauma. *Arrows* show these in the cardia and posteromedial wall of the gastric fundus. (Courtesy of J. Farman, MD, SUNY Downstate Medical Center, Brooklyn, New York)

(Fig. 2-10) to true rupture, may also be induced at this site by the fibergastroscope. The most frequent and characteristic endoscopic sign of gastric perforation is inability to inflate the stomach, since air escapes through the foramen of Winslow to produce pneumoperitoneum. Taylor cited an unusual case in which "the endoscopic view was of a tentlike cavity with a yellowish surface showing occasional fine vessels. One realized that this was the lesser sac of the peritoneal cavity" (26).

Water-soluble contrast studies may not demonstrate extravasation, and perforation has not been found in almost half of the patients undergoing laparotomy for this complication (25). This has given rise to the concept of "spontaneous postgastroscopy pneumoperitoneum" (27). Other observations have been cited in support of this (28,29). However, Calem (25) showed that the usual site of a gastric perforation is easily overlooked during routine exploratory laparotomy. The posterior wall of the stomach in the area of the fundus and gastroesophageal junction is comparatively inaccessible unless the stomach is well mobilized. He demonstrated that mechanical perforation of the stomach does indeed occur, often with a rent as large as 1.5 cm, but tends to be self-sealing. Thus it has become accepted that conservative therapy based on continuous gastric aspiration and prophylactic antibiotic administration is generally preferable to emergency laparotomy, since the stomach is empty at the time of perforation and the escaping gastric juice is nearly sterile (25). Usually the clinical course is surprisingly benign, without evidence of peritoneal irritation. At other times, however, extravasation into the lesser sac from a large posterior gastric perforation can be demonstrated radiologically (Fig. 2-11); these patients are best treated surgically.

Endoscopic perforation through the anterior wall of the stomach is usually the result of instrumental passage through a lesion or transmural penetration following biopsy (2) (Figs. 2-12 to 2-14). It typically presents more serious and immediate consequences. The rent is not self-sealing and leads to peritonitis or a localized abscess. Intramural hematoma may be seen as a less serious consequence (14) (Fig. 2-15). Fibergastroscopic perforation of the gastric remnant following a Billroth II procedure has also been reported (30).

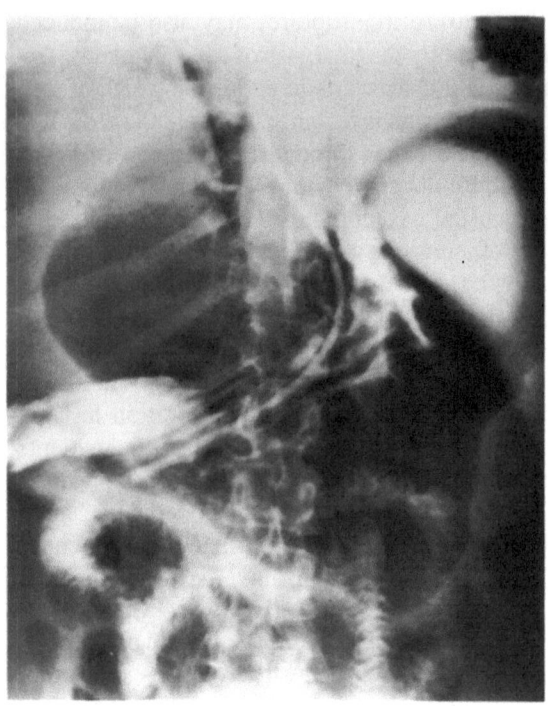

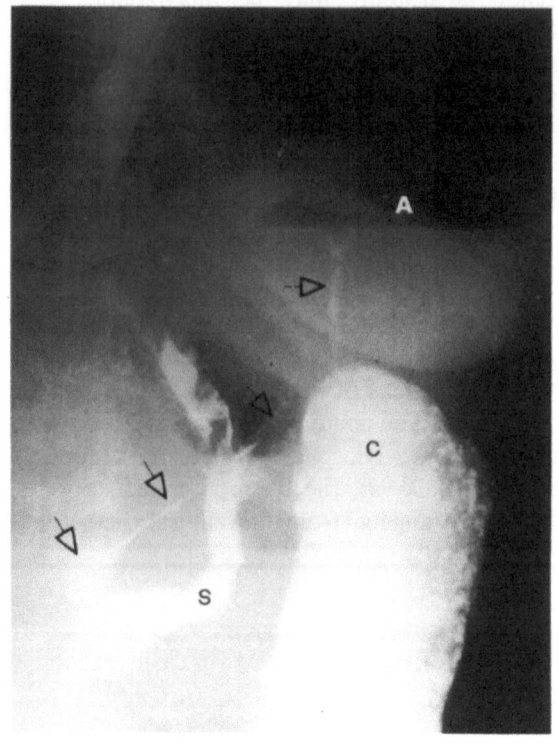

Fig. 2-11. Fibergastroscopy-induced perforation of stomach into lesser sac. Water-soluble contrast material introduced through the nasogastric tube demonstrates the position of the stomach. Extravasation posteriorly into the lesser sac has occurred via perforation near the cardia and gravitated to the area of the splenic bed at the site of a previous splenectomy. (Meyers MA, Ghahremani GG: Complications of fiberoptic endoscopy. I. Esophagoscopy and gastroscopy. Radiology 115:293–300, 1975)

Fig. 2-12. Left subphrenic abscess following fibergastroscopic perforation of anterior wall of stomach. In a patient with extensive linitis plastica, there is extravasation in a tract *(arrows)* leading from the stomach *(S)* to a large subdiaphragmatic abscess *(A)* above the colon *(C).* (Meyers MA, Ghahremeni GG: Complications of fiberoptic endoscopy. I. Esophagoscopy and gastroscopy. Radiology 115:293–300, 1975)

Fig. 2-13. Subphrenic air-fluid collection after gastric ▶ **perforation.** At fibergastroscopy and biopsy of a polypoid adenocarcinoma of the gastric fundus, perforation occurred anteriorly in the periphery of the tumor. In this erect film note that the subphrenic fluid level *(open arrow)* is on the same plane as that within the stomach *(closed arrows),* indicating communication between the gastric lumen and the incipient subphrenic abscess. The soft-tissue tumor mass is evident within the fundus. (Meyers MA, Ghahremani GG: Complications of fiberoptic endoscopy. I. Esophagoscopy and gastroscopy. Radiology 115:293–300, 1975)

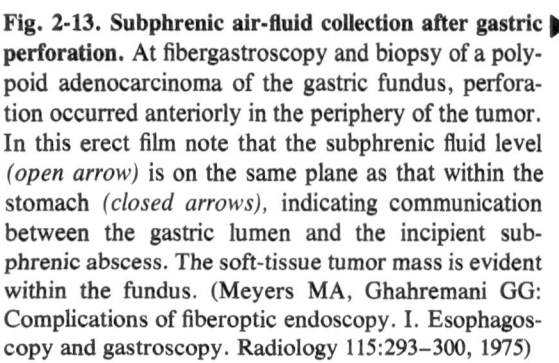

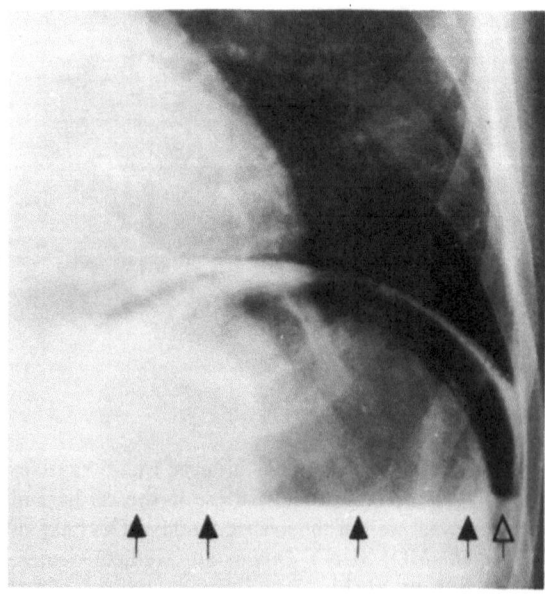

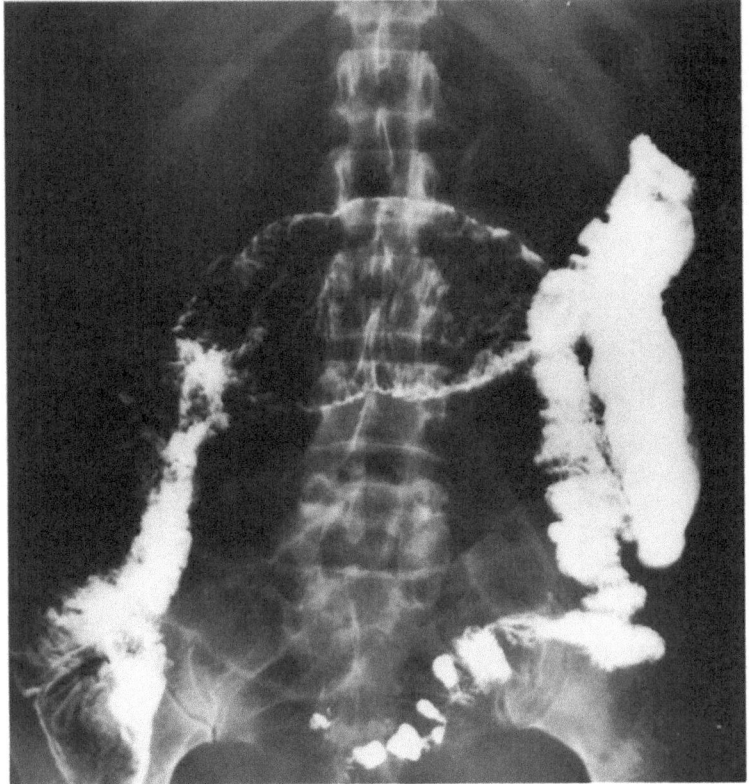

a

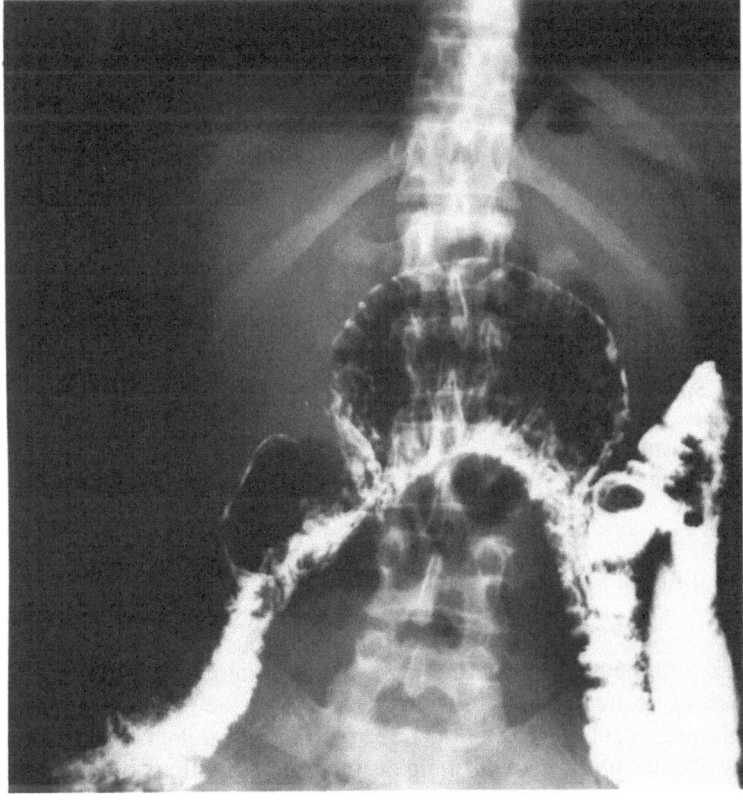

b

Fig. 2-14, a and b. Perforation of greater curvature of stomach following endoscopic biopsy of carcinoma. In supine (a) and erect (b) radiographs of the abdomen, residual contrast material in transverse colon demonstrates effects of paresis secondary to extension of perforation along the gastrocolic ligament. Free intraperitoneal air is also evident. (Meyers MA, Ghahremani GG: Complications of gastrointestinal fiberoptic endoscopy. Gastrointest Radiol 2:273–280, 1977)

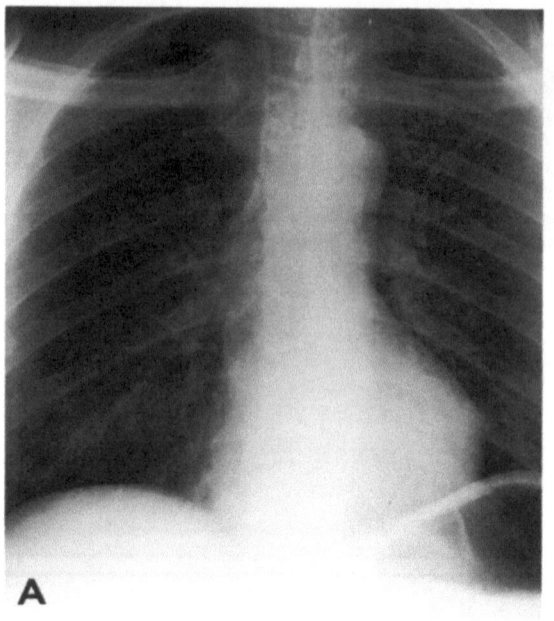

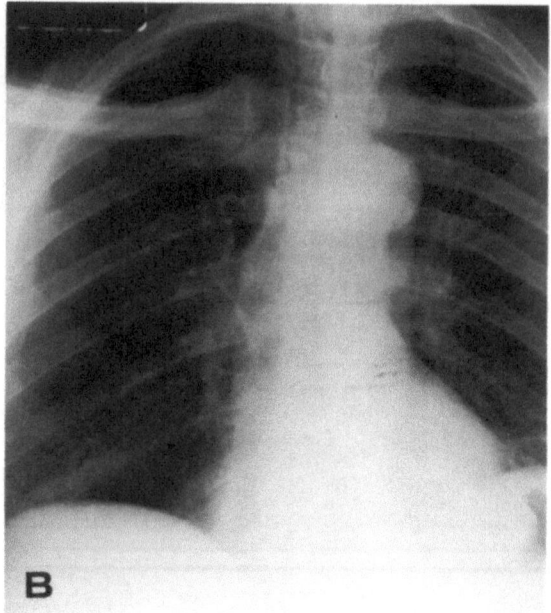

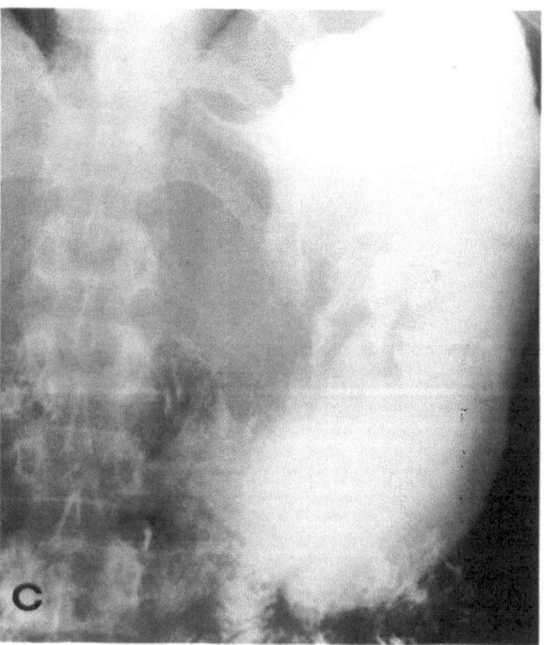

Fig. 2-15, A–C. Intramural gastric hematoma secondary to fiberoptic endoscopy. Emergency panendoscopy disclosed a bleeding duodenal ulcer in a 54-year-old man who had had previous cardiac surgery and who presented with melena. **A** Normal chest film on admission. **B** Semi-erect chest film 1 day after endoscopy shows a mass in the fundus. **C** Barium contrast examination shows deformity of the fundus and localized enlargement of the gastric rugae in the lesser curvature due to intramural hematomas. Spontaneous resolution was noted on subsequent studies. (Meyers MA, Ghahremani GG: Complications of gastrointestinal fiberoptic endoscopy. Gastrointest Radiol 2:273–280, 1977)

Pseudoacute Abdominal State Following Gastroscopy

New instruments with a powered air supply are capable of introducing large volumes of air during endoscopy, leading to considerable acute gaseous distention of the small bowel. The process is probably facilitated by the hypotonic effects of anticholinergic drugs, which are often used in premedication of patients undergoing gastrointestinal endoscopy. The dramatic clinical picture of severe abdominal pain, distention, and diffuse tenderness may be mistaken for perforation (31,32). Prompt radiologic evaluation should indicate the true condition, but Rastogi and Brown reported a case in which the patient underwent emergency laparotomy (32).

Submandibular and Parotid Swelling

Submandibular swelling is an unusual complication but deserves brief attention because of its rather confusing clinical presentation. In patients with persistent blind remnants of the fourth branchial cleft, insufflation of air during the procedure can result in bilateral swelling below the parotid glands. The air can easily be evacuated by manual compression of these branchial pouches (33). The submandibular glands may also swell because of ductal obstruction due to displacement of these organs during the endoscopic procedure (34). Spontaneous regression of symptoms usually occurs within a few hours.

Aspiration Pneumonia and Other Complications

Pharyngeal motor dysfunction of mild degree and short duration is not uncommon after gastrointestinal endoscopy and is usually due to topical anesthesia and the mild trauma induced. We have noted delayed clearing—up to 2 days—of contrast material from the hypopharynx of several patients after uncomplicated gastrointestinal fiberendoscopy (2); this may also explain the occasional development of aspiration pneumonia in such cases. Patients with obstructive lesions and functional disorders of the esophagus are prone to aspiration even without the contributory effects of traumatic endoscopy.

Hematemesis may be associated with perforation. Clinically significant hemorrhage very seldom occurs following biopsy of gastroesphageal lesions by means of a fiberendoscope since small samples are obtained under good visibility, in contrast to "blind" biopsy through a standard endoscope. Nevertheless, a bleeding diathesis, acute phlegmonous and corrosive esophagitis, and gastroesophageal varices are still contraindications to biopsy.

Colonoscopy

Fiberoptic colonoscopy is being used increasingly for endoscopic visualization of the large intestine, particularly in the removal of colonic polyps by means of an electrosurgical snare advanced through the biopsy channel of the colonoscope. Despite the relative flexibility of the instrument and the removal of polyps by cauterization under direct visualization, several complications have been encountered. Radiologic examination plays a decisive role in the initial identification and documentation of many complications (2,14,35). Most frequent and requiring prompt diagnostic evaluation is perforation of the colon.

Technical Considerations

Fiberoptic colonoscopes of various lengths permit endoscopic evaluation of the colon from the rectum to the cecum. Passage through the rectum is under direct vision, but negotiation through the sigmoid is usually accomplished without complete visualization of the lumen (36). Visualization of the entire wall of the colon is carried out primarily during withdrawal. Not infrequently some difficulty in passage of the instrument is encountered at the points of curvature of the rectosigmoid and the junction of the sigmoid and descending colon, and too much "persuasive pressure" (37) in advancing the colonoscope may result in mural perforation. Marked redundancy of the colon and narrowing or angulation due to diverticulosis, previous inflammatory processes, or extrinsic compression of the lumen by pelvic masses may make negotiation difficult (38).

Gaseous distention of the colon is used to facilitate passage of the instrument. Initially, because of the presence of the combustible gases hydrogen and methane in the colon, carbon dioxide was introduced to avoid colonic explosion during cautery. Room air is now generally used because the adequately cleansed colon is free of putrefactive gases, and the gas content of the bowel is exchanged several times during introduction of the colonoscope (39). Bond and Levitt confirmed experimentally that following colonic preparation the concentrations of hydrogen and methane are well below hazardous combustible levels (40).

While advancement of the colonoscope may be monitored fluoroscopically, most endoscopists employ fluoroscopy or abdominal radiography only when difficulty is encountered (36,39).

Colonoscopic Perforation

A survey by the American Society for Gastrointestinal Endoscopy has shown that the most common complication of diagnostic colonoscopy is perforation (0.22%). Furthermore, colonoscopic polypectomy resulted in perforation in 0.29% of cases, although its most common complication was hemorrhage (1.9%) (38). Others reported a perforation rate as high as 1.9% with initial experience in colonoscopy (41).

The most common sites of mural perforation during diagnostic colonoscopy include the rectosigmoid and the junction of the sigmoid and descending colon (35,38). Many occur during mechanical manipulations, including the techniques of slide-by, alpha maneuver, and straightening of the sigmoid loop. Friability of the wall from inflammatory colitis is a recognized hazard (35,38).

The colonoscope may also be advanced into a prominent diverticulum, causing its orifice to be mistaken for the proximal continuation of the colonic lumen. Insufflation of the colon with gas has also been incriminated in diverticular perforation.

Colonoscopic fulguration of polyps has wide application but may also result in serious complications. A loop of wire is advanced through the biopsy channel of the colonoscope, and electric current is applied while the snare is closed around the pedicle or base of the polyp. Large sessile lesions may have to be removed piecemeal (39). Overzealous application of heat, inadvertent inclusion of a portion of the colonic wall in the cautery snare, or unclear visualization of the snare in the center of the bowel lumen while touching a point on the opposite wall may produce coagulation necrosis and resultant perforation (35).

Free (intraperitoneal) perforation is about four times more frequent than closed (extraperitoneal) perforation, both in diagnostic colonoscopy and following polypectomy (38).

Clinically, perforation may be recognized immediately, or there may be considerable delay. Intraperitoneal rupture is usually immediately apparent but may be initially overlooked, particularly in an aged or infirm patient (35). Prompt surgical closure is generally indicated. A few reports suggest that some patients may be treated conservatively without emergency laparotomy (42,43). Extraperitoneal perforation may be masked for several hours or days (35) and is often not evident by the usual clinical methods of auscultation, palpation, and percussion. Indeed, it may not be until the extraperitoneal gas extends to the abdominal wall, mediastinum, or cervical tissues that it becomes clinically apparent. However, extraperitoneal rupture generally follows a more benign course and can be treated conservatively. We have recommended routine abdominal radiography following diagnostic and therapeutic colonoscopy (35). Because the colon is distended for easier endoscopic passage and visualization, considerable extraluminal gas is usually apparent if rupture has occurred.

Free intraperitoneal air is indicated on a supine film by increased radiolucency, visualization of the falciform ligament and perhaps the umbilical folds, and demonstration of both sides of the bowel wall (Figs. 2-16 to 2-19). The last may be the main finding but can be somewhat subtle, with the wall outlined as a white stripe. Erect or decubitus films readily demonstrate free intraperitoneal air. With procedures limited commonly to the left half of the colon, intraperitoneal gas indicates perforation of the sigmoid colon (usually at its junction with the rectum or the descending colon) or at the site of an anterior polypectomy.

Extraperitoneal perforation most commonly involves the rectum or the posterior wall of the descending colon. Since fully 75% of colonic diverticula face the extraperitoneal tissues (44), acute diverticular perforation usually gives rise to extraperitoneal gas (Fig. 2-20) and only occasionally to intraperitoneal air. Perforation of the sigmoid or transverse colon into the mesentery (Fig. 2-21) also extends posteriorly as extraperitoneal gas (45). Correlative anatomic-radiologic studies by Meyers have established the characteristic distribution and localization of extraperitoneal gas according to its source (45). The extraperitoneal structures are divided by fascial planes into three distinct compartments: anterior pararenal, perirenal, and posterior pararenal. Extraperitoneal gas within each compartment has been shown to have distinctive spread and localization. Radiographic findings may therefore reveal not only that a perforation has occurred but also the site of rupture.

Rectal perforation is indicated by gas ascend-

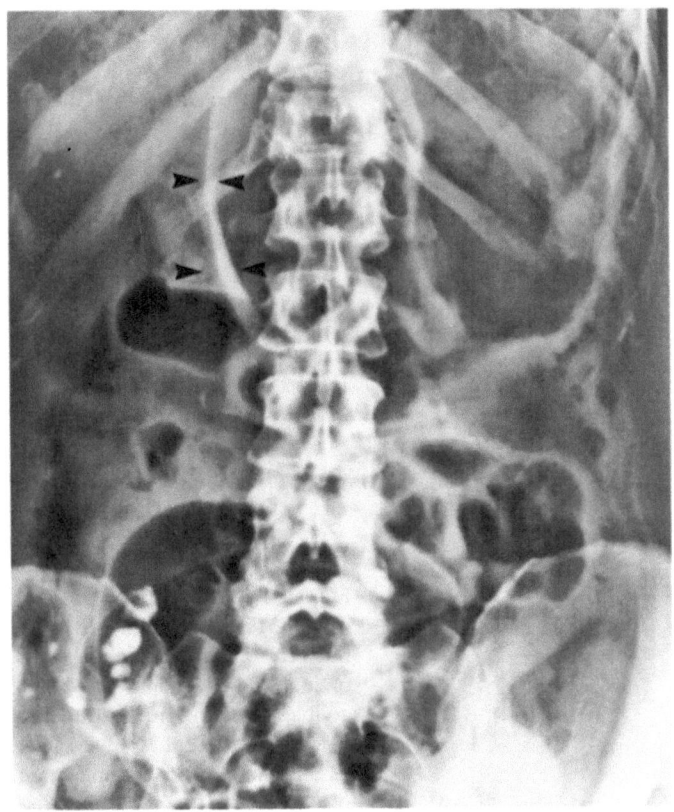

Fig. 2-16. **Sigmoid perforation secondary to coagulation necrosis of colonic wall at colonoscopic polypectomy.** Gross free intraperitoneal air causes lucent distention of the abdomen and allows visualization of the falciform ligament *(arrows).* (Meyers MA, Ghahremani GG: Complications of fiberoptic endoscopy. II. Colonoscopy. Radiology 115:301–307, 1975)

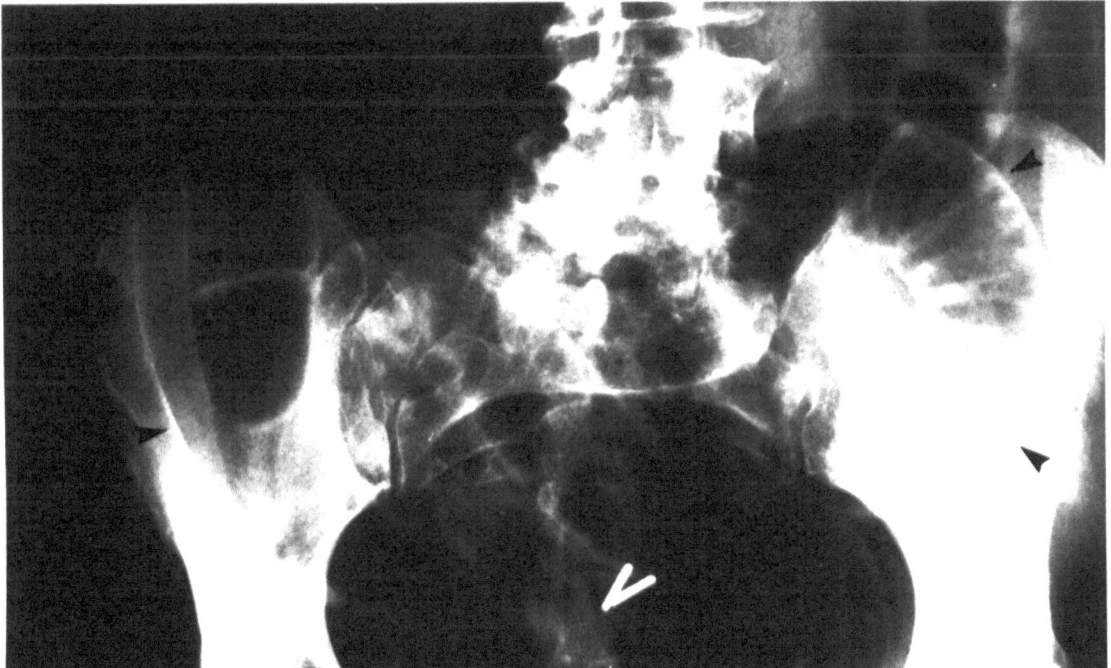

Fig. 2-17. Sigmoid perforation due to coagulation necrosis. This occurred despite creation of a pseudopedicle by colonoscopic traction on a sessile polyp. Free intraperitoneal air *(closed arrows)* is revealed with visualization of the bowel wall. (Meyers MA, Ghahremani GG: Complications of fiberoptic endoscopy. II. Colonoscopy. Radiology 115:301–307, 1975)

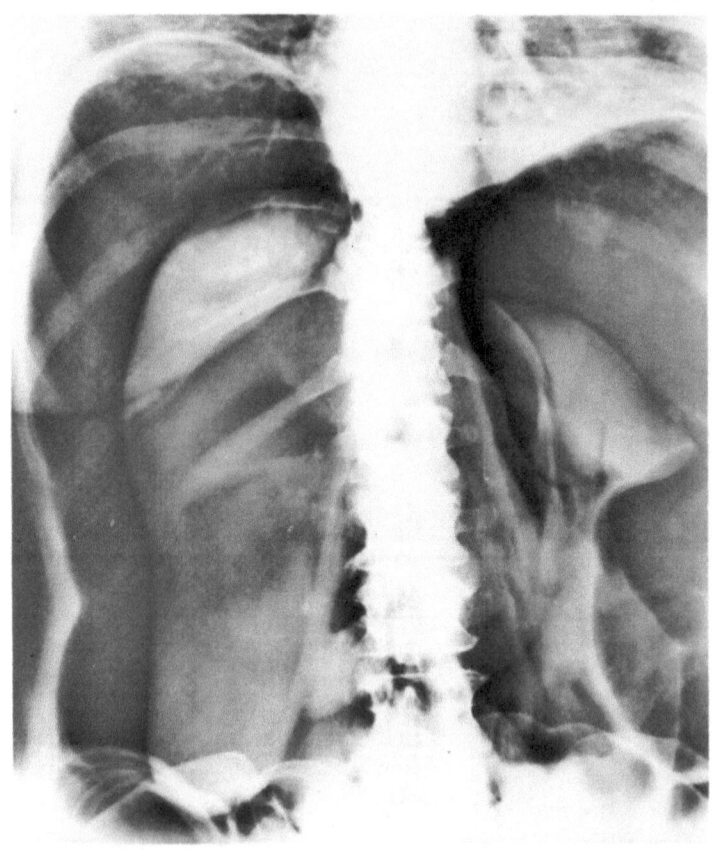

Fig. 2-18. Sigmoid perforation thought to be secondary to colonoscopic air insufflation. The patient had chronic ulcerative colitis. Massive free intraperitoneal air is present. (Meyers MA, Ghahremani GG: Complications of fiberoptic endoscopy. II. Colonoscopy. Radiology 115:301–307, 1975)

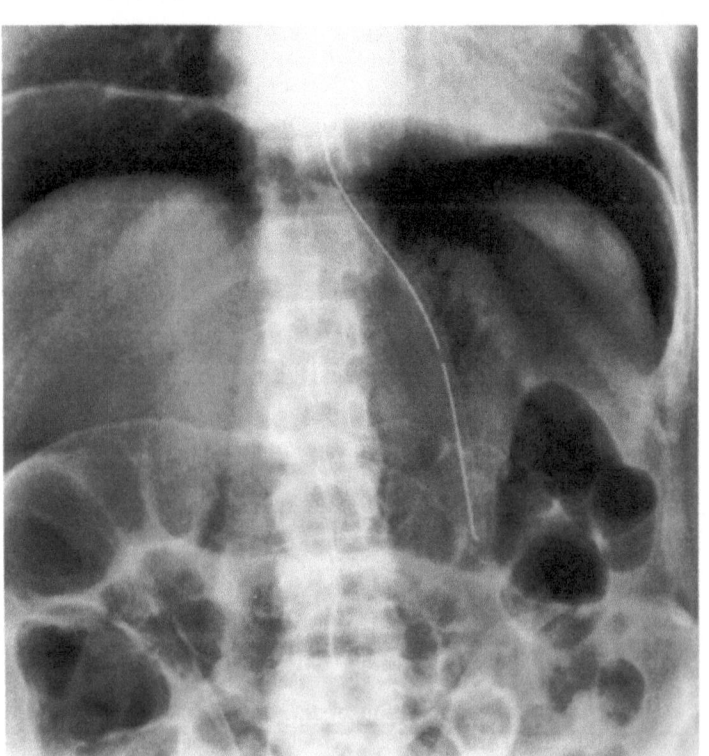

Fig. 2-19. Sigmoid perforation occurring during alpha maneuver. Erect abdominal film demonstrates free subdiaphragmatic gas bilaterally with visualization of the bowel wall. (Meyers MA, Ghahremani GG: Complications of fiberoptic endoscopy. II. Colonoscopy. Radiology 115:301–307, 1975)

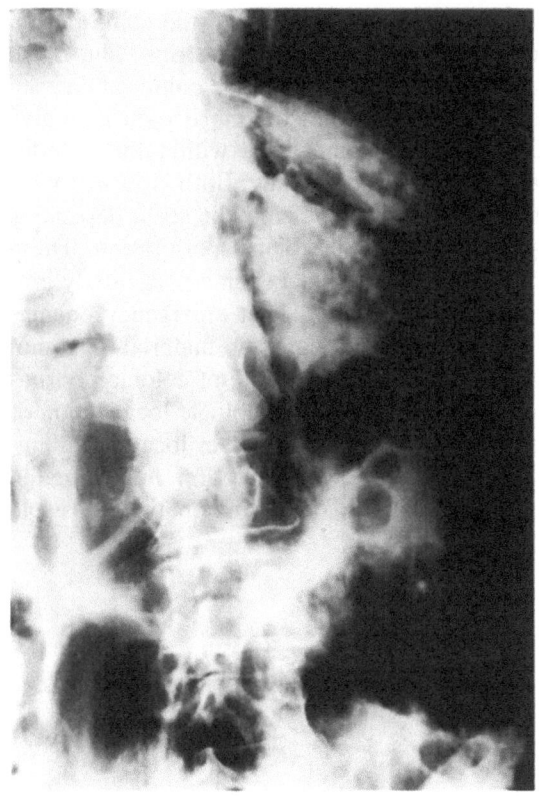

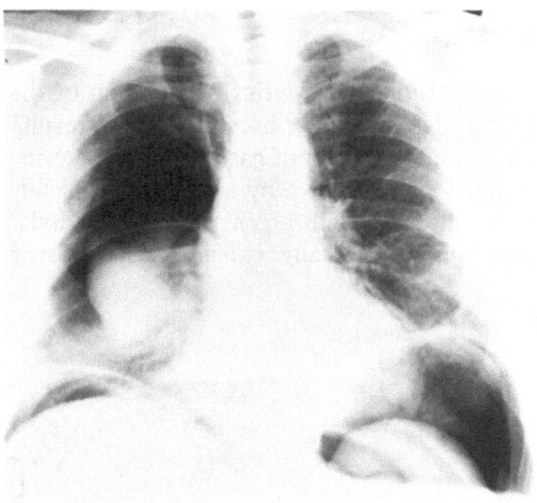

a

Fig. 2-20. Perforation of diverticulum of descending colon during colonoscopy. Extraperitoneal gas outlines the left kidney and the medial border of the spleen. Free air or extraperitoneal gas were not seen on the right side. (Meyers MA, Ghahremani GG: Complications of gastrointestinal fiberoptic endoscopy. Gastrointest Radiol 2:273–280, 1977)

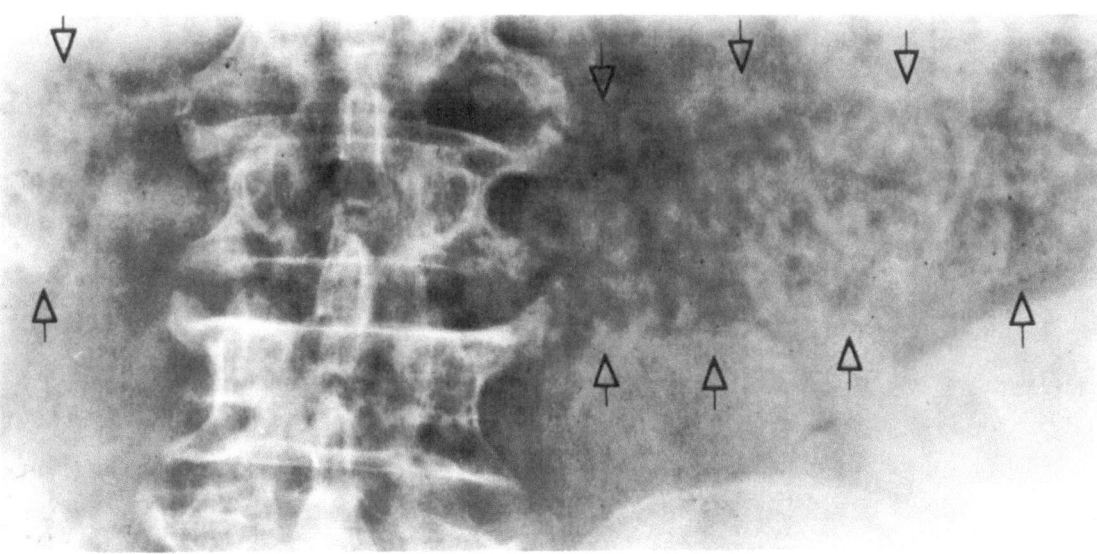

b

Fig. 2-21, a and b. Colonoscopic perforation of transverse colon into peritoneal cavity and extraperitoneal tissues. This occurred following electrosnare removal of a small polyp from the transverse colon. **a** Erect chest film shows a large amount of free intraperitoneal air. Bilaterally, extraperitoneal gas collects as lucent crescents immediately below the domes of the diaphragm. Note pneumomediastinum and massive right pneumothorax. **b** Supine abdominal film shows mottled lucent areas representing gas extending across the midline *(arrows)* in the plane of the transverse mesocolon. (Meyers MA, Ghahremani GG: Complications of fiberoptic endoscopy. II. Colonoscopy. Radiology 115:301–307, 1975)

ing the posterior pararenal spaces bilaterally, with lucent areas paralleling the lateral borders of the psoas muscles; superiorly it sometimes extends as high as the upper renal pole and adrenal gland, the medial border of the spleen and liver, the medial crus of the diaphragm, and the immediate subphrenic tissues (Figs. 2-22, 2-23). Extension into the flank fat stripes, anterior abdominal walls, scrotum, and mediastinum may occur.

Extraperitoneal (posterior) perforation of the sigmoid, descending, or ascending colon results in unilateral collection of gas within the anterior pararenal space, shown by a collection of mottled lucent areas with a generally vertical axis. These characteristically extend medially over

the psoas muscle to approach the spine but do not usually infiltrate the flank stripe (Fig. 2-24). Perforation of the sigmoid colon at a site between the leaves of the mesocolon may give rise to extraperitoneal gas within the anterior pararenal spaces bilaterally. Both intraperitoneal and extraperitoneal gas may be seen, depending upon the site of the colonic perforation. These plain-film observations become particularly crucial when one realizes that emergency enemas with water-soluble contrast material may not directly demonstrate the site of colonic perforation (46) (Fig. 2-23B). Radiologic localization of the precise site is important in locating a clinically uncertain site of perforation, indicating the proper treatment, and anticipating possible complications.

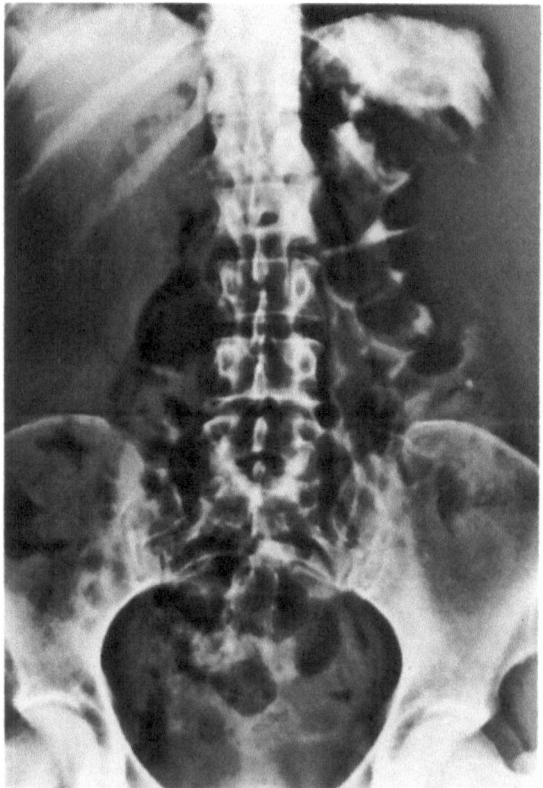

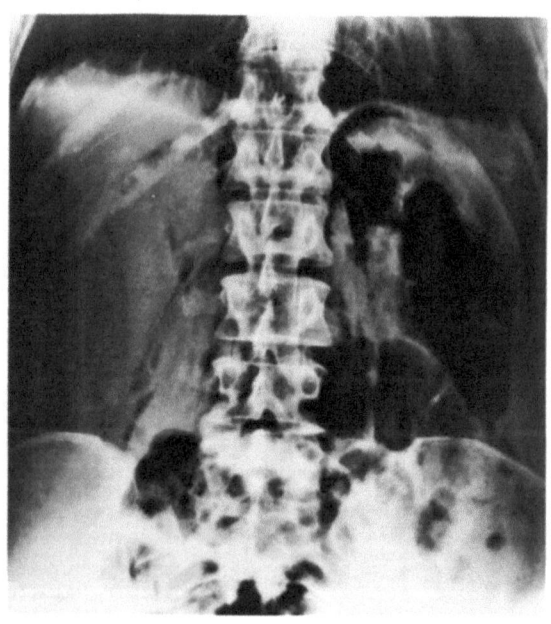

b

a

Fig. 2-22, a and b. Rectal perforation secondary to colonoscopy. Supine (a) and erect (b) films demonstrate extraperitoneal gas paralleling the lateral borders of the psoas muscles. Cephalad extension on the left outlines the upper pole of the kidney, the adrenal gland, the medial border of the spleen, the medial crus

of the diaphragm, and the immediate subphrenic tissues. These findings localize the gas to the posterior pararenal compartments. (Meyers MA: Radiologic features of the spread and localization of extraperitoneal gas and their relationship to its source. An anatomical approach. Radiology 111:17–26, 1974)

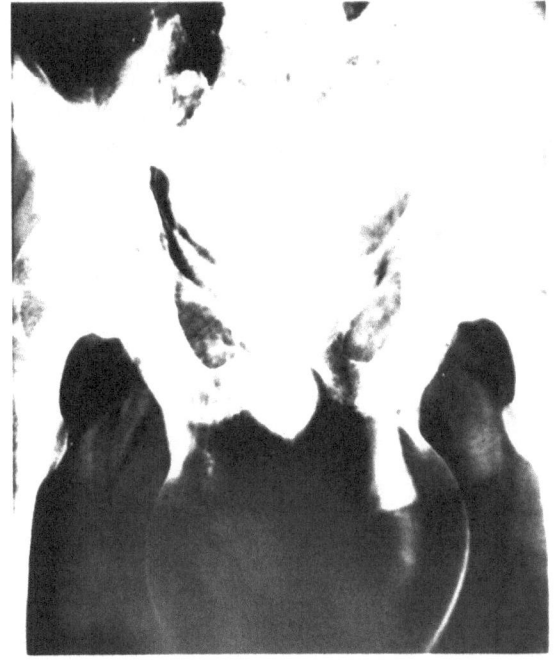

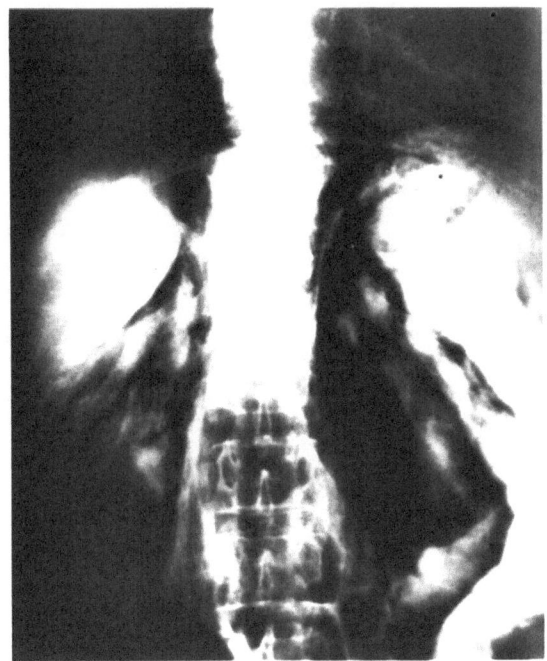

a   b

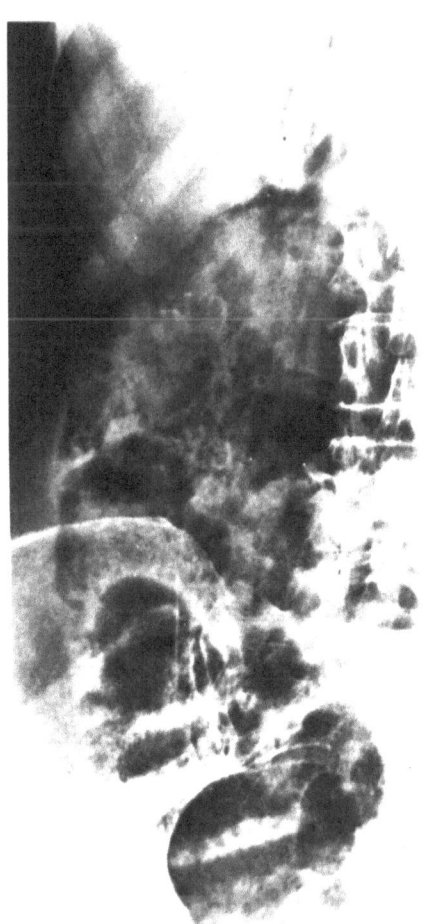

Fig. 2-23, a and b. Rectal perforation secondary to colonoscopy.

a Massive scrotal and extraperitoneal gas. (Lezak MB, Goldhamer M: Retroperitoneal emphysema after colonoscopy. Gastroenterology 66:118–120, 1974.)

b There is gas within both posterior pararenal spaces, outlining the lateral borders of the psoas muscles, the upper renal poles and adrenal glands, the medial borders of the liver and spleen, the medial crura of the diaphragm, and the immediate subphrenic tissues. The Gastrografin enema study of the left colon demonstrated no extravasation. (Meyers MA, Ghahremani GG: Complications of fiberoptic endoscopy. II. Colonoscopy. Radiology 115:301–307, 1975)

Fig. 2-24. Perforation of hepatic flexure following colonoscopic polypectomy. Mottled lucent areas on the right represent collections of gas extending medially over the psoas muscle and approaching the spine. The flank stripe is intact. These changes localize the extraperitoneal gas to the anterior pararenal space. (Meyers MA, Ghahremani GG: Complications of fiberoptic endoscopy. II. Colonoscopy. Radiology 115:301–307, 1975)

Other Complications

A spectrum of other complications has also been experienced. Insufflation of gas to facilitate passage of the colonoscope occasionally may cause massive and prolonged dilatation of the small intestine in patients with a patulous ileocecal valve (14) (Fig. 2-25). Mural perforation by the colonoscope at the site of a stricture may result in a localized abscess. A hematoma may develop

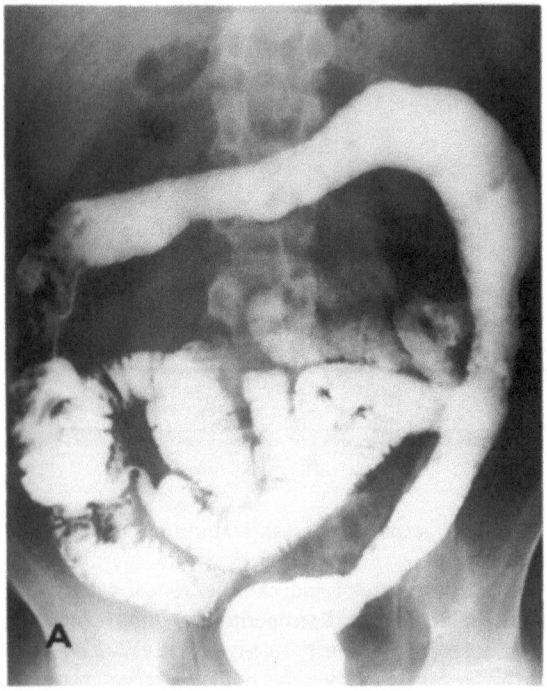

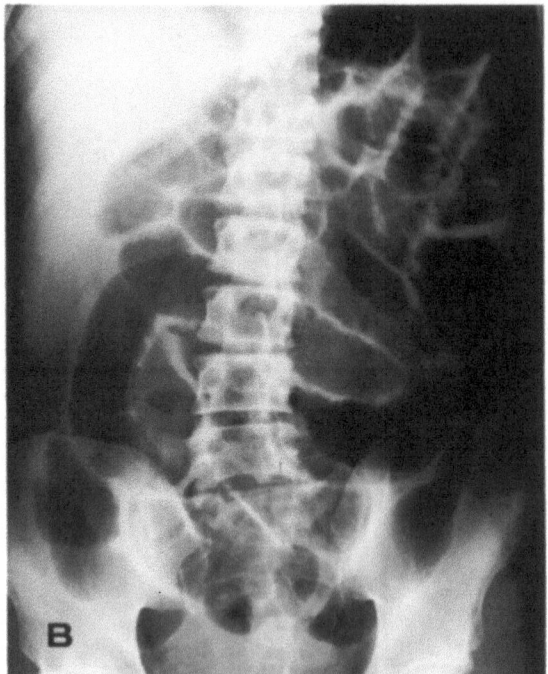

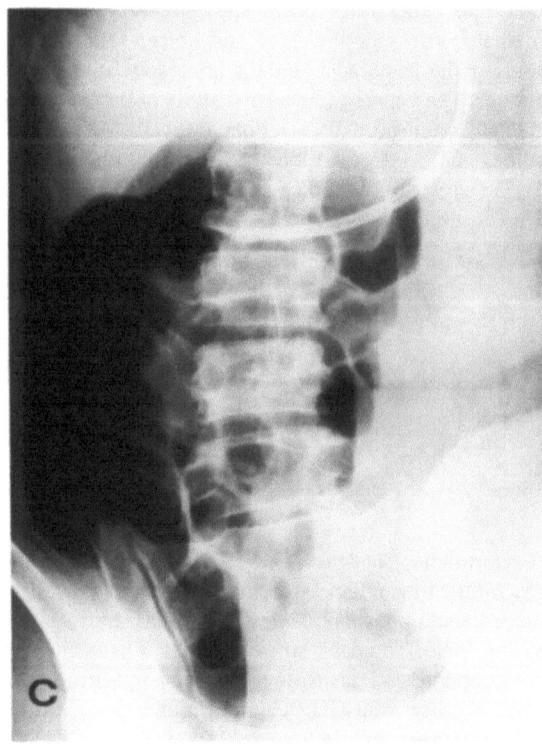

Fig. 2-25, a–c. Prolonged gaseous distention of small intestine following fiberoptic colonoscopy. a Barium enema examination shows diffuse chronic ulcerative colitis and a patulous ileocecal valve. b Supine radiograph of the abdomen immediately after colonoscopy demonstrates marked distention of the small intestine. c The left lateral decubitus film obtained 2 days later shows persistent dilatation and fluid levels within the small intestine. The bowel gas pattern became normal on the fourth day after colonoscopy. (Meyers MA, Ghahremani GG: Complications of gastrointestinal fiberoptic endoscopy. Gastrointest Radiol 2:273–280, 1977)

in the sigmoid mesentery as the result of difficulty in passing the instrument or attempts to
alter or bypass the redundant curvature of the
sigmoid loop (Fig. 2-26). Serosal lacerations or
seromuscular tears due to mechanical pressure
of the instrument or increased intraluminal pressures, and often clinically occult, have also been
encountered (47–49). Problems may also be
encountered during withdrawal of the instrument. Reported complications include incarceration of the colonoscope in an unsuspected
inguinal hernia and avulsion and rupture of the
spleen, presumably secondary to instrumental
intussusception of the colon (35).

Explosion of colonic gas has occurred during
anal surgery (50), colonic surgery on the unpre-
pared bowel (51), and during proctosigmoidos-
copic polypectomy (52), for which there is generally limited bowel preparation. Fatal colonic
explosion during colonoscopic polypectomy has
recently been reported in a patient in whom iso-
tonic mannitol solution was used for bowel preparation. It is presumed that the metabolism of a
part of the mannitol by colonic bacteria resulted
in an explosive concentration of hydrogen (53).

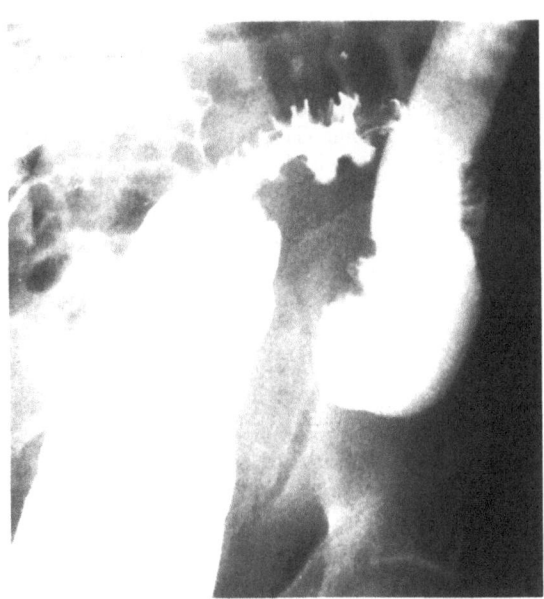

**Fig. 2-26. Intramural hematoma localized to segment
of sigmoid colon after colonoscopic removal of polyp.**
This is evident on barium enema examination 3 days
later. (Meyers MA, Ghahremani GG: Complications
of gastrointestinal fiberoptic endoscopy. Gastrointest
Radiol 2:273–280, 1977)

References

1. Mandelstam P, Sugawa C, Silvis SE, et al: Complications associated with esophago-gastroduo-
   denoscopy and with esophageal dilation. Gastrointest Endosc 23:16–19, 1976
2. Meyers MA, Ghahremani GG: Complications of
   fiberoptic endoscopy. I. Esophagoscopy and gastroscopy. Radiology 115:293–300, 1975
3. Palmer E: Discussion of Katz (4)
4. Katz D: Morbidity and mortality in standard and
   flexible gastrointestinal endoscopy. Gastrointest
   Endosc 15:134, 136, 138, 140–141, 1969
5. Berry BE, Ochsner JL: Perforation of the esophagus. A 30 year review. J Thorac Cardiovasc Surg
   65:1–7, 1973
6. Foster JH, Jolly PC, Sawyers JL et al: Esophageal perforation: Diagnosis and treatment. Ann
   Surg 161:701–709, 1965
7. Wychulis AR, Fontana RS, Payne WS: Instrumental perforations of the esophagus. Dis Chest
   55:184–189, 1969
8. Anselm K, Shartsis JM, Carandang NV, et al:
   Perforation of the esophagus with the gastrocamera fiberscope. Am J Dig Dis 15:311–315, 1970
9. Davis JS: Esophageal perforation by the gastrocamera gastroscope. Gastrointest Endosc 15:201–
   203, 1969
10. Sealy WC: Rupture of the esophagus. Am J Surg
    105:505–510, 1963
11. Leigh TF, Achord JL: Pharyngeal and esophageal

12. Gerard FP, Sabety AM, Trillo RA, et al: Esopha-
    geal perforation. Arch Surg 96:414–419, 1968
13. Youngs J, Nicoloff D: Management of esophageal
    perforation. Surgery 65:264–268, 1969
14. Meyers MA, Ghahremani GG: Complications of
    gastrointestinal fiberoptic endoscopy. Gastroin-
    test Radiol 2:273–280, 1977
15. Mosher HP: The lower end of the oesophagus at
    birth and in the adult. J Laryngol Otol 45:161–180,
    1930
16. Cohen G, Katz J: The importance of radiographic
    examination of the oesophagus and routine chest
    radiography after oesophagoscopy. S Afr Med J
    34:273–274, 1960
17. Abrams HS: Esophagorespiratory fistulae. Arch
    Otolaryngol 60:371–374, 1954
18. Kavin H, Schneider J: Impaction of fibre-optic
    gastroscope in the oesophagus: An unusual com-
    plication of gastroscopy. S Afr Med J 44:478–479,
    1970
19. Falkenstein DB, Hsu KD, Dagradi AE, et al:
    Repetitive endoscopic accidents and instrument
    malfunction. Gastrointest Endosc 23:206–208,
    1977
20. Parker LS: Impacted fibrescope in the oesopha-
    gus. J Laryngol Otol 83:1123–1125, 1969
21. Bralow SP: Fibrogastroscopic technic for exami-
    nation of the gastric fundus. Am J Dig Dis 12:653–
    656, 1967

perforations during instrumentation. Am J Roentgenol 91:757–765, 1964

22. Cohen NN: An unusual complication of the fiber-scope. Gastrointest Endosc 11:19, 1964

23. Braucher RE, Kirsner JB: Case report: Impacted fiberscope. Gastrointest Endosc 12:20–22, 1965

24. Burke EL, Roling GT: Reflections on retroflexions. Gastrointest Endosc 17:99–100, 1971

25. Calem WS: Perforation of the stomach during gastroscopy. Am J Surg 103:640–645, 1962

26. Taylor H: Difficulties and dangers in gastroscopy. Gastroenterology 35:79–91, 1958

27. Katz D, Selesnick S: Massive pneumoperitoneum and pneumoretroperitoneum after gastroscopy. Report of a case and review of the literature. Am J Dig Dis 1:512–520, 1956

28. Fierst SM, Robinson HM, Lasagna L: Interstitial gastric emphysema following gastroscopy. Its relation to syndrome of pneumoperitoneum and generalized emphysema with no evident perforation. Ann Intern Med 34:1202–1212, 1951

29. Myhre J, Wilson JA: A study on the occurrence of pneumoperitoneum after gastroscopy and the observance of intestinal emphysema of the stomach. Gastroenterology 11:115–119, 1948

30. Sanders MG, Schimmel EM: Perforation of a gastric remnant following fiber-optic gastroscopy. Gastrointest Endosc 17:186–187, 1971

31. Moldow R, Waye JD, Cohen N, et al: Pseudo-acute abdomen following gastroscopy. Gastrointest Endosc 17:117–118, 1971

32. Rastogi H, Brown CH: Pseudo acute abdomen following gastroscopy. Gastrointest Endosc 14:16–18, 1967

33. Palmer ED, Boyce HW Jr: Manual of Gastrointestinal Endoscopy. Baltimore: Williams & Wilkins 1964, p 74

34. Slaughter RL, Boyce HW Jr: Submaxilliary salivary gland swelling developing during peroral endoscopy. Gastroenterology 57:83–88, 1969

35. Meyers MA, Ghahremani GG: Complications of fiberoptic endoscopy. II. Colonoscopy. Radiology 115:301–307, 1975

36. Waye JD: Colonoscopy. Surg Clin North Am 52:1013–1024, 1972

37. Overholt BF: Flexible fiberoptic sigmoidoscopy. Technique and preliminary results. Cancer 28:123–126, 1971

38. Rogers BHG, Silvis SE, Nebel OT, et al: Complications of flexible fiberoptic colonoscopy and polypectomies. Gastrointest Endosc 22:73–77, 1975

39. Wolff WI, Shinya H: Polypectomy via the fiber-optic colonoscope. Removal of neoplasms beyond reach of the sigmoidoscope. N Engl J Med 288:329–332, 1973

40. Bond JH, Levitt MD: Factors affecting the concentration of combustible gases in the colon during colonoscopy. Gastroenterology 68:1445–1448, 1975

41. Spencer RJ, Coates HL, Anderson MJ Jr: Colonoscopic polypectomies. Mayo Clin Proc 49:40–43, 1974

42. Ecker MD, Goldstein M, Hoexter B, et al: Benign pneumoperitoneum after fiberoptic colonoscopy. Gastroenterology 73:226–230, 1977

43. Taylor R, Weakley FL, Sullivan BH Jr: Non-operative management of colonoscopic perforation with pneumoperitoneum. Gastrointest Endosc 24:124–125, 1978

44. Meyers MA, Volberg F, Katzen B, et al: Haustral anatomy and pathology: A new look. II. Roentgen interpretation of pathological alterations. Radiology 108:505–512, 1973

45. Meyers MA: Radiological features of the spread and localization of extraperitoneal gas and their relationship to its source. An anatomical approach. Radiology 111:17–26, 1974

46. Lezak MB, Goldhamer M: Retroperitoneal emphysema after colonoscopy. Gastroenterology 66:118–120, 1974

47. Livstone EM, Cohen GM, Troncale FJ, et al: Diastatic serosal lacerations: An unrecognized complication of colonoscopy. Gastroenterology 67:1245–1247, 1974

48. Wu TK: Occult injuries during colonoscopy. Gastrointest Endosc 24:236–238, 1978

49. Sjogren RW, Johnson LF, Butler ML, et al: Serosal laceration: A complication of intra-operative colonoscopy explained by transmural pressure gradients. Gastrointest Endosc 24:239–242, 1978

50. Lambling A, Truffert L: L'explosion des gas intestinaux au cours de l'électro-coagulation intra-rectale. Un cas de rupture sigmóidienne mortelle. Arch Mal Appl Dig 33:148, 1944

51. Stucker, FJ, Molzberger H: Die Darmgasexplosion als seltene Ursache einer traumatischen Dickdarmperforation. Chirurg 45:373–375, 1974

52. Bond JH, Levy M, Levitt MD: Explosion of hydrogen gas in the colon during proctosigmoidoscopy. Gastrointest Endosc 23:41–42, 1976

53. Bigard M-A, Gaucher P, Lassalle C: Fatal colonic explosion during colonoscopic polypectomy. Gastroenterology 77:1307–1310, 1979

3 Complications of Gastrointestinal Intubation

Gary G. Ghahremani

In 1790 the British physician John Hunter first introduced gastric intubation as an artificial means of feeding a paralyzed patient (1). During the last century William Beaumont's classic studies of gastric juice led to further utilization of such tubes in the analysis of digestive functions of the stomach (2). More recently, however, technical refinements have made gastrointestinal intubation a routine procedure in medical and surgical management of many abdominal disorders. The principal application of this technique is in intestinal decompression in patients with obstructive symptoms or paralytic ileus (3,4). Flexible tubes are also placed into the gastrointestinal tract for various other diagnostic or therapeutic purposes, including alimentation with liquefied food (5–7), hypotonic duodenography, enteroclysis, gastrointestinal secretory tests, and mucosal biopsy (8–13).

The commercially available tubes are made of polyethylene or other pliable synthetic materials and usually contain radiopaque marking (2–7). Their flexibility and blunt tips are generally considered to safeguard against induction of trauma during insertion into the body. Nevertheless, many instances of gastrointestinal perforation by feeding tubes have been reported in infants (14–21). A large variety of other tube-induced complications have also been experienced, particularly among adult patients (22–28) These observations indicate that the confidence in the safety of these devices may not be fully justified. Since the radiologist is often in a unique position to assess the precise location of these tubes, his or her awareness of the possible complications can play a crucial role in early diagnosis and management of iatrogenic gastrointestinal intubation injuries. Moreover, several problems to placement of tubes into the thorax or abdomen secondarily affect the digestive tract.

Nasopharyngeal

Most patients experience only minimal discomfort while being intubated through the nasopharynx. Local complications can arise, depending upon the tube's physical characteristics and duration of retention. Irritative rhinitis, epistaxis, pressure necrosis of the nasal wall, sinusitis and otitis media have been reported to result from indwelling tubes (22,23,25). Patients with severe maxillofacial trauma are particularly prone to iatrogenic injury during attempted nasogastric or nasotracheal intubation. In such cases the distorted soft tissues and associated fractures involving the base of the skull or walls of the paranasal sinuses may misdirect the tube (Fig. 3-1). Seebacher et al. reported a similar case in which a nasogastric suction tube blindly inserted in a victim of an automobile accident crossed the cribriform plate and curled within the cerebral cavity (29). These authors also noted that in the presence of fractures of the paranasal sinuses the nasogastric tube may enter the maxillary sinus or the orbits. Therefore it is recommended that patients with extensive maxillofacial injury be intubated through the mouth under direct vision.

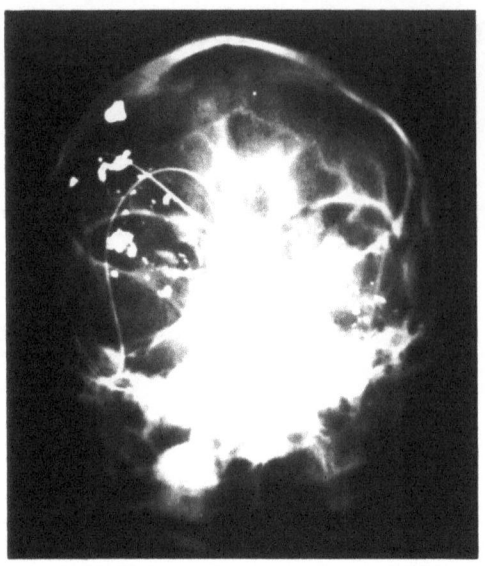 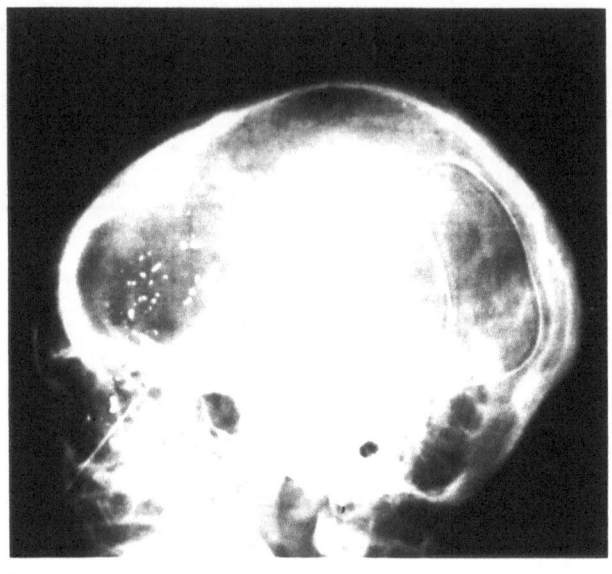

a   b

Fig. 3-1, a and b. Inadvertent intracranial insertion of nasogastric suction tube. Skull radiographs in an 18-year-old woman with gunshot injury to the orbits demonstrate that the tube has crossed the fractured cribriform plate and the dura, curling within the cerebral cavity. (Courtesy of F. S. Vines, MD, and M. A. Turner, MD, Richmond, Virginia)

Laryngotracheal and Pulmonary

In uncooperative or comatose patients the tube may coil within the larynx or enter the tracheobronchial tree. Malposition of the tube may not be apparent clinically until recognized on a subsequent chest radiograph. Laceration of the laryngeal mucosa and perforation of the pyriform sinuses may complicate passage of nasogastric tubes (22,23,25,30). This type of penetrating injury occurs particulary when the tube is iced to make it semirigid for ease of insertion (25,31,32).

Laryngitis is frequently noted after prolonged use of indwelling nasogastric tubes; patients may also develop pressure ulceration of the pharyngeal or laryngeal mucosa or both (23,31). In ten cases reported by Iglauer and Molt, stenosing lesions of the larynx complicated duodenal intubation and required treatment with tracheostomy (33).

Aspiration pneumonia is a well-recognized complication of gastrointestinal intubation for several reasons. The abnormal position of the tube in the upper airways or esophagus may be initially overlooked, and thus food and drugs may be administered directly into the lungs (22,-23) (Fig. 3-2). Even if correctly placed, nasogastric tubes promote gastroesophageal reflux and the chance of aspiration (34). Furthermore, many bedridden patients who have been intubated because of obstructive symptoms or other digestive problems often have nausea and vomiting, factors contributing to the potential for aspiration pneumonia (4,23).

Esophageal

The pharyngoesophageal region represents the most common site of significant trauma sustained either during insertion or as a result of continuous local irritation of nasogastric tubes. Wolff and Kessler studied the hypopharynx and cervical esophagus at autopsy of 103 patients who were subjected to intubation, endoscopy, or both during their final hospitalization; Mucosal ulceration, submucosal hemorrhage, or perforation was demonstrated in this region in 62 (60%) (31). Only 2% of these iatrogenic injuries were recognized clinically. Nasogastric intubation was a possible cause of trauma in 34 of 103 and resulted in postcricoid ulcers in 9 patients in

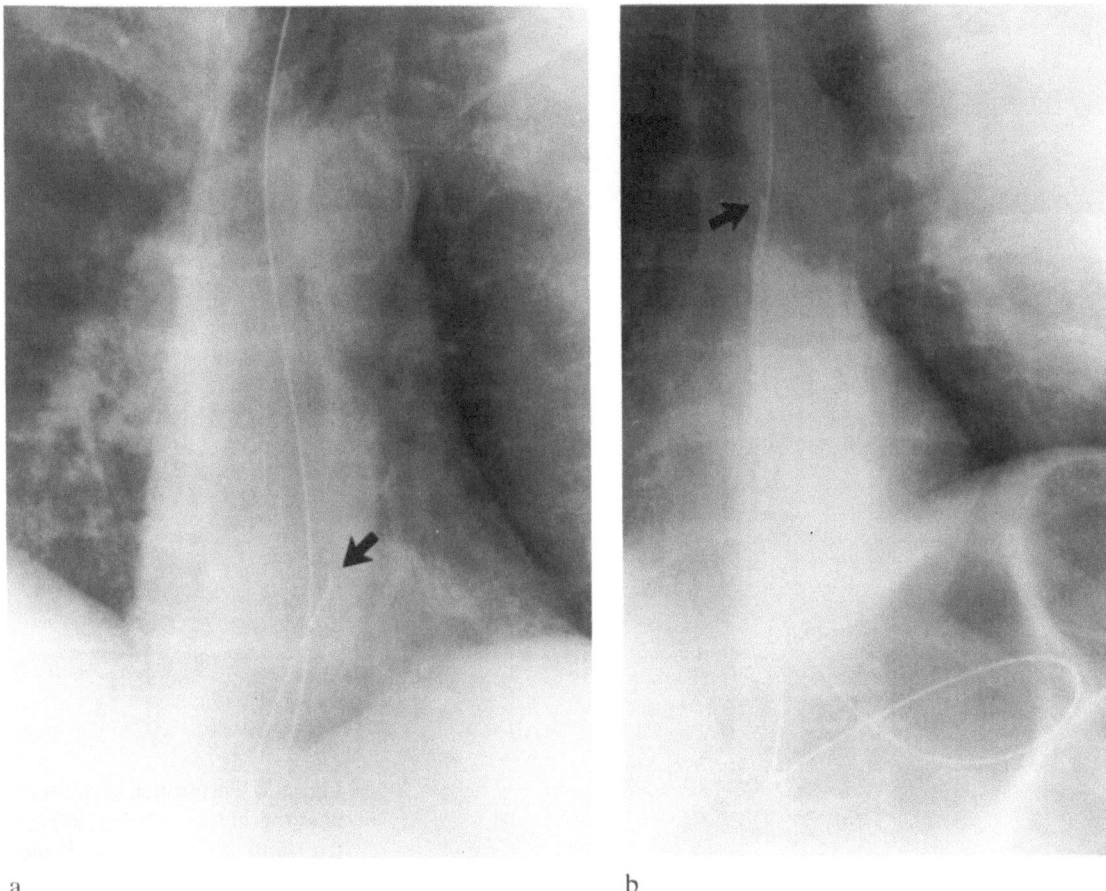

a   b

Fig. 3-2, a and b. Malposition of nasogastric feeding tubes. This is demonstrated on bedside chest films of two different patients (**a** and **b**). The distal end of both tubes is within the esophageal lumen *(arrows)*, and aspiration pneumonia involving the right lower lobe is noted in **a**.

whom the tube had been in place for an average of 5 days.

In newborn infants pharyngoesophageal perforations can occur during insertion of nasogastric tubes or suctioning of oral and upper-airway secretions (14,17–19) (Fig. 3-3). Lucaya et al (35) have analyzed the clinical and radiographic features of such trauma in 31 neonates and infants. Four other examples manifested by extraluminal passage of feeding tubes into the pleural space were described by Kassner et al. (18). Perforation of the hypopharynx or cervical esophagus of adult patients during routine intestinal intubation is rather unusual. However, several instances have occurred when the nasogastric tube was frozen to permit easy insertion, particularly in uncooperative patients (23,25,31,32). More frequently this type of injury complicates inadvertent placement of endotracheal tubes into the cervical esophagus (30,36,37) (Fig. 3-4).

The mechanisms of tube-induced perforation of the pharyngoesophageal region are similar to those of perforation by flexible fiberoptic endoscopes (38,39). The tip of tube may be engaged in the pyriform sinus or cause mucosal outpouching posteriorly just above the cricopharyngeus muscle. A type of "crush injury" with perforation may ensue as a result of compression of the posterior pharyngoesophageal wall against the cervical spine (19,38). The extraluminal protrusion of the tube can create a false passage into the posterior mediastinum or even the retroperitoneal space (18,19). The created sinus tract or pharyngeal pseudodiverticulum often closely resembles an esophageal duplication or a true pharyngeal diverticulum when opacified with contrast material (14,17,35) (Figs. 3-3, 3-4). The possibility of iatrogenic perforation of the pharynx or cervical esophagus should be considered when a patient develops respiratory distress,

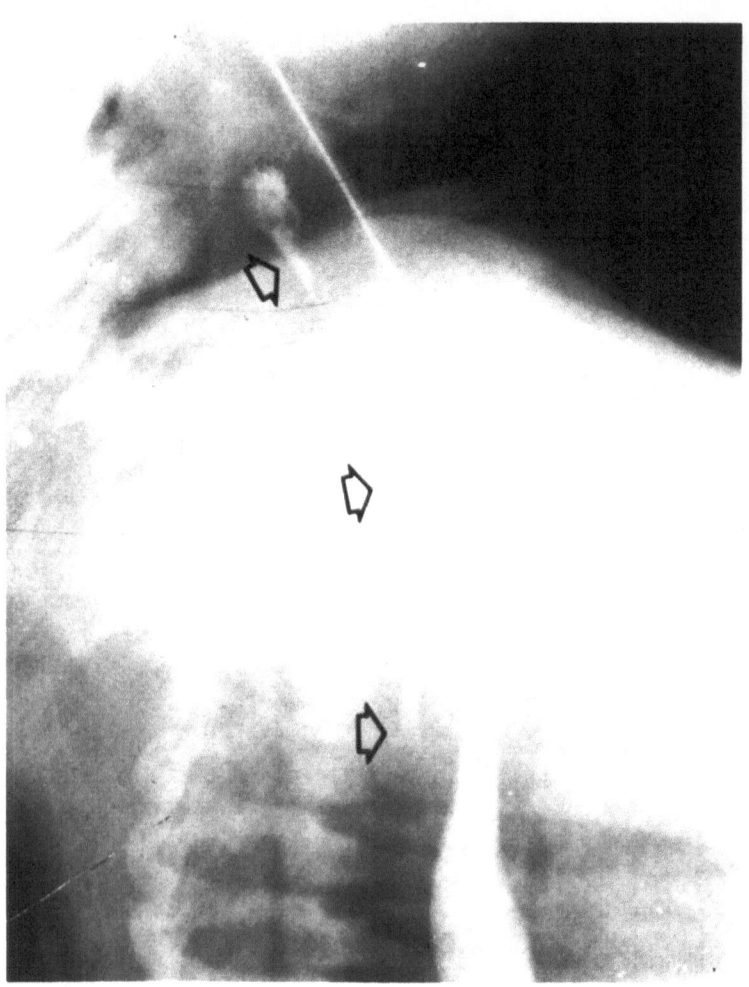

Fig. 3-3. Perforation of posterior pharyngeal wall during nasogastric intubation. A false channel *(arrows)* was created in the infant. (Courtesy of J. Kelleher, MD, and R. B. Port, MD, Chicago, Illinois)

increase in oral secretions, and dysphagia soon after a difficult or unsuccessful nasogastric or endotracheal intubation. Radiographs of the chest and neck may reveal cervical emphysema, pneumomediastinum, pneumothorax (usually right sided or bilateral), and ectopic location of the tube. Pneumopericardium or retroperitoneal air is also seen on rare occasions (35). Esophagography, endoscopy, or both may be used to identify the exact location of perforation before surgical closure or drainage is attempted. Several authors have advocated conservative treatment of traumatic pharyngeal pseudodiverticulum in infants, reserving surgery for cases further complicated by mediastinitis, cervical abscess, or pneumopericardium with cardiac tamponade (19,35,40,41).

Perforation or rupture of the esophagus has been associated with a variety of flexible tubes used mainly in adult patients (23,27,28,30–32).

The risk is further increased if the esophageal wall is involved by inflammatory or neoplastic lesions (Fig. 3-5). The Sengstaken-Blakemore tube utilized for decompression of bleeding esophageal varices is a well-recognized cause of such injury (23,42-45). In a series of 40 patients studied by Conn and Simpson, tube-induced complications were noted in 35% and associated mortality in 22% (43). Major problems encountered with use of the Sengstaken-Blakemore tube are pressure necrosis, submucosal hemorrhage or laceration of the esophagus, and fatal aspiration of bloody gastric contents (43). A variety of other complications have also been reported, including rupture of the balloons (44), obstruction of airways (43), extrinsic blockage of the innominate vein (46), and impaction of the tube by administered barium (47). The Linton tube appears to be safer because it has a single gastric balloon that is inflated and retracted

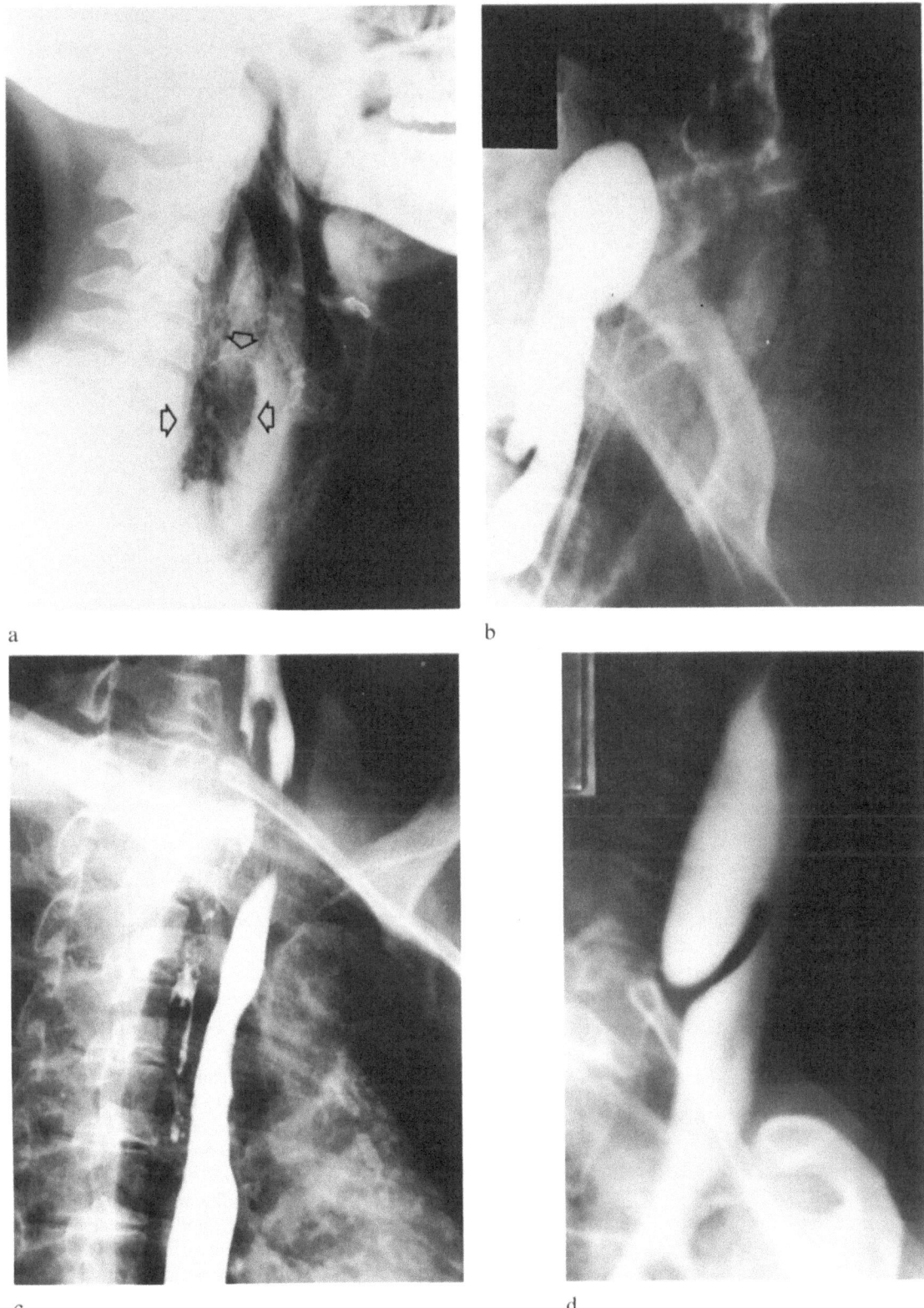

a

b

c

d

Fig. 3-4, a–d. Perforation of pharyngoesophageal junction by misdirected endotracheal tube. This occurred during induction of general anesthesia in a 40-year-old woman. **a** Lateral film of the neck shows an air-filled cavity *(arrows)* and emphysema of the prevertebral soft tissues. **b** Spot film demonstrates large collection of extravasated contrast material posterior to the cervical esophagus. **c** and **d** Esophagograms obtained 4 months and 8 months after surgical drainage of the upper mediastinum show gradual healing of the iatrogenic sinus tract and subsequent formation of a pseudodiverticulum.

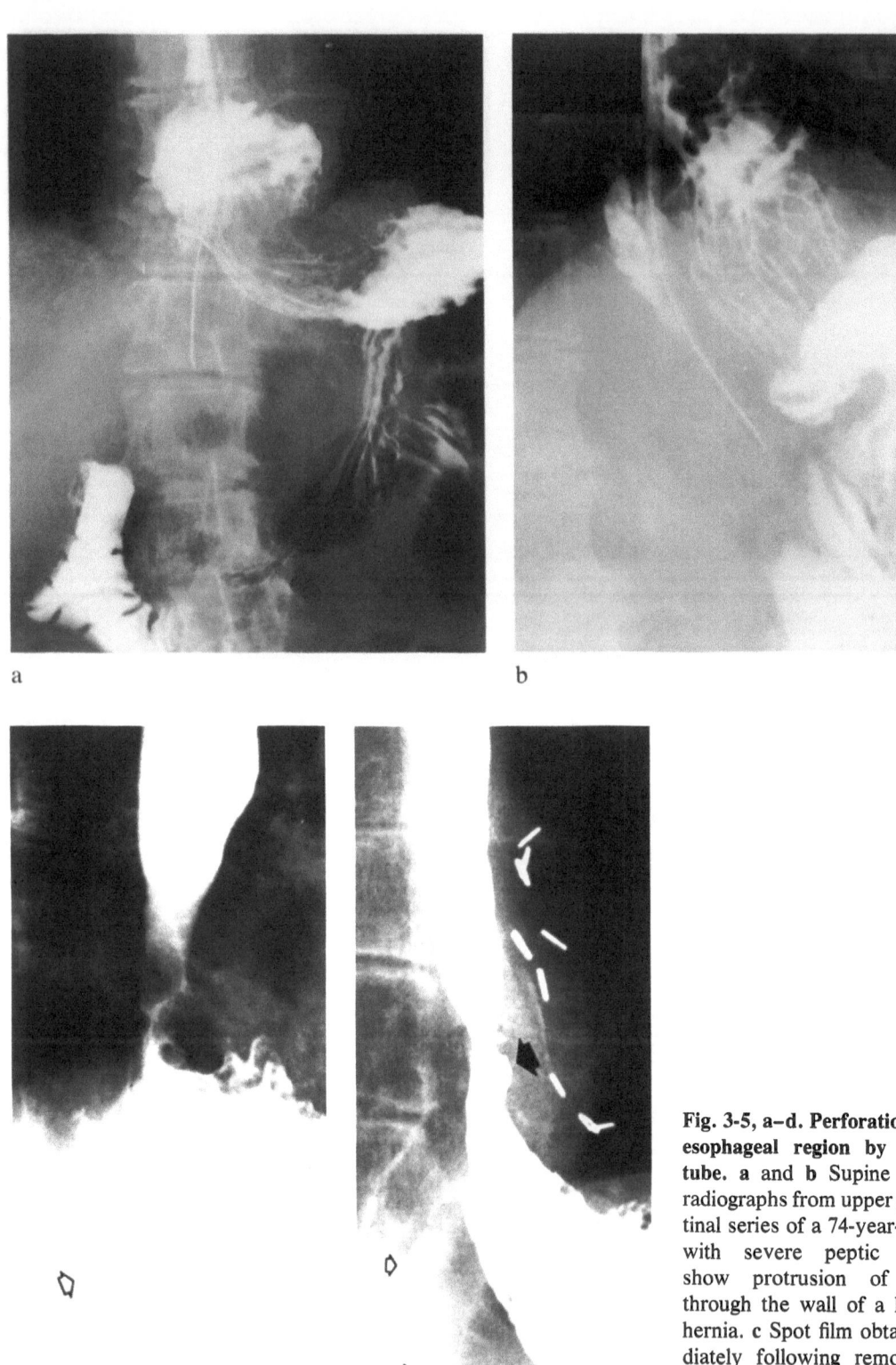

a

b

c

d

Fig. 3-5, a–d. Perforation of gastro-esophageal region by nasogastric tube. a and b Supine and lateral radiographs from upper gastrointestinal series of a 74-year-old woman with severe peptic esophagitis show protrusion of the tube through the wall of a large hiatus hernia. c Spot film obtained immediately following removal of the tube demonstrates extravasation of the contrast material *(arrows)*. d Reexamination 1 year after surgical repair of the perforated hernia shows barium retained in the iatrogenic sinus tract *(open arrows)*. A short esophageal stricture with an ulcer is also visible *(black arrow)*.

against the cardia to block blood flow to varices (48). Nevertheless, incorrect intraesophageal placement or regurgitation of the inflated balloon (Fig. 3-6) has repeatedly caused esophageal rupture (44,49).

Several types of plastic tubes are used for palliative treatment of nonresectable carcinoma or other obstructive lesions of the esophagus (50–52). Depending on the type of such prosthetic devices and the endoscopic or operative method of insertion, one-fourth of the patients develop complications (37,53). The incidence of esophageal perforation is approximately 10%. Dislodgment of the tube and its impaction by food particles are the most common problems, respectively accounting for 39% and 31% of all

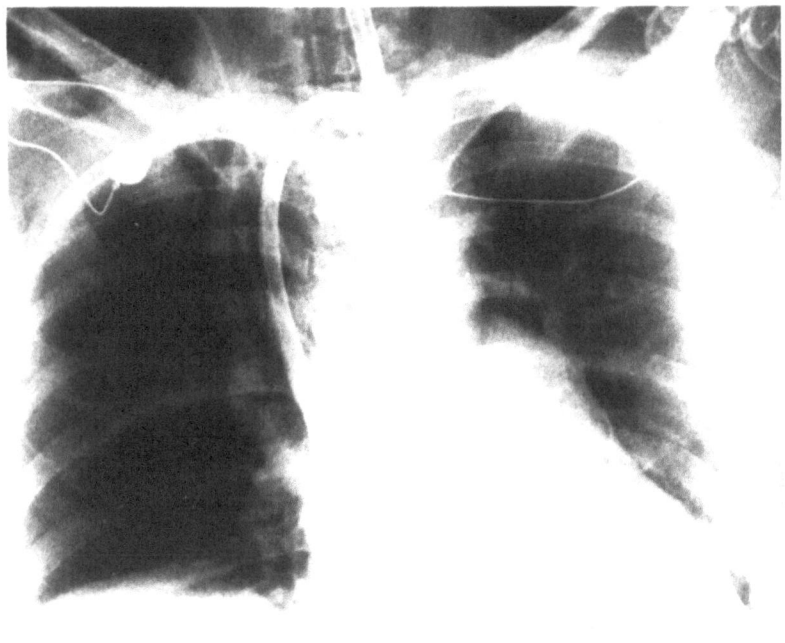

a

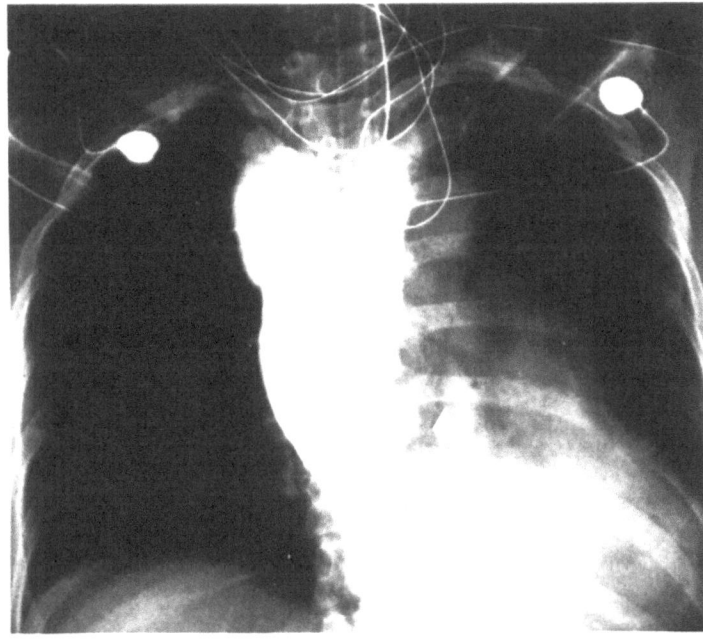

b

Fig. 3-6, a and b. Esophageal rupture complicating insertion of a Linton tube. The patient was being treated for bleeding varices. a Chest film demonstrates the coiled tube and its inflated balloon within the esophagus. b Esophagogram shows the irregularly dilated esophageal lumen and the site of its rupture (arrow). A nasogastric tube is in place.

reported complications (53) (Fig. 3-7). In one of our patients the dislodged polyethylene tube subsequently perforated the stomach (Fig. 3-8). Hemorrhage, ulceration, fistula formation, reflux esophagitis, and passage of the dislodged tube per rectum may also complicate prosthetic esophageal intubation (27,53,54). These devices are also being utilized in the treatment of benign esophageal strictures. Mackenzie et al. have described two patients in whom prolonged reten-

tion of a Celestin tube led to complications due to structural deterioration of the prosthesis (55).

As mentioned earlier, the esophagus is also subject to injury if an endotracheal tube is misdirected into the cervical esophagus (31,36,37). Furthermore, laryngeal or tracheal trauma from an endotracheal tube can secondarily involve the adjacent wall of the esophagus and produce tracheoesophageal fistula (56,57). I recently observed an unusual example of extrinsic injury

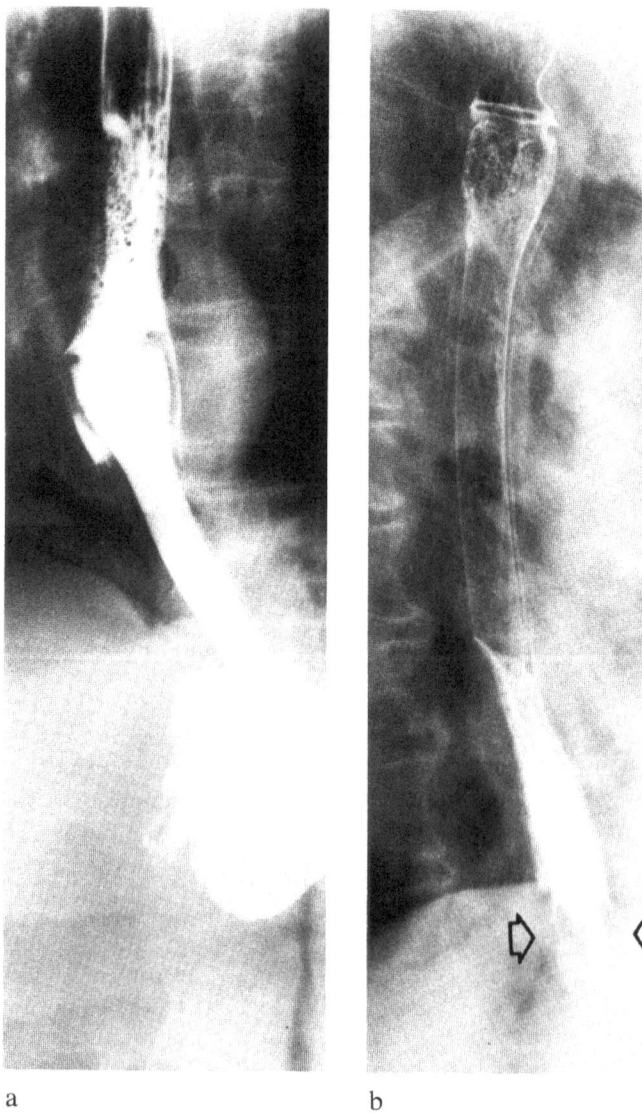

a   b

Fig. 3-7, a and b. Dislodgment of Celestin tube. The tube was inserted for palliative treatment of obstructing carcinoma of the gastroesophageal junction. **a** Initial postoperative study shows satisfactory position of the tube. **b** Three weeks later the tube is seen dislodged in midesophagus, far above the segment involved by carcinoma (*arrows*).

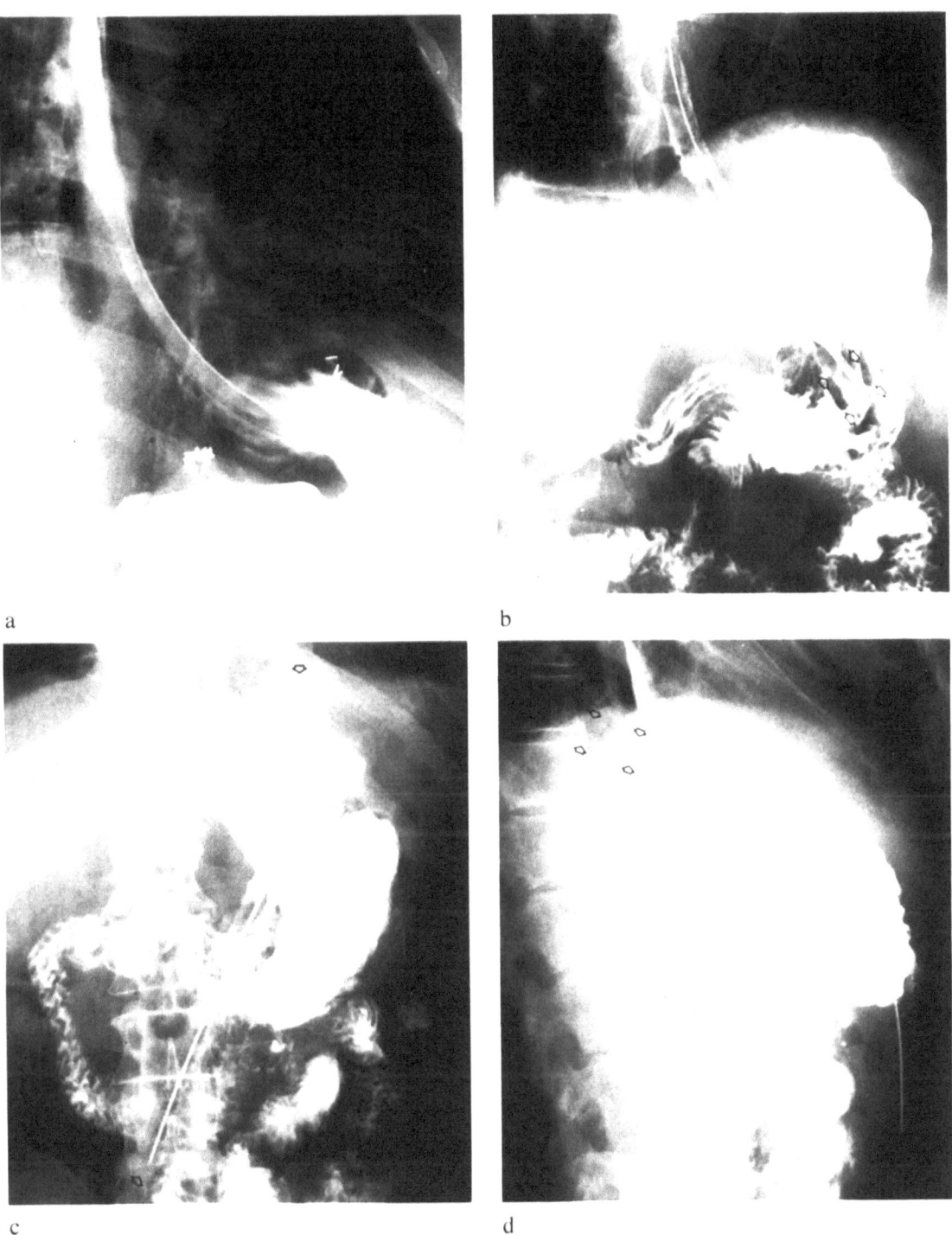

a

b

c

d

Fig. 3-8, a–d. Perforation of stomach by dislodged endoesophageal prosthetic tube. a Upper gastrointestinal series 2 weeks after palliative intubation for carcinoma of the lower esophagus shows satisfactory position of the tube, with its distal end sutured to the anterior gastric wall. **b** Four months later the distal half of the dislodged tube is seen protruding into the gastric lumen *(arrows)*. A small outpouching of the greater curvature is noted at the site of previous gastrostomy. **c** and **d** Supine and lateral films of an upper gastrointestinal series 2 months later demonstrate perforations of the stomach by both ends of the dislodged tube *(arrows)*. Gradual penetration of the gastric wall and marked desmoplastic reaction due to peritoneal metastasis had prevented leakage of contrast material.

to the esophagus, namely, its perforation by a polyethylene chest tube (Fig. 3-9). Others have shown that chest tubes, even when used at a low suction pressure, can aspirate adjacent.pulmonary tissue, resulting in subsequent focal infarction and perforation of the lung (58,59). Therefore the close relationship of the end hole of a suction chest tube to the esophagus or other mediastinal structures should be considered a potential cause of trauma to these organs.

The so-called esophageal obturator airway is another cause of pharyngeal or esophageal perforation (60–62). This tube is used by paramedical personnel during cardiopulmonary resuscitation and is introduced easily into the esophagus without direct vision. Balloon tamponade of the esophagus is then used for diverting the insufflated air into the lungs. During this procedure, 0.2%–2.0% of the patients sustain esophageal perforation (63). In a similar manner, tubes used for pneumatic dilatation of the lower esophageal sphincter in patients with achalasia can rupture

the esophagus in 4%–6% (64–66). The complication is usually recognized immediately on the basis of clinical and radiographic findings. However, Zegel et al. described two patients in whom esophageal perforation was not manifest until almost 24 hours after pneumatic dilatation (65).

Reflux esophagitis and its sequelae represent a relatively common iatrogenic complication of gastrointestinal intubation. Experimental and clinical studies have documented that the presence of any tube in the gastroesophageal junction promotes reflux of gastric secretions (34,67). Patients with a nasogastric tube in place for a prolonged time and who are kept generally in a recumbent position are particularly prone to develop severe peptic esophagitis (67–69). This may further lead to formation of long strictures involving the distal third or half of the esophagus (Fig. 3-10). Reconstructive surgery of the esophagus may become necessary to relieve the obstructive symptoms in such patients.

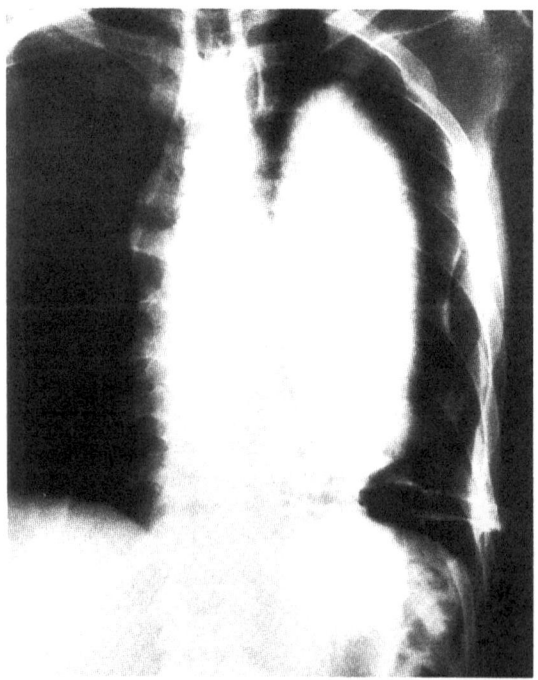

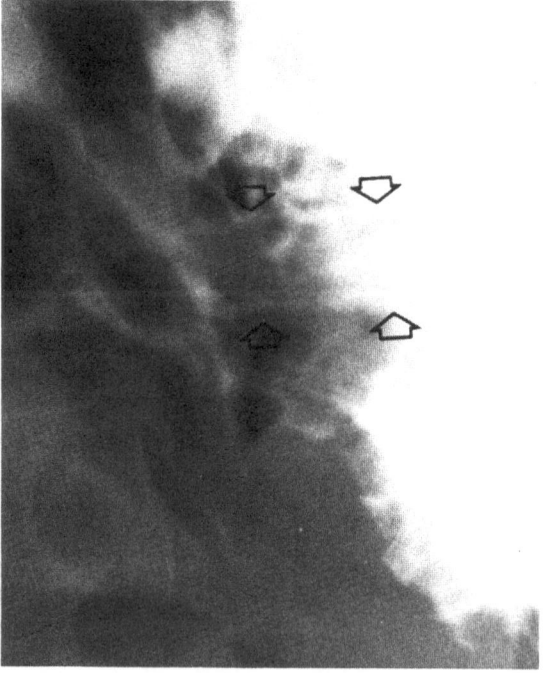

a

b

Fig. 3-9, a and b. Esophageal perforation by a suction chest tube. Left lower lobe pneumonia and pleural effusion had developed in a 49-year-old man after laparotomy for a perforated duodenal ulcer. Two days after insertion of the suction chest tube he complained of dysphagia and shortness of breath. Supine chest film (a) and a close-up (b) of the gastroesophageal junction were obtained during esophagography. The chest tube (arrows) has perforated the lateral wall of the distal esophagus, causing massive extravasation of contrast material into the left pleural space.

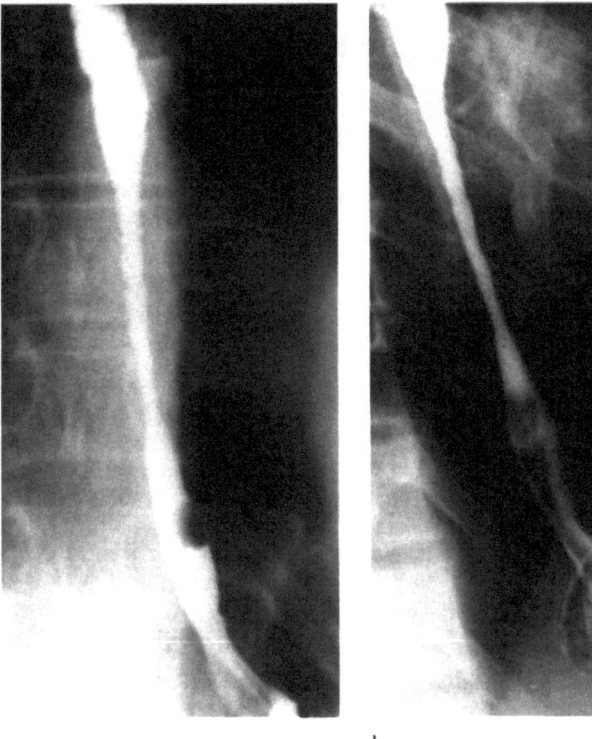

a   b

Fig. 3-10, a and **b. Long esophageal stricture.** Severe reflux esophagitis, induced by a nasogastric tube that had been in place for 10 days during treatment of acute pancreatitis, led to development of the stricture.

Gastric

Fortunately the widely utilized nasogastric tubes are a rare cause of perforation of the stomach, although this may occur, particularly if the gastric wall is inflamed and friable. Meyers and Ghahremani have emphasized that inflammatory or neoplastic involvement of the gastrointestinal tract significantly enhances the danger of perforation by flexible fiberoptic endoscopes (38,39). This is also a potential hazard of nasogastric tubes whose physical characteristics are somewhat similar to those of fiberoptic endoscopes. For example, in patients with sliding hiatus hernia the tip of a nasogastric tube can perforate the herniated part of the stomach (Fig. 3-5). The tube may also be a contributing factor in delayed perforation of the gastroesophageal region due to induced reflux esophagitis and mucosal ulcerations. In a patient who had previously had subtotal gastrectomy and a Billroth II procedure, insertion of a gastrointestinal suction tube led to tearing of the anastomotic suture line (Fig. 3-11). These examples clearly demonstrate that the distorted anatomy and preexisting inflammatory changes of the gastric wall can increase the risk of tube-induced injury.

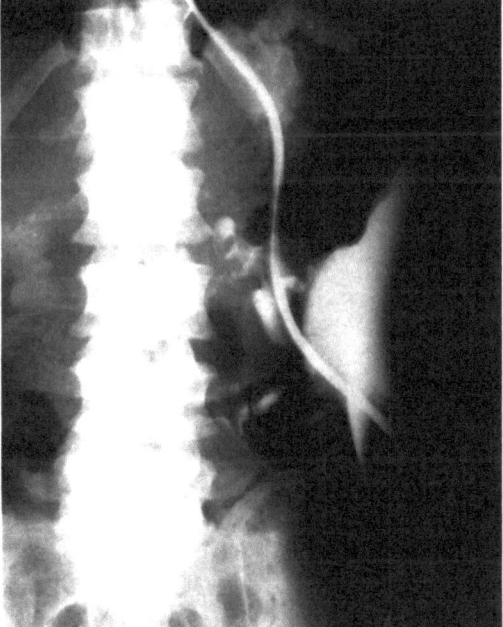

Fig. 3-11. Tube-induced tear of gastrojejunal anastomosis. The patient had recurrent epigastric pain and vomiting 6 months after partial gastrectomy for peptic ulcer disease. A polyethylene nasogastric suction tube was inserted without fluoroscopic control. After administration of contrast material a supine film of the abdomen reveals extravasation into the left paracolic gutter and subphrenic space.

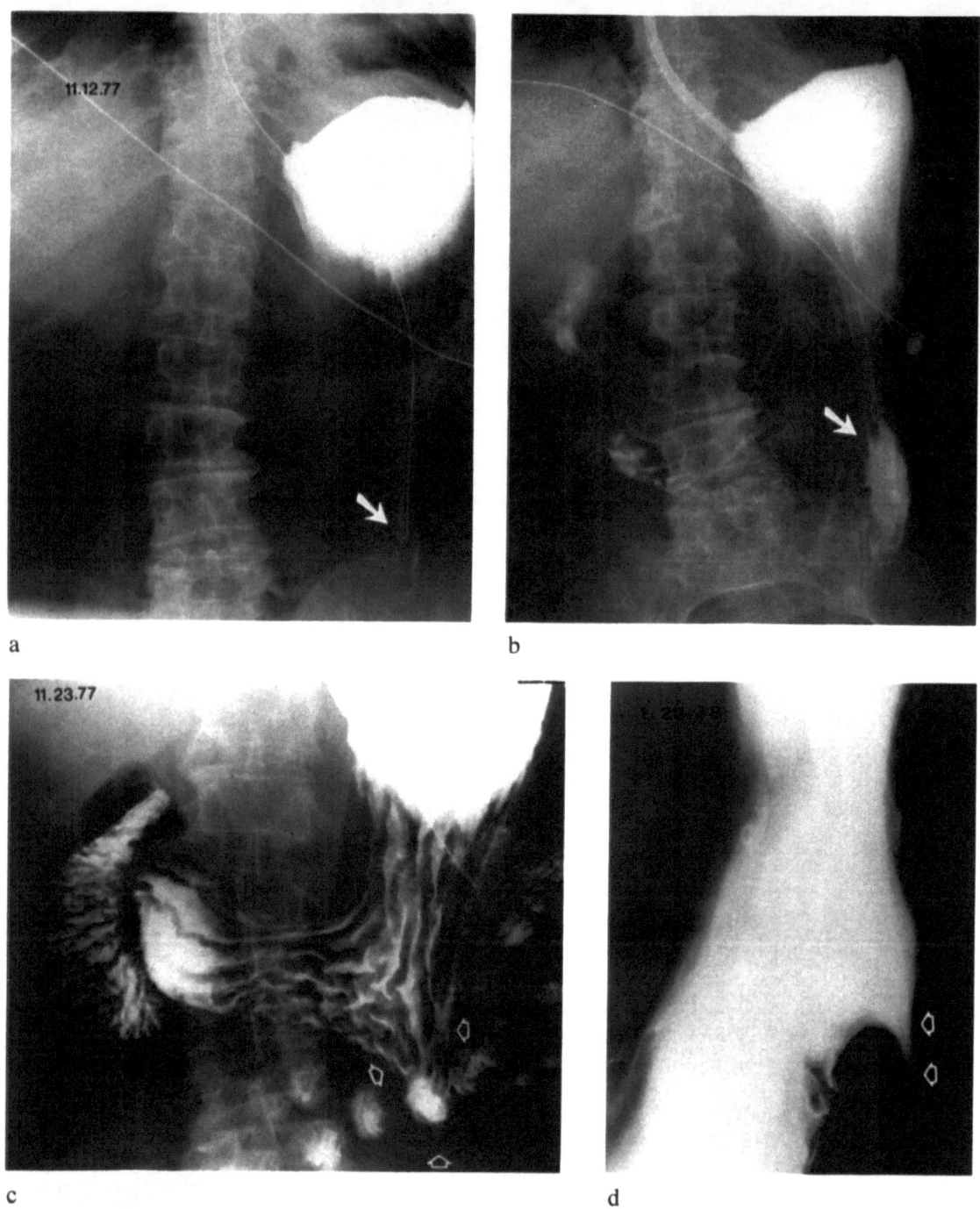

Fig. 3-12, a–d. Penetration of gastric wall by polyethylene suction tube. Gastric distention developed in a 63-year-old woman after insertion of a total hip prosthesis. Bedside supine radiographs of the abdomen (**a** and **b**) show the distal end of the nasogastric tube against the greater curvature of the stomach just above the left iliac crest *(arrows)*. Most of the contrast material has gravitated to the fundus, but no extravasation is evident. **c** Eleven days later a funnel-shaped deformity of the stomach is seen in the previous location of the tube *(arrows)*. **d** Two months later a tube-induced sinus tract *(arrows)* is demonstrated.

Ghahremani et al. have reported three cases in which the distal end of a nasogastric suction tube gradually penetrated the greater curvature of an otherwise normal stomach (Fig. 3-12) (70). In each instance the tube had been retained for more than 5 days. The continuous pressure exerted by the tip of the tube against the gastric mucosa apparently caused a decubitus ulcer with subsequent penetration through the wall, producing a sinus tract (Fig. 3-12). Others have described another important factor in the mechanism of this complication (15,16). They have noted that polyethylene tubes become discolored and increasingly more rigid after several days of use, probably because of the effects of gastrointestinal secretions. Drenick and Lipset pointed out that the plastic nasogastric tubes consist of a vinyl chloride resin made flexible by addition of bis (2-ethylhexyl) phthalate (71). The softening agent can be hydrolyzed and extracted from the plastic by the gastric hydrochloric acid or alkaline duodenal content that has flowed back into the stomach. This chemical interaction results in progressive stiffening of the tube. In such cases, injury to the wall of the gastrointestinal tract occurs usually in areas subject to pressure by the tube's distal end. However, needle-sharp corners developing at the sites of angulation of the tube may also erode the adjacent mucosa (71) (Fig. 3-13). Therefore it is advisable to either remove or replace the nasogastric tube after a few days.

Several other gastric complications have been described that are related to either the placement or subsequent removal of the tube. Metabolic alkalosis is a well recognized and potentially serious clinical problem resulting from drainage of gastric secretions through nasogastric suction tubes (72). To decrease the possibility of nutritional and electrolyte imbalance the material aspirated by continuous nasogastric suctioning is sometimes returned to the intestinal tract through another polyethylene feeding tube placed more distally. This procedure may lead to jejunal ulceration and perforation as described by Hafner et al. (23).

A relatively common problem is coiling and knot formation of the tube within the stomach (22,23,73,74). This may result in obstruction of the tube and trauma to the gastroesophageal junction or the nose during extubation (Fig. 3-14). Larsen recommends a simple fluoroscopic

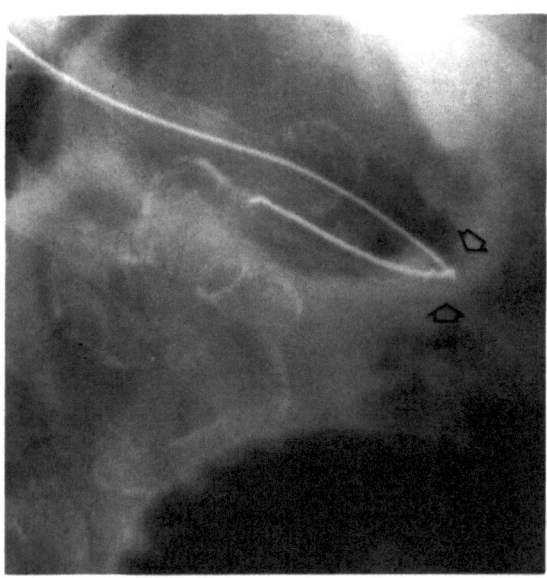

Fig. 3-13. Penetration of the gastric wall by a tube. Close-up view of the left upper abdomen shows marked angulation of the nasogastric tube, with needle-sharp corners penetrating the adjacent gastric wall (arrows). The polyvinyl tube had been retained for one week and was discolored and semirigid when removed.

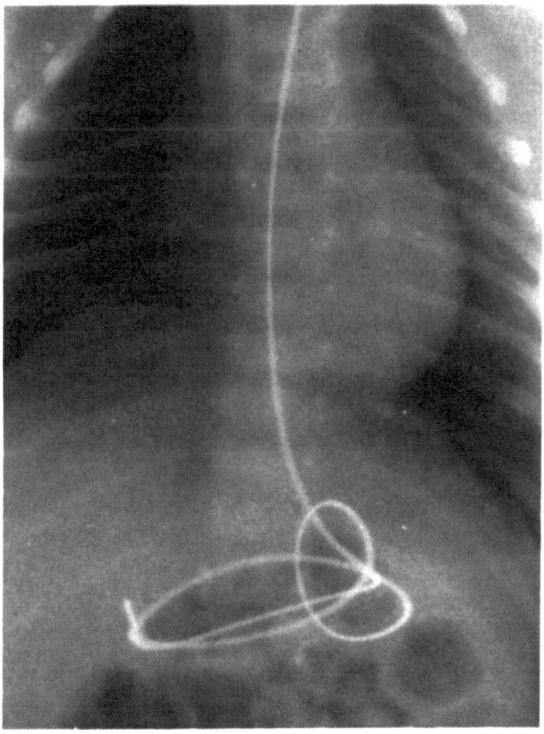

Fig. 3-14. Coiled and knotted feeding tube. Considerable difficulty was encountered during withdrawal of the knotted tube through the gastroesophageal junction of a newborn infant, but subsequent contrast examination did not show perforation.

technique to untie the tube by distending the stomach with water (73). He notes that even a large and complex knot in the tube will usually untie itself if allowed to float freely within the water-filled stomach.

In patients with a gastroenterostomy an inserted tube may loop and form a knot around the anastomosis (23,75,76). In the case reported by Shulman a Cantor tube passed into the duodenum twice reentered the stomach through the gastroenterostomy (75). Attempted withdrawal led to further tightening of the two coiled loops, but these were eventually unwound under fluoroscopy. At times, however, surgical removal has been necessary. Hafner et al. described a patient in whom a polyethylene feeding tube traversed the duodenojejunostomy but returned in an antiperistaltic manner back into the duodenum (23). The resultant locking loop lacerated the duodenum and superior mesenteric artery. Cantor noted that an altered technique of intubation is mandatory if the anatomic position of the gastric outlet has been changed by prior gastrectomy or gastrojejunostomy (76). He recommends intubating these patients in the erect position so that the greater curvature with the anastomotic stoma becomes the most dependent part of the stomach. This approach would permit passage of the tube directly into the efferent jejunal segment, thus preventing it from encircling the gastroduodenostomy loop. Careful fluoroscopic monitoring is necessary because blind insertion of the tube may lead to perforation of the anastomosis (Fig. 3-11). Routine use of fluoroscopy in gastrointestinal intubation of patients without previous surgery remains controversial (2,11,12). Nevertheless, proper attention to procedural details of tube placement should diminish the risk of significant trauma.

Complications related to gastrostomy tubes are described elsewhere (see Chap. 6). We have also pointed out earlier in this chapter that a prosthetic endoesophageal tube can become dislodged and subsequently perforate the stomach (Fig. 3-8).

Intestinal

During the past decade nasojejunal feeding tubes have been extensively utilized in alimenting premature and sick newborn infants. Continuous infusion of formula into the proximal jejunum is generally considered to be a safer and more physiologic approach than intravenous hyperalimentation (5–7). As with many other medical advances, however, a variety of complications have been experienced, the most important being esophageal and intestinal perforation by the feeding tubes (14–21,35,41). In the majority of the cases reported so far the distal end of the tube perforated the duodenum (15,20,21), and only rarely the jejunum (16). This complication occurred mostly with tubes made of polyvinyl rather than silicone rubber. There is now ample evidence that polyvinyl tubes change their consistency after 1 day or more of retention in the intestinal lumen (15,16,21). The initially soft and pliable plastic material becomes progressively discolored and hardened, thus converting a life-supporting tube to a semirigid and hazardous device (20,70,71). The persistent pressure of such a tube against the duodenal wall and its subsequent manipulation or repositioning can result in perforation. Therefore, several authors suggest that the tube be initially advanced beyond the third portion of the duodenum so that the distal end lies in a relatively straight jejunal loop (20,21). The tube should not be further manipulated, and, if there is need for repositioning, a new tube should be inserted. It has also been recommended that stools be examined frequently for occult fetal blood and, in cases of suspected perforation, radiographs of the abdomen be obtained to evaluate the position of the tube and presence of intraperitoneal air. However, tube-induced retroperitoneal perforation of the duodenum or jejunum occasionally does not manifest free air in the abdomen (16). In such cases, injection of water-soluble contrast material through the tube may be necessary to establish the diagnosis.

The use of long intestinal-decompression tubes in adult patients has caused a variety of iatrogenic problems (3,4,22–24,33,34,75,76). A relatively common finding is telescoping (accordion effect) of the small bowel upon the intraluminal indwelling tube (77) (Fig. 3-15). This may lead to cramping abdominal pain and vomiting and further progress to antegrade intussusception (Fig. 3-16), particularly if the proximal end of the tube is anchored securely to the nose (26,77–80). Conversely, retrograde intussusception may result during withdrawal of a tube.

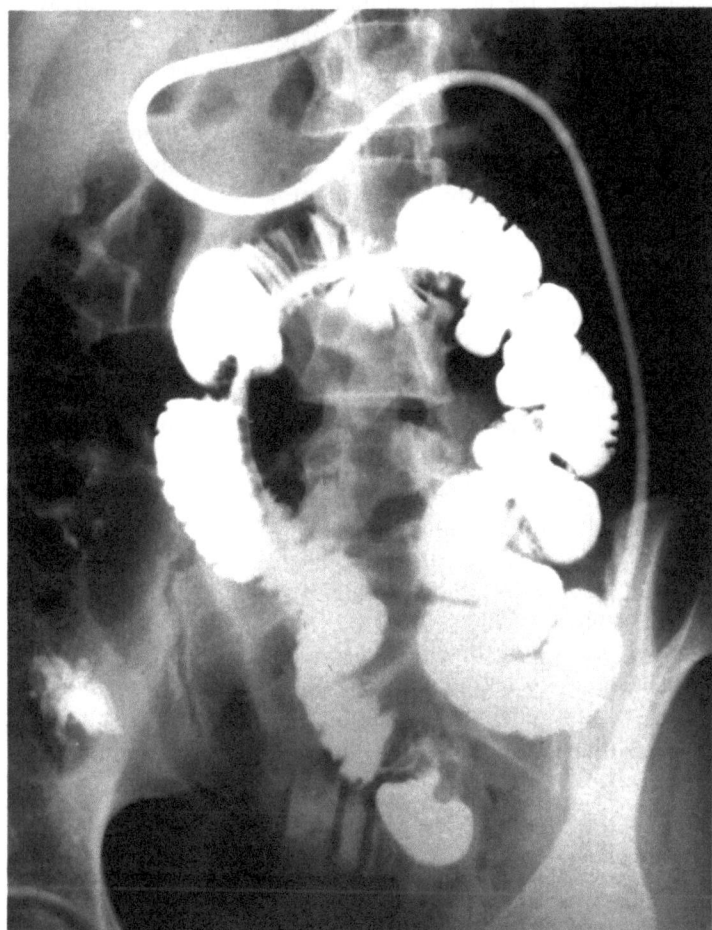

Fig. 3-15. Telescoping of the jejunum. This occurred around a Cantor tube. Resultant pleating and foreshortening of the small bowel are demonstrated.

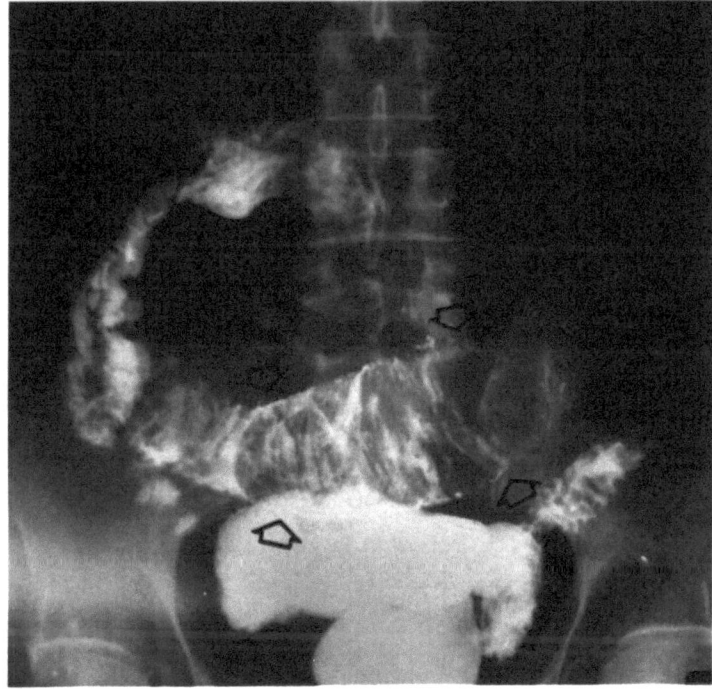

Fig. 3-16. Tube-induced antegrade jejunal intussusception. A 32-year-old man who had ileal resection and jejunocolic anastomosis for treatment of Crohn's disease developed crampy abdominal pain and vomiting immediately after removal of a Cantor tube on the eighth postoperative day. Gastrografin enema clearly demonstrates the antegrade intussusception *(arrows)*, which at laparotomy proved to involve 30 cm of jejunum. (Courtesy of D. Paloyan, MD, Evanston, Illinois)

Simonowitz and Paloyan reviewed 22 such cases from the English literature and added 3 of their own (79). The type of intussusception was jejunojejunal in 13, ileoileal in 9, colocolonic in 1, and unspecified in the remaining 2 cases. The death of 5 of the 25 patients in this series emphasizes the potential lethal outcome of this tube-induced complication.

A long intestinal tube may at times rapidly advance into the colon, making its withdrawal through the ileocecal valve either impossible or hazardous because of the inherent risk of inducing intussusception. In such cases the proximal end is transected with the expectation that the entire tube will pass per rectum. Hafner et al. reported an unusual complication whereby a Miller-Abbott tube could not be withdrawn and remained within the gastrointestinal tract for 9 months, eventually perforating the stomach (23).

Another potential complication of indwelling intestinal-decompression tubes is gaseous distention of the mercury bag (3,22–24). The thin-walled latex balloon is highly permeable to carbon dioxide and hydrogen sulfide present within the distended intestinal loops. Gas gradually diffuses into the mercury bag until the pressures are equalized on both sides of the membrane (Fig. 3-17). Because of the biluminal construction of the Miller-Abbott tube, any gas accumulated in its terminal balloon can be easily aspirated unless the tube is coiled or knotted. In single-lumen tubes devised by Cantor, Harris, Kaslow, and others, however, the inflated balloon becomes impacted and cannot be withdrawn nor will it pass. This complication tends to occur when the tube has been in place for a week or longer (24). It may require either surgical removal or percutaneous transabdominal-needle-puncture of the balloon under fluoroscopy (81,82). To prevent this complication several authors have recommended that the mercury bag be vented by introducing 21- or 22-gauge needle holes in its wall prior to intestinal intubation (82,83).

There are a few other rare complications of intestinal-decompression tubes that deserve brief mention. The tube itself may coil and result in knot formation within the gastrointestinal lumen (23,84) (Fig. 3-18). It may also negotiate

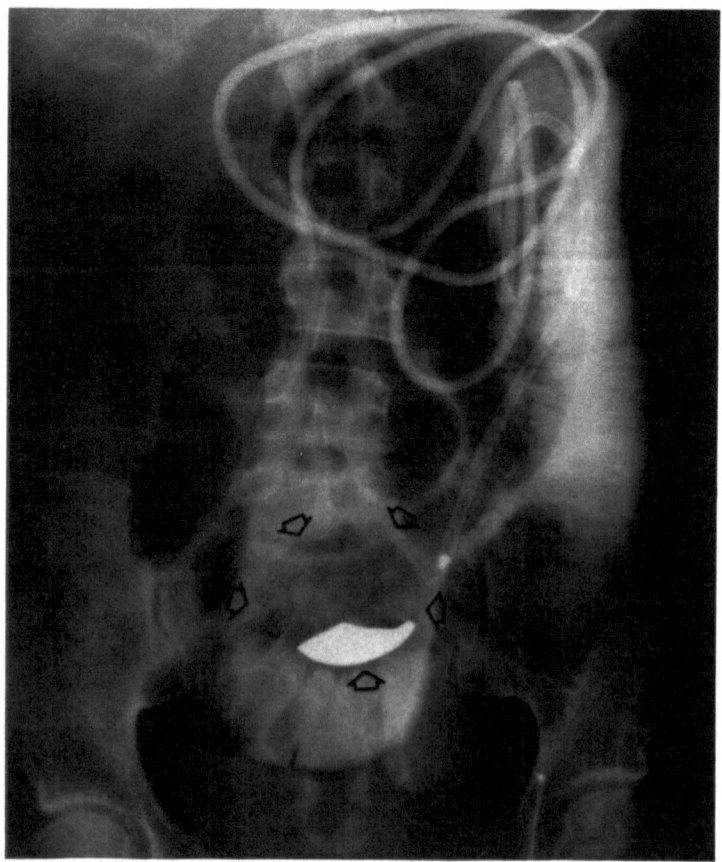

Fig. 3-17. Gaseous distention of mercury bag of indwelling intestinal tube. A Cantor tube was inserted for decompression of dilated small bowel in this patient with regional ileitis. Radiograph of the abdomen 6 days later shows the distended latex bag *(arrows)* obstructing antegrade flow of the injected contrast material. The mercury is in the dependent portion of the bag because of the semi-upright position of the patient.

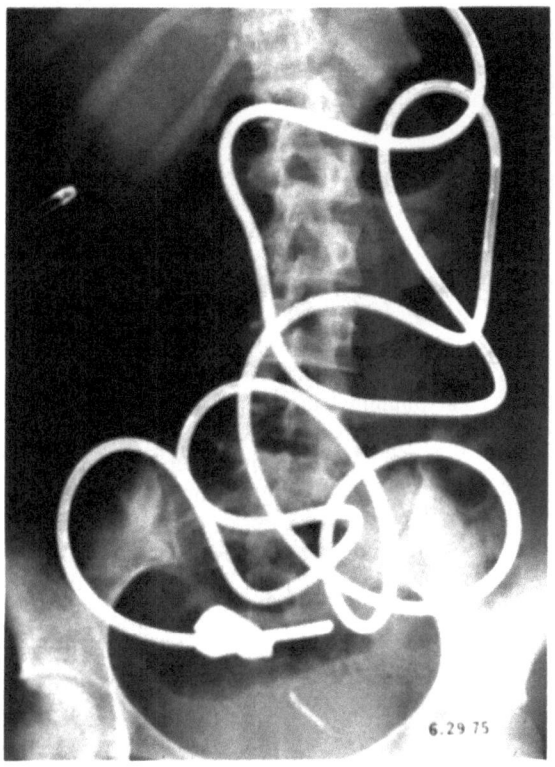 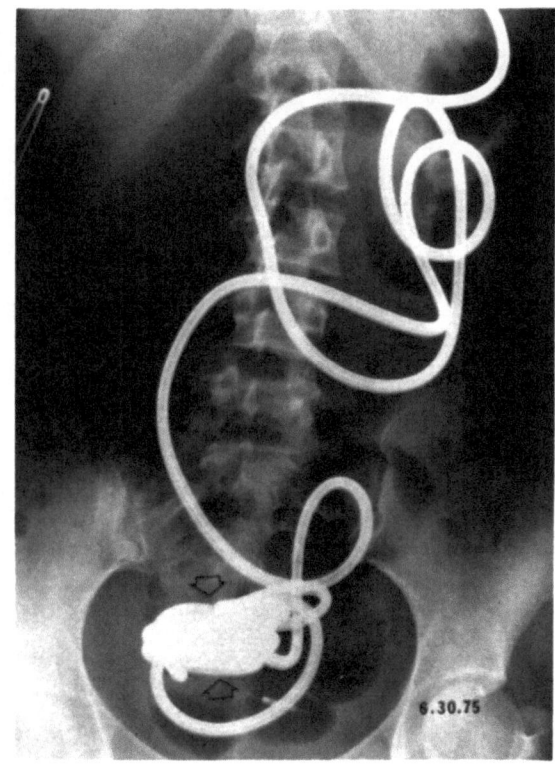

a   b

Fig. 3-18, a and **b. Knot formation in intestinal decompression tube. a** Radiograph of the abdomen initially shows the distal end of the Miller–Abbott tube within a moderately dilated ileal loop. **b** On the following day a considerable length of the tube is coiled in a complex knot *(arrows)*. The tube was removed during ileal resection for regional enteritis.

its way one or more times through enteroenteric fistulas or surgically created anastomotic sites, thus making operative removal necessary (75, 76,85,86). In a biluminal Miller-Abbott tube the channel connecting to the terminal bag may be mistakenly used for introduction of contrast material or medications. The balloon may become markedly distended (Fig. 3-19) and explode, and injury to the intestine may ensue (2,3,23). Conversely, the mercury may be injected into the bowel lumen through the wrong channel and be retained there for a prolonged time but without serious sequelae.

Hydraulically operated suction biopsy tubes are being used with increasing frequency for obtaining specimens of the intestinal mucosa (13). Dobbins et al. reported complications of this procedure in a series of 84 intubations (87). Clinically significant intestinal bleeding developed in 5% of their patients. Such hemorrhage was related to the number and depth of mucosal fragments or incomplete excision in which the partially transected vessel could not retract. The authors also described a "postbiopsy syndrome" consisting of transient fever, diffuse abdominal pain, and rebound tenderness. These findings are attributed to overly rapid withdrawal of the tube causing excessive traction on the mesenteric root.

Soft rubber tubes are frequently used for nonoperative reduction of sigmoid volvulus. Insertion of a long rectal tube allows immediate decompression of the twisted loop by the release of gas and fluid. A potential complication of this approach is detorsion of an already ischemic segment of the colon. Meyers et al. described four cases of ischemic colitis demonstrated on barium enema examination soon after successful reduction of sigmoid volvulus by rectal tubes (88) (Fig. 3-20). Mucosal injury and perforation of the rectum may also be caused by rectal tubes although such complications are more apt to occur during barium enema examination. In the latter procedure the inflated balloon of an inserted catheter

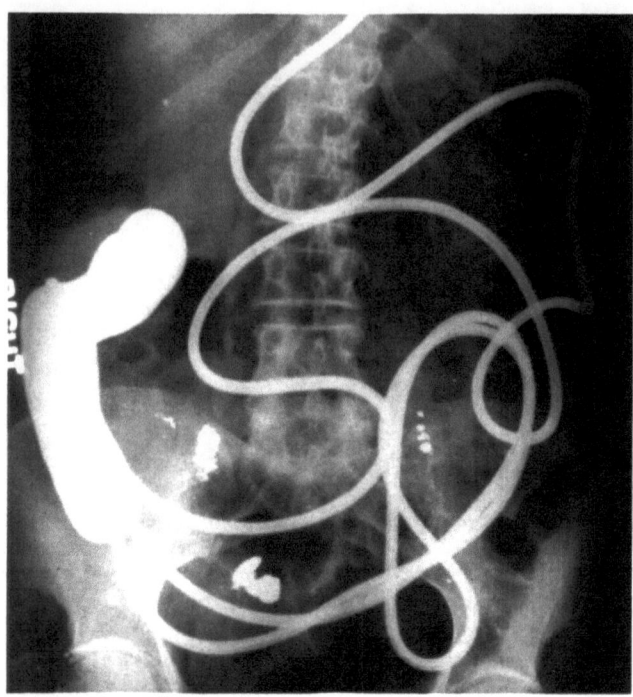

Fig. 3-19. Mistaken identification of channels of biluminal intestinal decompression tube. This radiograph of the abdomen was obtained a few minutes after injection of 100 ml diatrizoate meglumine and diatrizoate sodium (Gastrografin) through a Miller–Abbott tube to evaluate small bowel obstruction. It shows marked distention of the balloon within the distal ileum due to inadvertent injection of the contrast material through the wrong channel. Droplets of mercury are noted in the bowel lumen.

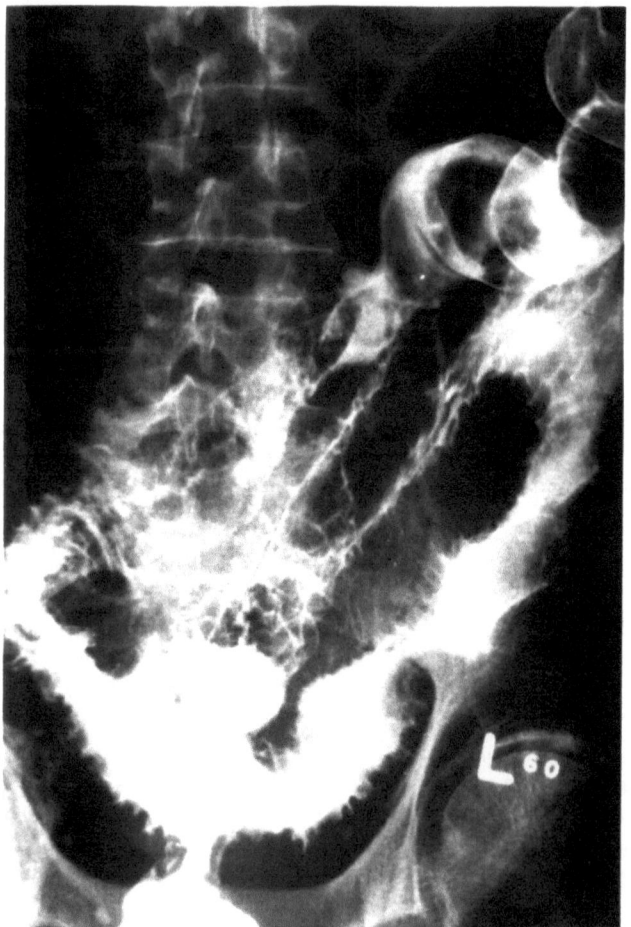

Fig. 3-20. Ischemic colitis complicating reduction of sigmoid volvulus with a rectal tube. Barium enema performed following conservative treatment of sigmoid volvulus with a long rectal tube shows diffuse mucosal ulcerations and submucosal hemorrhage in the redundant sigmoid. The use of rectal tube had resulted in detorsion of an already ischemic sigmoid colon. (Meyers MA, Ghahremani GG, Govoni AF: Ischemic colitis associated with sigmoid volvulus: New observations. Am J Roentgenol 128:591–595, 1977)

is usually responsible for the rectal injury (89). However, perforation of the colon may occasionally complicate even the use of a flexible rectal tube, barium enema tip, or catheter without inflatable balloon, particularly in the presence of underlying disease of the large intestine (90).

Complications Due to the T-Tube

Following cholecystectomy and bile duct exploration it is relatively common to note drainage of blood through the indwelling T-tube. This is generally considered to be related to the surgical procedure itself. However, Rabinovitch and Rabinovitch reported two patients who developed massive bleeding due to erosion of the wall of bile ducts by a T-tube (91). This complication occurred on the tenth postoperative day in one patient and 3 weeks after surgery in another patient. Mechanical irritation from an indwelling T-tube has also been implicated in production of hemobilia due to injury of blood vessels in the wall or adjacent to the bile ducts and later development of pseudoaneurysms (92–95). Even minor or occult hemorrhage induced by a T-tube can lead to formation of blood clots within the biliary system, closely simulating the appearance of a calculus on postoperative evaluation (Fig. 3-21). A clinical and experimental study by Sandblom et al. demonstrated that an intraductal filling defect noted on a T-tube cholangiogram may represent a fibrin deposit or blood clot (96). These tend to form particularly if the tube is unclamped for a prolonged time in the postoperative period, thereby shielding a coagulum below the draining point from the fibrinolytic effects of bile. Documentation of postoperative bile duct hemorrhage directly induced by T-tube rather than operative trauma is difficult. However, it may explain the appearance and subsequent disappearance of "retained stones," which are, in fact, blood clots in the common duct occasionally noted on T-tube cholangiograms (96).

Complications Due to Other Intraabdominal Tubes

Just as the esophagus may be injured by endotracheal and chest tubes (Figs. 3-4, 3-9), the gastrointestinal tract may be subject to trauma from

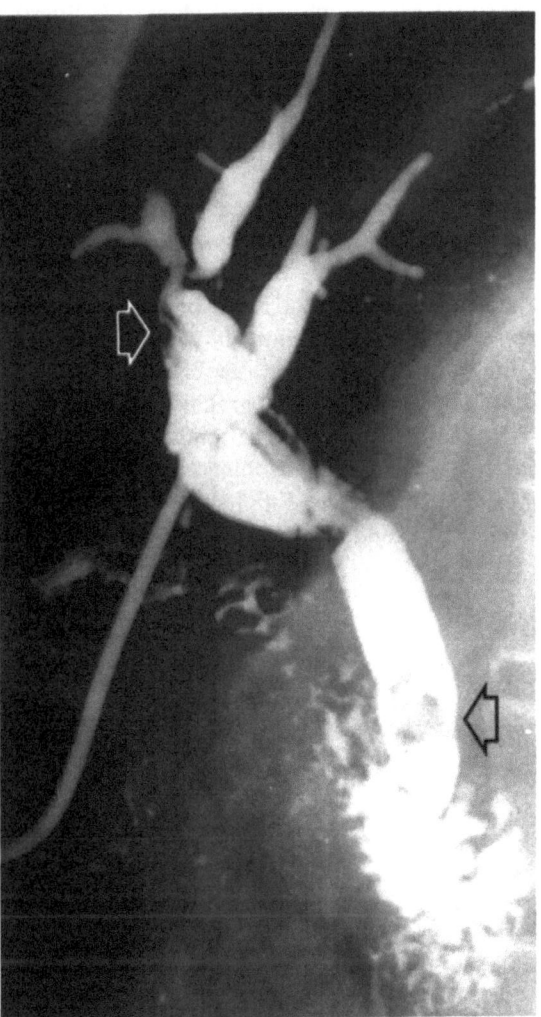

Fig. 3-21. Clot formation in the common bile duct. In a T-tube cholangiogram obtained 10 days after cholecystectomy and removal of impacted gallstones the large and irregular filling defect *(black arrow)* closely simulates a retained stone. Reexploration disclosed an intraductal blood clot, however, with hemorrhage due to erosion of the bile duct by the proximal branch of the T-tube *(white arrow).*

tubes placed extraluminally within the abdominal cavity.

Ventriculoperitoneal shunt has become a popular procedure for treatment of hydrocephalus. The use of tubes for intraperitoneal diversion of cerebrospinal fluid has led to a variety of complications. In a series reported by Grosfeld et al., 45 of 185 (24%) patients developed abdominal complications (97). The most frequent was inguinal hernia in 16.8% of the pediatric patients. This is due mainly to increased abdominal pressure and ascites when the volume of diverted cerebrospinal fluid exceeds the rate of peritoneal absorption. Intraperitoneal inflammatory reactions and omental or mesenteric adhesions may also develop and obstruct the shunt tip. Several authors have described formation of pseudocysts due to intraabdominal loculation of cerebrospinal fluid (97–99). This complication is manifested clinically by postoperative appearance of an abdominal mass or an increase in abdominal girth, occasionally with intestinal distention, pain, and fever. Such pseudocysts are best diagnosed by radiographic examinations, including plain films, gastrointestinal contrast studies, and computed tomography of the abdomen (Fig. 3-22). These methods also help to differentiate pseudocysts from solid masses that can develop as a result of metastatic spread of a brain tumor to the abdomen through the shunt tube (100).

One of the most significant complications of ventriculoperitoneal shunt tubes is perforation of the intestine, urinary bladder, and other viscera (97,101–103). Approximately 30 cases of tube-induced bowel perforation have been described in the literature. The clinical findings have been variable, ranging from acute fatal peritonitis, gram-negative ventriculitis and meningitis, to asymptomatic passage of the tube per rectum. Fortunately the newer silicone tubings are more pliable, less irritating, and cause fewer complications than the polyethylene catheters (101). Furthermore, fibrous encasement of the tube throughout its intraabdominal course and perhaps adhesions formed during gradual penetration of the tube into the intestinal lumen often prevent peritoneal spillage of the bowel contents (102). Injection of the shunt with a water-soluble contrast medium under fluoroscopic control can be most helpful in diagnosing intestinal perfora-

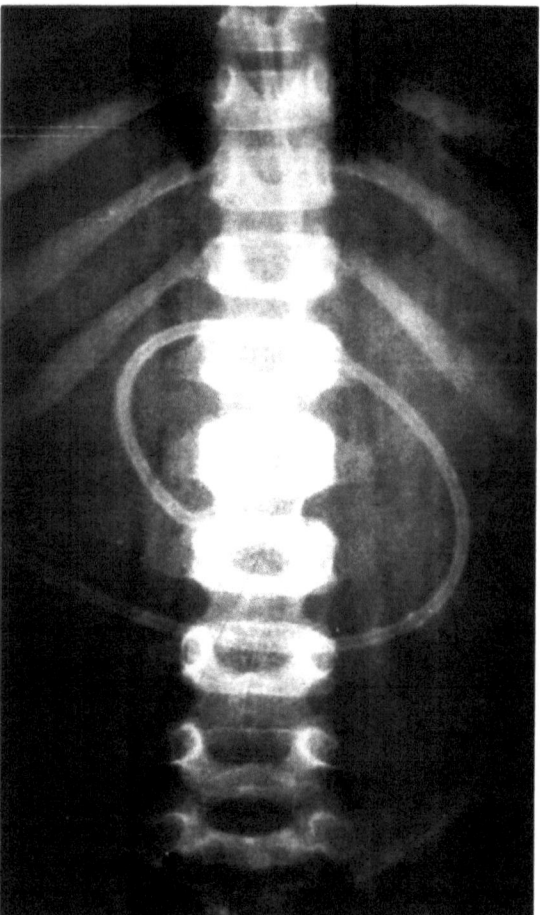

a

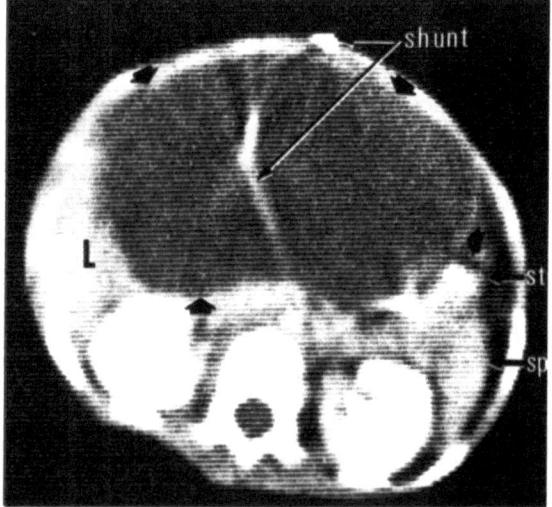

b

Fig. 3-22, a and b. Abdominal pseudocyst due to loculation of cerebrospinal fluid around ventriculoperitoneal shunt tube. a Plain film of the abdomen shows the distal part of the shunt tube coiled in the epigastrium. b CT section at the level of L-2 reveals a large cerebrospinal fluid pseudocyst (black arrows) with compression of the liver (L), stomach (st), and spleen (sp). The shunt catheter is seen both subcutaneously and within the pseudocyst. (Chuang VP et al: Abdominal CSF pseudocyst secondary to ventriculoperitoneal shunt. Diagnosis by computed tomography in two cases. JCAT 2:88–91, 1978)

tion (Fig. 3-23); antibiotic therapy and rapid surgical repair are required.

Tube-induced trauma to the abdominal viscera is not limited only to ventriculoperitoneal shunts. Complications, including intestinal perforation, peritonitis, and hemorrhage, can also develop after placement of tubes for other purposes such as peritoneal dialysis of uremic patients (104–108). Small-bowel volvulus around the intraperitoneally mobile tube may occur (97,102); if it is recognized early, immediate withdrawal of the tube can lead to detorsion of

the involved bowel loops without further sequelae. At times, however, peritoneal adhesions, formed as a result of the irritating effect of a tube within the peritoneal cavity, are the actual cause of intestinal obstruction and require surgical intervention (105) (Fig. 3-24). Furthermore, patients with chronic renal failure are prone to experience other gastrointestinal symptoms (e.g., peptic ulcer, hemorrhage, and spontaneous bowel perforation), which should be differentiated from complications directly related to peritoneal dialysis tubes (106–110).

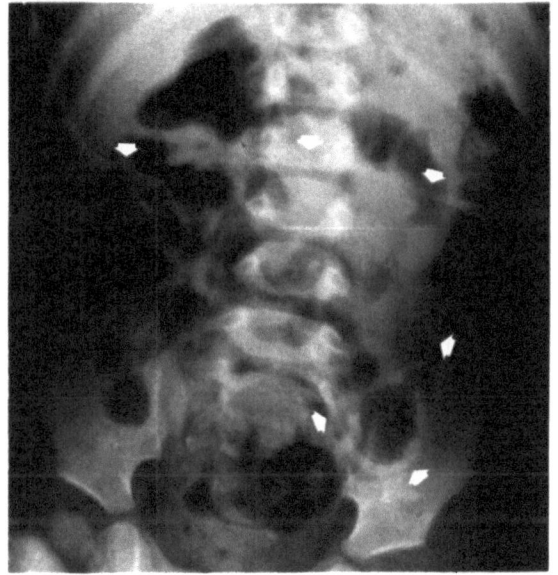

a

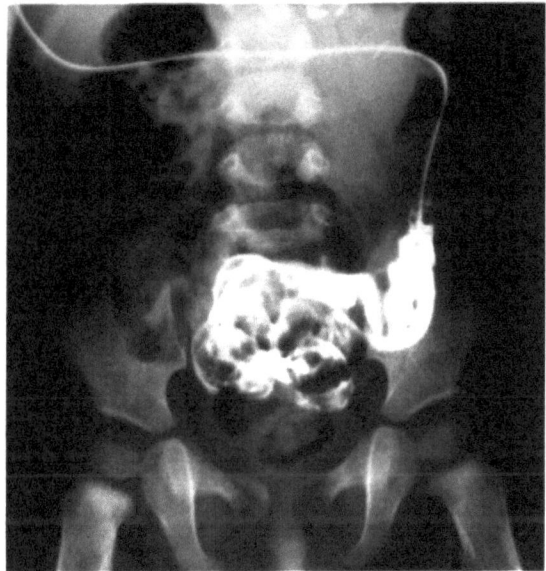

b

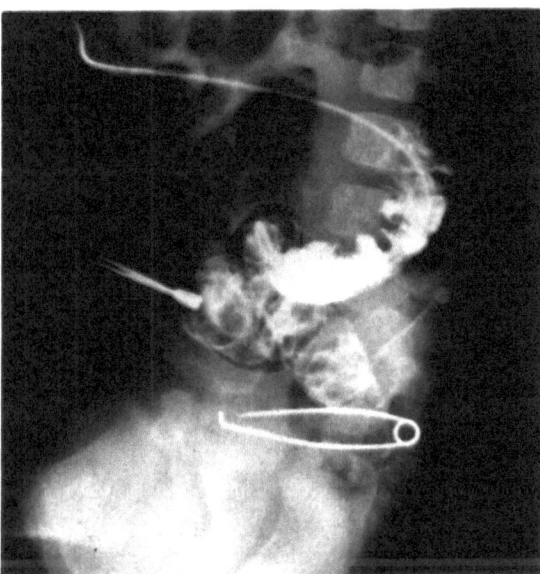

c

Fig. 3-23, a–c. Intestinal perforation by ventriculoperitoneal shunt tube. a Radiograph of the abdomen shows the shunt tube in unusual course through the transverse and descending colon *(arrows)*. b and c Supine and lateral films after injection of shunt with water-soluble contrast material reveal opacification of the sigmoid colon. (Azimi F et al: Intestinal perforation: An infrequent complication of ventriculoperitoneal shunts. Radiology 121:701–702, 1976)

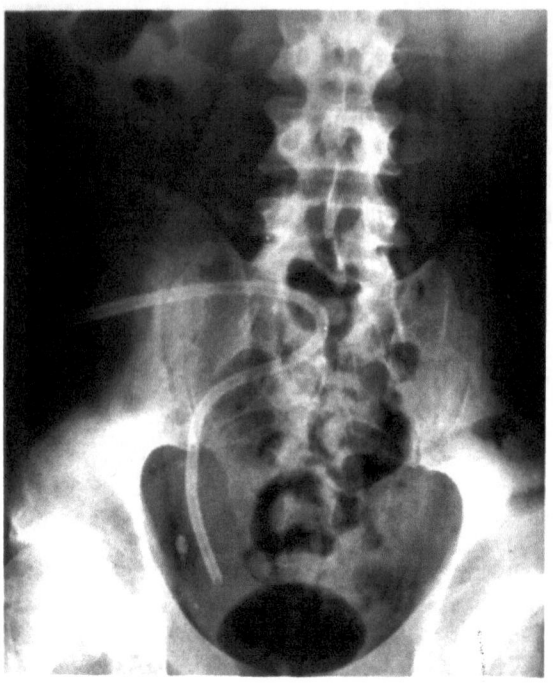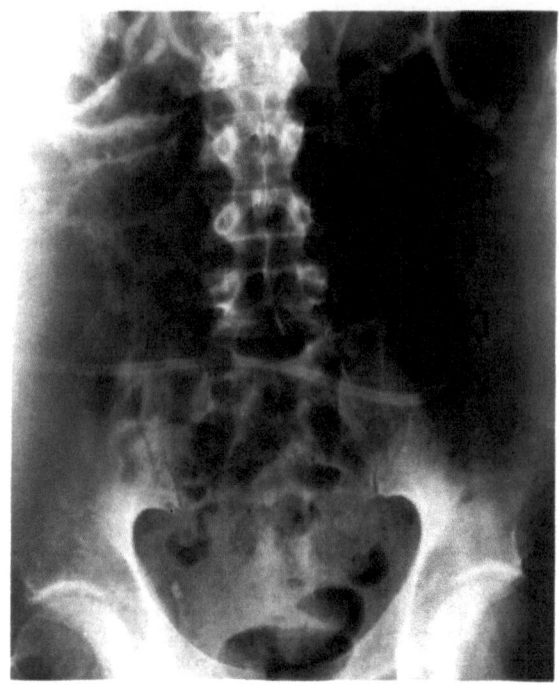

a   b

Fig. 3-24, a and b. Intraperitoneal tube causing intestinal obstruction. a Radiograph of the abdomen shows a peritoneal dialysis tube in the right lower quadrant. **b** Reexamination 3 weeks later demonstrates the altered position of the tube *(arrows)* and evidence of small-bowel distention.

References

1. Palmer JS: The Complete Works of John Hunter, vol 4. Philadelphia: Haswell, Barrington & Haswell 1841, p 185
2. Ingelfinger FJ: Tubes. Gastroenterology 74:310–318, 1978
3. Cantor MO: Intestinal Intubation. Springfield, Ill.: Thomas 1949
4. Harris FI, Gordon M: Intestinal intubation in small bowel distention and obstruction: Further experiences with the single lumen mercury weighted tube and analysis of complications. Surg Gynecol Obstet 86:647–658, 1948
5. Rhea JW, Ghazzawi O, Weidman W: Nasojejunal feeding: An improved device and intubation technique. J Pediatr 82:951–954, 1973
6. Pareira MD, Conrad EJ, Hicks W, et al: Therapeutic nutrition with tube feeding. JAMA 156:810–816, 1954
7. Fallis LS, Barron J: Gastric and jejunal alimentation with fine polyethylene tubes. Arch Surg 65:373–381, 1952
8. Bilbao MK, Frische LH, Dotter CT, et al: Hypotonic duodenography. Radiology 89:438–443, 1967
9. Eaton SB, Benedict KT, Ferrucci JT, et al: Hypotonic duodenography. Radiol Clin North Am 8:125–137, 1970
10. Herlinger H: A modified technique for the double-contrast small bowel enema. Gastrointest Radiol 3:201–207, 1978
11. Hall WH, Hodges SC: Effect of fluoroscopic tube placement on basal gastric secretion collections. South Med J 69:164–166, 1976
12. Palmer ED: Duodenal intubation. JAMA 233:818–819, 1975
13. Flick AL, Quinton WE, Rubin CE: A peroral hydraulic biopsy tube for multiple sampling at any level of the gastrointestinal tract. Gastroenterology 40:120–126, 1961
14. Astley R, Roberts KD: Intubation perforation of the esophagus in the newborn baby. Br J Radiol 43:219–223, 1970
15. Boros SJ, Reynolds JW: Duodenal perforation: A complication of neonatal nasojejunal feeding. J Pediatr 85:107–108, 1974
16. Chen JW, Wong PWK: Intestinal complications of nasojejunal feeding in low-birth-weight infants. J Pediatr 85:109–110, 1974
17. Girdany BR, Sieber WK, Osman MZ: Traumatic pseudodiverticulums of the pharynx in newborn infants. N Engl J Med 280:237–240, 1969
18. Kassner EG, Baumstark A, Balsam D, et al: Passage of feeding catheters into the pleural space: A radiographic sign of trauma to the pharynx and esophagus in the newborn. Am J Roentgenol 128:19–22, 1977

19. Lee SB, Kuhn JP: Esophageal perforation in the neonate. A review of the literature. Am J Dis Child 130:325–329, 1976
20. Siegle RL, Rabinowitz JG, Sarasohn C: Intestinal perforation secondary to nasojejunal feeding tubes. Am J Roentgenol 126:1229–1232, 1976
21. Sun SC, Samuels S, Lee J, et al: Duodenal perforation: A rare complication of neonatal nasojejunal tube feeding. J Pediatr 55:371–375, 1975
22. Bruny SJA: Hazards of intestinal intubation. Am J Roentgenol 79:862–865, 1958
23. Hafner CD, Wylie JH Jr, Brush BE: Complications of gastrointestinal intubation. Arch Surg 83:147–160, 1961
24. Rozanski J, Kleinfeld M: A complication of prolonged intestinal intubation: Gaseous distention of the terminal balloon. Am J Dig Dis 20:1067–1070, 1975
25. Siemers PT, Reinke RT: Perforation of the nasopharynx by nasogastric intubation: A rare cause of left pleural effusion and pneumomediastinum. Am J Roentgenol 127:341–343, 1976
26. Sower N, Wratten GP: Intussusception due to intestinal tubes. Case reports and review of literature. Am J Surg 110:441–444, 1965
27. Adams CL: The complications of endoesophageal tubes. J Thorac Cardiovasc Surg 51:685–693, 1966
28. Zeid SS, Young PD, Reeves JT: Rupture of the esophagus after introduction of the Sengstaken-Blakemore tube. Gastroenterology 36:128–131, 1959
29. Seebacher J, Nozik D, Mathieu A: Inadvertent intracranial introduction of a nasogastric tube, a complication of severe maxillofacial trauma. Anesthesiology 42:100–102, 1975
30. Stauffer JL, Petty TL: Accidental intubation of the pyriform sinus. A complication of "roadside" resuscitation. JAMA 237:2324–2325, 1977
31. Wolff AP, Kessler S: Iatrogenic injury to the hypopharynx and cervical esophagus: An autopsy study. Ann Otolaryngol 82:778–783, 1973
32. Tubes in the oesophagus (editorial). Lancet 1:491–492, 1974
33. Iglauer S, Molt WF: Severe injury to the larynx resulting from indwelling duodenal tube. Ann Otol 48:886–892, 1939
34. Nagler R, Spiro HM: Persistent gastroesophageal reflux induced during prolonged gastric intubation. N Engl J Med 269:495–500, 1963
35. Lucaya J, Herrera M, Salcedo S: Traumatic pharyngeal pseudodiverticulum in neonates and infants. Two case reports and review of the literature. Pediatr Radiol 8:65–69, 1979
36. Hirsch M, Abramowitz HB, Shapira S, et al: Hypopharyngeal injury as a result of attempted endotracheal intubation. Radiology 128:37–39, 1978
37. Wolff AP, Kuhn FA, Ogura JH: Pharyngeal-esophageal perforations associated with rapid oral endotracheal intubation. Ann Otolaryngol 81:258–261, 1972
38. Meyers MA, Ghahremani GG: Complications of fiberoptic endoscopy. I. Esophagoscopy and gastroscopy. Radiology 115:293–300, 1975
39. Meyers MA, Ghahremani GG: Complications of gastrointestinal fiberoptic endoscopy. Gastrointest Radiol 2:273–280, 1977
40. Eklöf O, Löhr G, Okmian L: Submucosal perforation of the esophagus in the neonate. Acta Radiol (Diagn) 8:187–192, 1969
41. Lynch FP, Coran AG, Cohen SR, et al: Traumatic esophageal pseudodiverticula in the newborn. J Pediatr Surg 9:675–681, 1974
42. Sengstaken RW, Blakemore AH: Balloon tamponade for the control of hemorrhage from esophageal varices. Ann Surg 131:781–789, 1950
43. Conn HO, Simpson JA: Excessive mortality associated with balloon tamponade of bleeding varices. A critical reappraisal. JAMA 202:587–591, 1967
44. Conn HO: Hazards attending the use of esophageal tamponade. N Engl J Med 259:701–707, 1958
45. Hermann RE, Traul D: Experience with the Sengstaken-Blakemore tube for bleeding esophageal varices. Surg Gynecol Obstet 130:879–885, 1970
46. Juffe A, Tellez G, Eguaras MG, et al: Unusual complication of the Sengstaken-Blakemore tube. Gastroenterology 72:724–725, 1977
47. Bouchier IAD: Impaction of the Sengstaken-Blakemore tube. Gastroenterology 45:274–278, 1963
48. Linton RR: The emergency and definitive treatment of bleeding esophageal varices. Gastroenterology 24:1–9, 1953
49. Rosoff L, White EJ: Perforation of the esophagus. Am J Surg 128:207–215, 1974
50. Carter R, Hinshaw DB: Use of the Celestin indwelling plastic tube for inoperable carcinoma of the esophagus and cardia. Surg Gynecol Obstet 117:641–644, 1963
51. O'Connor T, Watson R, Lepley D Jr, et al: Esophageal prosthesis for palliative intubation. Arch Surg 87:257–279, 1963
52. Peura DA, Heit HA, Johnson LF, et al: Esophageal prosthesis in cancer. Am J Dig Dis 23:796–800, 1978
53. Girardet RE, Ransdell HT Jr, Wheat MW Jr: Palliative intubation in the management of esophageal carcinoma. Ann Thorac Surg 18:417–427, 1974
54. Palmer ED: Peroral prosthesis for management of incurable esophageal carcinoma. Am J Gastroenterol 59:487–498, 1973
55. Mackenzie AS, Whyte AS, Tankel HI: Structural deterioration in Celestin tubes. Br J Surg 63:851–852, 1976
56. Bartlett RH: A procedure for management of acquired tracheoesophageal fistula in ventilator patients. J Thorac Cardiovasc Surg 71:89–95, 1976
57. Thomas AN: Management of tracheoesophageal fistula caused by cuffed tracheal tubes. Am J

Surg 124:181–189, 1972

58. Moessinger AC, Driscoll JM Jr, Wigger HJ: High incidence of lung perforation by chest tube in neonatal pneumothorax. J Pediatr 92:635–637, 1978
59. Stahly TL, Tench WD: Lung entrapment and infarction by chest tube suction. Radiology 122:307–309, 1977
60. Johnson KR, Genovesi MG, Lassar KH: Esophageal obturator airway: Use and complications. J Am Coll Emerg Physician 5:36–39, 1976
61. Pilcher DB, DeMeules JE: Esophageal perforation following use of esophageal airway. Chest 69:377–380, 1976
62. Scholl DG, Tsai SH: Esophageal perforation following the use of the esophageal obturator airway. Radiology 122:315–316, 1977
63. Carlson WJ, Hunter SW, Bonnabeau RC Jr: Esophageal perforation with obturator airway. JAMA 241:1154–1155, 1979
64. Stewart ET, Miller WN, Hogan WJ, et al: Desirability of roentgen esophageal examination immediately after pneumatic dilatation for achalasia. Radiology 130:589–591, 1979
65. Zegel HG, Kressel HY, Levine GM, et al: Delayed esophageal perforation after pneumatic dilatation for the treatment of achalasia. Gastrointest Radiol 4:219–221, 1979
66. Berry BE, Ochsner JL: Perforation of the esophagus. A 30 year review. J Thorac Cardiovasc Surg 65:1–7, 1973
67. Banfield WJ, Hurwitz AL: Esophageal stricture associated with nasogastric intubation. Arch Intern Med 134:1083–1086, 1974
68. Waldman I, Berlin L: Stricture of the esophagus due to nasogastric intubation. Am J Roentgenol 94:321–324, 1965
69. Douglas WK: Esophageal strictures associated with gastroduodenal intubation. Br J Surg 43:404–409, 1955
70. Ghahremani GG, Turner MA, Port RB: Iatrogenic intubation injuries of the upper gastrointestinal tract in adults. Gastrointest Radiol 5:1–10, 1980
71. Drenick EJ, Lipset M: Difficulty with removal of plastic nasogastric tube (letter). JAMA 218:1573, 1971
72. Barton CH, Vaziri ND, Ness RL, et al: Cimetidine in the management of metabolic alkalosis induced by nasogastric drainage. Arch Surg 114:70–74, 1979
73. Larsen PD: Knotted nasogastric tubing. JAMA 238:211–212, 1977
74. Morris HH: Nasogastric intubation: A potentially knotty problem (letter). JAMA 237:1432, 1977
75. Shulman H: Passing the Cantor tube in a patient with a gastroenterostomy: An unusual complication. Am J Roentgenol 110:332–333, 1970
76. Cantor MO: Intestinal intubation (letter). JAMA 205:251, 1968

77. Rennel CL: Intubation with telescoping of small bowel. Radiology 97:155–156, 1970
78. McGoon DC: Intussusception: Hazard of intestinal intubation. Surgery 40:515–519, 1956
79. Simonowitz D, Paloyan D: Intussusception associated with intestinal intubation. Illinois M J 155:21–23, 1979
80. Poppel MH, Brinsley B: Ileal intussusception as result of intestinal intubation. JAMA 169:1189–1190, 1959
81. Coffey ME, Gordon MJ, Mayes GR: Gaseous distention of an intestinal tube bag relieved by transabdominal puncture. Ann Intern Med 85:480–481, 1976
82. Coleman SL, Miller WE, Stroehlein JR, et al: Nonoperative retrieval of an impacted long intestinal tube. Am J Dig Dis 22:462–464, 1977
83. Fricke FJ, Niewodowski MA: Hazardous gaseous distention of intestinal balloons. JAMA 235:2611–2613, 1976
84. Herschman A, Phillips JC: Knotted intestinal decompression tube (letter). JAMA 204:634, 1968
85. Khan JH, Cooper HF: Intestinal intubation (letter). JAMA 205:251–252, 1968
86. De Barros SG, Lane MF, Trotman BW: Long-tube coiling in enterocolonic fistula. JAMA 241:2636, 1979
87. Dobbins WO, Trier JS, Parkins RA, et al: A warning regarding the dangers of hydraulic biopsy in gastrointestinal research. Gastroenterology 45:335–340, 1963
88. Meyers MA, Ghahremani GG, Govoni AF: Ischemic colitis associated with sigmoid volvulus: New observations. Am J Roentgenol 128:591–595, 1977
89. Nelson JA, Daniels AU, Dodds WJ: Rectal balloons: Complications, causes, and recommendations. Invest Radiol 14:48–59, 1979
90. Ansell G: Complications in Diagnostic Radiology. Oxford: Blackwell 1974, pp 339–350
91. Rabinovitch J, Rabinovitch P: Massive bleeding from common bile duct caused by indwelling T-tube. Arch Surg 69:849–852, 1954
92. Grove WJ: Biliary tract hemorrhage as a cause of hematemesis. Arch Surg 83:67–72, 1961
93. Campbell DA: Discussion of Guynn VL, Reynolds JT: Surgical management of hemobilia. Arch Surg 83:73–80, 1961
94. Moreaux J, Bismuth H, Lagneau P: Les hémobilies post-opértoires par lésion artérielle pédiculaire. Ann Chir 20:368–375, 1966
95. Boijsen E, Göthlin J, Hallbook T, et al: Preoperative angiographic diagnosis of bleeding aneurysms of abdominal viscera. Radiology 93:781–791, 1969
96. Sandblom P, Mirkovitch V, Saegesser F: Formation and fate of fibrin clots in the biliary tract: A clinical and experimental study. Ann Surg 185:356–366, 1977
97. Grosfeld JL, Cooney DR, Smith J, et al: Intra-

abdominal complications following ventriculo-peritoneal shunt procedures. Pediatrics 54:791–796, 1974

98. Chuang VP, Fried AM, Oliff M, et al: Abdominal CSF pseudocyst secondary to ventriculoperitoneal shunt: Diagnosis by computed tomography in two cases. J Comput Assist Tomogr 2:88–91, 1978

99. Norfray JF, Henry HM, Givens JD, et al: Abdominal complications from peritoneal shunts. Gastroenterology 77:337–340, 1979

100. Wood BP, Haller JO, Berdon WE, et al: Shunt metastases of pineal tumors presenting as a pelvic mass. Pediatr Radiol 8:108–109, 1979

101. Azimi F, Dinn WM, Naumann RA: Intestinal perforation. An infrequent complication of ventriculo-peritoneal shunts. Radiology 121:701–702, 1976

102. Lee FA, Gwinn JL: Complications of ventriculo-peritoneal shunts. Ann Radiol 18:471–478, 1975

103. Schulhof LA, Worth RM, Kalsbeck JE: Bowel perforation due to peritoneal shunt. A report of seven cases and a review of the literature. Surg Neurol 3:265–269, 1975

104. Krebs RA, Burtiss BB: Bowel perforation. A complication of peritoneal dialysis using a permanent peritoneal cannula. JAMA 198:486–487, 1966

105. Mion CM, Boen ST: Analysis of factors responsible for the formation of adhesions during chronic peritoneal dialysis. Am J Med Sci 250:675–679, 1965

106. Rubin J, Oreopoulos DG, Lio TT, et al: Management of peritonitis and bowel perforation during chronic peritoneal dialysis. Nephron 16:220–225, 1976

107. Simkin EP, Wright FK: Perforating injuries of the bowel complicating peritoneal catheter insertion. Lancet 1:64–67, 1968

108. Vaamonde CA, Michael UF, Metzger RA, et al: Complications of acute peritoneal dialysis. J Chron Dis 28:637–659, 1975

109. Wiener SN, Vertes V, Shapiro H: The upper gastrointestinal tract in patients undergoing chronic dialysis. Radiology 92:110–114, 1969

110. Lipschutz DE, Easterling RE: Spontaneous perforation of the colon in chronic renal failure. Arch Intern Med 132:758–762, 1973

4 Gastrointestinal Complications of Radiologic Procedures

David W. Gelfand, David J. Ott, and Thomas H. Hunt

Complications of Routine Fluoroscopic Studies

Barium Sulfate as a Contrast Medium

Barium studies of the gastrointestinal tract are the contrast examinations most frequently performed by radiologists. The inert nature of barium sulfate and its use as a suspension of insoluble particles make the routine examination of the gastrointestinal tract the safest of radiologic contrast examinations. Complications of these studies are very infrequent considering the vast numbers performed—more than 10 million in 1964 (1).

Barium sulfate is almost totally inert because of its insolubility in water. This property makes it an almost perfect contrast material for the gastrointestinal tract. Modern commercial barium sulfate suspensions are generally prepared to standards equaling or exceeding those set by the United States Pharmacopeia. This has virtually eliminated toxicity due to impurities.

Substitution of the wrong substance for barium sulfate in preparation of a suspension has resulted in severe poisoning (2–4). Barium sulfide, barium chloride, and barium carbonate have been mistakenly administered. Barium poisoning apparently results in a rapid and severe decrease of the serum potassium due to a shift of fluid from extracellular to intracellular compartments, and intravenous infusion of potassium may have been crucial in promoting recovery during one such instance (4).

Substitution of other white powders present in a radiology department has also resulted in poisoning (5,6). A bizarre instance was reported by Felson (6). Plaster of Paris was stored in a container previously used for barium sulfate, and a plaster suspension was mistakenly administered to four patients. The plaster "set," forming casts of the patients' stomachs. Fortunately the plaster crumbled after several days and was eventually passed. The trend toward use of commercially prepackaged barium in plastic cups and enema bags diminishes the potential for inadvertent administration of a dangerous but benign-appearing white powder.

Contamination of barium by bacteria or other organisms is a possibility when barium sulfate suspensions are stored unrefrigerated and mechanical mixers are not cleaned, or when nondisposable tips, tubing, and reservoirs are employed for barium enemas. Growths of *Streptococcus faecalis*, *Pseudomonas*, *Klebsiella*, *Clostridium*, and *Escherichia coli* have been recovered from mixers and reservoirs and in stored barium sulfate powders and suspensions (7). It has been demonstrated that a normal contraction of the colon may be sufficient to propel a mixture of barium and feces into a reservoir several feet above the x-ray table (8,9). The development of the disposable barium enema bag with attached tubing and tip has been the specific result of clinical investigations of this problem (8,10).

Oral Studies Employing Barium Sulfate

Administration of barium sulfate orally for diagnostic purposes carries risks that are primarily related to the disease process present. Hazards include perforation, obstruction, impaction, aspiration, and embolization.

Perforation

The effect of barium outside the gastrointestinal tract is always deleterious, but it varies considerably, depending upon the location and circumstances of the perforation. If a perforation or laceration of the esophagus or gastric or duodenal perforation due to ulcer disease is suspected, a water-soluble contrast medium should be employed for the examination.

Reports of a few cases of perforation of gastric and duodenal ulcers during x-ray examinations attribute this to the effects of compression or to weakening of the wall of the viscus by therapeutic agents such as steroids.

Obstruction or Impaction

Orally administered barium sulfate may accumulate proximal to a constricting lesion of the bowel, causing obstruction or impaction (13,14). This rarely occurs in the upper gastrointestinal tract and small bowel because the fluidity of the suspension is maintained. In the colon, however, progressive dehydration of the barium may cause impaction proximal to even an incomplete obstruction, with the possibility of perforation (15). Barium may also be impacted in the colon because of prolonged stasis, without an underlying obstructing lesion. Bowel evacuation may then be successfully induced by administration of 50% solutions of lactulose (16).

Barium appendicitis due to stasis has also been reported 9–105 days subsequent to barium meal examinations (17). Another report describes a large barolith persistent in the cecum 2 years after an oral barium study and requiring operative removal (18).

The likelihood of barium impaction can be diminished by several measures. Use of well-suspended, isosmotic barium suspensions decreases the possibility of significant dehydration of the barium in the distal small bowel or colon. Maintenance of good hydration of the patient further decreases the resorbtion of water. Use of cathartics, particularly saline cathartics, greatly decreases the chance that the barium will become dehydrated in the distal bowel. Awareness that drugs inhibiting peristalsis may contribute to impaction is also important in its prevention.

Esophageal Obstruction Due to Barium Tablets

The use of fresh barium tablets for diagnosis of esophageal obstruction or dysmotility is advocated; a case of obstruction of the esophagus by an aged barium table, in which disintegration was delayed has been reported (19).

Aspiration

The introduction of uncontaminated barium sulfate into the bronchial tree is for most practical purposes harmless if the barium aspirated does not obstruct major bronchi or contain certain regurgitated gastric contents (20). Ciliary action and phagocytosis will almost always clear this trapped barium. However, remaining barium particles can be expected to stimulate a granulomatous foreign-body reaction (20,21).

Radiologists are often asked to perform contrast examinations of the upper gastrointestinal tract using iodinated water-soluble materials when patients are known to be aspirating or vomiting or are thought to have obstruction proximal to the ligament of Treitz. It is wrongly assumed that aspiration of these water-soluble materials is less harmful than aspiration of barium sulfate suspension (22). In actual fact, aspiration of hyperosmotic iodinated contrast materials results in acute pulmonary edema (23–24). In this type of case one is well advised to use barium suspension because of its relatively benign effects on the lung, care being taken that the patient is not allowed to aspirate large quantities.

Barium Embolization

A single case of barium embolization following an upper gastrointestinal examination has been reported in a patient with Hodgkin's disease who was experiencing massive upper gastrointestinal bleeding (25). It is postulated that extensive mucosal ulcerations of the duodenum and upper small bowel allowed barium to enter the portal venous circulation.

Complications Peculiar to Hypotonic Duodenography

Complications of hypotonic duodenography are associated primarily with the use of anticholinergic drugs. These cause side effects that include difficulty in micturition, tachycardia, and mydriasis. Administration of these agents is contraindicated in patients with glaucoma, many forms of heart disease, prostatic hypertrophy, and bowel obstruction. Advent of the use of glucagon as a substitute for anticholinergic agents has largely eliminated these considerations.

Acute gastric dilatation has been recorded in three instances as a complication of hypotonic duodenography performed with 30 mg of propantheline bromide (Pro-Banthine) intramuscularly (26). In one case, gross dilation of the stomach occurred, the stomach occupying most of the abdomen 36 hours later when detected (Fig. 4-1). The patient died shortly thereafter from pulmonary embolism. In the second and third cases, gastric dilatation was detected several hours after the study and successfully treated with nasogastric suction. In two of these cases the duodenum was partially obstructed by carcinoma of the pancreas. It was suggested that hypotonic duodenography using Pro-Banthine not be performed on patients suspected of having partial obstruction and that food be withheld for several hours after the study to allow the stomach to regain its inherent muscular tone prior to feeding. Similar complications have not been reported with scopolamine bulylbromide (Buscopan) or glucagon.

Oral Studies Employing Aqueous Media

Available Media

Derivatives of the diatrizoate moiety form the basis of most aqueous iodinated contrast materials used for investigation of the gastrointestinal tract. Most commonly employed in the United States is Gastrografin, a 76% solution of sodium methylglucamine diatrizoate. A wetting agent and flavors are present as well. The major ingredient, sodium methylglucamine diatrizoate, is essentially identical to materials employed for intravenous urography and angiography.

The singular advantage of the iodinated aqueous contrast materials is that they are readily absorbed from the peritoneal cavity, pleural cavities, and interstitial tissues and are thus useful in examination of patients with suspected perforation of a viscus (27,28). Their dangers relate primarily to two of their physical characteristics: hypertonicity and the potential for precipitation in certain circumstances.

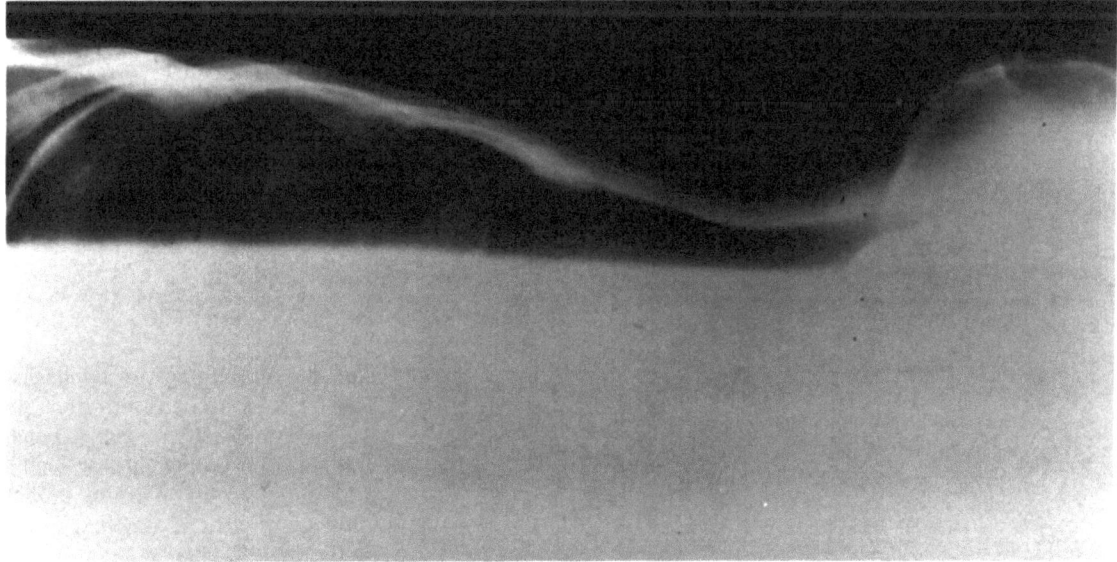

Fig. 4-1. Massive gastric dilatation complicating hypotonic duodenography performed with propantheline bromide (Pro-Banthine). Right lateral decubitus view shows the fluid level extending from diaphragm to lower abdomen in the massively dilated stomach 36 hours after the study. (Gelfand DW, Moskowitz M: Massive gastric dilatation complicating hypotonic duodenography. A report of three cases. Radiology 114: 301–302, 1974)

Aspiration

Aspiration is probably the most frequent and serious consequence of oral administration of aqueous contrast materials. These agents are hyperosmolar, with 1900 mosmols/liter, approximately 6 times more than normal serum. Within the lungs this hyperosmolarity draws fluid into the alveoli, causing pulmonary edema. When water-soluble contrast materials must be employed because of the possibility of perforation and the threat of aspiration is also present, every effort should be made to minimize the amount employed in an effort to prevent substantial apsiration (Fig. 4-2).

Precipitation

Precipitation of aqueous contrast materials may occasionally occur (29–31). Hydrochloric acid is known to precipitate meglumine diatrizoate 76% (Gastrografin) in strengths of 0.1N (29,30). This

event does not often occur in patients. However, Gastrografin is recorded as having formed a putty-like mass in one patient's stomach (29) and having precipitated within the balloon of a Sengstaken-Blakemore tube that had been in another patient's stomach for 6 days (30). In the latter instance there was considerable difficulty in withdrawing the tube from the stomach. Hydrogen ions from the gastric hydrochloric acid were presumed to have migrated across the rubber membrane into the balloon, precipitating the diatrizoate.

Obstruction may also cause precipitation of Gastrografin in patients who are achlorhydric (31). Precipitation of Gastrografin occurred in an obstructed gastric stump, the solid mass of Gastrografin causing gastric erosions and hematemesis. Figure 4-3 demonstrates harmless precipitation of small amounts of Gastrografin in a patient with gastric outlet obstruction.

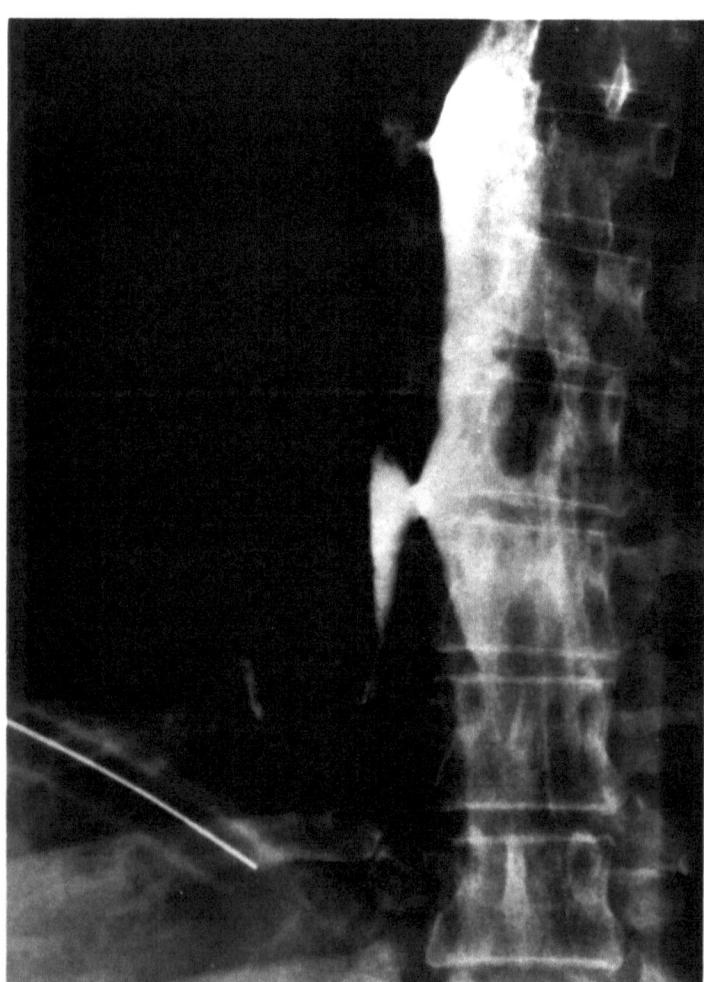

Fig. 4-2. Lacerations of esophagus. Two lacerations occurred after the patient swallowed a chicken bone. The lower one communicates with a bronchus (arrow). Because it was anticipated that the esophagus was perforated the examination was performed with a water-soluble material. When it became apparent that small amounts of contrast material were entering a bronchus, the examination was terminated to avoid provoking pulmonary edema.

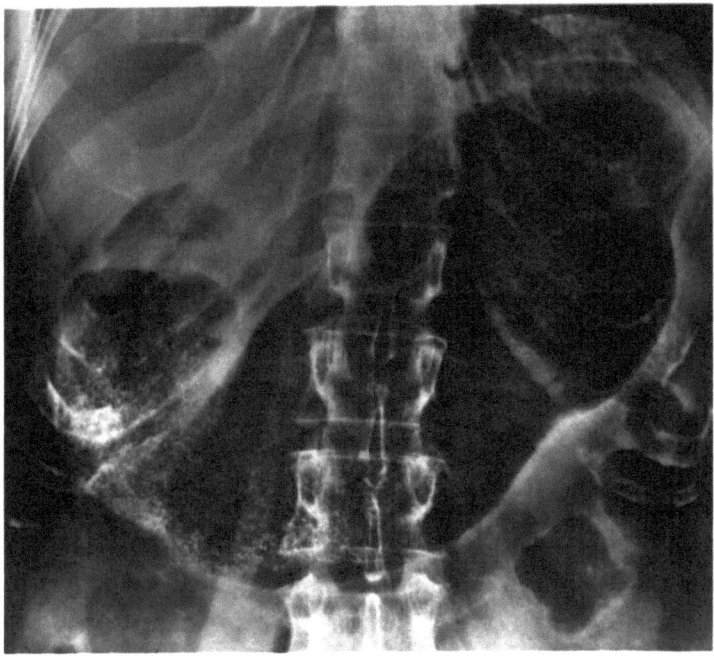

Fig. 4-3. Precipitation of water-soluble contrast material in stomach with outlet obstruction. Small amounts are seen on a film of the abdomen taken 24 hours after administration.

Hypovolemia

A further consequence of the use of water-soluble contrast materials is hypovolemia. The six-fold tonicity of Gastrografin compared to serum causes fluid to be drawn into the lumen of the gastrointestinal tract in large quantities, with resulting loss of plasma volume (32). These changes have been most marked in infants receiving Gastrografin orally, although similar changes have been noted in adults (33). Usually there is no deleterious effect, but if the patient is initially dehydrated and plasma volume is low, cardiovascular collapse may occur.

Barium Enema

Perforation

Incidence. Perforation is the most frequent serious complication of barium enema examinations. The complication is infrequent but not rare, and published reports are legion (34–85). The reported incidence ranges from 1 in 2,250 examinations (54) to 1 in 12,000 (43). However, in evaluating these reports, it is apparent that there is considerable variance in the detection and reporting mechanisms from institution to institution. The type of perforation—intraperitoneal, retroperitoneal, or intramural—depends on the site and depth of colonic laceration. It is not certain from available reports whether intra-peritoneal or retroperitoneal perforation is more common. Intramural perforation may be less common.

Mechanisms. Four general causes of perforation can be cited: laceration of the rectum by the enema tip, rupture of the wall of the rectum or colon by an overinflated balloon (Fig. 4-4), necrosis or weakening of the colonic wall as a result of underlying disease processes, and bursting due to hydrostatic pressure.

Laceration of the rectum by the enema tip has been attributed to a number of factors. Use of rigid enema tips allows exertion of considerable pressure against a small area of the anterior rectal wall during insertion, leading to laceration. This is particularly likely if the rectal wall is deviated from its normal position by extrinsic factors or made rigid by a disease process. Improper insertion is a specific hazard, even with nonrigid plastic tips. Balloon tips increase the hazards, and a majority of recorded cases of barium enema perforation have occurred with their use.

Simple overinflation, inflation of a balloon within the less distensible rectosigmoid or anal regions (64), and eccentric inflation of the small balloons often attached to disposable tips (58) all may cause tears. A particular hazard is the use of a balloon-equipped enema tip in a patient with severe colitis or rectal neoplasms.

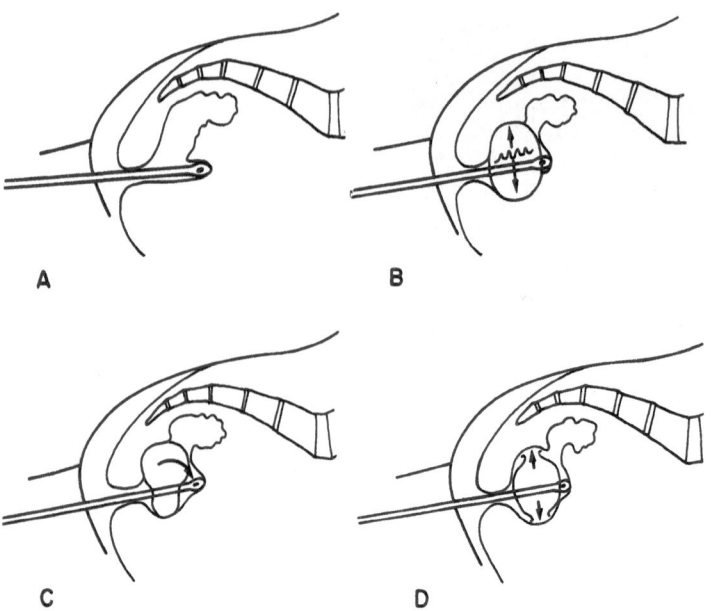

Fig. 4-4, a–d. Causes of rectal perforation related to enema tips and balloons. a Continued anterior direction of the tip after traversing the anus impales the anterior rectal wall. **b** Overdistention of a balloon tears the rectum. **c** Eccentric inflation of the small rectal balloon on a disposable tip levers the tip into the rectal wall. **d** Balloon bursts in rectum, causing tear.

Bursting of the colon from excessive pressure has received investigative attention. Burt (86) and Noveroske (87) established that the pressure generated by a column of barium from a reservoir several feet above the table may be sufficient to rupture the colon. The cecum is the portion of the colon most likely to burst, rupturing in autopsy specimens at a pressure as low as 40 mm Hg. This corresponds to a reservoir height of just over 2 ft above the rectum for a 20% wt/v barium sulfate suspension of low viscosity. Thus the reservoir should probably not be set more than this distance above the rectum or approximately 2.5 ft above the table. An additional considerable safety factor results from a complex interaction of flow rate, viscosity, and resistance to flow and from the great distensibility of the colon itself. Indeed, with the extremely viscous materials employed for double-contrast barium enema, the reservoir may be safely raised 4 or 5 ft above the table.

Necrosis of the bowel wall or its weakening by disease processes, particularly colonic tumors, contributes to perforation of the colon, and this may occur at the "safe" pressures routinely employed (42,51,72). Acute ulcerative colitis, particularly when associated with toxic megacolon (43), also predisposes the colon to rupture by barium enema. Because of the danger of perforation in toxic megacolon, or of exacerbating the disease process in acutely ill patients (34), barium enema is contraindicated in patients with severe, active ulcerative colitis (Fig. 4-5). Gen-

eral weakening of tissues by steroid therapy has also been incriminated (82).

Performance of a barium enema through a colostomy, particularly examination of a distal defunctionalized loop, presents certain unique hazards (34,43,68,69,82). Colostomies are placed in portions of the colon less distensible than the rectal ampulla. As a result, inflation of a balloon within the colon adjacent to a colostomy is more likely to result in a tear. Examination of a defunctionalized loop via a colostomy is unusually hazardous in that such loops have generally assumed a small diameter and temporarily lost their normal distensibility.

Consequences. The course of events following perforation of the colon during barium enema is largely dictated by the site of the perforation and whether the barium makes its way into the peritoneal cavity, the retroperitoneal tissues, or the wall of the colon itself. With double-contrast enemas there is the unique possibility of massive quantities of air entering the peritoneum, retroperitoneal tissues, or both (Fig. 4-6) (36,80).

Barium peritonitis occurs when feces-contaminated barium suspension flows into the peritoneal cavity. This complication has a high fatality rate if not promptly and properly managed (88–92). The usual treatment is laparotomy with diverting colostomy, repair or resection of the ruptured colon segment, lavage of the peritoneal cavity, and administration of fluids and antibiotics.

Diagnosis of the extracolonic presence of bar-

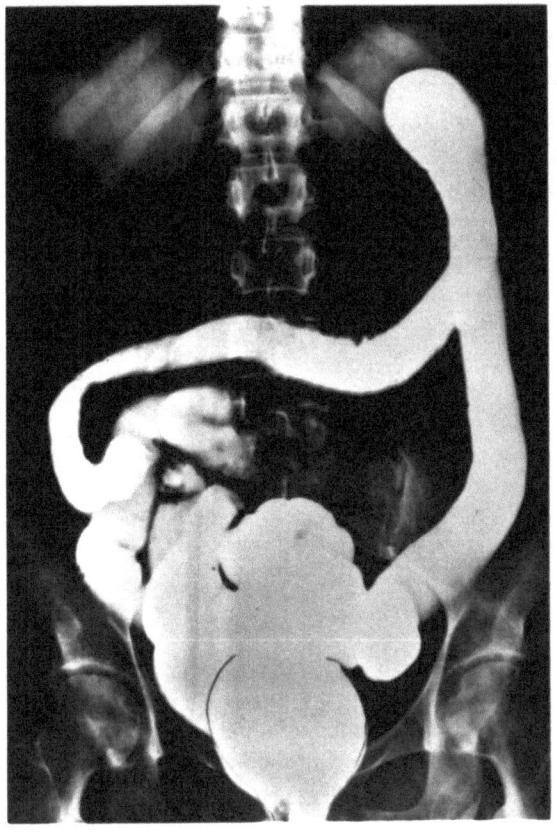

a

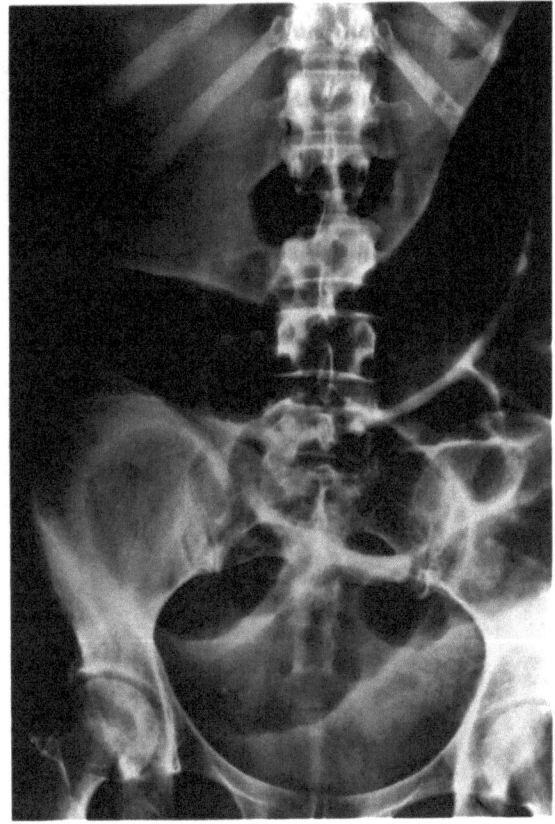

b

Fig. 4-5, a and b. Barium enema associated with development of toxic megacolon in acute ulcerative colitis. a Barium enema study shows ahaustral colon with atypically large rectum. **b** Toxic megacolon is seen 6 days later. (Courtesy of I. Meschan, MD, Winston-Salem, North Carolina)

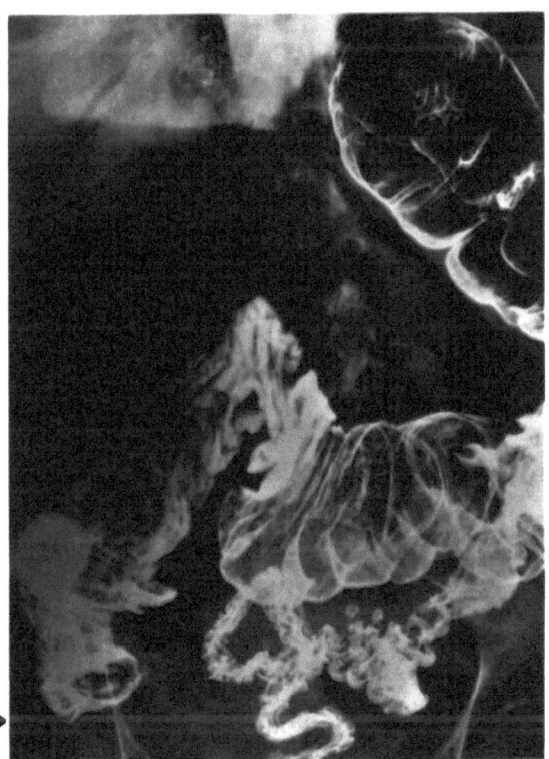

Fig. 4-6. Perforation of colon during double-contrast ▶ enema. Large quantities of air escaped from the colon into the retroperitoneal and peritoneal spaces.

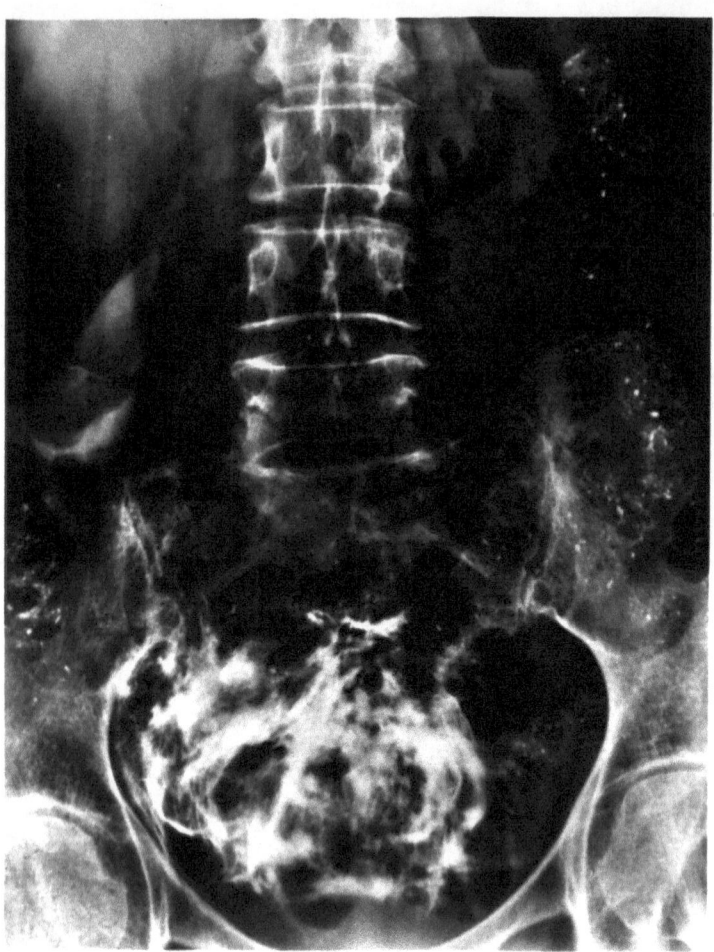

Fig. 4-7. Barium in peritoneal cavity, outlining bowel loops, and in retroperitoneal tissues 3 years after perforation of colon during barium enema. The perforation was not recognized at the time of the examination, and no specific treatment was ever instituted. The extracolonic presence of barium was detected on this film.

ium is less certain than one might suspect. Many cases are reported in which extravasation of barium—peritoneal, extraperitoneal, or intramural—was not diagnosed at the time of fluoroscopy (Fig. 4-7). In peritoneal spillage sudden cardiovascular collapse may occur several hours later, apparently due to loss of extracellular fluid components into the peritoneal cavity. The colon itself is relatively insensitive to forms of pain other than those caused by stretching or distention, and laceration or rupture may be totally undetected by the patient. The presence of barium in the peritoneum or extraperitoneal spaces also may be unaccompanied by any particular initial discomfort.

The first severe effect of barium peritonitis is hypovolemia, which occurs after several hours, from massive exudation of serum components into the peritoneal space (88,91). If the patient survives and surgical intervention and administration of antibiotics are not undertaken, suppu-

rative peritonitis eventually becomes the dominant factor. This may progress to shock because of endotoxin effects (92). Eventually, the foreign body reaction which inevitably surrounds intraperitoneal barium sulfate particles ensures a severe fibrotic reaction in the area of any remaining barium sulfate.

Barium extravasation into interstitial tissues (Fig. 4-8), if extensive, has many of the same risks as barium peritonitis. The risk of severe infection due to fecal contamination of the extravasated barium is high. Barium sulfate particles in the interstitial tissues cause a foreign-body reaction that may result in any infection being difficult to eradicate and in severe fibrosis with strictures of the bowel and barium granuloma of the rectum (53,55,76–78).

Barium Enema after Endoscopy. Controversy exists over the timing of barium enemas after sigmoidoscopy or colonoscopy, particularly if a biopsy has been performed (72,93,94). It is prob-

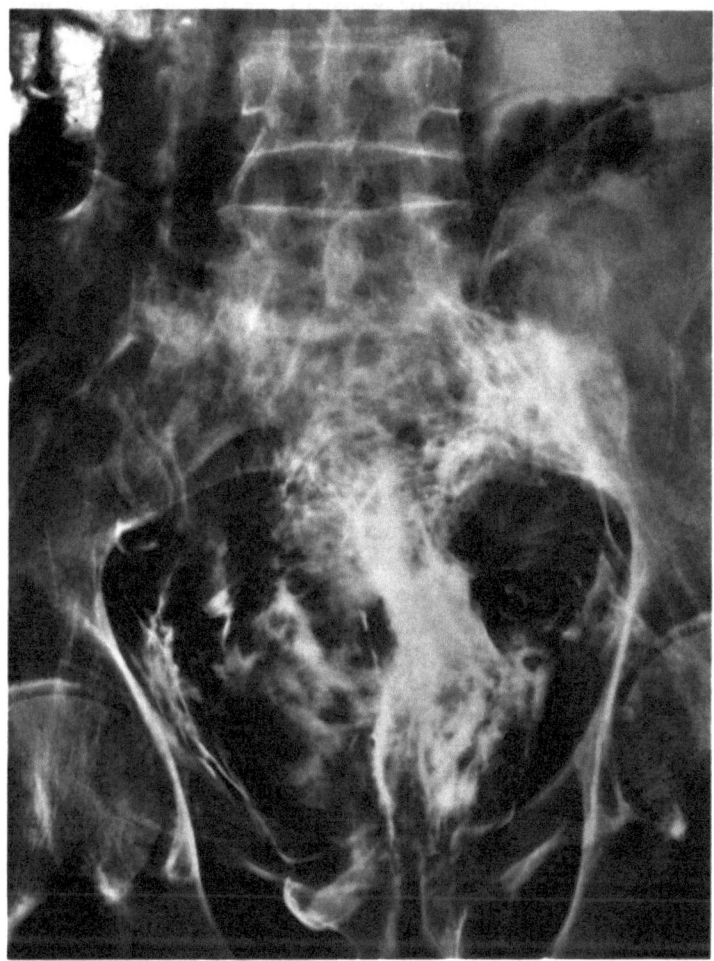

Fig. 4-8. Barium in retroperitoneal tissues after rectal perforation during barium enema. The streaky and granular appearance is typical of barium located interstitially.

able that a biopsy compromising the muscular layers predisposes the colon to perforation during barium enema, particularly if the biopsy location is above the peritoneal reflection. A sensible approach is to wait several days or a week if possible, since moderate healing of the biopsy site will occur during that interval.

Venous Intravasation

The most lethal complication of a barium enema is venous intravasation (43,95–97). In most reported cases, barium made its way via the inferior mesenteric veins and inferior vena cava to the heart and pulmonary circulation. The resulting massive pulmonary embolism has usually been fatal. In two cases, however, recovery was reported, with no residual cardiovascular symptoms. In another case a liver abscess developed, implying intravasation into the portal venous system (96). This patient also survived.

Vaginal Perforation

Inadvertent insertion of an enema tip into the vagina carries many of the same risks outlined above (43,98). In all cases of vaginal rupture during barium enema recorded to date, a balloon catheter was employed. Several have resulted in fatality, most commonly from venous intravasation.

Water Intoxication

Since the barium suspensions used for most barium enemas consist mainly of water and are quite hypotonic, the danger of water intoxication is inherent (48,99–101). The typical history is retention of the barium enema or tap-water cleansing enema. The colonic mucosa is capable of absorbing water efficiently, and the result may be hyponatremia and eventual cerebral edema (102). Children with Hirschsprung's disease are particularly susceptible to this complication (100).

Tannic Acid Toxicity

To promote evacuation of the colon and enhance coating of the evacuated colon with barium, tannic acid was used for many years in both cleansing enemas and barium enemas (103). Its use was considered safe until reports in the early 1960s of fatal liver damage from tannic acid toxicity (104,105). Subsequently animal and human investigations confirmed that tannic acid is absorbed from the colonic mucosa and is capable of damaging both the liver and the kidneys (106–108). The degree of organ damage is dependent upon the concentration of tannic acid employed and the time it is retained in the colon.

In contrast, others have found no evidence that tannic acid presents a danger (109), particularly if its concentration does not exceed 1.0% (110) or 0.25% (111). Nevertheless, the sale of pure tannic acid for use in barium enemas or cleansing enemas was banned by the U.S. Food and Drug Administration.

Portal Venous Gas

The performance of barium enemas, both single contrast and double contrast, has been associated with the appearance of portal venous gas in the liver (112–113). In all cases the patients have had either granulomatous colitis or ulcerative colitis and have recovered without significant morbidity. Compromise of the mucosal integrity in these cases may allow air within the colon to enter portal venous channels.

Bacteremia Due to Barium Enema

Routine barium enema as a cause of bacteremia has been documented (114–115). However, this finding is contradicted by investigations unable to demonstrate bacteremia after barium enema (116). Nevertheless, its occurrence during other manipulative procedures, such as sigmoidoscopy and colonoscopy (117), suggests that the hazard is indeed real, although self-limited. There is no evidence that the transient bacteremia induced warrants special measures except in highly susceptible individuals.

Impaction of Barium

Since barium administered during enema may become impacted, it is common practice to avoid instilling significant quantities proximal to a severely constricting tumor or other stricture of the colon. Impaction is particularly likely when the colon proximal to the lesion is filled with feces. Then the admixture of barium particles and fecal material may become progressively dehydrated into a rock-hard mass.

Silicone Foam Enema

A unique approach to the diagnosis of distal colon tumors was advocated for a time and involved production of semisolid silicone foam in the distal colon and rectum, the reaction producing the foam taking place within the colon itself (118–120). The foam cast yielded negative impressions visible at points where polypoid or circumferential tumors existed. Colonic contraction was allowed to expel the foam cast. Suspicious areas could be brushed for histologic sampling to confirm the presence of cancer. Unfortunately perforation of the colon resulted as a complication of retention of the foam cast (121). Because of its apparent danger and its limitation to diagnosis only in the distal colon the procedure has fallen from use.

Water-Soluble Contrast Enemas

Occasionally it is necessary to perform diagnostic enemas with water-soluble contrast materials. Most complications are related to the hypertonicity of the commonly used contrast agents, which have been described in detail in earlier portions of this chapter. A specific danger of water-soluble contrast enemas is hypernatremic dehydration (122–123).

Laxatives and Preparatory Enemas

The vigorous catharsis required for preparatory cleansing of the colon for barium enema carries the danger of dehydration of the patient due to the resulting diarrhea. Accordingly, virtually all currently advocated barium enema preparations suggest compensatory hydration of the patient. Further dangers of cleansing enemas are those of water intoxication due to retention of a voluminous hypotonic enema, colitis caused by a soapsuds enema (124–125), thermal burn of the colon (Fig. 4-9), laceration of the rectum by an improperly inserted enema tip, and rupture of the colon due to excess pressure or volume. Finally, vigorous catharsis and administration of large enemas are contraindicated in patients with severe ulcerative or granulomatous colitis.

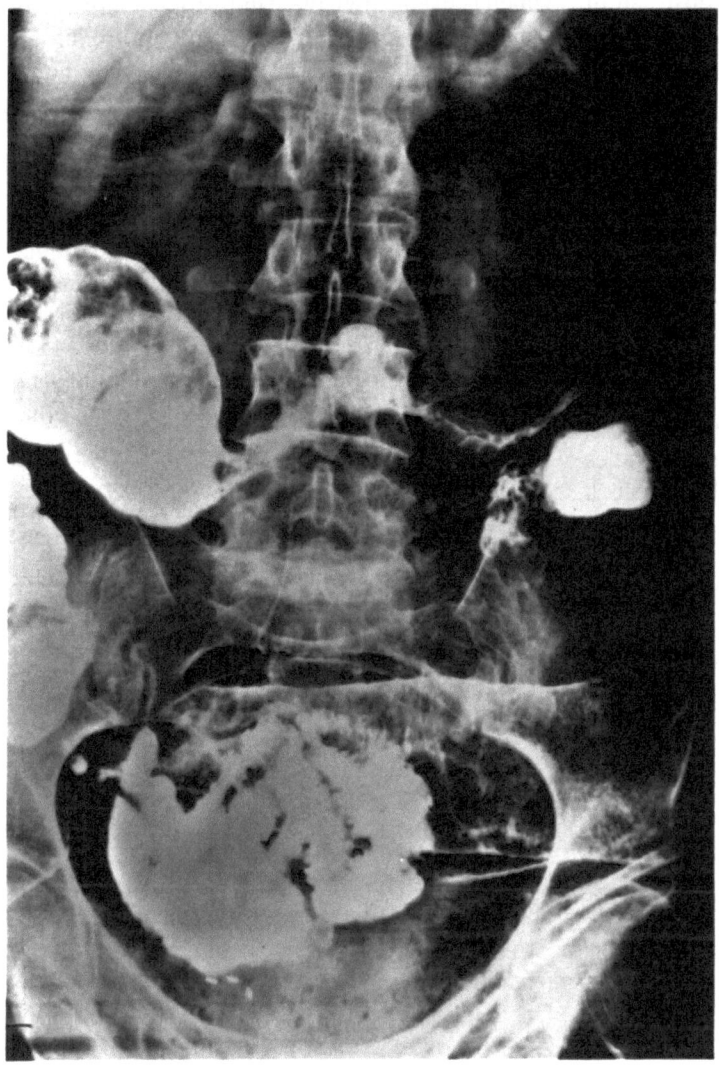

Fig. 4-9. Thermal burn of the colon following cleansing enema administered through a colostomy. Irregular stenosis of the colon has resulted.

Complications of Radiologic Procedures Related to the Biliary Tract

Oral Cholecystography

Iopanoic acid (Telepaque) remains the most widely used contrast medium for gallbladder studies; over 40 million doses have been given (126). Other cholecystographic agents used in the United States include sodium tyropanoate (Bilopaque), ipodate sodium (Oragrafin), and iocetamic acid (Cholebrine). All are based on the triiodinated benzene ring.

Minor Reactions to Oral Cholecystographic Agents

The oral cholecystographic agents are relatively innocuous, with serious side effects occurring rarely. Minor reactions, however, have a reported incidence of 3%–57%, including most commonly nausea and vomiting, as well as abdominal cramping, diarrhea, dysuria, headache, and skin rash (127–132).

Major Reactions to Oral Cholecystographic Agents

As mentioned, serious or life-threatening reactions are distinctly rare. Major reactions include anaphylactic shock, cardiovascular complications, hepatorenal toxicity, and overdose, all of which may cause death. Anaphylactic shock is rare; its incidence has been reported to be 1/600,000 doses of ipodate sodium (133).

Renal toxicity has been the most frequent serious reaction to oral cholecystographic agents. The etiology is not clear (134–143). Most patients have had no underlying renal disease. Certainly factors that promote high blood levels of contrast agent would appear to be important. These include excessive dosage, enhanced gastrointestinal absorption, and decreased hepatic clearance caused by liver derangement (134,-135,138,139,143). Other proposed mechanisms include a direct toxic effect on the renal tubules (137,142), crystalluria with intratubular block (137,138), and constriction of the preglomerular vessels with subsequent renal ischemia (135,-136). The last could be further potentiated by dehydration, leading to hypovolemia and hypotension. More recently a potent uricosuric effect of these agents has been noted, and intratubular uric acid precipitation may play a role (144). However, direct evidence for this hypothesis is lacking.

Massive overdoses have been reported, the largest amount being 75 g of iopanoic acid accidentally ingested without permanent ill effects (145). On the other hand, death from overdose has been reported. Fortunately fatal reactions from routine oral cholecystography are almost nonexistent. In an extensive review by Shehadi in 1966, only 7 deaths in 22 million doses of Telepaque were noted; 4 resulted from renal damage, while 1 each was related to myocardial insufficiency, hepatic disease, and overdose (133).

Intravenous Cholangiography

In 1954 meglumine iodipamide (Cholografin; Squibb, USA) was introduced as a radiographic contrast material for intravenous cholangiography. The compound is a dimer composed of two triiodinated benzoate rings interconnected by a polymethylene chain. Iodipamide meglumine is a relatively strong dibasic acid and is highly soluble in aqueous solution.

Other cholangiographic agents have been developed but are either not available in the United States or undergoing extensive clinical trials. These include ioglycamide (Biligram), which is used extensively in Europe, iodoxamate (Cholovue), and most recently iotroxamide (147). All of these newer compounds are chemically similar to Cholografin except for variations in the interconnecting polymethylene chain.

Minor Reactions to Cholografin

When compared to the reactions to urographic contrast agents, minor and major reactions to Cholografin are more frequent (148). Minor reactions, varying from 4.1% to 23.9% (149–151), have primarily included nausea and vomiting and skin reactions. Use of a test dose has been of no value in predicting either minor or serious reactions (152). However, several factors have been shown to decrease the frequency of reactions to Cholografin: (1) use of a single dose (i.e., 20 cc of Cholografin) (151); (2) slow infusion rate (i.e., 10 min or more) (148,151); and (3) use of an antihistamine (149,150); controversy remains, however, regarding the overall value of premedication (152). Johnson and Wise observed an increased reaction rate in dehydrated and fasting patients (149).

Major Reactions to Cholografin

More serious reactions to iodipamide are infrequent and include more severe cutaneous reactions, cardiorespiratory manifestations, hypotension, hepatorenal toxicity, and anaphylaxis. Death has been observed in 1 of 3000–5000 cases (148, 153). Pretesting is of no value in predicting either major or lethal reactions. Furthermore, premedication with antihistamines or steroids has no proven effect on preventing major reactions or death.

Liver damage has occurred rarely. Current evidence would indicate that iodipamide is a predictable, albeit infrequent, hepatotoxin (154,155).

Renal failure may rarely follow the use of Cholografin (141,156–158). The pathogenesis remains unknown, but current considerations include: (1) a dose-related phenomenon (158); (2) simultaneous administration of other contrast agents; (3) direct effect on the kidney due to either tubular toxicity or preglomerular vasoconstriction; (4) contribution of enhanced uric acid excretion (142,159) and possibility of urate nephropathy; and (5) other less well understood factors such as protein binding.

Endoscopic Retrograde Cholangiopancreatography

Endoscopic retrograde cholangiopancreatography (ERCP) has become a widely used procedure for evaluating suspected biliary tract and pancreatic disease. Complications include not only those of routine upper gastrointestinal endoscopy but also problems arising from the cannulation and injection of the biliary and pancreatic ductal systems (160–166). The reported rate of symptomatic complications has been 0.6%–5.0% (163,166). A low mortality of 0–0.2% has been observed and reflects the relative safety of the procedure (162,163). Fatalities have resulted primarily from cholangitis with sepsis, pancreatic sepsis, and pseudocyst injection and less frequently from instrument injury.

Hyperamylasemia

A transient asymptomatic rise in serum amylase occurs frequently and is nearly always related to injection of the pancreatic duct.

Pancreatitis

The most common clinically important complication of ERCP, pancreatitis has been observed in 0.5%–1.3% of cases (160,163). Typically there is epigastric pain associated with an increase in serum and urinary amylase. The disorder is usually mild and self-limiting. More severe forms of hemorrhagic or necrotizing pancreatitis, including fatality, have been sporadically reported (167,168).

Pancreatitis occurs only after successful injection of the pancreatic duct and presumably relates to overdistention of the ductal system. Although the exact pathogenesis is unknown, proposals have included parenchymal acinarization (Fig. 4-10), ductal rupture, and pancreatic enzyme activation. Close fluoroscopic monitoring has been recommended to prevent ductal overfilling and excessive parenchymal opacification (161,169,170).

Pseudocyst Abscess and Sepsis

The incidence of sepsis following pancreatography is 0.3% in the survey by Bilbao et al. (161).

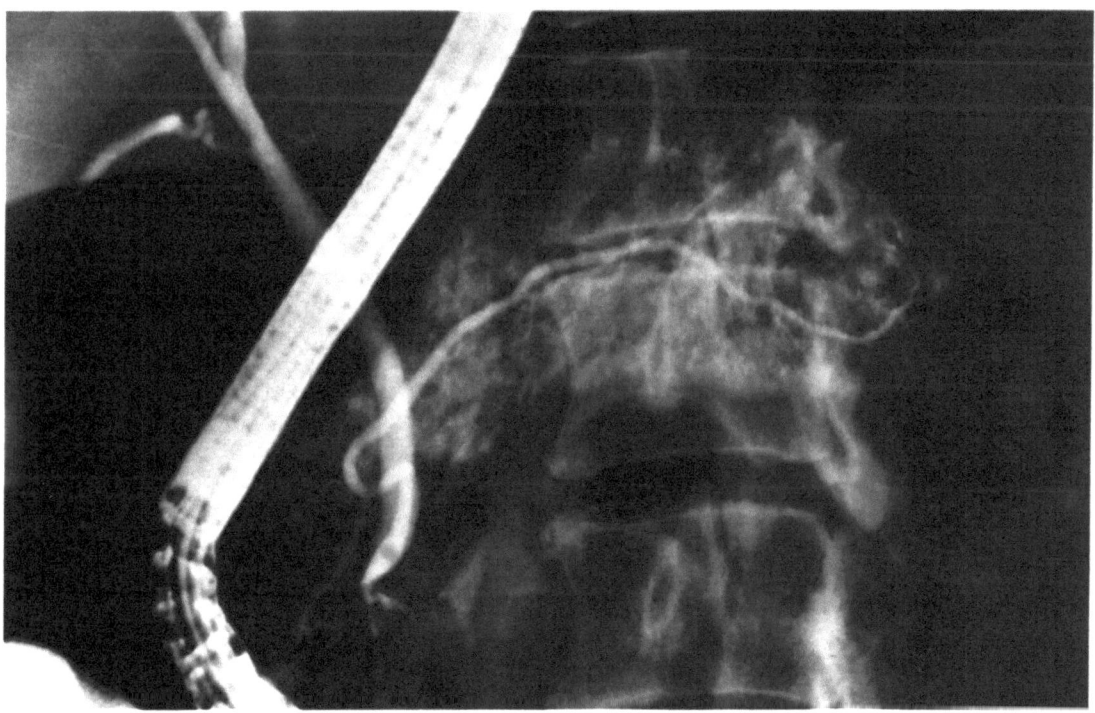

Fig. 4-10. Pancreatic acinarization from ductal overfilling during ERCP. Chemical or less commonly clinical pancreatitis may result from this situation. Careful fluoroscopic monitoring of ductal filling helps to avoid this problem.

Of 25 patients with pancreatic sepsis, 8 had pancreatic ductal obstruction, and 17 developed an abscess following pseudocyst injection. Mortality in this group of patients was 20%. The 17 pseudocyst abscesses developed from a total of 193 injected pseudocysts, an incidence of 8.8%. Thus, although injection of a pancreatic pseudocyst is a potentially serious complication (Fig. 4-11), the risk is not as great as previously believed (161,165,171,172). Therefore suspicion of a pancreatic pseudocyst is not an absolute contraindication to ERCP, but the following precautions have been suggested: (1) avoid complete filling of a pseudocyst discovered at pancreatography; (2) provide antibiotic coverage; (3) consider prompt operative drainage.

Cholangitis with Sepsis

This was noted in 72 cases (0.8%) by Bilbao et al. with a corresponding mortality of 11% (8 of 72) (161). Obstruction of ducts was present in 90% of these patients and in all 8 patients who died. A similar incidence of cholangitis (0.6%) was noted by Nebel et al. with a fatality rate of 8% (2 of 25) (160). Importantly, this complication did not occur in the presence of a normal biliary

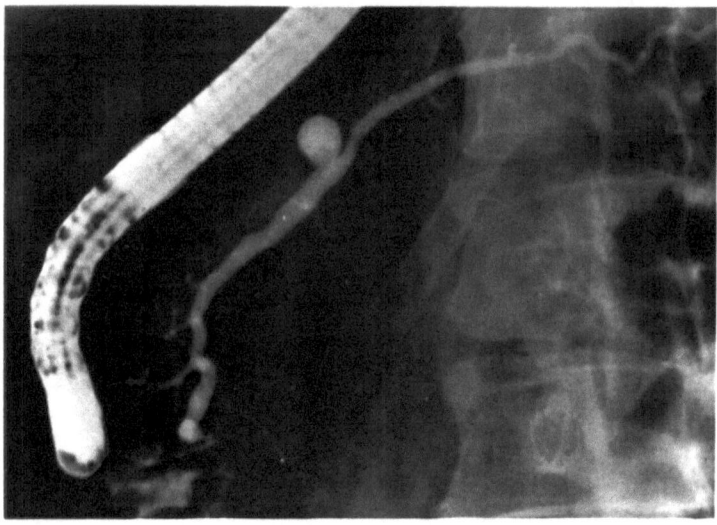

a

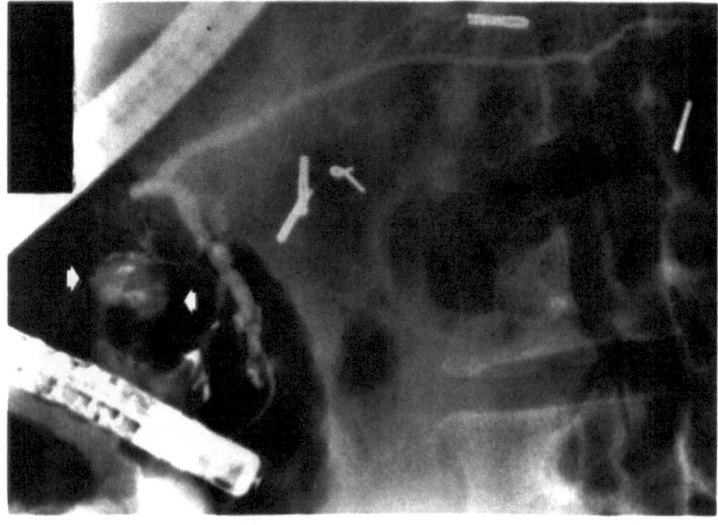

b

Fig. 4-11, a and b. Injection of pancreatic pseudocyst.

a A small pseudocyst fills off midportion of main pancreatic duct in a patient with recurrent pancreatitis. The cyst remained stable in size on repeated examinations, and no serious complications resulted. (Stewart ET, Vennes JA, Geenen JE: Atlas of Endoscopic Retrograde Cholangiopancreatography. St. Louis: Mosby 1977. Used by permission of Edward Stewart, MD, and the publisher)

b A cystic space near the head of the pancreas (arrows) is partially filled in another patient with acute pancreatitis. Because of the risk of inducing pancreatic sepsis, further filling of the pseudocyst was not attempted. (Courtesy of Edward Stewart, MD, Milwaukee, Wisconsin)

tract. Thus cholangitis with sepsis has been the most common cause of death resulting from ERCP.

The pathogenesis of cholangitis following ERCP remains unknown. Certainly stasis from an obstructed biliary tract is nearly always present. This, associated with preexisting infection in the biliary tree or possibly the introduction of pathogens via ductal cannulation, could contribute to the development of cholangitis and sepsis (173,174). The following precautions have been suggested to reduce the risk of septic cholangitis: (1) avoid overfilling of the biliary tree when obstruction is found; (2) provide antibiotic coverage; (3) consider prompt surgical drainage; (4) use clean endoscopic instruments; and (5) use sterile contrast solutions.

Instrument Injury

Problems related to instrumentation occur infrequently. In two large surveys (12,565 examinations) of ERCP complications a total of 22 (0.18%) injuries caused by instrumentation was tabulated (160,161). These included 13 extraluminal injections due to faulty cannulation, 6 perforations, and 3 gastrointestinal bleeding. Submucosal or intramural injection of contrast material was rarely a serious complication. On the other hand, 1 patient in 6 with bowel perforation and 1 patient in 3 with bleeding died. Certainly experience, careful cannulation of the papilla of Vater, and fluoroscopic monitoring of the injection reduce the potential hazards for mechanical injury.

Reactions to Contrast Media

Although both minor and serious reactions to commonly used analgesic and hypotonic drugs have occurred during ERCP, contrast media reactions have been virtually absent. Sterile urographic contrast agents (50%–76%) are generally employed. Both undiluted and diluted solutions (25%–30%) should be available, the latter being used in the presence of dilated ducts.

Transhepatic Cholangiography

Percutaneous transhepatic cholangiography (PTC) is a valuable procedure in differentiating cholestatic jaundice from extrahepatic obstructive jaundice and in localizing the site and nature of the obstruction. Traditionally patients were operated upon immediately after the procedure if biliary obstruction was found (175–177). Innovations in technique, particularly spearheaded by introduction of the Chiba (Japanese) needle, have created a renewed interest in PTC.

Non-Chiba-Needle Techniques

Preceding introduction of the Chiba needle the major improvement in technique for percutaneous cholangiography was the use of sheathed needles in which the nonflexible portion was removed immediately after insertion into the liver, leaving the flexible catheter in place (178–180). Both cholangiography and temporary biliary drainage were possible. Complications decreased, particularly in cases of obstruction, when temporary use of biliary drainage and prompt surgical relief of obstruction were found to be important.

The major complications included bile leakage and bile peritonitis, intraperitoneal hemorrhage, sepsis (181), formation of various types of intrahepatic fistula (182), and hemobilia (183). Death also occurred. Other less common problems included puncture of a hollow viscus such as the gallbladder, pneumothorax, and subphrenic or subhepatic abscess formation. Reactions to contrast media have been nearly nonexistent.

The overall complication rate with the sheath systems has been 3.8%–12.7% (178,179) and the mortality 0.25%–0.5% (177,184). Nearly all of the morbidity and mortality occurred in patients with obstruction of the biliary tract, often due to inoperable neoplasms.

Bile extravasation and, less frequently, bile peritonitis are the most common complications of sheath-needle cholangiography. The reported incidence is 1.9%–6.9% (179,184,185). Nearly all patients with these complications have had biliary tract obstruction requiring external drainage or operative intervention.

Steps recommended to reduce the incidence and hazards of bile leakage and peritonitis include: (1) aspiration of bile in the presence of obstruction, (2) use of the cholangiographic catheter to drain and decompress the biliary tract, (3) use of broad-spectrum antibiotics, and (4) prompt surgical intervention. Major precautions to prevent hemorrhage are: (1) exclusion of the presence of a bleeding diathesis, (2) correction of abnormal bleeding values, and (3) routine performance of clotting tests such as the prothrombin time. In fact, the last is an absolute prerequisite to PTC regardless of technique. Systemic antibiotic coverage is warranted when obstruction is shown. Indeed, prophylactic administration of antibiotics has been suggested in all patients having PTC (176).

Chiba-Needle Cholangiography

With introduction of the Chiba needle from Japan increased enthusiasm for percutaneous cholangiography has emerged. The so-called Chiba, Japanese, or skinny needle is a flexible thin needle that has simplified diagnostic evaluation of jaundice. More recently the development of external biliary drainage methods following percutaneous cholangiography has expanded the technique into a therapeutic role (186,187).

A major reason for enthusiasm over Chiba-needle cholangiography is the ability of the technique to opacify not only dilated but also normal-caliber biliary tracts. The success rate in visualizing a dilated ductal system averages 97%, while nondilated ducts can be opacified 73% of the time (188–194). Indeed, inability to opacify the biliary tree in an icteric patient has been used as a criterion for diagnosis of nonobstructive jaundice.

The complications reported with skinny-needle cholangiography are similar in kind to those discussed above with the sheath-needle techniques (188–197). The overall complication rate has been 4%–13%, with most large series being under 10% (188–195). Complications occur almost solely in those patients with obstructive jaundice. In 1662 cases collected by us from the literature (188–195), only 1 death (from sepsis) was recorded, a remarkably low mortality of 0.06%.

Fever and bacteremia were the most common important complications, with an incidence of 2.5%. Cholangitis and sepsis occurred in 1.1% of patients, and a 1.8% incidence of bile leakage and peritonitis was noted. Hemorrhage resulted infrequently (0.3%). Nearly all of these complications occurred in patients with obstruction of the biliary tree. Indeed, the rarity of deleterious effects following skinny-needle cholangiography in the presense of normal bile ducts has made surgical standby unnecessary. The same precautions and recommendations discussed above with the sheath-needle systems for lessening the hazards in those with biliary obstruction apply here.

Operative and T-Tube Cholangiography

Mirizzi is given credit for first performing operative cholangiography in 1932 (198). Since then, wide experience indicates that adverse effects due to operative cholangiography are extremely rare (199). Potential problems include liver damage or abscess formation, sepsis, pancreatitis, and contrast reactions. Despite these possibilities, Schulenburg (200), in reviewing 1000 personal cases, reported complete absence of complications and stated that no definite contraindication exists to performing the procedure.

T-tube cholangiography also has little hazard (198,199). Potential problems include pain with injection, nausea and vomiting, fever, cholangitis and sepsis in obstructed biliary tracts, pancreatitis, and contrast reactions. Except for occasional pain and infrequent nausea, these adverse effects are extremely rare.

Nonoperative Extraction of Biliary Tract Stones

Nonsurgical methods have been developed for removing residual stones from the biliary tract following cholecystectomy.

Mazzariello has reported extensive personal experience with a variety of extraction instruments, primarily different types of forceps, in 570 patients (201). A successful extraction rate of 95.3% was achieved with an overall complication incidence of 9.7%. No deaths were reported.

In the early 1970s Burhenne developed an additional method for removal of residual stones via the T-tube tract (202,203). Using a steerable catheter system and wire basket he achieved results similar to those of the forceps technique. Stone extraction with this method has been 95% successful, although more than one attempt has been required in up to 36% of patients. In 717 patients compiled from the reports of Burhenne (204) and Garrow (205), the incidence of complications has been 4.9%. Although creation of a false sinus tract was noted in 1.3% of cases (Fig. 4-12), no bile duct perforations have occurred. Most important, no deaths have been reported.

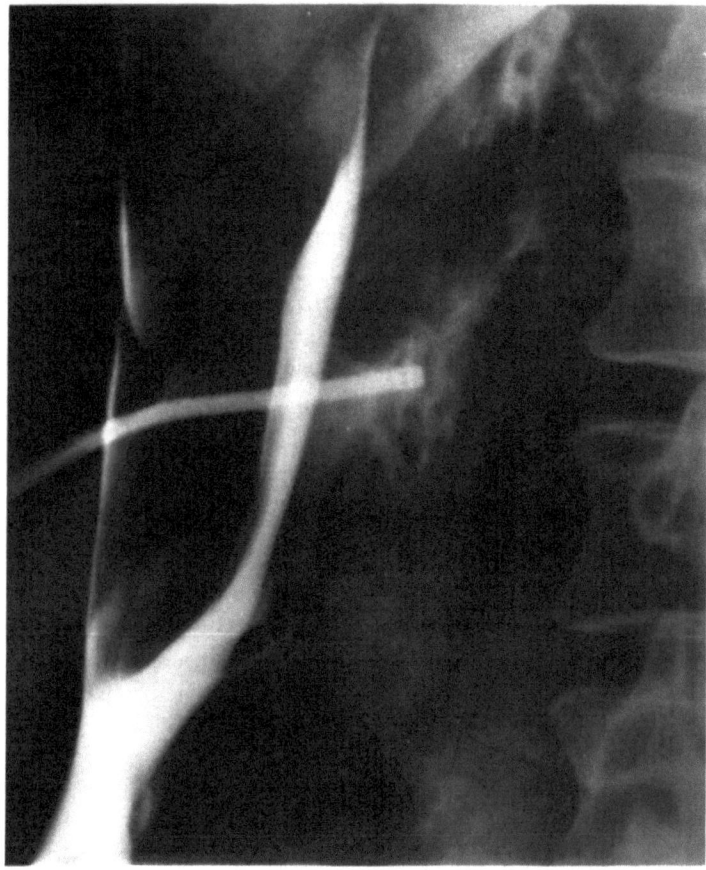

Fig. 4-12. Sinus tract perforation following removal of retained common-duct stone. Intraperitoneal extravasation has occurred with contrast medium outlining the hepatic angle and extending down the right paracolic gutter. The patient had no apparent complications. (Burhenne HJ: Complications of nonoperative extraction of retained common duct stones. Am J Surg 131:260–262, 1976)

Complications of Diagnostic and Interventional Angiographic Procedures

Angiography has firmly established itself as a diagnostic procedure in the evaluation of many diseases. Interventional techniques include transcatheter embolization and transcatheter infusion of vasoactive or chemotherapeutic agents. These procedures are increasingly popular in management of gastrointestinal bleeding and therapy of neoplasms. Both diagnostic and interventional procedures have morbidity and mortality that have been the subject of investigation and review. Extensive data are available on complications of catheter angiography, translumbar aortography, and splenoportography. Information is sporadic and anecdotal for other procedures.

By convention, any complication occurring within 48 hours of a vascular study is regarded as secondary to that procedure (206); complications may be classified as minor, serious, and fatal (207). A minor complication results in no significant alteration in therapy or hospitalization, whereas a major complication is accompanied by a threat to life, limb, or visceral integrity. Examples of a minor complication include small hemorrhages at the puncture site and temporary vascular spasm. Arterial thrombosis is the most common major complication. Current data confirm the overall safety of these procedures, indicating serious complications of catheter angiography or translumbar aortography of less than 1.0%, with fatalities extremely rare (207–209).

It is convenient to classify these complications as: (1) complications of percutaneous catheter and translumbar angiography in general; (2) complications peculiar to diagnostic angiography of the gastrointestinal tract; and (3) complications of interventional procedures.

Catheter Angiography and Translumbar Aortography in General

Reactions to Intravascular Contrast Agents

An ideal intravascular contrast agent should blend high opacity, low viscosity, and low toxicity. This is best approximated by the currently employed sodium and methylglucamine salts of iothalamate and diatrizoate. The relative safety of these media over former agents is well established (210). However, their use is infrequently associated with minor, serious, or even fatal complications and side effects: nausea; vomiting; flushing; urticaria; transient; usually inconsequential, alterations in blood pressure; renal dysfunction; angioneurotic edema; and cardiovascular collapse (209–214).

The most common serious contrast-related complication is renal dysfunction. Recent data suggest an incidence of 10%–12% following angiographic studies (212,213). Although usually self-limited, a significant minority progress to severe renal failure. The etiologic basis is unclear, but prestudy dehydration is a likely factor in combination with a possible direct toxic effect of the contrast medium on the kidney. Patients particularly at risk are those with preexisting renal or hepatic insufficiency, hypertension, and diabetes mellitus.

Brief mention should be made of thorium dioxide (Thorotrast), an intravascular agent extensively used in the 1930s and 1940s for arteriography and hepatolienography. Visualization of the liver and spleen was possible because of localization of the contrast agent in those organs, as well as in the bone marrow and lymph nodes (Fig. 4-13). Its use was subsequently curtailed, however, because of its low-grade radioactivity and tendency to form indurations at the sites of injection (214). More significant has been its association with the late induction of hepatic tumors (hemangioendothelioma, cholangiocarcinoma, hepatoma), liver fibrosis, and fatal blood dyscrasias (215,216).

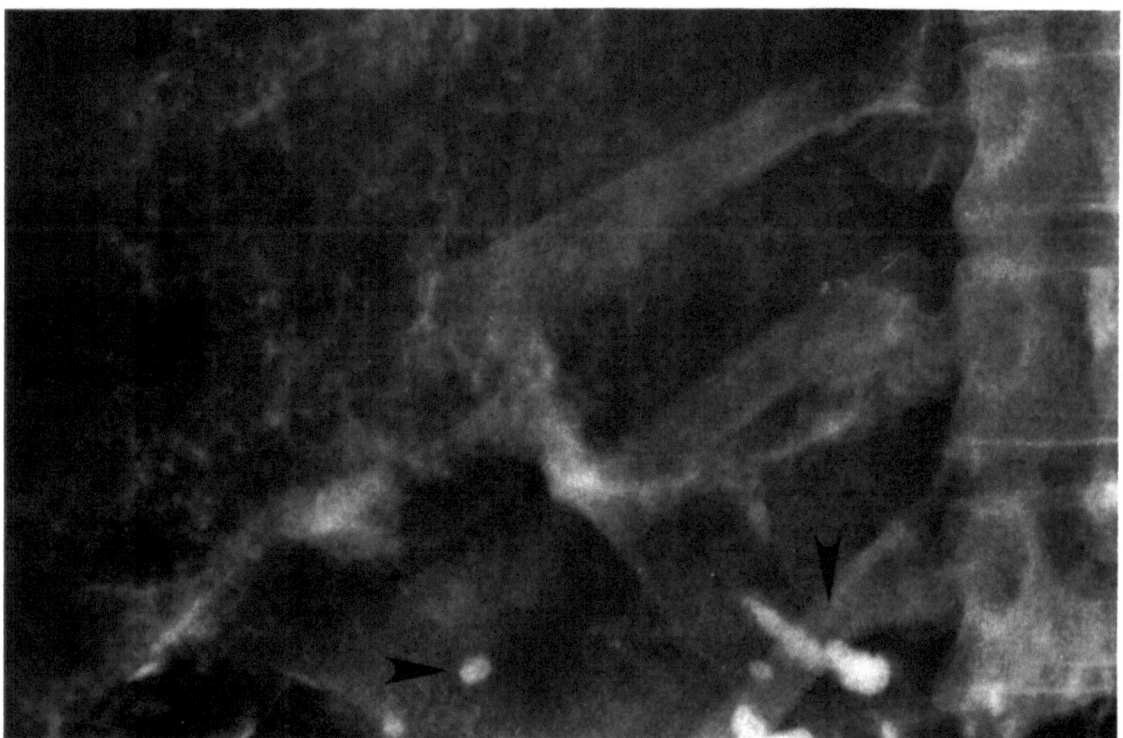

Fig. 4-13. Longstanding hepatic thorium dioxide. Plain film demonstrates lacy, reticulated appearance. Note migration of agent to regional lymph nodes *(arrowheads)*. (Courtesy of I. Meschan, MD)

Catheter Angiography

Angiographic catheterization in general entails risks of two types: (1) those at the site of puncture, and (2) those occurring elsewhere due to manipulation of the guide wire and catheter.

Complications occurring at the site of introduction of the catheter are the most frequent and include hematoma formation, local vascular thrombosis, delayed bleeding, local infection, arteriovenous fistulas, and pseudoaneurysm formation. Local hematoma formation is the most common, occurring in approximately 4% of transfemoral punctures (209) and 10% of transaxillary studies (217). Although usually inconsequential, compression of adjacent neurovascular structures can cause venous spasm and thrombophlebitis (206) and, in transaxillary angiography, compromise of the brachial plexus.

Thrombosis of the punctured vessel represents the most feared and most common serious local complication (218,219).

Complications due to manipulations of the guide wire or catheter or both are uncommon but include intimal injury (209,220,221) (Fig. 4-14), vascular dissection, vascular perforation (219) (Fig. 4-15), vascular spasm, embolism (207,219, 222–225), and breaking (219) or knotting (226) of guide wires and catheters. Embolizations are thought to result from fibrin debris formed on the catheter surface and subsequently stripped off during removal or exchange of the catheter (Fig. 4-16). Embolization may occur in selectively catheterized vessels from dislodged atheromatous material, clots within the catheter, cotton-fiber or glove-powder debris, and air from ill-fitting connections or improperly prepared injection syringes.

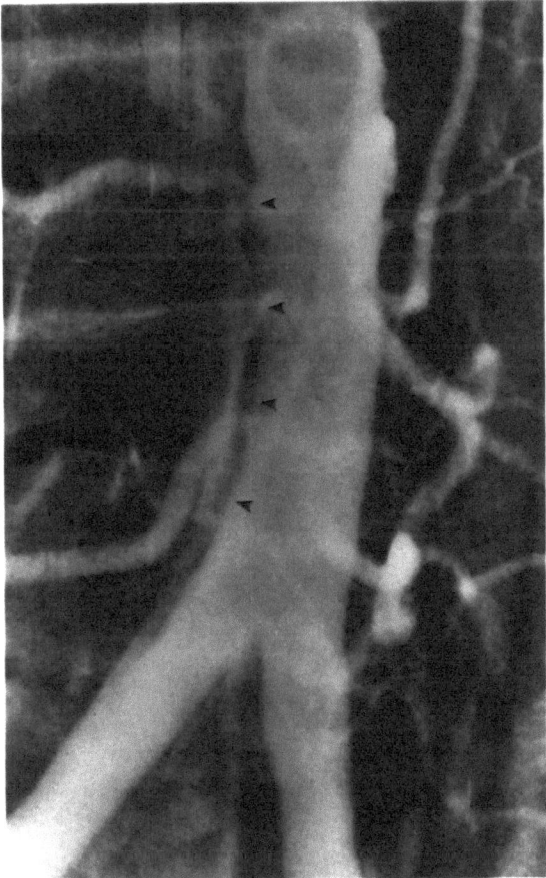

Fig. 4-14. Complication of catheter angiography. Abdominal aortogram shows intimal flap *(arrowheads)* projecting into lumen.

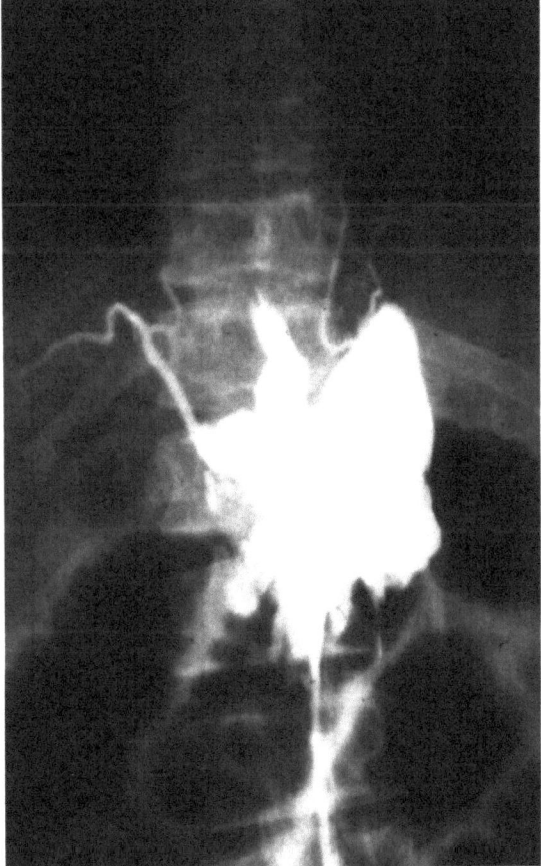

Fig. 4-15. Complication of catheter angiography. Perivascular injection occurred during attempted abdominal aortography. (Courtesy of V. D'Souza, MD)

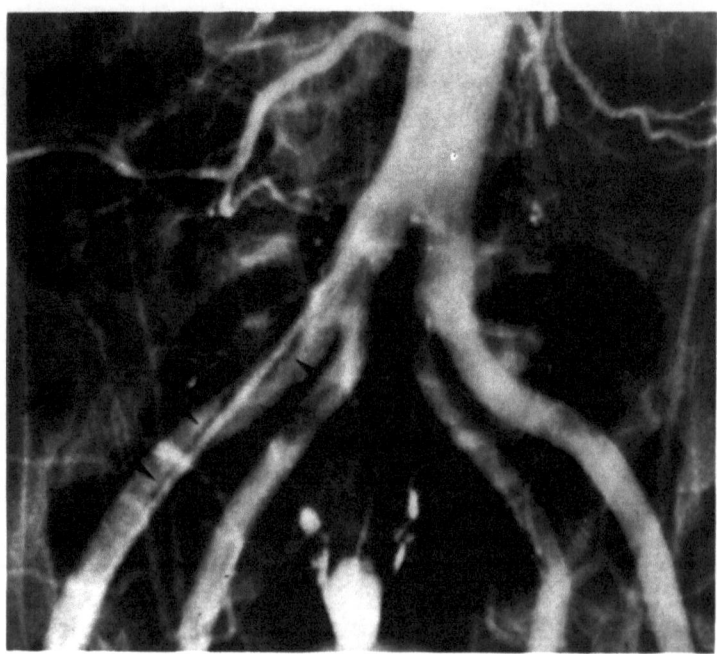

Fig. 4-16. Complication of catheter angiography. Pelvic angiogram demonstrates extensive thrombus buildup on outer surface of catheter *(arrowheads)* as outlined by contrast agent in catheter and vessel.

Translumbar Aortography

Although most gastrointestinal angiography is performed by selective catheter technique, translumbar aortography may be necessary in patients with advanced peripheral vascular disease. Despite the documented safety of this technique, systemic and local complications occasionally occur, but the present incidence of such complications is less than in earlier years.

The major complication has been spinal cord injury, with occasional paralysis. This unfortunate complication most often occurs with injection of an excessive volume of concentrated contrast medium into or about a major spinal feeding vessel. It is rare with the currently used, less neurotoxic contrast media (219).

Most complications associated with translumbar aortography are related to the local puncture and include retroperitoneal hemorrhage (227) (Fig. 4-17); intramural aortic injection (227,228); misdirection of the needle with injection of a neighboring organ, cavity, or vessel (227,228); and more rarely hemothorax, pneumothorax, chylothorax, and retroperitoneal infection.

Small retroperitoneal hemorrhages are usual following routine translumbar aortography, and it has been estimated that approximately 50 cc of blood is typically present about the site of the aortic puncture (229). Computed tomographic

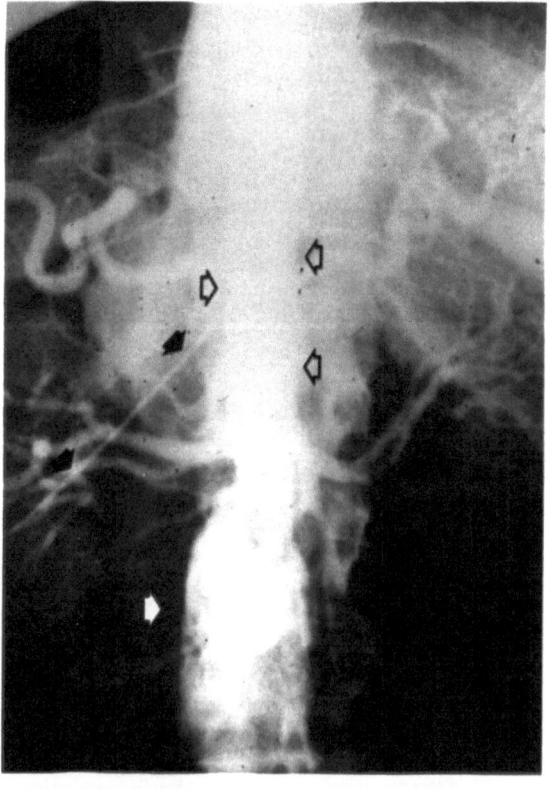

Fig. 4-17. Complication of translumbar aortography. Translumbar aortogram shows perivascular injection of contrast medium: *black arrowheads,* sheath; *open arrowheads,* normal aortic outline; *white arrowhead,* aortic aneurysm. (Courtesy of V. D'Souza, MD)

studies of the retroperitoneum following translumbar aortography have confirmed the presence of small, clinically inconsequential hematomas in the majority of cases (230,231) (Fig. 4-18). However, symptomatic retroperitoneal hematomas occur much less commonly (up to 0.2% [227]), and the majority are in patients with either hypertension or a hemorrhagic diathesis.

Intramural aortic injection and subintimal dissection are unusual with modern fluoroscopic guidance of the needle and are usually without clinical significance. Rarely such injections may result in formation of false extraluminal passages or occlusion of branch vessels (228).

Gastrointestinal Angiography in Particular

In addition to those complications inherent to angiography in general, selective visceral angiography, transhepatic portography, and splenoportography are associated with unique gastrointestinal complications. Translumbar aortography also may be associated with gastrointestinal complications despite its nonselective nature.

Selective Visceral Catheterization
Infrequently, selective gastrointestinal angiography is associated with complications other than those common to all angiographic procedures. The majority are related to the manipulations of the catheter and guide wire necessary for selective and superselective studies. Direct gastrointestinal complications include intimal vascular injury, vascular spasm, thromboembolism, and untoward effects of the contrast medium on the perfused viscera.

The most common gastrointestinal vascular complication of selective catheterization is intimal injury (209), the incidence of which significantly increases with progressively superselective catheterizations (221). These injuries are usually the result of direct damage to the vascular wall by the catheter tip, catheter recoil, or contrast jet. Following injection of contrast, intimal injuries are recognized as lingering, sharply demarcated subintimal accumulations of contrast material within or adjacent to the opacified vascular outline (Fig. 4-19).

The acute result of such injury is usually vascular occlusion. Immediate collateralization typically develops, as has been documented in acute mesenteric (232) and common hepatic arterial occlusions (233). However, in certain instances collaterals are not readily available, as in occlusion of the proper hepatic artery. Distal ischemia or infarction is then possible (233). Hepatic arterial injuries are potentially most harmful in patients with cirrhosis, as portal blood flow may already be diminished or reversed (209).

Most intimal lesions are of little consequence, but occasionally serious sequelae occur, particularly with injury of the superior or inferior mesenteric arteries. Injury of these vessels may be associated with residual damage and local aneurysm formation (209,221). The incidence of intimal injury, however, can be minimized by gentle manipulation of guide wires and catheters, use of flexible-tipped wires and end-hole-only cathe-

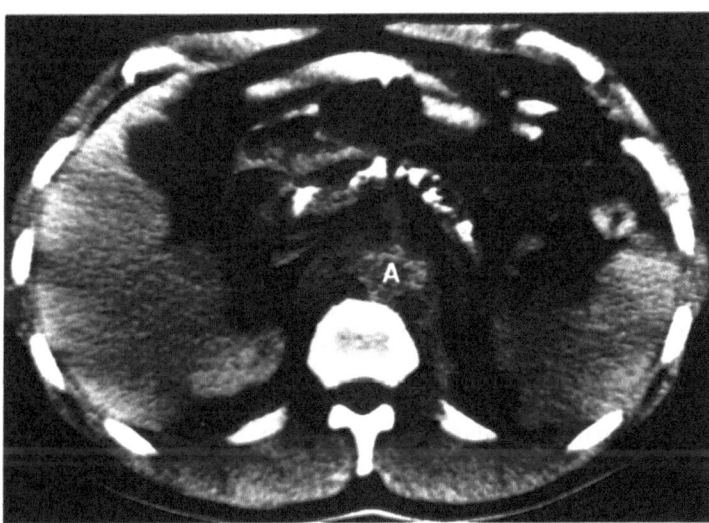

Fig. 4-18. Complication of translumbar aortography. Computed tomographic scan of aortic puncture site following translumbar aortography demonstrates nearly complete obliteration of aortic contour (*A*) and slight thickening of adjacent retrocrural space indicative of small retroperitoneal hematoma.

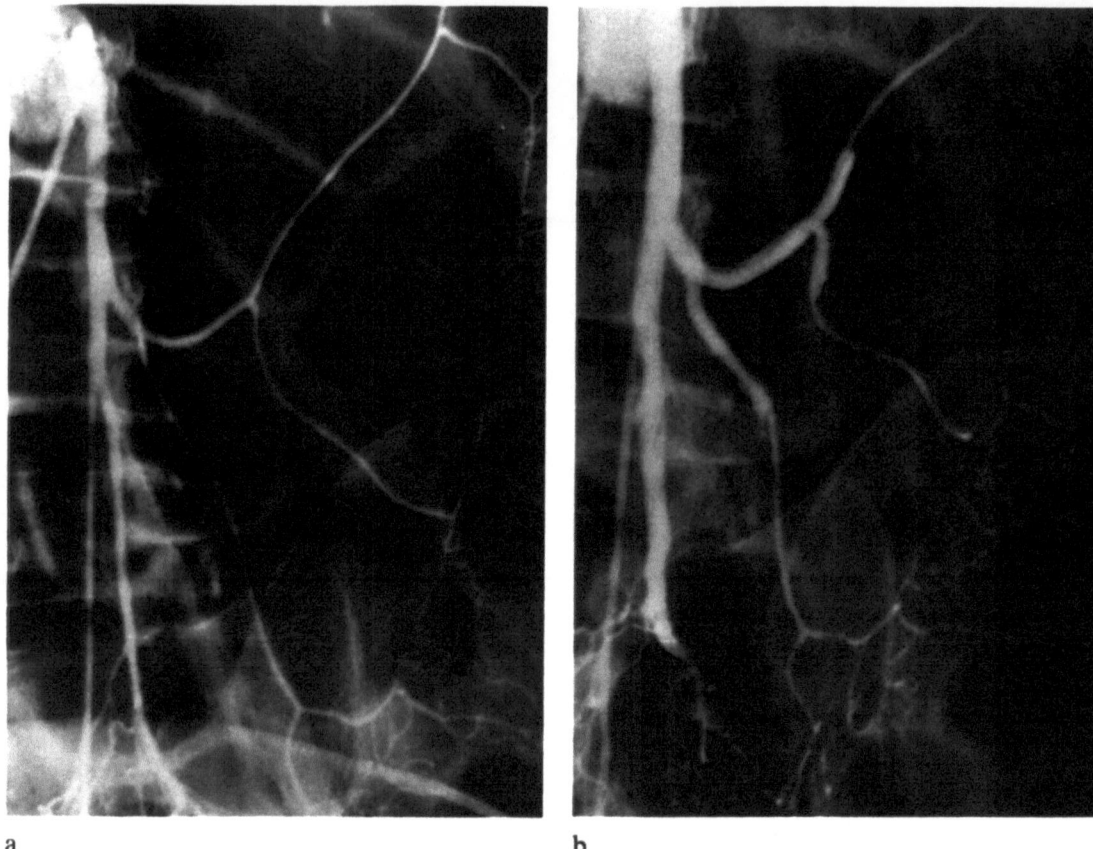

a   b

Fig. 4-19, a and **b. Complication of selective catheterization.** Inferior mesenteric arteriograms before (**a**) and after (**b**) extensive subintimal dissection by contrast medium. (Courtesy of V. D'Souza, MD)

ters, and prudent use of superselective angiography.

Vascular spasm represents a normal response of vascular contractile elements to stimulation of the wall by the catheter tip, guide wire, or contrast jet (234). Although usually inconsequential, severe spasm may result in stasis and subsequent thrombosis of the vessel. If spasm is severe or if there is uncertainty about its possibly representing a fixed stenotic or encased area, intraarterial injection of a vasodilator such as procaine or tolazoline will usually be helpful (235).

Selective visceral catheterization may also be complicated by embolization of catheter-induced thrombi (232), dislodged atheromatous debris (219), air, or contaminating particulate matter (222,236). In each instance the clinical consequences depend on the type and quantity of embolic material and on the region in which embolization occurs. Among gastrointestinal vessels the superior mesenteric artery is at great-

est risk (225). Superior mesenteric artery emboli are usually of no consequence but may result in large zones of intestinal infarction with radiographic evidence of mucosal edema, intramural bleeding, and ultimately intestinal stenosis (225,232). Significant emboli are usually secondary to either catheter-induced thromboembolism or, in the elderly, atheroembolism.

Wedged hepatic venography, frequently employed in evaluating portal hypertension and parenchymal liver disease, has been associated with occasional transient increase in serum transaminase activity when multiple injections are performed (237). It is recommended that the number of wedged injections in an individual case be minimized and that the injection be performed slowly and with small quantities of contrast agent (238).

Translumbar Aortography
Gastrointestinal complications of translumbar aortography are unusual with the newer contrast

agents and techniques and with fluoroscopic guidance of the needle. Inadvertent puncture of visceral vessels, particularly the celiac, superior mesenteric, and renal arteries, may occur, but is easily recognized and usually of no consequence. In rare instances vascular injury with subsequent arterial thrombosis and organ injury may occur (220). Furthermore, intimal injury of the abdominal aorta has been reported to cause occlusion of the visceral arteries (228).

Direct Portography

Most commonly the portal venous system is visualized indirectly by study of the venous phases of celiac and superior mesenteric arterial injections (arterial portography). However, occasional use is made of direct portography, i.e., percutaneous transhepatic portography or splenoportography. The percutaneous transhepatic portal approach has been extended, using catheters, to include selective pancreatic venous sampling for detecting pancreatic endocrine tumors (239) and transcatheter obliteration of enlarged gastroesophageal varices (240,241).

The major complication of direct portography is poststudy bleeding at the site of organ puncture, which, with splenoportography, may necessitate emergency splenectomy. Such studies are therefore contraindicated in patients with a hemorrhagic diathesis or ascites, in which case the tamponade effect of the abdominal wall may be diminished. Significant poststudy hemorrhage is reported as 2%–3% (242–244) with splenoportography and 0–1% (242,245,246) with transhepatic portography. Placement of a small plug of occluding material, e.g., gelatin sponge, at the periphery of the hepatic needle track greatly reduces the frequency of this complication in transhepatic portography (241).

Percutaneous transhepatic portography may rarely be associated with intraperitoneal leakage of bile (240,246), but this likewise is controlled by plugging. Inadvertent punctures of the colon and duodenum have also been noted, but without consequence (241,245). Traumatic hepatic aneurysm and arteriovenous fistula have not been reported (240).

Splenoportography may occasionally be associated with bacteremia, extrasplenic puncture, and pneumothorax (243,244). Intrasplenic arterial aneurysms in areas coinciding with the previous needle track have been noted in approximately 20% of patients having repeat splenoportograms (247); all of these patients have had elevated portal venous pressure, and degenerative vascular changes secondary to this may be responsible for aneurysm formation.

Interventional Gastrointestinal Angiography

Selective catheterization and superselective catheterization also offer means for therapeutic intervention through embolization of occluding materials and infusion of vasoactive and chemotherapeutic agents. Such techniques are applied to control arterial and variceal bleeding and to infuse chemotherapeutic agents directly into malignant hepatic tumors. These interventional techniques may produce complications related to the catheterization and to the interventional procedure.

Virtually all pharmacologic attempts at controlling gastrointestinal bleeding use vasopressin (Pitressin) and depend on its intense vasoconstrictor effect on small vessels. Vasopressin is infused regionally for arterial bleeding. Direct infusion into a peripheral vein or the superior mesenteric artery is employed to diminish portal blood flow and pressure for control of gastroesophageal variceal bleeding. Both intraarterial and intravenous infusions have been associated with systemic toxicity, and intraarterial infusions may also be associated with local organ or vascular injury.

Regional complications due to visceral arterial infusion of vasopressin to control bleeding are extremely uncommon. They consist mainly of occasional vascular thrombosis, including the superior mesenteric artery (248), superior mesenteric vein (249), and portal vein (250), at times with bowel necrosis. These rare occurrences are probably due to the combined effects of reduction in arterial flow and diminished portal pressure, often compounded by hypotension.

To avoid too great a vasoconstrictive effect from the vasopressin it is wise to obtain another angiogram of the infused vessel approximately 20 min after initiation of vasopressin therapy. The initial rate of infusion can then be adjusted according to the observed degree of vasoconstriction. Thereafter, careful monitoring of the infusion and periodic checking of catheter position can alleviate regional complications.

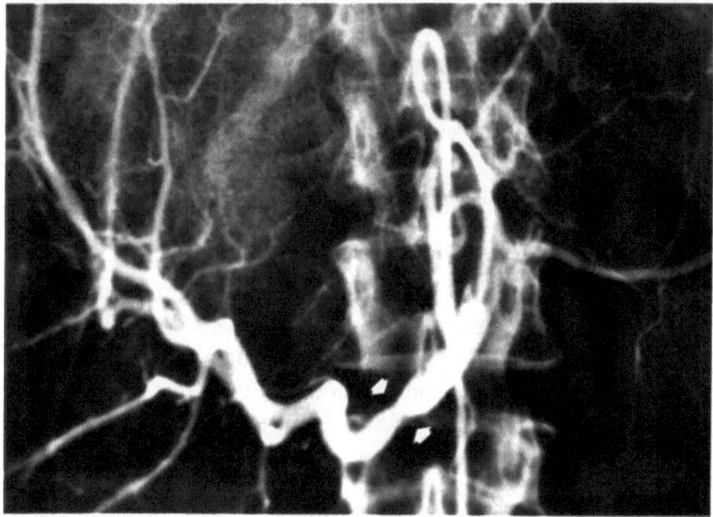

a

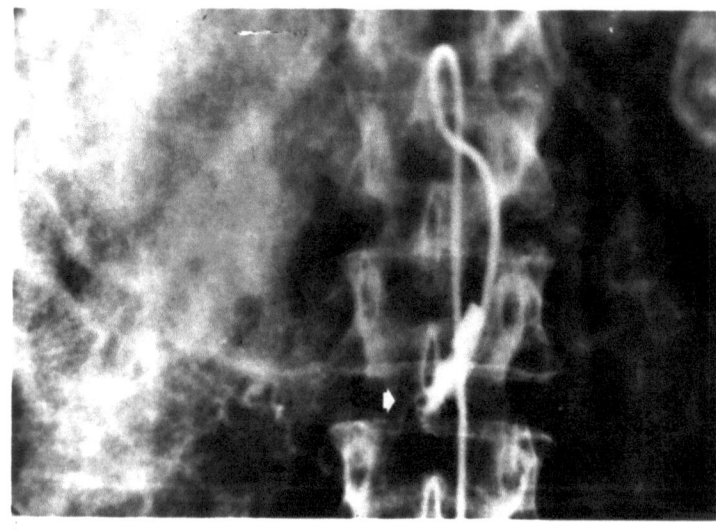

Fig. 4-20, a and b. Complication of interventional angiography. Hepatic arteriogram demonstrates (a) narrowing *(arrowheads)* and (b) eventual thrombosis *(arrowheads)* of hepatic artery during chemotherapeutic infusion.

b

Transcatheter arterial embolization is employed in cases of upper gastrointestinal hemorrhage unresponsive to more conventional treatment, including vasopressin infusion, and in entities particularly amenable to such management such as the Mallory-Weiss lesion and focal gastroduodenal hemorrhage. To a lesser extent embolization is utilized in lower gastrointestinal bleeding in patients who are unresponsive to vasopressin therapy and are poor surgical risks (251,252). Hepatic arterial embolization is used for tumor palliation and management of hepatic bleeding, trauma, and hemobilia. Direct transhepatic obliteration of gastroesophageal varices through catheterization of the portal vein is like-

wise occasionally employed as an adjunct to the medical treatment of bleeding varices (240,253). Each of these procedures, in addition to its target-organ effects, has potential complications inherent to the visceral catheterization and the transhepatic portal study.

Embolic materials are numerous and include absorbable gelatin sponge (Gelfoam), autogenous blood clots, coils, polyvinyl alcohol sponge (Ivalon), balloons, and tissue adhesives such as isobutyl 2-cyanoacrylate (Bucrylate). Temporary occluding agents such as absorbable gelatin sponge and autogenous blood clot are used most frequently.

A major concern in embolization is related to

effects of the induced ischemia on the target organ. Experience has shown that it is unlikely that embolization for upper gastrointestinal bleeding will result in significant ischemia or infarction of the intact stomach or duodenum (254). However, gastric or duodenal necrosis has been reported in patients in whom potential collateral pathways have been disrupted by a previous splenectomy or gastroduodenal surgical procedure (255) or in whom the ischemic effects of embolization have been compounded by subsequent infusion of vasopressin (256). Embolization distal to the duodenum is more dangerous because of the diminished number of collateral pathways, and occasional small bowel or colonic infarctions occur. Lower gastrointestinal embolization should be performed as subselectively as possible, and generally only on patients who are poor surgical risks in whom other treatment, including vasopressin infusion, has failed.

Hepatic arterial embolization has been shown experimentally to produce variable and usually transient liver dysfunction (257), hepatic infarcts and abscesses (258), and sterile intrahepatic bile duct cysts (258,259). Most hepatic complications occur with peripheral small-branch occlusions. Occlusion of the proximal hepatic artery allows more collateral development (259,260).

Complications of splenic embolization include splenic abscess (261–263) and inadvertent gastric and pancreatic infarctions (262). Also, embolization of pancreatic and peripancreatic false aneurysms has resulted in their rupture (264).

Transbrachial, transaxillary, and transfemoral catheters have been placed for long-term infusion of chemotherapeutic agents in primary and secondary malignant hepatic tumors (265). Specific gastrointestinal complications are not uncommon. Thrombosis of the catheterized branch of the celiac artery has been reported in approximately 15% of cases (266,267), but usually is well tolerated (Fig. 4-20). However, the superior mesenteric artery is specifically avoided because of the high incidence of local thrombosis (266). Local intimal injury and pseudoaneurysm formation have been reported at the catheter tip, the latter complication being potentially serious because of the threat of rupture (266). Finally, gas-forming hepatic abscesses have been noted in patients undergoing infusion therapy for hepatic cancer. This may be related to the hypoxic environment in a necrotic tumor (265). The presence of a mottled gas pattern in the hepatic area of such a patient should alert one to this complication.

References

1. Gitlin JN, Lawrence PS: Population exposure to x-rays. Washington: USPHS Publ 1519, 1964
2. Govindiah D, Bhaskar GR: An unusual case of barium poisoning. Antiseptic 69:675–677, 1972
3. McNally WD: Two deaths from the administration of barium salts. JAMA 84:1805–1807, 1925
4. Berning J: Hypokalemia of barium poisoning. Lancet 1:110, 1975
5. Corby C, Camps FF: Therapeutic accidents during the administration of barium enemas. J Forensic Med 7:206–220, 1960
6. Felson B: Radiologist on the rocks. Semin Roentgenol 4:361–363, 1973
7. Amberg JR, Unger JD: Contamination of barium sulfate suspension. Radiology 97:182–183, 1970
8. Meyers PH: Contamination of barium enema apparatus during its use. JAMA 173:1589–1590, 1960
9. Steinbach HL, Rousseau R, McCormack KR, et al: Transmission of enteric pathogens by barium enemas. JAMA 174:1207–1208, 1960
10. Steinbach HL, Burhenne HJ: Performing the barium enema: Equipment, preparation and contrast medium. Am J Roentgenol 87:644–654, 1962
11. Puyleart CBAJ: Barium perforation of a peptic ulcer and barium granuloma of the colon. Radiol Clin Biol 38:84–95, 1969
12. Schilling JA: Perforation of a duodenal ulcer during roentgen examination. Surgery 20:730–743, 1946
13. Killingback M: Acute large bowel obstruction precipitated by barium x-ray examination. Med J Aust 2:503–508, 1964
14. Ansell G (ed): Complications in Diagnostic Radiology. Oxford: Blackwell 1976, p 334
15. Serjeant JCB, Raymond JA: Perforation of apparently normal colon after a barium meal. Lancet 263:1245–1246, 1952
16. Prout BJ, Datta SB, Wilson TS: Colonic retention of barium in the elderly after barium meal examination and its treatment with lactulose. Br Med J 4:530–533, 1970
17. Young MO: Acute appendicitis following retention of barium in the appendix. Arch Surg 77:1011–1014, 1958
18. Dixon GD, Ferris DO, Hodgson JR: Unusual complications of barium studies: Report of a case of adherent cecal barolith. Am J Roentgenol 99:106–111, 1967
19. Schabel SI, Skucas J: Esophageal obstruction following administration of "aged" barium sulfate tablets—A warning. Radiology 122:835–836, 1977

20. Willson JKV, Rubin PS, McGee TM: The effects of barium sulfate on the lungs. A clinical and experimental study. Am J Roentgenol 82:84–94, 1959

21. Huston J, Wallach DP, Cunningham GJ: Pulmonary reaction to barium sulfate in rats. Arch Pathol 54:430–438, 1952

22. Nelson SW: Facts versus folklore. Am J Surg 109:543–545, 1965

23. Chiu CL, Gambach RR: Hypaque pulmonary edema. Radiology 111:91–92, 1974

24. Ansell G: A national survey of radiological complications: Interim report. Clin Radiol 19:175–191, 1968

25. Mahboubi S, Gohel VK, Dalinka MK, et al: Barium embolization following upper gastrointestinal examination. Radiology 114:301–302, 1974

26. Gelfand DW, Moskowitz M: Massive gastric dilatation complicating hypotonic duodenography. A report of three cases. Radiology 97:637–639, 1970

27. Jacobson G, Berne CJ, Meyers HI, et al: The examination of patients with suspected perforated ulcer using a water soluble contrast medium. Am J Roentgenol 86:37–49, 1961

28. Margulis AR: Contrast media. The present status of water-soluble iodine-containing material in the examination of acute abdominal disease. Calif Med 110:193–199, 1969

29. Ross LS: Precipitation of meglumine diatrizoate 76% (Gastrografin) in the stomach. Radiology 105:19–22, 1972

30. Hugh TB, Hennessey WB, Sunner BW, et al: Precipitation of contrast medium causing impaction of Sengstaken Blakemore oesophageal tube. Med J Aust 1:60–61, 1970

31. Gallitano AL, Kondi ES, Phillips E, et al: Near fatal hemorrhage following Gastrografin studies. Radiology 118:35–36, 1976

32. Harris PD, Neuhauser EDB, Gerth R: The osmotic effect of water-soluble media on circulating plasma volume. Am J Roentgenol 91:694–698, 1964

33. Elman S, Palayew MJ: Assessment of biochemical and hematologic changes to oral administration of an iodinated contrast medium. Invest Radiol 8:322–325, 1975

34. Seaman WB, Wells J: Complications of the barium enema. Gastroenterology 48:728–737, 1965

35. Norland CC, Kirsner JB: Toxic dilatation of the colon (toxic megacolon): Etiology, treatment and prognosis in 42 patients. Medicine 48:229–250, 1969

36. Lorinc P, Brahme F: Perforation of the colon during examination by the double contrast method. Gastroenterology 37:770–773, 1959

37. Welin S, Welin G: The double contrast examination of the colon. Experiences with the Welin modification. Stuttgart: Thieme 1976, p 17

38. Santulli TV: Perforation of the rectum or colon in infancy due to enema. Pediatrics 23:972–975, 1959

39. DeCarlo J: Complications associated with diagnostic barium enema. Surgery 47:965–969, 1960

40. Spector GW, Susman N: The roentgen recognition of intramural perforation following barium enema examination in obstructing lesions of the sigmoid. Am J Roentgenol 89:876–879, 1963

41. Spiro RK: Perforation of the rectum following barium enema. Am J Gastroenterol 30:540–543, 1958

42. Zheutlin N, Lasser EC, Rigler LG: Clinical studies on the effect of barium in the peritoneal cavity following rupture of the colon. Surgery 32:967–979, 1952

43. Masel H, Masel JP, Casey KV: A survey of colon examination techniques in Australia and New Zealand with a review of complications. Aust Radiol 15:140–147, 1971

44. Westfall RH, Nelson RH, Musselman MM: Barium peritonitis. Am J Surg 112:760–763, 1966

45. Winsky AD, Robinson FW: Barium peritonitis, Kans Med Soc J 112:426–428, 1966

46. Yudis M, Cohen A, Pearce AE: Perforation of the transverse colon during barium enema examination and air contrast studies. Am Surg 34:334–336, 1968

47. Becker MH, Genieser NB, Clark H: Perforation of the colon during barium enema. NY State J Med 67:278–282, 1967

48. Pyle R, Samuel E: An evaluation of the hazards of barium enema examinations. Clin Radiol 11:192–196, 1960

49. Kiser JL, Spratt JS, Johnson CA: Colon perforations occurring during sigmoidoscopic examinations and barium enemas. Mo Med 65:969–974, 1968

50. DeBoer HHM, Speyer B: Perforatie van het rectum tijdens het maken van colon-inloopfotos. Ned Tidschr Geneeskd 112:1026–1029, 1968

51. Vieta JO, Bell-Thomson J: Barium peritonitis. Am J Gastroenterol 63:414–419, 1975

52. Kleinsasser LJ, Warshaw H: Perforation of the sigmoid colon during barium enema. Am Surg 135:560–565, 1952

53. Seaman WB, Bragg DB: Colonic intramural barium: A complication of the barium enema examination. Radiology 89:250–255, 1967

54. Gardiner H, Miller RE: Barium peritonitis. A new therapeutic approach. Am J Surg 125:350–352, 1973

55. Cameron HC: Barium proctitis. Proc Soc Med 57:399–400, 1964

56. Porter EC: The risk of barium enema. J Maine Med Assoc 51:422–423, 1960

57. Dubarry JJ, Martin PL, Broussin J, et al: Un accident imprevu du lavement baryte: l'infiltration parietale et lymphatique du rectum. J Radiol Electrol Med Nucl 46:800–802, 1965

58. Nelson JA, Daniels AV, Dodds WJ: Rectal balloons: Complications, causes and recommendations. Invest Radiol 14:48–59, 1979

59. Pratt JH, Jackman RJ: Perforation of the rectal wall by enema tips. Proc Mayo Clin 20:277, 1945

60. Burrows EH: An unusual pelvic opacity. Br J Radiol 35:287–289, 1962

61. Brown S, Fine A: Diffuse emphysema following a double-contrast enema. Radiology 37:228–229, 1941

62. Shapiro JH, Rifkin H: Perforation of the colon during a barium-enema study. Development of retroperitoneal mediastinal and cervical emphysema. Am J Dig Dis 1:430–436, 1956

63. Neveroske RJ: Perforation of a normal colon by too much pressure. J Indiana State Med Assoc 65:23–25, 1972

64. Neveroske RJ: Perforation of the rectosigmoid by a Bardex balloon catheter. Am J Roetgenol 96:326–331, 1966

65. Hartman AW, Hills WJ: Rupture of the colon in infants during barium enema: Report of two cases. Ann Surg 154:712–717, 1957

66. Dibbell DG, Cohn R: Perforation of the colon during hydrostatic reduction. Am J Surg 111:715–717, 1966

67. Geigle CF: Rectal perforations during administration of barium enemas: Report of three cases. Dis Colon Rectum 13:29–30, 1970

68. Berk JE: Perforation following barium enema. JAMA 148:766, 1952

69. Goldston AB, Blast L, Hands S: Perforation of the large bowel during routine barium enema studies. Tex Med 64:52–56, 1968

70. Portin BA, Bernhoft WH: Colon perforation during barium enema: Report of a case. Dis Colon Rectum 6:308–310, 1963

71. Hamit HF: Perforation of the colon after barium enema and air contrast studies. Am Surg 21:1226–1234, 1955

72. Isaacs I: Intraperitoneal escape of barium enema fluid. Perforation of sigmoid colon. JAMA 150:645–646, 1952

73. Koucky J, Beck WC: Acute nonmalignant perforations of the colon. Surgery 7:674–685, 1940

74. Greentree LB, Wesley F: Perforation of normal colon by barium enema. Report of a case with uncomplicated survival. Ohio State Med J 58:1150–1151, 1966

75. Desaulniers M: Intramural perforation of barium—Transverse colon. J Can Assoc Radiol 29:194, 1978

76. Carter RW: Barium granuloma of the rectum: A complication of diagnostic barium enema examination. Am J Roentgenol 89:880–882, 1963

77. Carney JA, Stephens DH: Intramural barium (barium granuloma) of colon and rectum. Gastroenterology 65:316–320, 1973

78. Broadfoot E, Martin G: Barium granuloma of the rectum. Australas Radiol 21:50–52, 1977

79. Fielding JF, Lumsden K: Large bowel perfora-

tions in patients undergoing sigmoidoscopy and barium enema. Br Med J 1:471–473, 1973

80. Mowat PD: Pneumoperitoneum following double contrast enema. Br J Radiol 40:230–231, 1967

81. Gross MD, Howard MA: Perforations of the colon from barium enema. Am Surg 38:583–585, 1972

82. Ansell G (ed): Complications in Diagnostic Radiology. Oxford: Blackwell 1976, p 340–344

83. Staple TW, McAllister WH: Perforation of an atretic colon during barium enema examination. Am J Roentgenol 101:325–328, 1967

84. Spiro RH, Hertz RE: Colostomy perforation. Surgery 60:590–597, 1966

85. Zatzkin HR, Irwin AL: Nonfatal intravasation of barium. Am J Roentgenol 92:1169–1172, 1964

86. Burt CAV: Pneumatic rupture of the intestinal canal. Arch Surg 22:875–902, 1931

87. Noveroske RJ: Intracolonic pressures during barium enema examination. Am J Roentgenol 91:852–863, 1964

88. Nahrwold DL, Isch JH, Benner DA, et al: Effect of fluid administration and operation on the mortality rate in barium peritonitis. Surgery 70:778–781, 1971

89. Almond CH, Cochran DQ, Shucart WA: Comparative study of the effects of various radiographic contrast media on the peritoneal cavity. Ann Surg 154:219–224, 1961

90. Cochran DQ, Almond CH, Shucart WA: An experimental study of barium and intestinal contents on the peritoneal cavity. Am J Roentgenol 89:883–887, 1963

91. Westfall RH, Nelson RH, Musselman MM: Barium peritonitis. Am J Surg 112:760–763, 1966

92. Cuevas P, Fine J: Role of intraintestinal endotoxin in death from peritonitis. Surg Gynecol Obstet 134:953–957, 1972

93. Mullin HJ, Thoeni RF, Quan SH: Timing of barium enema studies following sigmoidoscopy (letter and replies). JAMA 241:941, 1979

94. Matek W, Fruhmorgen P, Fuchs HF: Barium enema with subsequent perforation of the rectum following rectoscopic biopsy. Endoscopy 10:132–136, 1978

95. Cave JK, Snyder RN: Fatal barium intravasation during barium enema. Radiology 112:9–10, 1974

96. Isaacs I, Nisser R, Epstein BS: Liver abscess resulting from barium enema in a case of chronic ulcerative colitis. NY State J Med 50:332–334, 1950

97. Truemner KM, White S, Vanlandingham H: Fatal embolization of pulmonary capillaries. Report of a case associated with routine barium enema. JAMA 173:1089–1092, 1960

98. Kaufman SA: Retrograde vaginal filling during barium enema. Am J Dig Dis 10:732–736, 1965

99. Peterson CA, Cayler CG: Water intoxication. Report of a case following a barium enema. Am J Roentgenol 77:69–70, 1957

100. Steinbach HL, Rosenberg RH, Grossman M, et

al: The potential hazards of enemas in patients with Hirschsprung's disease. Radiology 64:45–50, 1955

101. Richards MR, Hiatt RB: Untoward effects of enemata in congenital megacolon. Pediatrics 12:253–256, 1953

102. Wasterlain CG, Posner JB: Cerebral edema in water intoxication. I. Clinical and chemical observations. Arch Neurol 19:71–78, 1968

103. Hamilton JB: The use of tannic acid in barium enemas. Am J Roentgenol 56:101–103, 1946

104. McAlister WH, Anderson MS, Bloomberg GR, et al: Lethal effects of tannic acid in the barium enema. Report of three fatalities and experimental studies. Radiology 80:765–773, 1963

105. Lucke HH, Hodge KE, Patt NL: Fatal liver damage after barium enema containing tannic acid. Can Med Assoc J 89:1111–1114, 1963

106. Rambo ON, Zboralske FF, Harris PA, et al: Toxicity studies of tannic acid administered by enema. I. Effects of the enema-administered tannic acid on the colon and liver of rats. Am J Roentgenol 96:488–497, 1966

107. Harris PA, Zboralske FF, Rambo ON, et al: Toxicity studies on tannic acid administered by enema. II. The colon absorbtion and intraperitoneal toxicity of tannic acid and its hydrolytic products in rats. Am J Roentgenol 96:498–504, 1966

108. Zboralske FF, Harris PA, Riegelman S, et al: Toxicity studies of tannic acid administered by enema. III. Studies on the retention of enemas in humans. IV. Review and conclusions. Am J Roentgenol 96:505–509, 1966

109. Janower ML, Robbins LL, Tomchik FS, et al: Tannic acid and the barium enema. Radiology 85:887–894, 1965

110. Kemp Harper RA, Pemberton J. Tobias JS: Serial liver function tests following barium enemas containing 1% tannic acid. Clin Radiol 24:315–317, 1973

111. Staab EV, Vix VA: Serum glutamic oxalacetic transaminase levels following tannic acid enemas. Radiology 84:1087–1089, 1965

112. Kees CJ, Hester CL: Portal vein gas following barium enema exam. Radiology 102:525–526, 1972

113. Sadhu VK, Brennan RE, Nadan V: Portal vein gas following air-contrast barium enema in granulomatous colitis: Report of a case. Gastrointest Radiol 4:163–164, 1979

114. Butt J, Hentges D, Pelican G, et al: Bacteremia during barium enema study. Am J Roentgenol 130:715–718, 1978

115. Le Frock JL, Ellis CA, Klainer AS, Transient bacteremia associated with barium enema. Arch Intern Med 135:835–837, 1975

116. Schimmel DH, Hanelin LG, Cohen S, et al: Bacteremia and the barium enema. Am J Roentgenol 128:207–208, 1977

117. Pelican G. Hentges D, Butt J, et al: Bacteremia during colonoscopy. Gastrointest Endosc 23:33–35, 1976

118. Cook GB, Margulis AR: Silicone-foam diagnostic enema. I. Assessment with surgical specimens of human sigmoid colon. Surgery 50:513–518, 1961

119. Cook GB, Margulis AR: Use of silicone foam for examining the human sigmoid colon. Am J Roentgenol 87:633–643, 1962

120. Spjut HJ, Margulis AR, Cook CB: Silicone foam enema: Source for exfoliative cytologic specimens. Acta Cytol 7:79–84, 1963

121. Amberg JR: A hazard of silicone foam diagnostic enema. Report of a case with perforation of the colon. Am J Roentgenol 99:96–97, 1967

122. Rowe MI, Seagram G, Weinberger M: Gastrografin-induced hypertonicity. Am J Surg 125:183–188, 1973

123. Harris PD, Neuhauser EBD, Gerth R: The osmotic effect of water-soluble media on circulating plasma volume. Am J Roentgenol 91:694–698, 1964

124. Pike BF, Phillipi PJ, Lawsen EH: Soap colitis. N Engl J Med 285:217–218, 1971

125. Bendit M: Gangrene of the rectum as a complication of an enema. Br Med J 1:664, 1945

126. Berk RN, Loeb PM, Goldberger LE, et al: Oral cholecystography with iopanoic acid. N Engl J Med 290:204–210, 1974

127. White WW, Fischer HW: A double blind study of oragrafin and telepaque. Am J Roentgenol 87:745–748, 1962

128. Juhl JH, Cooperman LR, Crummy AB: Oragrafin, a new cholecystographic medium. Radiology 80:87–91, 1963

129. Russell JG, Frederick PR: Clinical comparison of tyropanoate sodium, ipodate sodium and iopanoic acid. Radiology 112:519–523, 1974

130. Parks RE: Double-blind study of four oral cholecystographic preparations. Radiology 112:525–528, 1974

131. Stanley RJ, Melson GL, Cubillo E, et al: A comparison of three cholecystographic agents. Radiology 112:513–517, 1974

132. Krook PM, Bush Jr WH: Single dose oral cholecystography. Radiology 127:643–644, 1978

133. Shehadi WH: Clinical problems and toxicity of contrast agents. Am J Roentgenol 97:762–771, 1966

134. Teplick JG, Myerson RM, Sanen FJ: Acute renal failure following oral cholecystography. Acta Radiol 3:353–369, 1965

135. Sanen FJ, Myerson RM, Teplick JG: Etiology of serious reactions to oral cholecystography. Arch Intern Med 113:241–247, 1964

136. Rene RM, Mellinkoff SM: Renal insufficiency after oral cholecystography of a double dose of a cholecystographic medium. N Engl J Med 261:589–592, 1959

137. Setter JG, Maher JF, Schreiner GE: Acute renal failure following cholecystography. JAMA 184:102–110, 1963

138. Harrow BR, Sloane JA: Acute renal failure following oral cholecystography. Am J Med Sci 249:26–35, 1965

139. Harrow BR, Winslow OP: Renal toxicity following oral cholecystography with oragrafin (Ipodate calcium). Radiology 87:721–724, 1966

140. Duggan FJ Jr, Rohner TJ Jr: Acute renal insufficiency following oral cholecystography. J Urol 109:156–159, 1973

141. Ansari Z, Baldwin DS: Acute renal failure due to radio-contrast agents. Nephron 17:28–40, 1976

142. Malt RA, Olken HG, Goade Jr WJ: Renal tubular necrosis after oral cholecystography. Arch Surg 87:743–746, 1963

143. Fink Jr HE, Roenigk WJ, Wilson GP: An experimental investigation of the nephrotoxic effects of oral cholecystographic agents. Am J Med Sci 247:201–216, 1964

144. Postlethwaite AE, Kelley WN: Uricsuric effect of radiocontrast agents. Ann Intern Med 74:845–852, 1971

145. Gelfand DW, Ott DJ, Klein A: Massive iopanoic acid (Telepaque) overdose without ill effects. Am J Roentgenol 130:1174–1175, 1978

146. Robbins AH, Earampamoorthy S, Koff RS, et al: Successful intravenous cholecystocholangiography in the jaundiced patient using meglumine iodoxamate (Cholovue). Am J Roentgenol 126:70–76, 1976

147. Loeb PM, Barnhart JL, Berk RN: Iotroxamide—A new intravenous cholangiographic agent. Radiology 125:323–329, 1977

148. Shehadi WH: Adverse reactions to intravascularly administered contrast media. Am J Roentgenol 124:145–152, 1975

149. Johnson JH Jr, Wise RE: Intravenous cholangiography: A study of reactions to iodipamide methylglucamine. Lahey Clin Bull 13:245–250, 1964

150. Peters GA, Hodgson JR, Donovan RJ: The effect of premedication with chlorpheniramine on reactions to methylglucamine iodipamide. J Allergy 38:74–83, 1966

151. Scholz FJ, Johnston DO, Wise, RE: Intravenous cholangiography. Optimum dosage and methodology. Radiology 114:513–518, 1975

152. Cogen FC, Zweiman B: Adverse radiographic contrast media reactions. Compr Ther 4:50–56, 1978

153. Ansell G: Adverse reactions to contrast agents. Invest Radiol 5:374–391, 1970

154. Stillman AE: Hepatotoxic reaction to iodipamide meglumine injection. JAMA 228:1420–1421, 1974

155. Sutherland LR, Edwards LA, Medline A, et al: Meglumine iodipamide (Cholografin) hepatotoxicity. Ann Intern Med 86:437–439, 1977

156. Craft IL, Swales JD: Renal failure after cholangiography. Br Med J 2:736–738, 1967

157. Gold CH, Abrahams C, Cohen I: Acute renal failure following intravenous cholangiography. S Afr Med J 45:1400–1402, 1971

158. Brown RC, Cohen WN: Acute renal failure following intravenous cholangiography. South Med J 66:1142–1144, 1973

159. Sargent EN, Barbour BH, Espinosa N, et al: Evaluation of renal function following double dose infusion intravenous cholangiography. Am J Roentgenol 117:412–418, 1973

160. Nebel OT, Silvis SE, Rogers G, et al: Complications associated with endoscopic retrograde cholangiopancreatography. Gastrointest Endosc 22:34–36, 1975

161. Bilbao MK, Dotter CT, Lee TG, et al: Complications of endoscopic retrograde cholangiopancreatography (ERCP). Gastroenterology 70:314–320, 1976

162. Kessler RE, Falkenstein DB, Clemett AR, et al: Indications, clinical value and complications of endoscopic retrograde cholangiopancreatography. Surg Gynecol Obstet 142:865–870, 1976

163. Seifert E: Endoscopic retrograde cholangiopancreatography. Am J Gastroenterol 68:542–549, 1977

164. Ihre T, Hellers G: Complications and endoscopic retrograde cholangiopancreatography. Acta Chir Scand 143:167–171, 1977

165. Standerskjöld-Nordenstam CG, Fräki OI: Endoscopic retrograde cholangiopancreatography in a surgical unit. Ann Clin Res 10:30–37, 1978

166. Zimmon DS, Falkenstein DB, Riccobono C, et al: Complications of endoscopic retrograde cholangiopancreatography. Gastroenterology 69:303–309, 1975

167. Ammann RW, Deyhle P, Butikofer E: Fatal necrotizing pancreatitis after peroral cholangiopancreatography. Gastroenterology 64:320–323, 1973

168. Tseng A, Sales DJ, Simonowitz DA, et al: Pancreas abscess: A fatal complication of endoscopic cholangiopancreatography (ERCP). Endoscopy 9:250–253, 1977

169. Goldberg HI, Bilbao MK, Stewart ET, et al: Endoscopic retrograde cholangiopancreatography (ERCP). Am J Dig Dis 21:270–278, 1976

170. Cotton PB: Progress report ERCP. Gut 18:316–341, 1977

171. James EC, Collin DB: Sepsis complications in endoscopic retrograde cholangiopancreatography. Am Surg 42:229–232, 1976

172. Wind GG, Rubin P, Waye JD, et al: Pancreatic pseudocyst: Is endoscopic retrograde cholangiopancreatography contraindicated? Mt Sinai J Med 43:558–564, 1976

173. Davis JL, Milligan FD, Cameron JL: Septic complications following endoscopic retrograde cholangiopancreatography. Surg Gynecol Obstet 140:365–367, 1975

174. Lam SK, Tsui JKC, Chan PKW, et al: How often does bacteraemia occur following endoscopic retrograde cholangiopancreatography (ERCP)? Endoscopy 9:231–234, 1977

175. Joseph WL, Golding AL, Mulder DG: Complications of percutaneous transhepatic cholangiography. Am Surg 31:679–682, 1965

176. Flemma RJ, Shingleton WW: Clinical experience with percutaneous transhepatic cholangiography. Am J Surg 111:13–19, 1966

177. Mujahed Z, Evans JA: Percutaneous transhepatic cholangiography. Radiol Clin North Am 4:535–545, 1966

178. Göthlin J, Tranberg K: Complications of percutaneous transhepatic cholangiography (PTC). Am J Roentgenol 117:426–431, 1973

179. Burcharth F, Christiansen L, Efsen F, et al: Percutaneous transhepatic cholangiography in diagnostic evaluation of 160 jaundiced patients. Am J Surg 133:559–561, 1977

180. Cahow CE, Burrell M, Greco R: Hemobilia following percutaneous transhepatic cholangiography. Ann Surg 185:235–241, 1977

181. Keighley MRB, Wilson G, Kelly JP: Fatal endotoxic shock of biliary track origin complicating transhepatic cholangiography. Br Med J 3:147–148, 1973

182. Koch RL, Gorder JL: Bile-blood fistula: A complication of percutaneous transhepatic cholangiography. Radiology 93:67–68, 1969

183. Redman HC, Joseph RR: Hemobilia and pancreatitis as complications of a percutaneous transhepatic cholangiogram. Am J Dig Dis 20:691–698, 1975

184. Hines C Jr, Ferrante WA, Davis WD Jr, Tutton RA: Percutaneous transhepatic cholangiography. Am J Dig Dis 17:868–874, 1972

185. Seldinger SI: Percutaneous transhepatic cholangiography. Acta Radiol (Suppl) 253:1–134, 1966

186. Nakayama T, Ikeda A, Okuda K: Percutaneous transhepatic drainage of the biliary tract. Gastroenterology 74:554–559, 1978

187. Ring EJ, Oleaga JA, Freiman DB, et al: Therapeutic applications of catheter cholangiography. Radiology 128:333–338, 1978

188. Fraser GM, Cruikshank JG, Sumerling MD, et al: Percutaneous transhepatic cholangiography with the Chiba needle. Clin Radiol 29:101–112, 1978

189. Ferrucci JT Jr, Wittenberg J: Refinements in Chiba needle transhepatic cholangiography. Am J Roentgenol 129:11–16, 1977

190. Ariyama J, Shirakabe H. Ohashi K, et al: Experience with percutaneous transhepatic cholangiography using the Japanese needle. Gastrointest Radiol 2:359–365, 1978

191. Goldstein LI, Kadell BM, Weiner M: Thin needle cholangiography. Ann Surg 186:602–606, 1977

192. Pereiras R Jr, Chiprut RO, Greenwald RA, et al: Percutaneous transhepatic cholangiography with the "skinny" needle. Ann Intern Med 86:562–568, 1977

193. Jain S. Long RG, Scott J, et al: Percutaneous transhepatic cholangiography using the "Chiba" needle—80 cases. Br J Radiol 50:175–180, 1977

194. Okuda K, Tanikawa K, Emura T, et al: Nonsurgical, percutaneous transhepatic cholangiography—Diagnostic significance in medical problems of the liver. Am J Dig Dis 19:21–35, 1974

195. Juler GL, Conroy RM, Fuelleman RW: Bile leakage following percutaneous transhepatic cholangiography with the Chiba needle. Arch Surg 112:954–958, 1977

196. Moskowitz H, Polivy C. Hackford AW, et al: Complications of "Chiba" needle transhepatic cholangiography. Br J Radiol 51:541–543, 1978

197. Okuda K, Musha H, Nakajima Y, et al: Frequency of intrahepatic arteriovenous fistula as a sequela to percutaneous needle puncture of the liver. Gastroenterology 74:1204–1207, 1978

198. Burhenne HJ: Direct cholangiography. In Miller RE, Skucas J: Radiographic Contrast Agents. Baltimore: University Park Press 1977, pp 251–259

199. Weigen JF, Thomas SF: Complications of Diagnostic Radiology. Springfield, Ill.: Thomas 1973, p 325

200. Schulenburg CAR: Operative cholangiography: 1,000 cases. Surgery 65:723–739, 1969

201. Mazzariello RM: Residual biliary tract stones: Nonoperative treatment of 570 patients. Surg Annu 8:113–144, 1976

202. Burhenne HJ: Nonoperative retained biliary tract stone extraction. Am J Roentgenol 117:388–399, 1973

203. Burhenne HJ, Richards V, Mathewson C Jr, et al: Nonoperative extraction of retained biliary tract stones requiring multiple sessions. Am J Surg 128:288–291, 1974

204. Burhenne HJ: Complications of nonoperative extraction of retained common duct stones. Am J Surg 131:260–262, 1976

205. Garrow DG: The removal of retained biliary tract stones: Report of 105 cases. Br J Radiol 50:777–782, 1977

206. Lang EK: Prevention and treatment of complications following arteriography. Radiology 88:950–956, 1967

207. Lang EK: A survey of the complications of percutaneous retrograde arteriography: Seldinger technic. Radiology 81:257–263, 1963

208. Moore CH, Wolma FJ, Brown RW, et al: Complications of cardiovascular radiology: A review of 1,204 cases. Am J Surg 120:591–593, 1970

209. Sigstedt B, Lunderquist A: Complications of angiographic examinations. Am J Roentgenol 130:455–460, 1978

210. Pollard JJ, Nebesar RA: Abdominal angiography. N Engl J Med 279:1035–1042, 1968

211. Fischer HW: Hemodynamic reactions to angiographic media: A survey and commentary. Radiology 91:66–73, 1968

212. Older RA, Miller JP, Jackson DC, et al: Angiographically induced renal failure and its radiographic detection. Am J Roentgenol 126:1039–1045, 1976

213. Swartz RD, Rubin JE, Leeming BW, et al: Renal

failure following major angiography. Am J Med 65:31–37, 1978

214. Looney WB: An investigation of the late clinical findings following Thorotrast (thorium dioxide) administration. Am J Roentgenol 83:163–185, 1960

215. Gondos B: Late clinical and roentgen observations following Thorotrast administration. Clin Radiol 24:195–203, 1973

216. Mann NS, Chaudhry A, Thaler S, et al: Hepatoma induced by thorium dioxide. South Med J 69:510–512, 1976

217. Antonovik R, Rosch J, Dotter CT: Complications of percutaneous transaxillary catheterization for arteriography and selective chemotherapy. Am J Roentgenol 126:386–393, 1976

218. Bolasny BL, Killen DA: Surgical management of arterial injuries secondary to angiography. Ann Surg 174:962–964, 1971

219. Meaney TF: Complications of percutaneous femoral angiography. Geriatrics 29:61–64, 1974

220. Grainger RG: Complications of cardiovascular radiological investigations. Br J Radiol 38:201–215, 1965

221. Jonsson K, Lunderquist A, Pettersson H, et al: Subintimal injection of contrast medium as a complication of selective abdominal angiography. Acta Radiol 18:55–64, 1977

222. Adams DF, Olin TB, Kosek J: Cotton fiber embolization during angiography: A clinical and experimental study. Radiology 84:678–681, 1965

223. Jacobsson B, Schlossman D: Angiographic investigation of formation of thrombi on vascular catheters. Radiology 93:355–359, 1969

224. Jacobsson B, Schlossman D: Thromboembolism of leg following percutaneous catheterization of femoral artery for angiography: Predisposing factors. Acta Radiol 8:109–118, 1969

225. Schwartz S, Waters L: Cholesterol embolization. Radiology 106:37–41, 1973

226. Holder JC, Cherry JF: The use of a tip deflecting guide in untying a knotted arterial catheter. Radiology 128:808–809, 1978

227. Szilagyi DE, Smith RF, Elliott JP Jr, et al: Translumbar aortography: A study of its safety and usefulness. Arch Surg 112:399–408, 1977

228. Gammill S, Craighead C: Translumbar aortography updated. Surg Gynecol Obstet 140:59–64, 1975

229. White RI Jr: Fundamentals of vascular radiology. Philadelphia: Lea & Febiger 1976, p 64

230. Bergman AB, Neiman HL: Computed tomography in the detection of retroperitoneal hemorrhage after translumbar aortography. Am J Roentgenol 131:831–833, 1978

231. Sagel SS, Siegel MJ, Stanely RJ, et al: Detection of retroperitoneal hemorrhage by computed tomography. Am J Roentgenol 129:403–407, 1977

232. Lande A, Meyers MA: Iatrogenic embolization of the superior mesenteric artery: Arteriographic observations and clinical implications. Am J Roentgenol 126:822–828, 1976

233. Reuter SR: Development of collateral vessels in an acute occlusion of the common hepatic artery. Am J Roentgenol 97:473–476, 1966

234. Harwood-Nash DC, Fitz CR: Complications of pediatric arteriography. In Gyepes MT (ed): Angiography in Infants and Children. New York: Grune & Stratton 1974, p 342

235. Howland WJ, Curry JL, Wheeler PP: Intra-arterial administration of procaine hydrochloride after angiography. Potential value in preventing arteriospasm and thrombosis. JAMA 201:135–138, 1967

236. Yunis EJ, Landes RR: Hazards of glove powder in renal angiography. JAMA 193:304–305, 1965

237. Goldstein HM, Bookstein JJ: Biochemical evaluation of liver and pancreas following selective and subselective angiography. Radiology 111:293–295, 1974

238. Castanede-Zuniga WR, Jauregui H, Rysavy JA, et al: Complications of wedge hepatic venography. Radiology 126:53–56, 1978

239. Lunderquist A, Eriksson M, Ingemansson S, et al: Selective pancreatic vein catheterization for hormone assay in endocrine tumors of the pancreas. Cardiovasc Radiol 1:117–124, 1978

240. Viamonte M Jr, Pereiras R, Russell E, et al: Transhepatic obliteration of gastroesophageal varices: Results in acute and nonacute bleeders. Am J Roentgenol 129:237–241, 1977

241. Widrich WC, Johnson WC, Robbins AH, et al: Esophagogastric variceal hemorrhage: Its treatment by percutaneous transhepatic coronary vein occlusion. Arch Surg 113:1331–1338, 1978

242. Burcarth F, Nielbo N, Andersen B: Percutaneous transhepatic portography. II. Comparison with splenoportography in portal hypertension. Am J Roentgenol 132:183–185, 1979

243. Foster JH, Conkle DM, Crane JM, et al: Splenoportography: An assessment of its value and risk. Ann Surg 179:773–781, 1974

244. Panke WF, Bradley EG, Moreno AH, et al: Technique, hazards, and usefulness of percutaneous splenic portography. JAMA 169:1032–1037, 1959

245. Burcarth F: Percutaneous transhepatic portography. I. Technique and application. Am J Roentgenol 132:177–182, 1979

246. Viamonte M Jr, LePage J, Lunderquist A, et al: Selective catheterization of the portal vein and its tributaries: Preliminary report. Radiology 114:457–460, 1975

247. Boijsen E, Efsing HO: Intrasplenic arterial aneurysms following splenoportal phlebography. Acta Radiol 6:487–496, 1967

248. Roberts C, Maddison FE: Partial mesenteric arterial occlusion with subsequent ischemic bowel damage due to Pitressin infusion. Am J Roentgenol 126:828–831, 1976

249. Renert WA, Button KF, Fuld SL, et al: Mesenteric venous thrombosis and small-bowel infarction following infusion of vasopressin into the superior mesenteric artery. Radiology 102:299–302, 1972

250. Berardi RS: Vascular complications of superior mesenteric artery infusion with pitressin in treatment of bleeding esophageal varices. Am J Surg 127:757–761, 1974

251. Bookstein JJ, Naderi MJ, Walter JF: Transcatheter embolization for lower gastrointestinal bleeding. Radiology 127:345–349, 1978

252. Goldberger LE, Bookstein JJ: Transcatheter embolization for treatment of diverticular hemorrhage. Radiology 122:613–617, 1977

253. Viamonte M Jr: Abdominal visceral venography. Radiol Clin North Am 14:255–264, 1976

254. Reuter SR, Redman HC: Gastrointestinal Angiography. Philadelphia: Saunders 1977, p 262

255. Bradley EL III, Goldman ML: Gastric infarction after therapeutic embolization. Surgery 79:421–424, 1976

256. Prochaska JM, Flye MW, Johnsrude IS: Left gastric artery embolization for control of gastric bleeding: A complication. Radiology 107:521–522, 1973

257. Cho KJ, Reuter S, Schmidt R: Effects of experimental hepatic artery embolization on hepatic function. Am J Roentgenol 127:563–567, 1976

258. White RI Jr, Strandberg JV, Gross GS, et al: Therapeutic embolization with long-term occluding agents and their effects on embolized tissues. Radiology 125:677–687, 1977

259. Doppman JL, Dunnick NR, Girton M, et al: Bile duct cysts secondary to liver infarcts: Report of a case and experimental production by small vessel hepatic artery occlusion. Radiology 130:1–5, 1979

260. Doppman JL, Girton M, Kahn ER: Proximal versus peripheral hepatic arterial embolization: Experimental study in monkeys. Radiology 128:577–588, 1978

261. Anderson JH, VuBan A, Wallace S, et al: Transcatheter splenic arterial occlusion: An experimental study in dogs. Radiology 125:95–102, 1977

262. Castaneda-Zuniga WR, Hammerschmidt DE, Sanchez R, et al: Nonsurgical splenectomy. Am J Roentgenol 129:805–811, 1977

263. Goldstein HM, Wallace S. Anderson JH, et al: Transcatheter occlusion of abdominal tumors. Radiology 120:539–545, 1976

264. Lina JR, Jaques P, Mandell V: Aneurysm rupture secondary to transcatheter embolization. Am J Roentgenol 132:553–556, 1979

265. D'Orsi CJ, Ensminger W, Smith EH, et al: Gasforming intrahepatic abscess: A possible complication of arterial infusion chemotherapy. Gastrointest Radiol 4:1–5, 1978

266. Clouse ME, Ahmed R, Ryan RB, et al: Complications of long term transbrachial arterial infusion chemotherapy. Am J Roentgenol 129:799–803, 1977

267. Lucas RJ, Tumacder O, Wilson GS: Hepatic artery occlusion following hepatic artery catheterization. Ann Surg 173:238–243, 1971

Acknowledgment

We express our immense gratitude to Mrs. Carolyn Shaver for her aid in preparing the preceding material.

5 Esophageal Complications of Surgery and Lifesaving Procedures

Leonid Calenoff and Lee F. Rogers

The esophagus, although well protected by other organs and structures in the posterior mediastinum, is easily accessible to endoscopy through the mouth. The same anatomic factors, however, make surgical approach difficult, necessitating thoracotomy, laparotomy, or both. Each is a major surgical procedure. The dual function of the esophagus as conduit for food and draining path for saliva makes complete removal of this organ impossible. Therefore, to provide a substitute esophagus by means of reconstruction has been the aim of surgeons for decades. New methods and improvement of old procedures are described frequently in surgical publications.

Esophageal surgery, by virtue of its complexity, is often followed by iatrogenic complications, some of them expected, and others creating major problems of recovery. To understand the cause and natural history of such iatrogenic complications it will be necessary to have a basic knowledge of the radiologic anatomy of esophageal surgery and potential complications and their effects upon other organs. Only then does radiologic evaluation of the postsurgical esophagus become meaningful and contribute significantly to management of the patient.

Radiologic Evaluation

Radiologic evaluation of the postsurgical esophagus is sometimes different from routine studies preceding surgery. The patient's inability to stand or move freely may necessitate improvisation of examinations. Distinction has to be made also between radiologic examination of an esophagus with no complications postoperatively and one in which complications are anticipated or have been already diagnosed.

Radiologic examination of an uncomplicated reconstructed esophagus will require detailed information about the nature of the esophageal surgery, particularly the organ used to achieve the reconstruction (1). A barium swallow will yield most of the information about the radiographic anatomy and relative function of the reconstructed organ. If there is any suspicion that the vascular supply of the reconstructed esophagus is not adequate, arteriography is appropriate (Fig. 5-1).

When postsurgical complications are anticipated, plain radiographs of the neck, chest, and possibly abdomen should be taken and evaluated for unusual collections of air in soft tissue, mediastinum, and peritoneal space. Abnormal air-fluid levels may indicate an abscess. Such can also be searched for by ultrasonography and computed tomography.

Contrast Media

When contrast studies are needed in the postoperative period the question of what medium to use will of necessity arise. When a leak in the esophagus itself or at any one anastomosis is expected, iodinated water-soluble contrast media are recommended. Barium is not used because of the widespread belief that it is potentially dangerous and produces inflammatory changes in the mediastinum. James et al. have

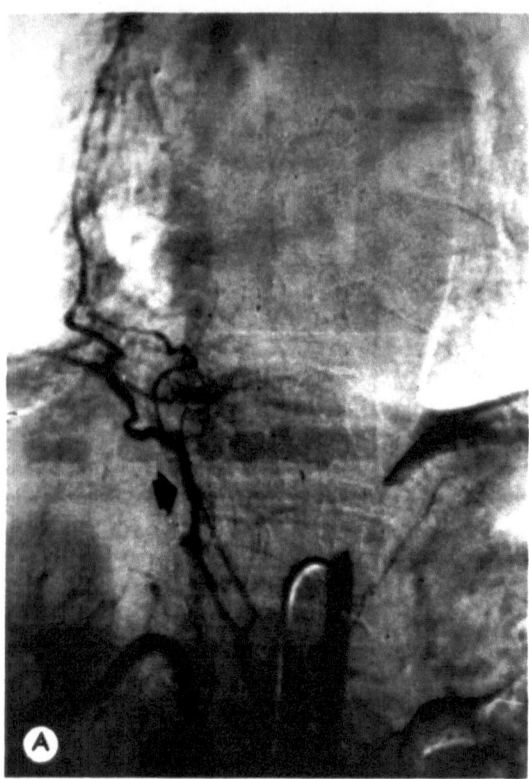

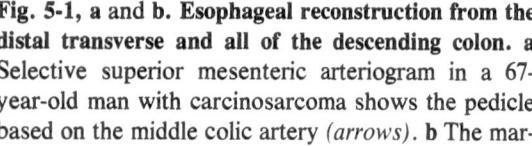

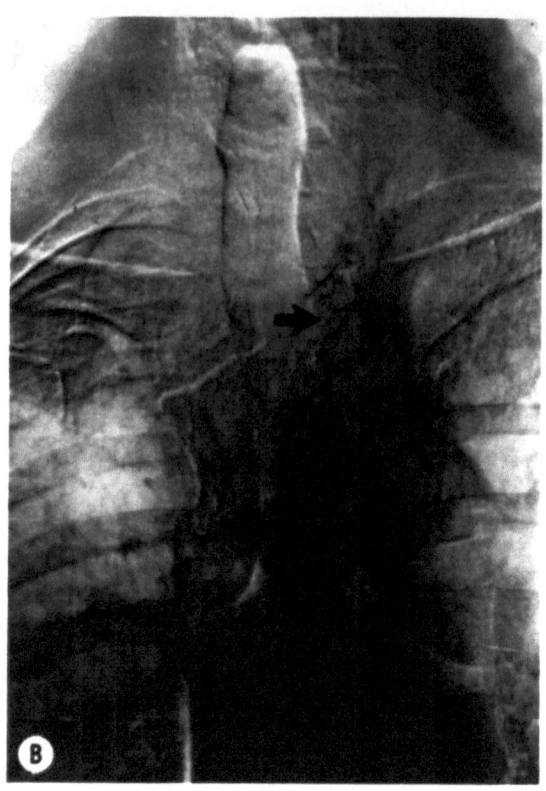

Fig. 5-1, a and b. Esophageal reconstruction from the distal transverse and all of the descending colon. a Selective superior mesenteric arteriogram in a 67-year-old man with carcinosarcoma shows the pedicle based on the middle colic artery *(arrows)*. **b** The mar-

ginal artery that courses in the anterior mediastinum *(arrows)* terminates above the thoracic inlet at the site of anastomosis. (Calenoff L, Norfray J: The reconstructed esophagus. Am J Roentgenol 125:864–876, 1975)

found that water-soluble contrast media injected into the mediastinum of an animal model caused no significant histologic reaction and were no longer visible 1 day after the injection (2). Barium, on the other hand, is known to have the superior physical properties of mucosal coating and radiographic density. When injected in the mediastinum of the same animal model, barium showed as localized, white, chalky deposits in the paraesophageal structures.

Histologically barium causes granuloma formation. When mixed with flora, barium in some circumstances has an inhibitory effect on the growth of bacteria. When barium is used in an iatrogenically damaged esophagus, it may remain for years in the neighboring organs, a telltale sign of iatrogenic damage and a hurried radiologic examination. (Fig. 5-2)

Potential Hazards

Potential hazards exist in the use of contrast material in postsurgical evaluation of the esophagus, the leading hazard being aspiration. Aspiration will introduce contrast material into the bronchial tree and alveoli. The contrast agent can reach the same structures via fistula and leaks of anastomoses. In investigating effects of opaque contrast media on the lung, Dunbar et al. concluded that of several agents studied (Lipoidol, aqueous Dionosil, and barium sulfate) no one appeared to be clearly more damaging to lung parenchyma than the others (3).

A real hazard is pulmonary edema, which may develop when a water-soluble contrast medium used for postsurgical examination of the esophagus enters the bronchial tree and reaches the

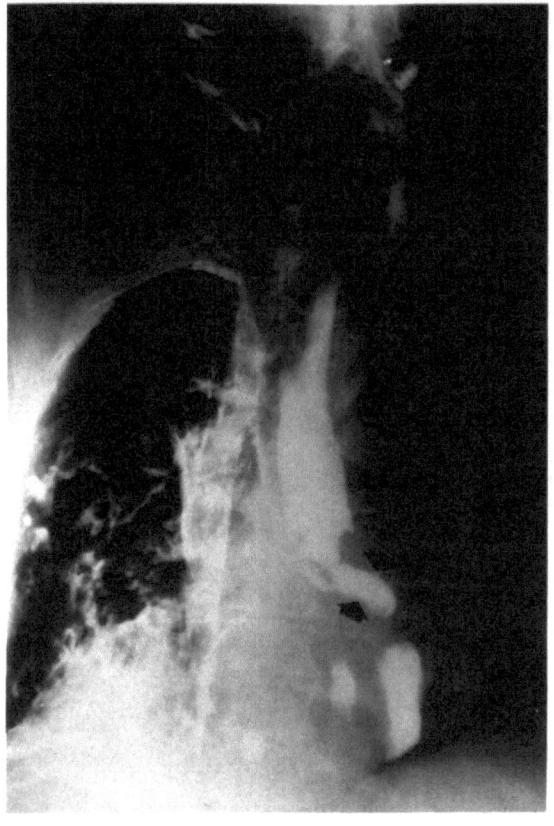
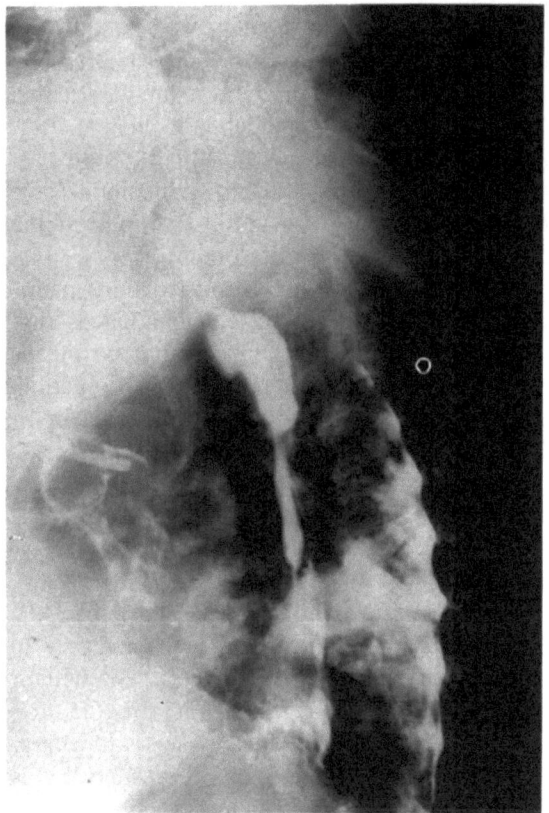

a   b

Fig. 5-2, a and b. Barium study after perforation of the esophagus during endoscopy. a A 62-year-old woman with hiatus hernia had undergone endoscopic evaluation of peptic ulceration *(arrows)* in the hernia. After barium swallow the barium spread from the per- forated pyriform sinus to the mediastinum, neck, and pleural space. **b** It remained visible at the same loca- tions 4 years later. (Calenoff L, Rogers LF: Radiologic manifestations of iatrogenic changes of the esophagus. Gastrointest Radiol 2:229–237, 1977)

alveoli (4). When a water-soluble contrast medium is used in small children or in patients with a decrease in circulating plasma, although the agent was introduced to examine the esoph- agus only, the subsequent retention in the bowel can cause severe hypovolemia (5).

Radiographic Anatomy of Esophageal Surgery

It is good practice to be aware of the radio- graphic anatomy of the esophagus postsurgically to perform an adequate radiologic evaluation (6). This may not be possible, however, because a description of the surgical procedure is not usu- ally available to the radiologist at the time of the examination. Movement of patients from one institution to another makes it even more diffi- cult to obtain precise information. If an opera- tion is designated by an eponym, the one per- formed may not be precisely the operation indicated by the eponym. Surgeons often modify a procedure in the presence of unexpected find- ings, particularly during cancer surgery.

Esophageal Reconstruction

Reconstruction of an obstructed or poorly func- tioning esophagus has been the aim of thoracic and gastrointestinal surgeons for the past seven decades. After an early series of failures, with the advent of antibiotics visceral replacement of the esophagus became relatively successful. Various viscera were placed subcutaneously in efforts to solve technical problems: skin tube by Bircher in 1894, jejunum by Roux and Herzen in 1907, large bowel by Vulliet and Kelling in 1911, and stomach by Kirschner in 1920 (7). In the past two decades, colon, stomach, and jejunum have been widely used with reconstructions in the anterior or posterior mediastinum.

In spite of successful reconstruction, palliation has never been completely abandoned. Simple gastrostomy permits feeding but no means for draining saliva. To remedy this, a polyethylene or silastic tube, such as the Celestin or Mousseau-Barbin, is inserted across the lesion to maintain a lumen (8) (Fig. 5-3).

Indications

In general, indications for reconstruction of the esophagus are poor function and obstruction. In infants and children these include atresia with or without tracheoesophageal fistula, strictures following chemical burns, and varices with extrahepatic obstruction. In adults the esophagus is usually reconstructed for benign conditions such as achalasia, scleroderma, tumors, fistula, and strictures due to instrumentation, chemical burns, or peptic esophagitis. However, the most common single indication for reconstruction is esophageal carcinoma.

The task of reconstruction is not simple; the viscus or viscera to be used for the procedure depend on circumstances. Numerous criteria have to be fulfilled before a reconstructed esophagus can be considered to be properly functioning. In addition to provision of a near-normal swallowing mechanism, there should be "normal" vomiting and no significant reflux of gastric or intestinal contents into the reconstructed esophagus as well as absence of dumping, anemia, diarrhea, and malabsorption. The reconstructed esophagus should not be digested by hydrochloric acid or by duodenal or jejunal contents.

Many terms are used to designate reconstruction procedures such as esophageal bypass, colon interposition, esophageal transplant, esophageal reconstruction, esophagoplasty, and neoesophagus. These terms, however, do not specify the exact procedure and how it was performed.

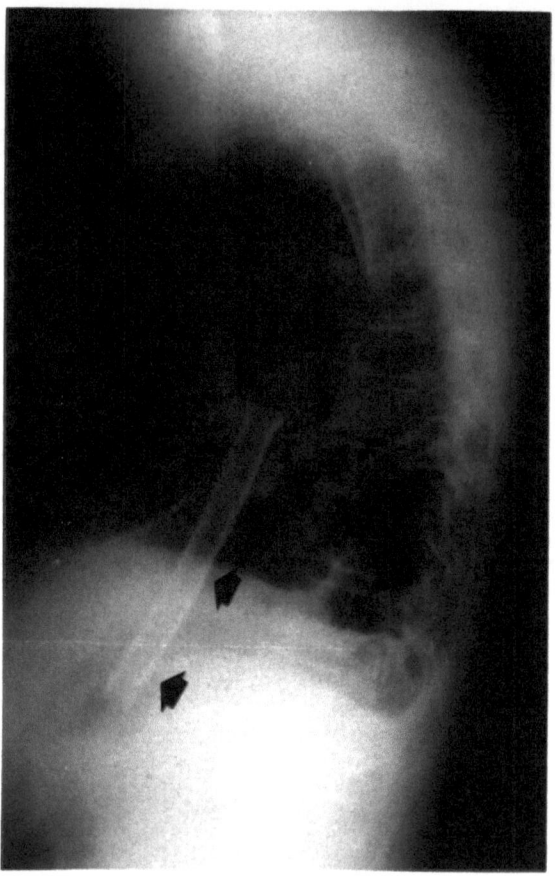

Fig. 5-3. **Palliative restoration of esophageal lumen.** A no. 8 polyethylene tube *(arrows)* was inserted across the lesion in a 70-year-old woman with obstructing carcinoma. (Calenoff L, Rogers LF: Radiologic manifestations of iatrogenic changes of the esophagus. Gastrointest Radiol 2:229–237, 1977)

Reconstruction of Thoracic Esophagus

Colonic Transplant

The colon has long been the leading choice of organs used in reconstruction of the esophagus. The term transplant is used to designate the mobilization of the viscus from its usual location, while retaining its blood supply, and its subsequent placement into the chest. Colon has been used to replace the entire esophagus, via subcutaneous placement or in the anterior mediastinum (Fig. 5-4), or to replace only part, as an interposed segment usually in the posterior mediastinum (Fig. 5-5).

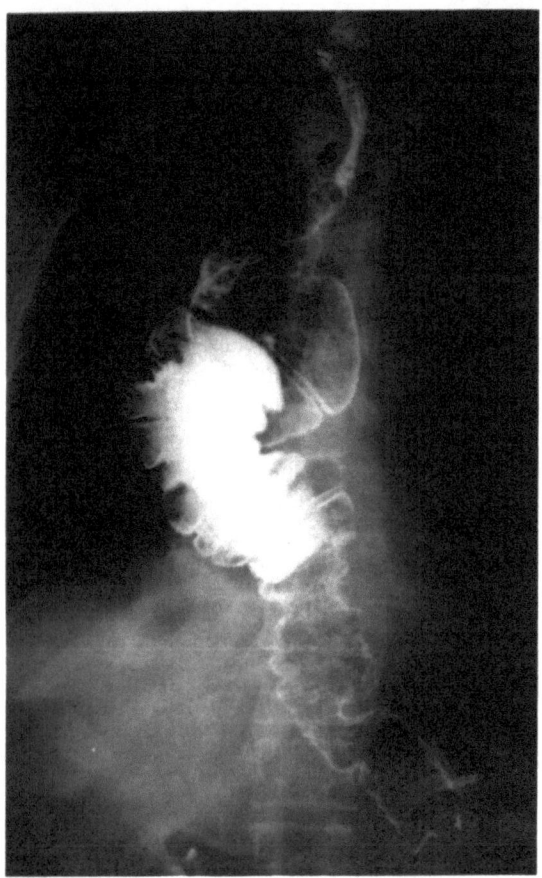

Fig. 5-4. Esophageal reconstruction from right colon and terminal ileum. Done in the anterior mediastinum in an 87-year-old woman with carcinoma, the proximal anastomosis *(small arrows)* is end to side, and the distal anastomosis *(large arrow)* is high at the lesser curvature of the stomach. (Calenoff L, Norfray J: The reconstructed esophagus. Am J Roentgenol 125:864–876, 1975)

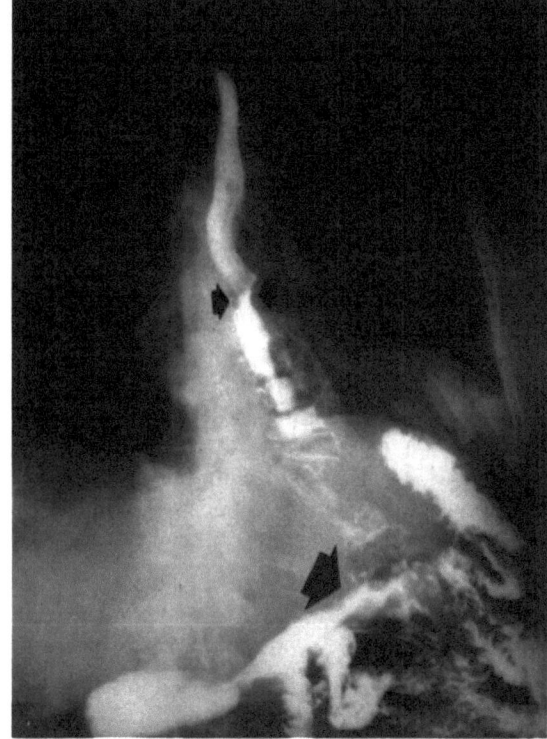

a

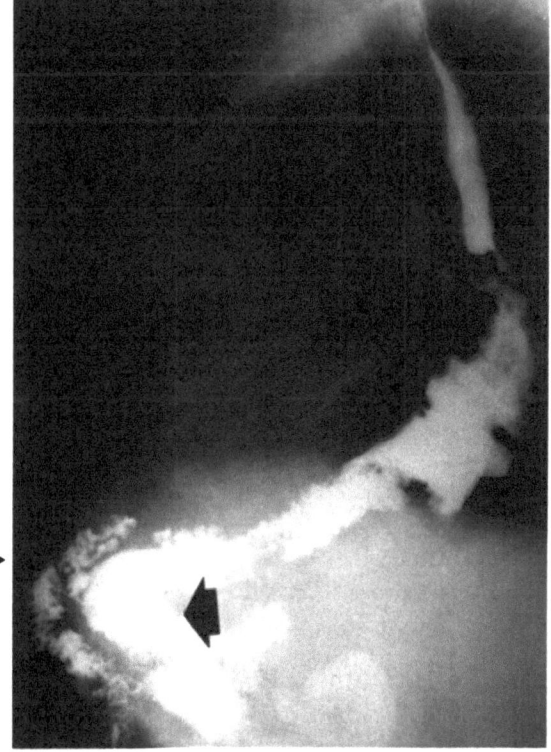

b

Fig. 5-5, a and b. Esophageal reconstruction from an 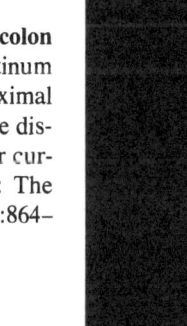 **interposed segment of colon.** In a 74-year-old man with esophageal carcinoma the lower esophagus and proximal stomach were resected and a segment of right colon interposed between the remaining esophagus and the distal stomach. **a** The upper anastomosis is end to end *(small arrows)*. **a** and **b** The lower anastomosis is end to side *(large arrow)*. (Calenoff L, Norfray J: The reconstructed esophagus. Am J Roentgenol 125:864–876, 1975)

Various segments of colon are being used for reconstruction: right colon and terminal ileum in isoperistaltic position; right colon in isoperistaltic position without terminal ileum and cecal pole; right colon in antiperistaltic position with the terminal ileum preserved or interposed; transverse colon in isoperistaltic position; left colon in isoperistaltic position; left colon in antiperistaltic position (9–12).

The popularity of the colon for reconstruction is due to its inherent qualities: adequate length, good marginal blood supply, and some resistance to digestion by hydrochloric acid. The right colon is used by most surgeons because it is easily mobilized and has an adequate blood supply provided by the middle colic artery. When the right colon is used with the terminal ileum preserved, the isoperistaltic nature of the segment prevents reflux. The inclusion of terminal ileum permits easy crossing of the thoracic inlet and a cervical anastomosis of the same caliber. When the right colon is used without the terminal ileum or cecal pole, the latter segments are resected and discarded because cecum, ileocecal valve, and terminal ileum are supplied by the ileocecal artery with its poor collateral circulation. The cecal pole is frequently too thick for a good cervical anastomosis. When the right colon is used in an antiperistaltic fashion the cecal pole and terminal ileum are preserved, and the ileum is anastomosed to the stomach. A segment of ileum or jejunum can be interposed so that the cecum is anastomosed to the stomach, with the intention to have the ileocecal valve function as cardia. The use of transverse colon has been justified by two facts: the left colic artery is 2–4 mm wide from its origin to the marginal artery, and there is a good venous network, which is considered important for the survival of the transplant. The use of the left colon has been justified because it is sufficiently long and has good blood supply and because its smaller caliber is closer to that of the esophagus.

Anastomoses

The first area to be evaluated radiographically is the upper anastomosis, usually end-to-end or end-to-side above the thoracic inlet. The colon segment should be straight and short to avoid redundancy. In children there is no need to use a long redundant colonic segment since the colon used for reconstruction grows as the child grows.

The lower anastomosis should also be evaluated. It is usually placed high on the lesser curvature of the stomach. A pyloroplasty is often necessary to prevent retention.

Function

Some investigators claim that the colonic segment fills and empties by gravity and that no peristalsis is detected during radiologic examination (13). On the other hand, esophageal motility studies have shown occasional contractions propagated throughout the colonic segment (14). Continuous colonic peristalsis was demonstrated in a reconstructed esophagus by Jones et al. (15). They infused the colonic segment with hydrochloric acid as a stimulus and recorded contractions with amplitudes of 14–15 mm Hg that lasted 25–30 seconds. They postulated that colonic contractions in a reconstructed esophagus are a response to acid reflux from the stomach. Colonic excretion and bicarbonate usually act as a buffer to the refluxed acid and prevent damage. It is, however, generally accepted that these peristaltic waves are not very effective in propagation of food particles.

Gastric Transplant

A simple and least sophisticated way of using the stomach for esophageal reconstruction is the pull-up procedure whereby the stomach is pulled through the hiatus into the chest and anastomosed to the cervical esophagus (Fig. 5-6). A more sophisticated approach is the fashioning of a gastric tube from the greater curvature. Such reversed gastric tube operations were initially described in 1905 by Beck and reintroduced in 1955 simultaneously by Gavriliu in Romania and Heimlich in the United States (16).

Heimlich Gastric Tube

In the Heimlich operation a pedicle tube 30 cm long and 2.5 cm wide is constructed from the greater curvature of the stomach, using the Izukura stapling instrument (17). The staples are visible on postoperative radiographs. The base of the tube remains attached to the gastric fundus. A splenectomy is performed to reinforce the blood supply to the gastric tube, which is then reversed and anastomosed to the cervical esophagus.

The advantages of a reversed gastric tube are that it provides a physiologic method for recon-

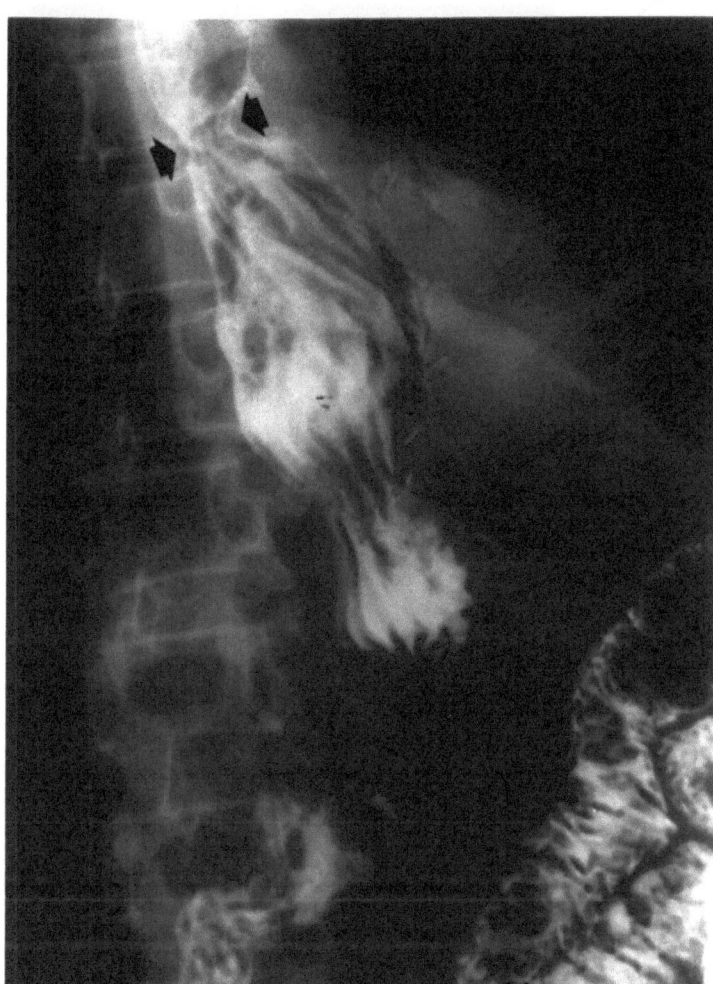

Fig. 5-6. **Esophageal reconstruction by means of the pull-up procedure.** after partial esophagogastrectomy for Barrett's ulcer in a 57-year-old man the remaining stomach was pulled into the chest to achieve anastomosis with the esophagus (*arrows*). (Calenoff L, Rogers LF: Radiologic manifestations of iatrogenic changes of the esophagus. Gastrointest Radiol 2:229–237, 1977)

struction; a distal organ is not interposed between the esophagus and the stomach; the new esophagus grows normally in children; the blood supply is excellent; and secondary peptic esophagitis does not occur. The reversed gastric tube can be placed subcutaneously, retrosternally, or in the posterior mediastinum.

Beck Gastric Tube

In the Beck operation the gastric tube remains attached to the gastric antrum (18) (Fig. 5-7). Splenectomy is not performed. Postoperative radiographic evaluation of the Beck type of reversed gastric tube focuses on two major points: the upper anastomosis (Fig. 5-8) and the lower aspect of the reversed gastric tube. The proximal tip of the gastric tube is brought out to the skin in the neck as a controlled fistula, which is closed later under local anesthesia (Fig. 5-9).

Barium can pass from the gastric tube into the gastric antrum and duodenum but also may reflux into the remaining diseased esophagus that is left in place (Fig. 5-10).

Jejunal Transplant

Surgeons who use jejunum for reconstruction of the esophagus believe that it is the only segment of the gastrointestinal tract devoid of inherent diseases (19). Others, however, believe that the anatomic arrangement of the jejunal vessels does not provide adequate vascularization for the length of segment needed for total reconstruction. Jejunum is therefore used to replace the distal esophagus by means of a variety of esophagogastrojejunostomies (Fig. 5-11). A Segment of jejunum can also be interposed between the distal esophagus and the duodenum (Fig. 5-

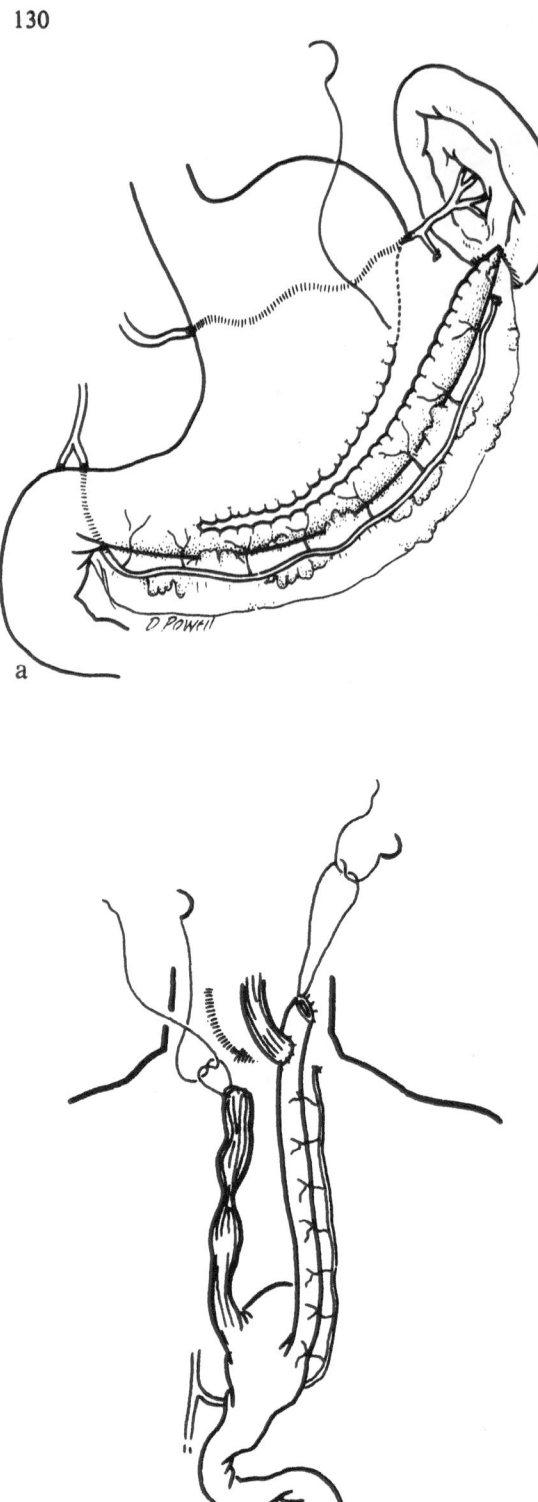

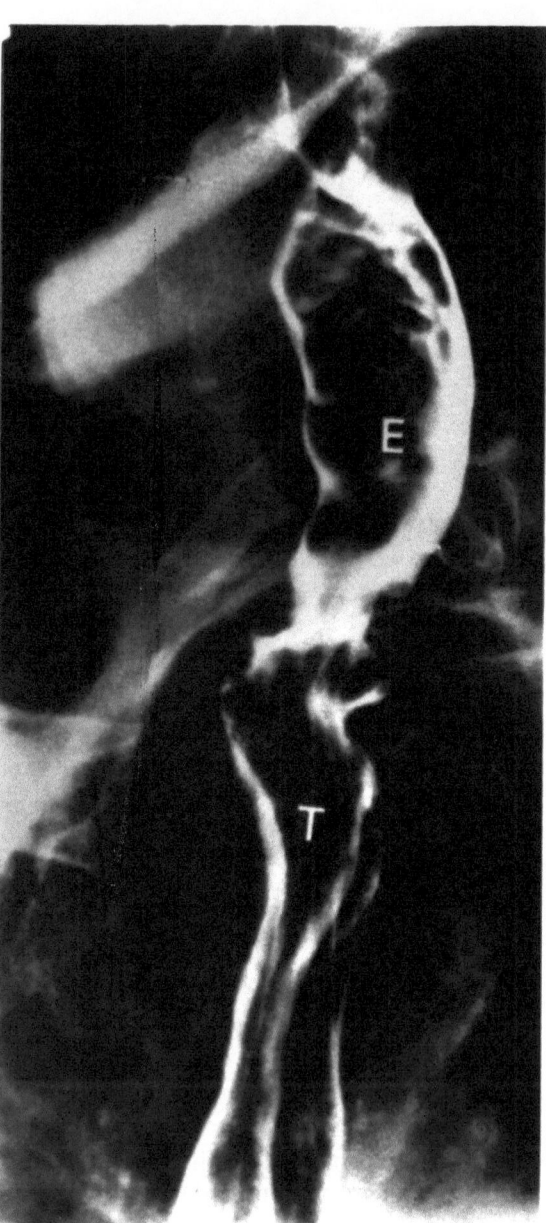

Fig. 5-8. **Beck reversed gastric tube** (*T*). Radiograph shows the postoperative appearance of the upper anastomosis. *E*, upper esophagus. (Fetouh SA et al: Radiologic aspects of Beck gastric tube in esophageal reconstruction. Am J Roentgenol 129:425–431, 1977)

Fig. 5-7, a and b. Beck operation for formation of a reversed gastric tube. a The gastric tube is formed from the greater curvature. **b** It is reversed and anastomosed to the cervical esophagus. The diseased esophagus is usually left in place. (Fetouh SA et al: Radiologic aspects of Beck gastric tube in esophageal reconstruction. Am J Roentgenol 129:425–431, 1977)

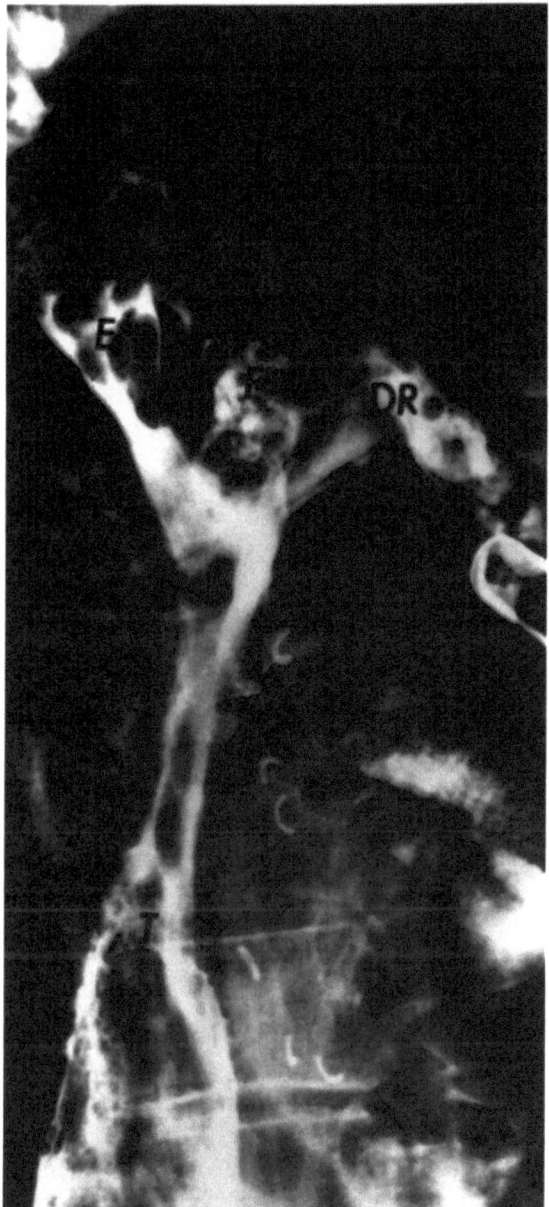

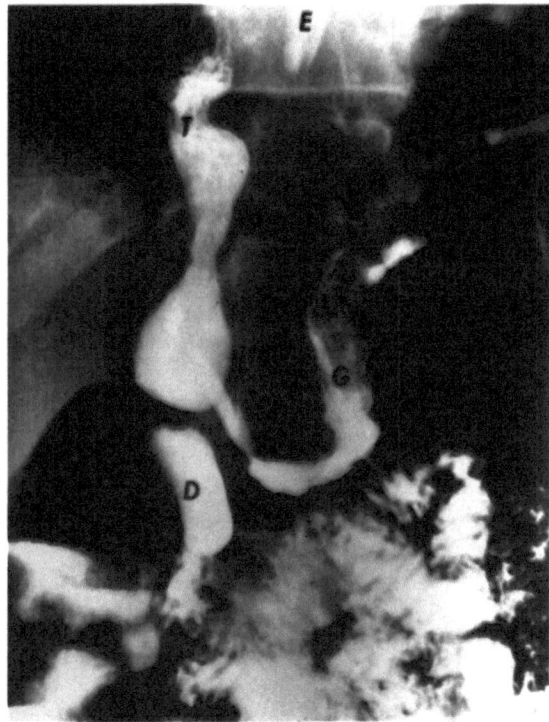

a

Fig. 5-9. Beck reversed gastric tube (*T*). Radiograph shows the postoperative appearance. A draining cutaneous fistula has been left in place (*F*). Penrose drain placed for leaking anastomosis (*DR*). *E*, upper esophagus. (Fetouh SA et al: Radiologic aspects of Beck gastric tube in esophageal reconstruction. Am J Roentgenol 129:425–431, 1977)

b

Fig. 5-10, a and b. Beck reversed gastric tube. Anteroposterior (**a**) and lateral (**b**) views demonstrate gastric remnant (*G*), reversed Beck gastric tube (*T*), remaining esophagus (*E*), duodenum (*D*). The gastric tube is located in the anterior mediastinum. (Fetouh SA et al: Radiologic aspects of Beck gastric tube in esophageal reconstruction. Am J Roentgenol 129:425–431, 1977)

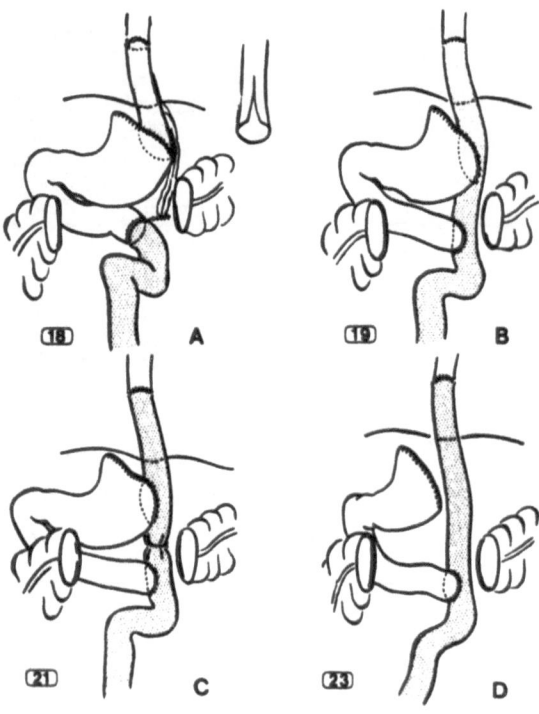

Fig. 5-11, A–D. Esophageal replacement with jejunum. Surgical techniques employing jejunum *(dotted segments)* in 81 patients are shown. **a** Esophagojejunogastrotomy; **b** Roux-en-Y procedure; **c** Roux-en-Y with heavy nonabsorbable ligature tied loosely around jejunal loop; **d** Roux-en-Y with the stomach excluded. (Dave KS et al: Esophageal replacement with jejunum for nonmalignant lesions: 26 years' experience. Surgery 72:466–473, 1972)

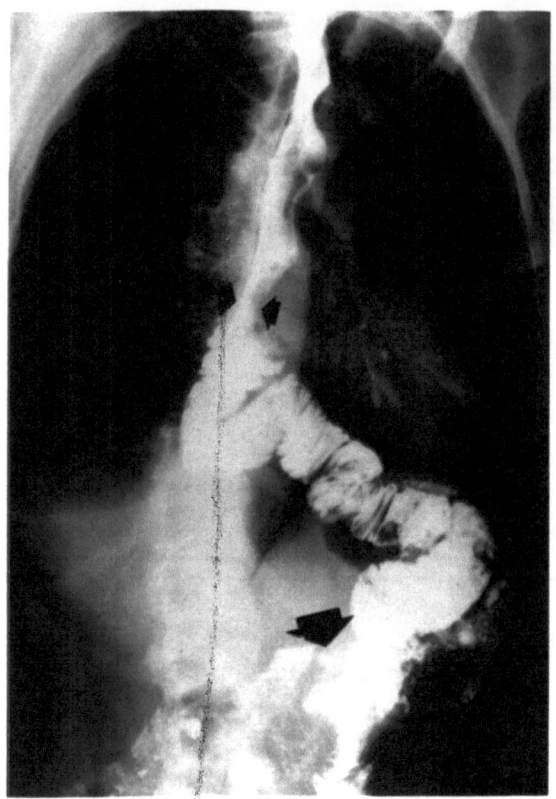

Fig. 5-12. Esophageal reconstruction with jejunal interposition. A segment of jejunum has been placed between the midesophagus *(upper arrows)* and the duodenum *(lower arrow)* in a 61-year-old woman. Total gastrectomy was performed. (Calenoff L, Norfray J: The reconstructed esophagus. Am J Roentgenol 125:864–876, 1975)

12). The radiological assessment of an esophagojejunostomy is easy, real difficulties being encountered only if the exact nature of a complex procedure is not known.

Reconstruction of Cervical Esophagus

Reconstruction of the cervical esophagus has always been more difficult than reconstruction of the thoracic esophagus. This is particularly true if a pharyngolaryngectomy had been performed.

Gastric Pull-up

Gastric pull-up operations are performed in one stage by two surgeons, one working at the neck, the other in the abdomen (20). The stomach and the thoracic esophagus are mobilized and pulled

through the enlarged hiatus into the posterior mediastinum. When the gastric fundus reaches the stump of the oropharynx, the lower esophagus is transected, the cardioesophageal junction is closed, and the gastric fundus is anastomosed to the pharynx. In a modification of the operation the gastric apex is invaginated over the anastomosis to prevent leakage (21).

Free Intestinal Graft

Free, unattached jejunal or ileal grafts have been successful since the advent of microvascular surgery, permitting rapid and dependable venous and arterial anastomoses of minute vessels. A stapling apparatus such as Inokuchi's (22) permits joining of two everted vessel ends together, intima to intima, with stainless staples, thus maintaining the tubular shape of the vessel.

Skin Flap Reconstruction

Rotated skin flaps from the neck and chest have been used to reconstruct the cervical esophagus after extensive resection for cancer. In the Wookey operation (23) a rectangular cervical flap is placed between the stumps of the oropharynx and cervical esophagus, and then a tubing of intervening skin segment. As a result the neoesophagus is skin-lined. With a single or double deltopectoral flap a tubed skin-lined cervical esophagus is also formed that could look almost normal on barium swallow (24).

Esophageal Surgery Other Than Reconstruction

Many mostly benign esophageal lesions require specific surgical intervention other than reconstruction. In most of these cases the radiographic anatomy of the esophagus is altered, and specific complications are prone to occur.

Repair of Congenital Tracheoesophageal Fistula

Surgical repair of congenital tracheoesophageal fistula could leave a residual "diverticulum" in the area of the previous fistula (Fig. 5-13) and result in motility disorders distal to the anastomosis. A residual diverticulum is usually of no clinical significance, however.

Esophageal Myotomy

Myotomy of the cervical and lower esophagus is performed for cricopharyngeal dysphagia and achalasia respectively.

Cricopharyngeal Myotomy

Cricopharyngeal dysphagia, often accompanied by a small pulsion diverticulum, is the result of dysfunction of the cricopharyngeus muscle, seen on barium swallow as a radiopaque bar across the hypoglottis on the frontal projection and as a posterior indentation at the level of C-6 on the lateral view. After myotomy the symptoms, the pulsion diverticulum, and the radiographic finding are no longer present (25).

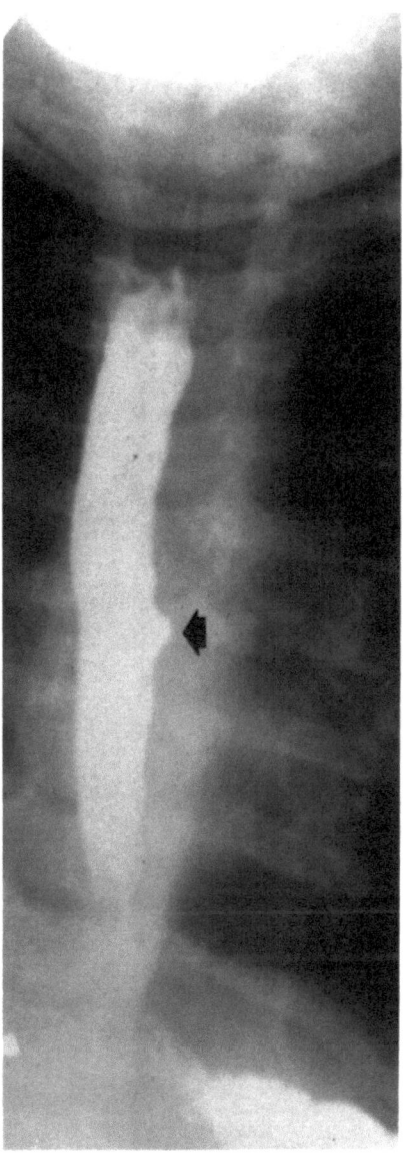

Fig. 5-13. Residual "diverticulum." This occurred in the midesophagus *(arrow),* following surgical repair of tracheoesophageal fistula. (Calenoff L, Rogers LF: Radiologic manifestations of iatrogenic changes of the esophagus. Gastrointest Radiol 2:229–237, 1977)

Heller Myotomy for Achalasia

This procedure consists of a single longitudinal incision of the esophageal wall down to the mucosa, extending from the dilated segment of the esophagus to the stomach. The lower esophageal sphincter is divided completely. It is done by a transthoracic approach. The incision is never less than 5 cm in length and usually is about 7 or 10 cm. If the esophageal mucosa is accidentally perforated it is sutured immediately. If the Heller myotomy fails, other esophageal reconstruction surgery is performed (26).

Management of Epiphrenic Diverticulum

Fewer than 10% of esophageal diverticula are epiphrenic in location. They are false diverticula of the pulsion type and are easily demonstrable on barium swallow. Occasionally they are mis-

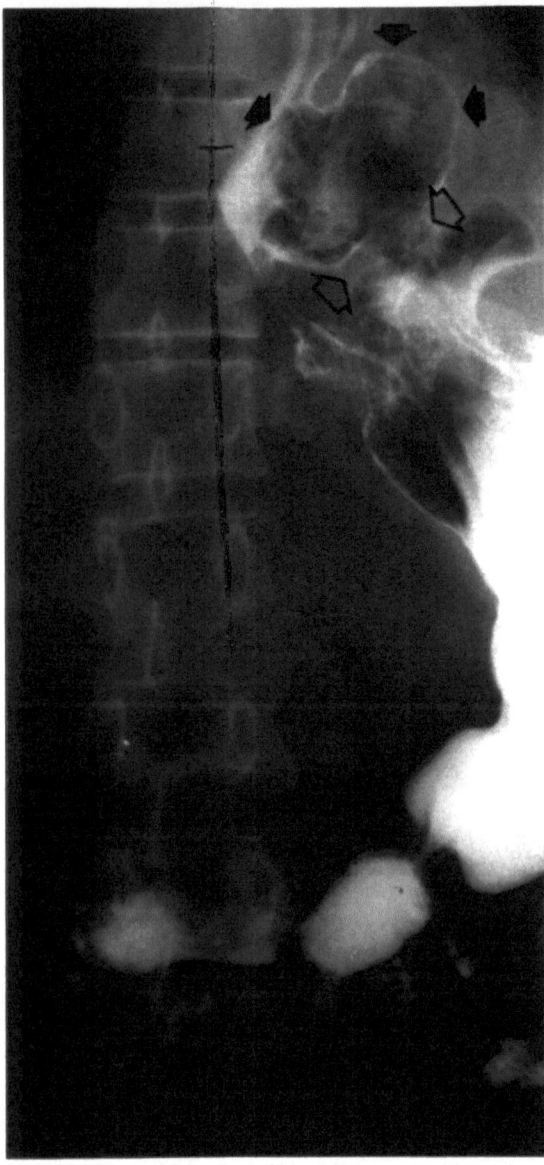

Fig. 5-14. Large epiphrenic diverticulum. Drainage was established in this 60-year-old man by anastomosis of the diverticulum *(black arrows)* to the gastric fundus *(open arrows)*.

taken for hiatal hernia, and sometimes the two coexist.

A constant finding in patients with epiphrenic diverticulum is hypertrophy of circular muscle distal to the diverticulum. Therefore, in addition to excision of such small diverticula, esophageal myotomy is performed. Postoperative barium contrast studies will show a slight bulge of the mucosa at the myotomy site (27). When the epiphrenic diverticulum is large it may be diverted to the gastric fundus (Fig. 5-14).

Treatment of Esophageal Varices

Transection of the esophagus, instead of the usual vascular shunts, is being employed to treat esophageal varices. Using a suture device, Takasaki et al. excise a zone about 1 cm wide from the whole circumference of the esophageal wall (28). This interrupts all three vasculature channels connected to the venous system (Fig. 5-15). Splenectomy and pyloroplasty are also done. Other procedures for varices include partial gastrectomy and gastroesophageal resection.

Antireflux Operations

Operations for gastroesophageal reflux with or without accompanying hiatus hernia alter significantly the radiographic anatomy of the distal esophagus and gastric fundus. The two most popular procedures are the Nissen and the Belsey Mark IV fundoplications.

Nissen Fundoplication
In this fundoplication the gastric fundus is wrapped around both sides of the esophagus, and the two segments of stomach are sutured together anteriorly (29) (Fig. 5-16). Postoperatively there is a definite filling defect at the gastroesophageal juntion. This filling defect is usually smoothly outlined and symmetrically placed on both sides of the esophagus (30). The filling defect is best seen by air-contrast study of the gastric fundus (Fig. 5-17). When the gastric fundus is completely filled with barium the distal esophagus appears as if it were passing through a tunnel, with a concave mass impression upon the stomach in this area (Fig. 5-17).

Belsey Mark IV Fundoplication
In the Belsey Mark IV fundoplication the distal esophagus is invaginated into the gastric fundus, which is then wrapped around and secured by

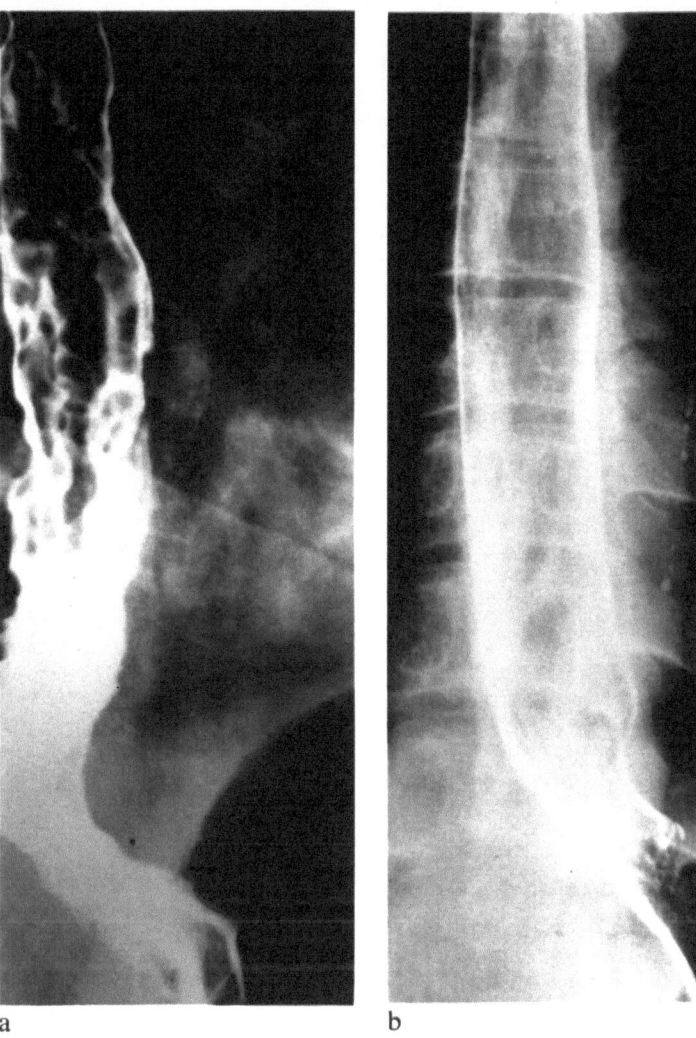

a   b

Fig. 5-15, a and b. Transabdominal esophageal transection for
esophageal varices. Radiographs
were obtained following barium
swallow before (a) and after (b)
the procedure. (Takasaki T et al:
Transabdominal esophageal transection by using a suture device in
case of esophageal varices. Int
Surg 62:426–478, 1977)

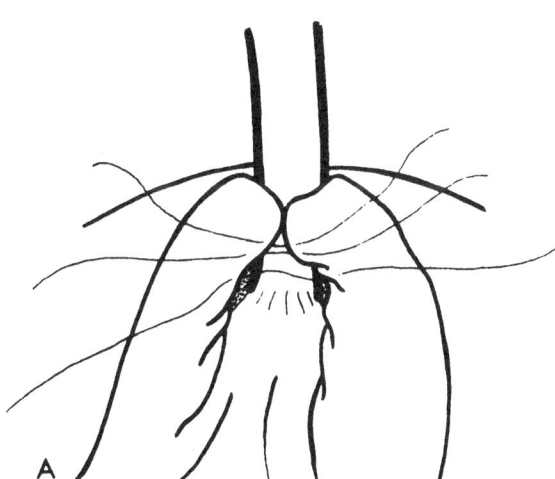

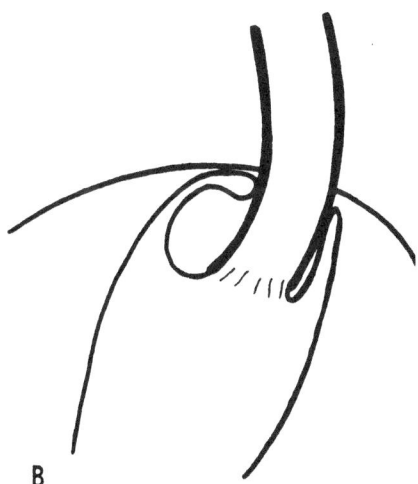

Fig. 5-16, a and b. Nissen fundoplication. The folds of
the fundus are wrapped around the esophagus (a).
Sagittal section of the final stage shows the relationship of the fundus to the esophagus (b). (Teixidor HS,

Evans JA: Roentgenographic appearance of the distal
esophagus and the stomach after hiatal hernia repair.
Am J Roentgenol 119:245–258, 1973)

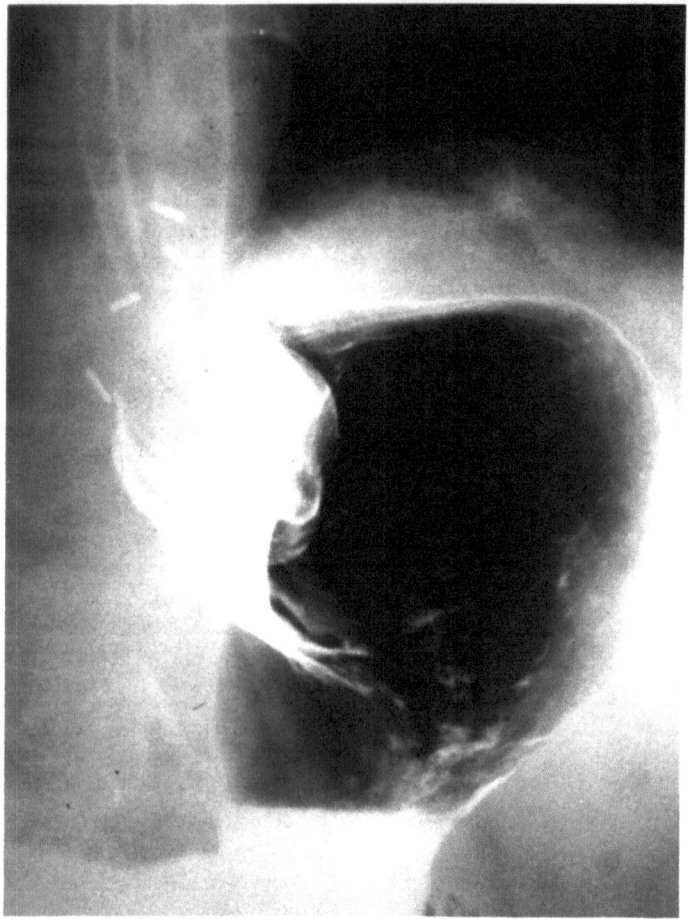

a

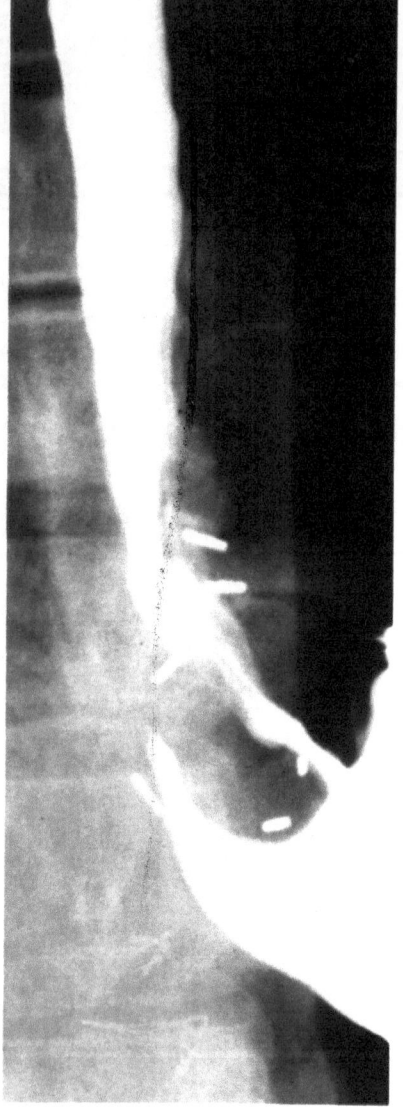

b

Fig. 5-17, a and **b. Nissen fundoplication.** The "typical" 13th post-operative day appearance shows the symmetrical fundal defect (**a**) and the esophagus passing through a "tunnel" (**b**). Note vagotomy clips. (Skucas J et al: An evaluation of the Nissen fundoplication. Radiology, 118:539–543, 1976)

sutures. The sutures are placed so that the esophagus remains fixed to the stomach and the diaphragm (Fig. 5-18). Postoperative barium contrast examination shows a fundal filling defect, which is slightly irregular in contour, and the esophagus tunnels through rather than alongside. It enters the gastric fundus at a somewhat sharper angle than in the Nissen fundoplication (Fig. 5-19).

Hiatus Hernia Repair

The most popular hiatal hernia repair, the Allison procedure, consists of reducing the hernia below the diaphragm and suturing the phreno-

esophageal ligament to the undersurface of the diaphragm in front and to the left of the cardia. The hiatus is then narrowed by suturing the right crus of the diaphragm behind the diaphragm. Variations of the procedure often result in excessive narrowing of the hiatus.

Management of Distal Esophageal Perforation and Stricture

In surgical management of distal esophageal perforation and stricture the gastric fundus is utilized as a patch or wrapped around the distal esophagus. The Thal procedure is the most popular (31). A longitudinal incision is made in the

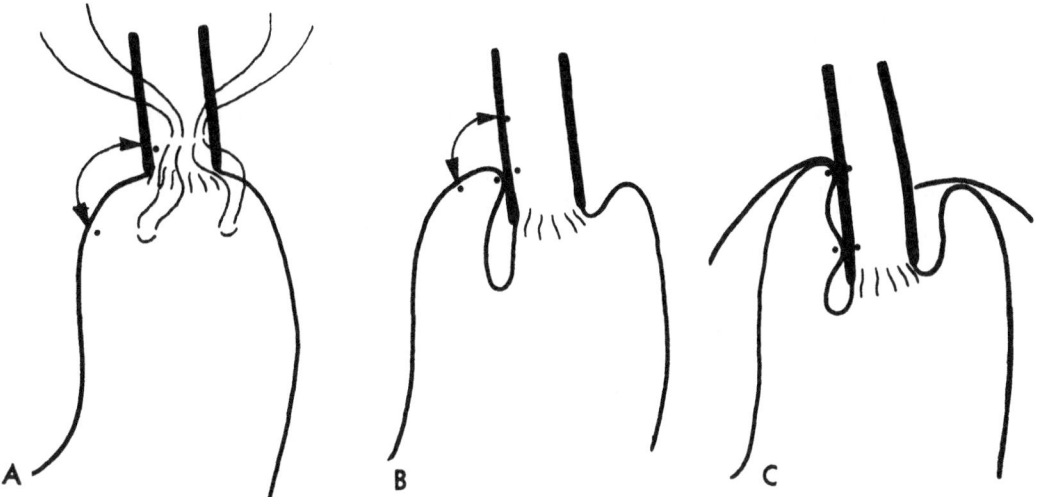

Fig. 5-18, a–c. Belsey Mark IV fundoplication. Stages of the operation are shown: **a** placement of sutures; **b** distal esophagus invaginated into fundus; **c** sagittal section of final stage. (Teixidor HS, Evans JA: Roentgenographic appearance of the distal esophagus and the stomach after hiatal hernia repair. Am J Roentgenol 119:245–258, 1973)

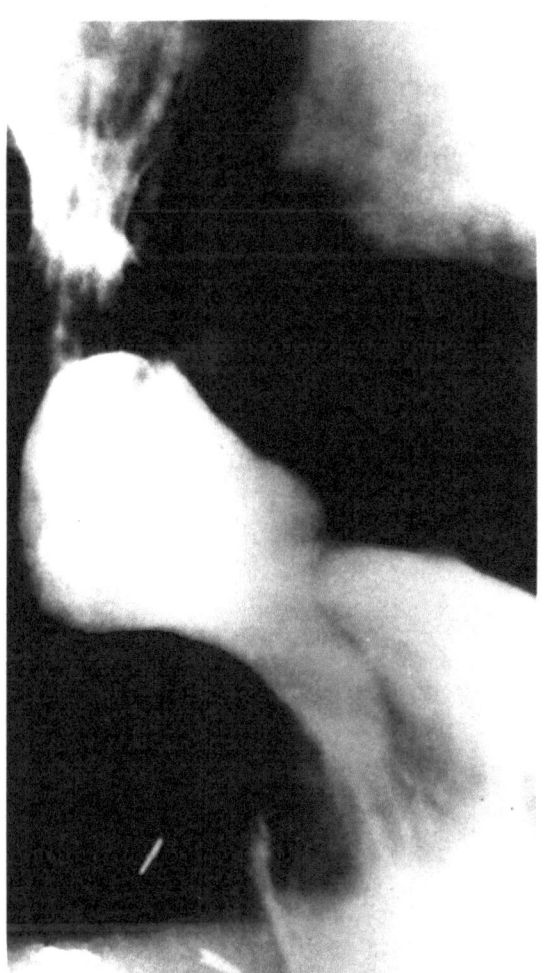

wall of the distal esophagus if a stricture is present, then the incision or the perforation defect is covered by suturing the serosa of the gastric cardia over it. Thus a patch is created.

The postsurgical chest radiographic manifestations are noteworthy. There is a large air-filled structure overlying the cardiac silhouette. This air cavity communicates only with the intraabdominal gastric lumen and is a positive-pressure sac within the negative intrathoracic cavity (31). The findings are often confused with paraesophageal hiatus hernia, epiphrenic diverticulum, or localized eventration.

Complications of Esophageal Surgery

Complications range from temporary leaks at the site of anastomosis, to chronic and debilitating failure of transplant, to a mortality of 40% in repair of congenital tracheoesophageal fistula

◀ **Fig. 5-19. Belsey Mark IV fundoplication.** One year later the distal esophagus tunnels through a large filling defect. (Teixidor HS, Evans JA: Roentgenographic appearance of the distal esophagus and the stomach after hiatal hernia repair. Am J Roentgenol 119:245–258, 1973)

(32). The complications of esophageal surgery can be divided into two major groups: complications common to all procedures and complications of specific procedures.

Esophageal Complications Common to Most Procedures

Complications common to almost all esophageal interventions are fistula, stricture, perforation, gangrene, abscess, obstruction, and, in cases of carcinoma, recurrence. Some of these complications are temporary, and the reconstruction will eventually hold. Vascular insufficiency of the transplant resulting in gangrene or obstruction (Fig. 5-20) is usually hopeless. Minimal perforation leaks can be insignificant, but they can lead to an abscess of graver consequence. Perforation at the distal esophageal stump can be fatal (33).

Leakage and Fistula

The leading complication in esophageal reconstruction is leakage at the upper anastomosis, which can be in the thorax (Fig. 5-21) or in the neck (Fig. 5-22). Minimal leakage is often noted, is temporary, and may subside rapidly without causing any additional complications. The incidence of leakage in the cervical anastomosis and resulting fistula is 35%–41% according to various reports (34–37).

A major factor in the high incidence of leakage and fistula is the tenuous blood supply at the anastomosis. A sudden drop in blood pressure in the postoperative period, even for a very short time, can temporarily disrupt the blood flow to the upper anastomosis, resulting in thrombosis of vessels and subsequent leakage and fistula. In addition, disruption and leakage occur because the upper esophagus has to be angulated anteriorly and around the trachea in order to meet

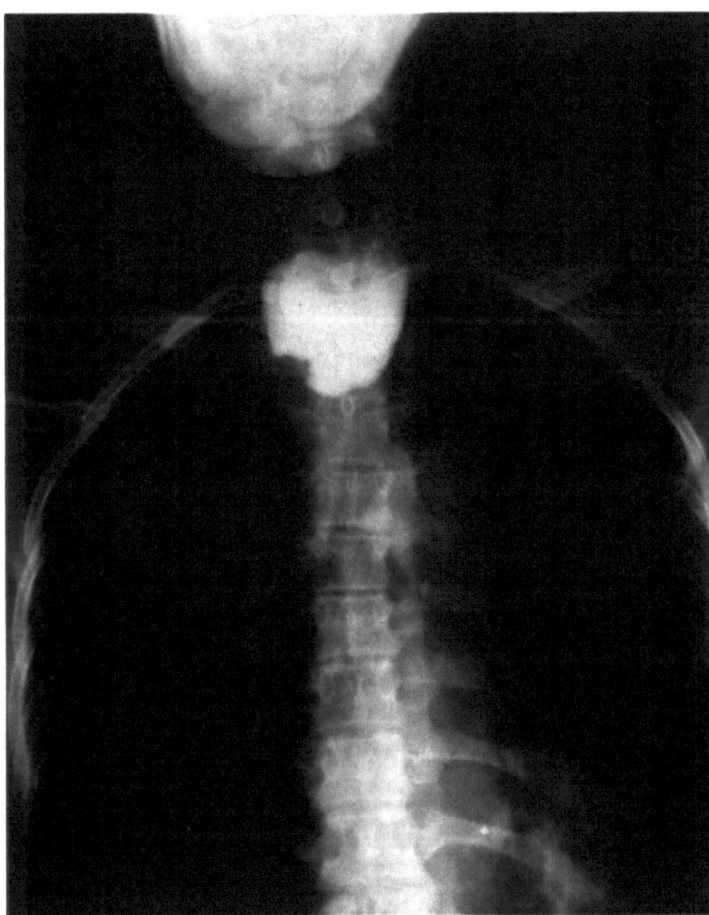

Fig. 5-20. Obstruction of the reconstructed esophagus. In a 46-year-old man with longstanding lye stricture the obstruction is below the level of the anastomosed colon and probably resulted from vascular insufficiency.

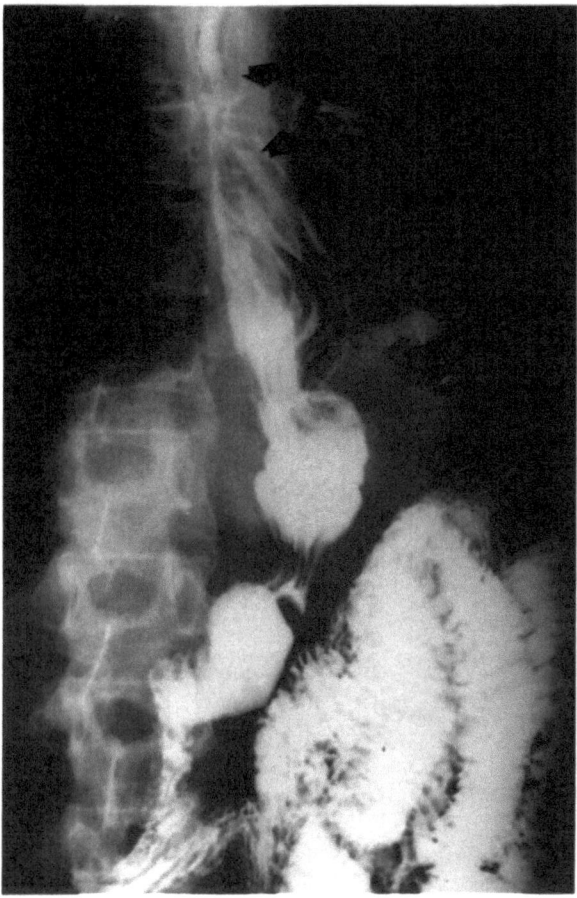

Fig. 5-21. Postoperative leakage. Minimal leakage occurred at the anastomosis *(arrows)* 1 week after esophageal reconstruction in the patient in Fig. 5-6. Leakage stopped 10 days later.

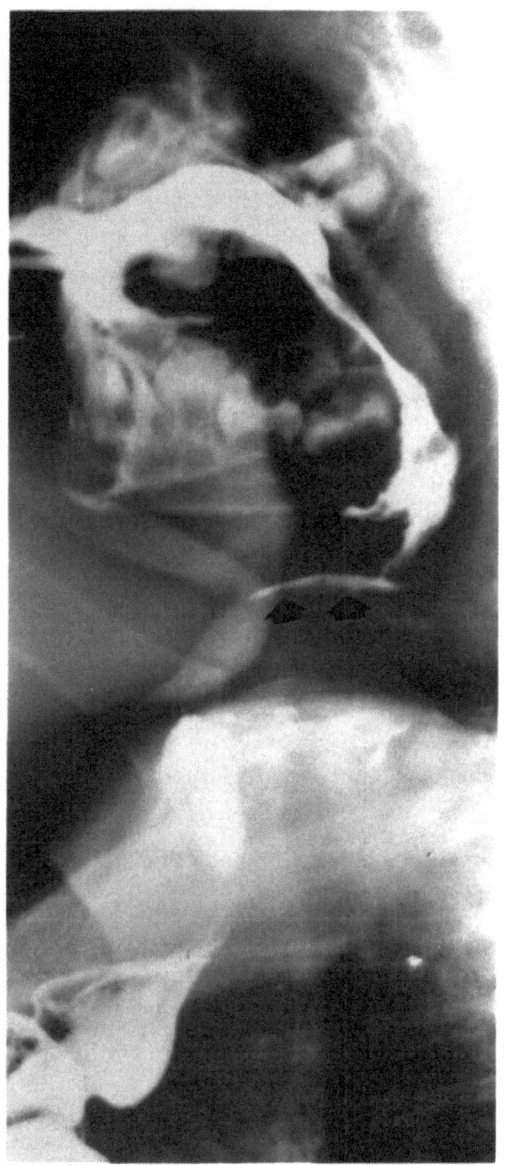

Fig. 5-22. Postoperative fistula. Fistula *(arrows)* developed after esophageal reconstruction from transverse colon in a 3-year-old boy with esophageal atresia at birth. The fistula closed spontaneously 2 months later. (Calenoff L, Norfray J: The reconstructed esophagus. Am J Roentgenol 125:864–876, 1975)

the transplant (Fig. 5-23); the upper esophagus passes through the narrow tunnel of the thoracic inlet; and every swallow creates movement of the anastomosis, interfering with healing. To minimize leakage an end-to-side anastomosis is used.

It has been postulated that an upper esophageal fistula develops because the esophagus lacks a protective serosal surface in the area of anastomosis. When a fistula does not find an easy path to the skin, an abscess can develop, usually at the lower anastomosis, and it can in itself give rise to a cutaneous fistula (Fig. 5-24).

Strictures

A stricture can form while the fistula is still present (Fig. 5-23), or it can be a late complication

(38) (Fig. 5-25). No specific type of fistula necessarily results in stricture. The upper and lower anastomoses are involved equally. Once stricture has developed, reoperation is necessary. Stricture at the lower anastomosis of an esophagus reconstructed for carcinoma is usually due to recurrent tumor (Fig. 5-26).

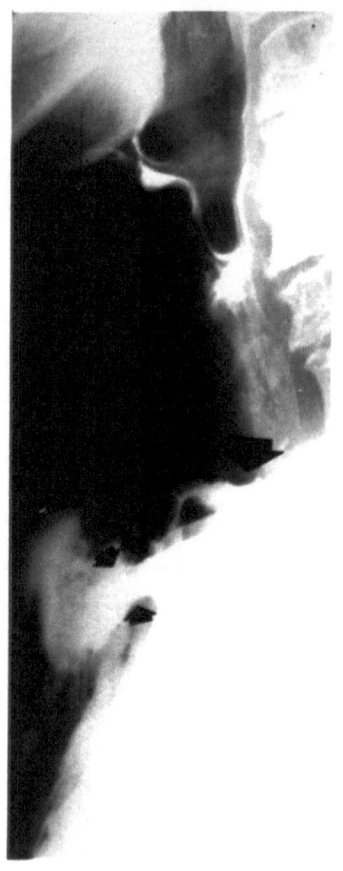
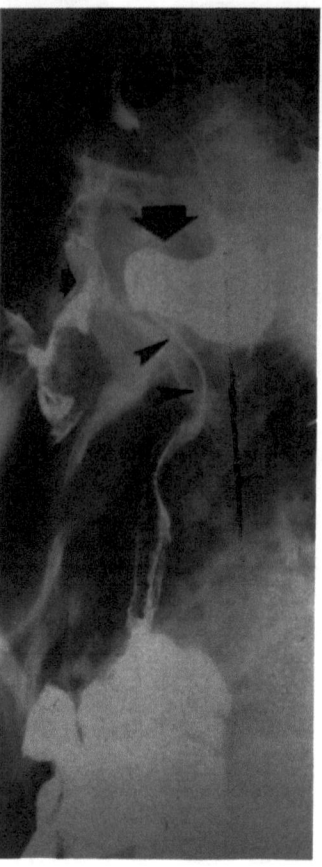

a   b

Fig. 5-23, a and b. Postoperative fistula. During esophageal reconstruction from cecum and terminal ileum in a 65-year-old man with squamous cell carcinoma of the midesophagus, the upper thoracic esophagus was brought forward for the anastomosis (*large arrows,* **a** and **b**). **a** One week after surgery there is a fistula at the upper anastomosis *(small arrows).* **b** Two months later persistent fistula *(small arrows)* and a stricture *(arrowheads)* are noted, but barium passes into the reconstructed segment. (Calenoff L, Norfray J: The reconstructed esophagus. Am J Roentgenol 125:864–876, 1975)

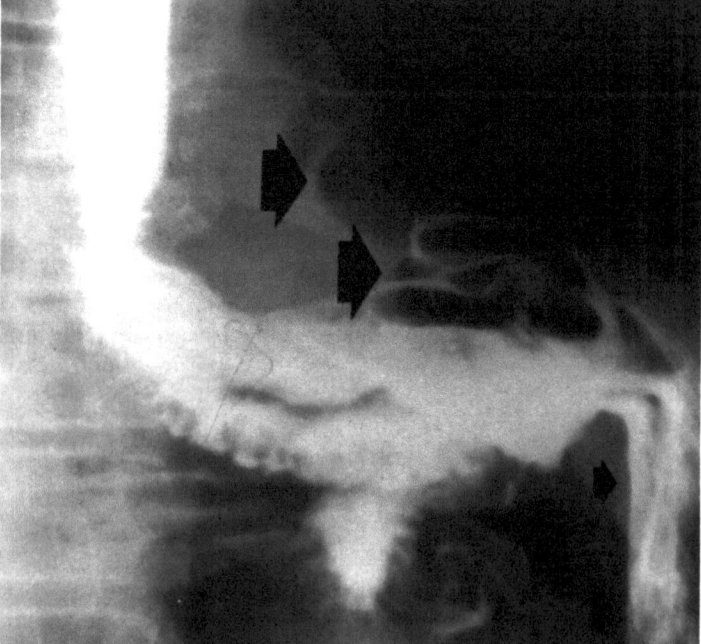

Fig. 5-24. Postoperative abscess and cutaneous fistula. After esophagojejunostomy in a 49-year-old man with carcinoma of the stomach, abscess *(large arrows)* and cutaneous fistula *(small arrows)* developed. (Calenoff L, Rogers LF: Radiologic manifestations of iatrogenic changes of the esophagus. Gastrointest Radiol 2:229–237, 1977)

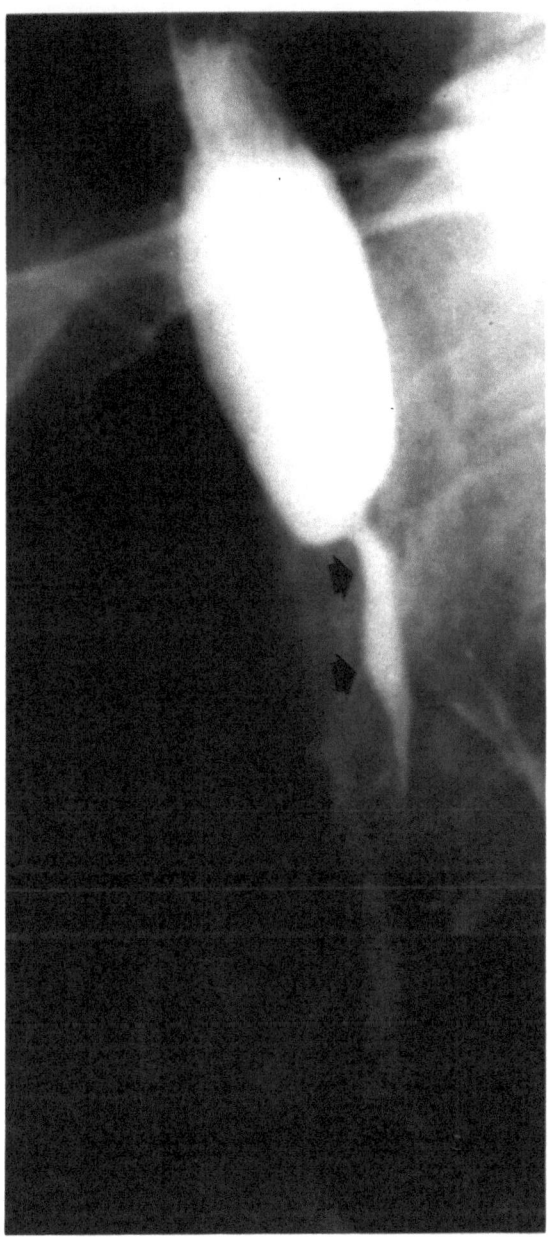
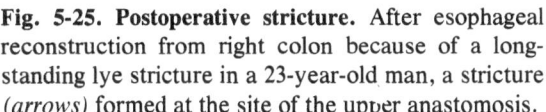

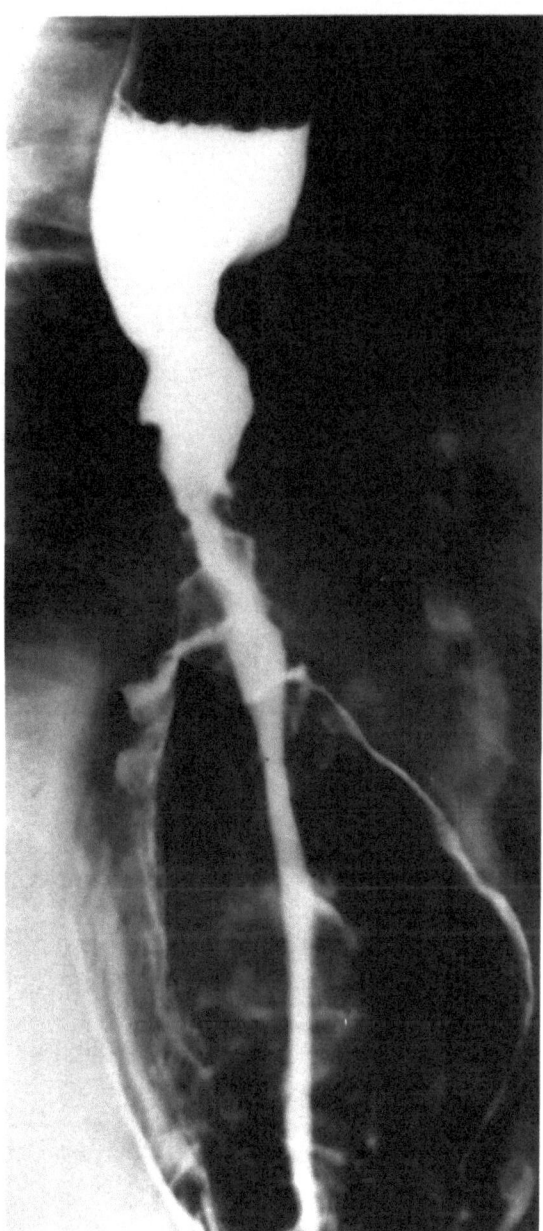

Fig. 5-25. Postoperative stricture. After esophageal reconstruction from right colon because of a long-standing lye stricture in a 23-year-old man, a stricture *(arrows)* formed at the site of the upper anastomosis.

Fig. 5-26. Recurrence of carcinoma at site of esophagogastrostomy. Six months after surgery in a 49-year-old man with carcinoma of the distal esophagus a radiograph obtained after barium swallow shows a narrow lumen, nodular mucosa, and a "jet-phenomenon" during passage of barium through the narrow segment. (Courtesy of G. G. Ghahremani, MD, Evanston, Illinois)

Esophageal Complications of Specific Procedures

Some of the complications are specific for the segment of gastrointestinal tract used as a transplant; others are characteristic of a particular surgical intervention involving a segment or the whole esophagus.

Colonic Transplant

Late complications in colonic transplant are halitosis, which is difficult to overcome, and colitis or other diseases inherent to the large bowel.

Ischemic Colitis

Ischemic colitis with a fatal outcome has been reported by Pradhan and Ikins (39). The typical thumbprinting of ischemic colitis was noted in the interposed colonic segment. The diagnosis was made by angiography. Death was due to massive bleeding.

Redundancy

When colon transplant is used for reconstruction the segment should be as short as possible to prevent redundancy. Redundancy causes delay in emptying (Fig. 5-27), which can result in malnutrition (40). A long colonic segment in the chest after reconstruction can be the result of

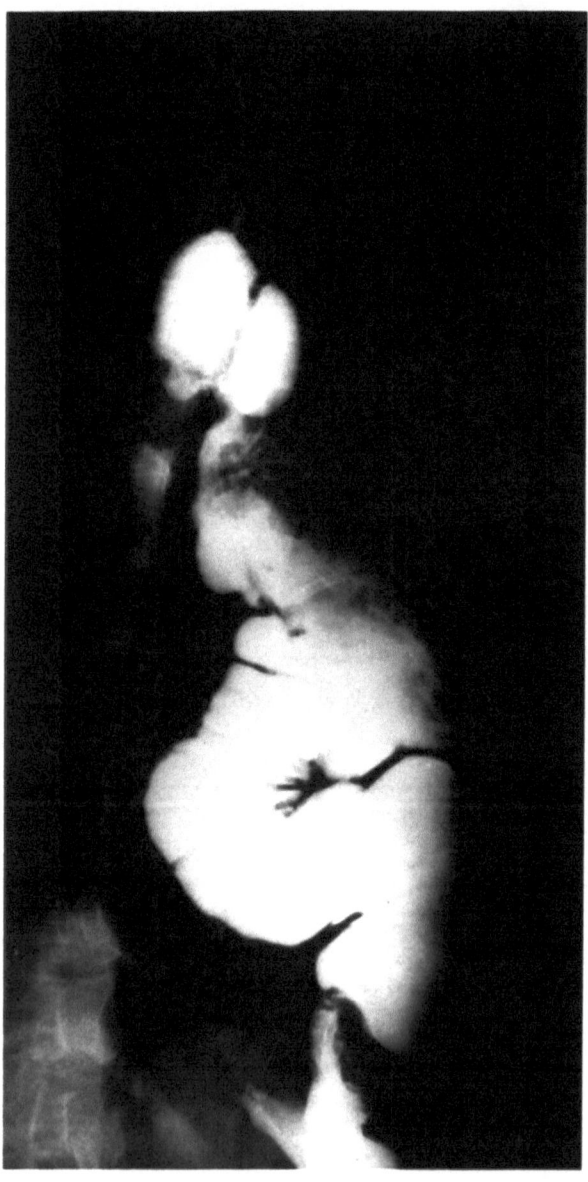

a

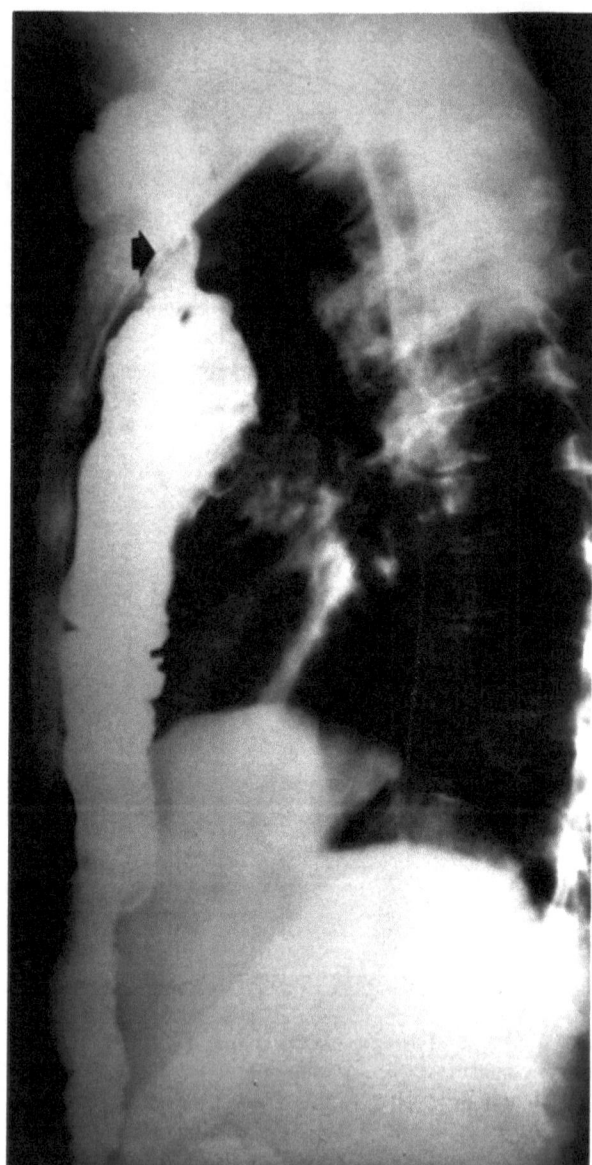

b

Fig. 5-27, a and b. Marked redundancy of reconstructed esophagus. This accounted for significant retention of food in the neoesophagus of the 49-year-old woman who had had stricture of the distal esophagus. The esophagus was reconstructed from the right colon used in isoperistaltic fashion. Two years after surgery she developed a stricture at the upper anastomosis *(arrows)* that required repeated dilatation. (Calenoff L, Norfray J: Radiologic manifestations of iatrogenic changes of the esophagus. Am J Roentgenol 125:864–876, 1975)

migration of the abdominal colon into the chest, which can result in dysphagia. When redundancy or some other complication is present, detection of recurrent tumor on follow-up studies may be difficult (Fig. 5-28).

Peptic Ulcerations
Peptic ulceration in the colonic transplant is rare. Eleven such cases were collected by Malcolm (41). In most of them the reason for peptic ulceration was the lack of an adequate drainage procedure such as vagotomy and pyloroplasty.

Diverticular Disease
Diverticular disease of the transplanted colon is rare but two cases were reported by Raia et al. (42). In both instances the appearance of the diverticula coincided with development of dys-

phagia. The diagnosis is done by a barium swallow. It is preferable, however, not to use a colonic transplant with preexisting diverticula.

Gastric Transplant
The entire stomach can be pulled into the chest or posterior mediastinum and anastomosed to the cervical esophagus, or a reversed gastric tube can be fashioned out of the greater curvature of the stomach. When the entire stomach is pulled up and pyloroplasty has not been done, gastroesophageal reflux can give rise to a very unpleasant cervical type of heartburn (Fig. 5-29). Peptic ulcers occur usually at the anastomosis (Fig. 5-30). Gastric ulcers in a transplant can be difficult to treat (Fig. 5-31). Ulcers of the stomach below the anastomosis could be secondary to ischemia (43).

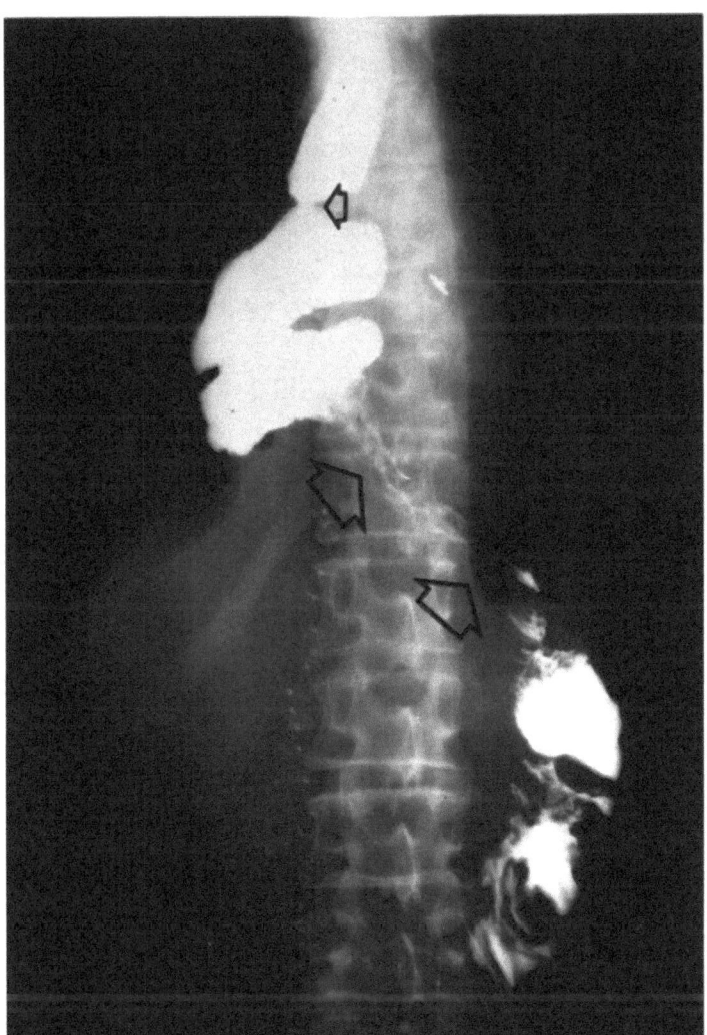

Fig. 5-28. Stricture formation and recurrence of carcinoma. Five years after colon interposition for carcinoma of the gastric fundus in a 57-year-old man there is a stricture of the upper anastomosis *(small arrow)* and recurrence of carcinoma of the distal colonic segment *(large arrows).* The stricture prevented early diagnosis of the recurrence.

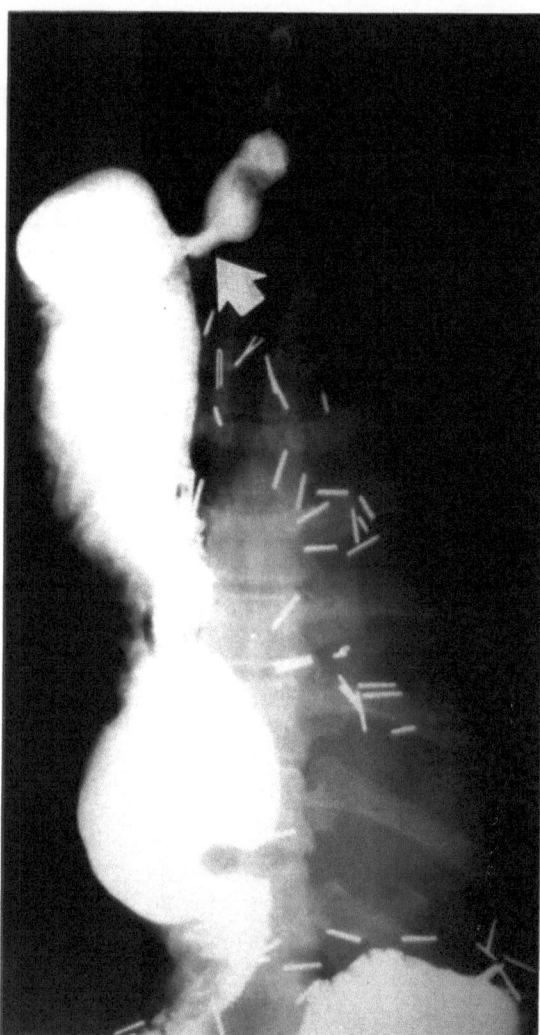

Fig. 5-29. Postoperative gastroesophageal reflux. The entire stomach was pulled up and anastomosed to the cervical esophagus in a 56-year-old man with carcinoma of the esophagus. A film obtained with the patient in the prone position after a barium meal shows gastroesophageal reflux *(arrow)*, which explains the patient's cervical heartburn. (Courtesy of J. Norfray, MD, Chicago, Illinois)

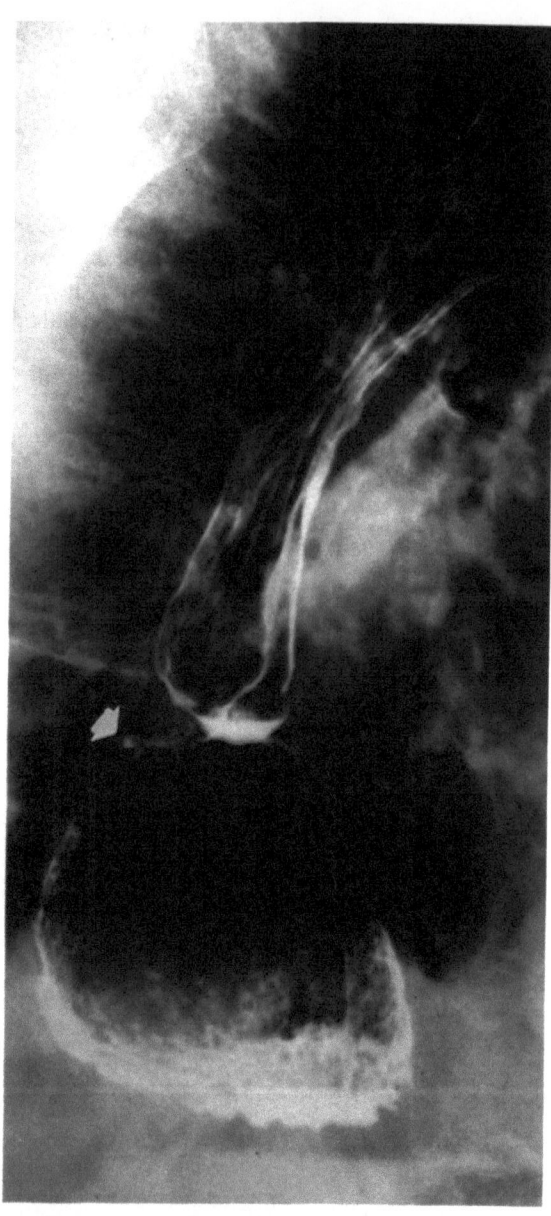

Fig. 5-30. Small postoperative peptic ulcer. The ulcer *(arrow)* developed in the inferolateral margin of an esophagogastrostomy 4 months after surgery for peptic stricture. (Courtesy of G. G. Ghahremani, MD, Evanston, Illinois)

The complication rate in reversed gastric tube operations is lower when compared to colonic transplant. Leakage at the upper anastomosis is the most frequent complication. Occasionally a leak can have grave consequences, particularly if the anastomosis is not holding well (Fig. 5-32). Narrowing of the reversed gastric tube seldom occurs but is easily amendable (Fig. 5-33).

Jejunal Transplant

Alkaline Stricture
Esophagojejunostomies have the potential problems of stricture formation. In a clinical experimental study reported in 1961, Helsingen concluded that regurgitation of duodenal content is the cause of the alkaline-induced stricture of the

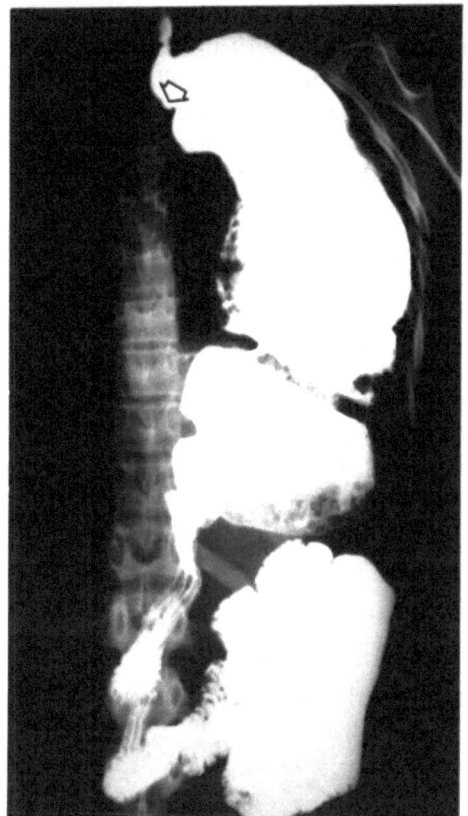

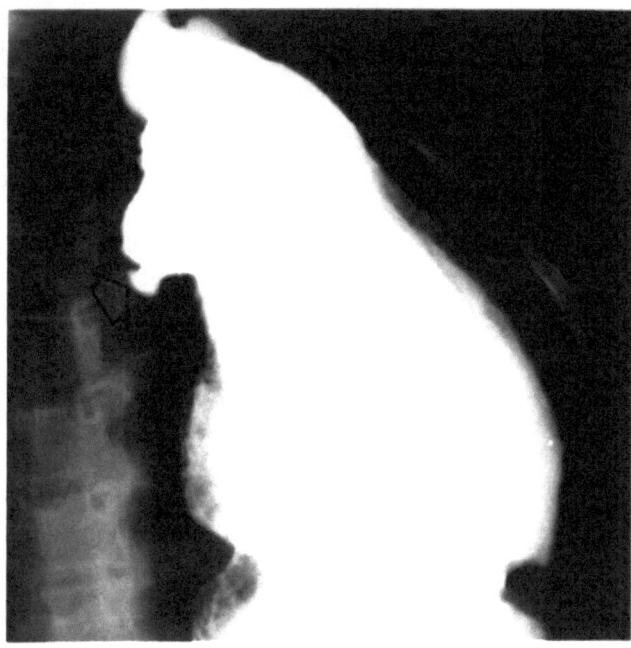

a

b

Fig. 5-31, a and **b. Postoperative peptic ulcer.** The entire stomach was anastomosed to the cervical esophagus in esophageal reconstruction for lye stricture in a 35-year-old man. A peptic ulcer developed at the lesser curvature of the gastric fundus *(arrows)*. (Courtesy of J. Norfray, MD, Chicago, Illinois)

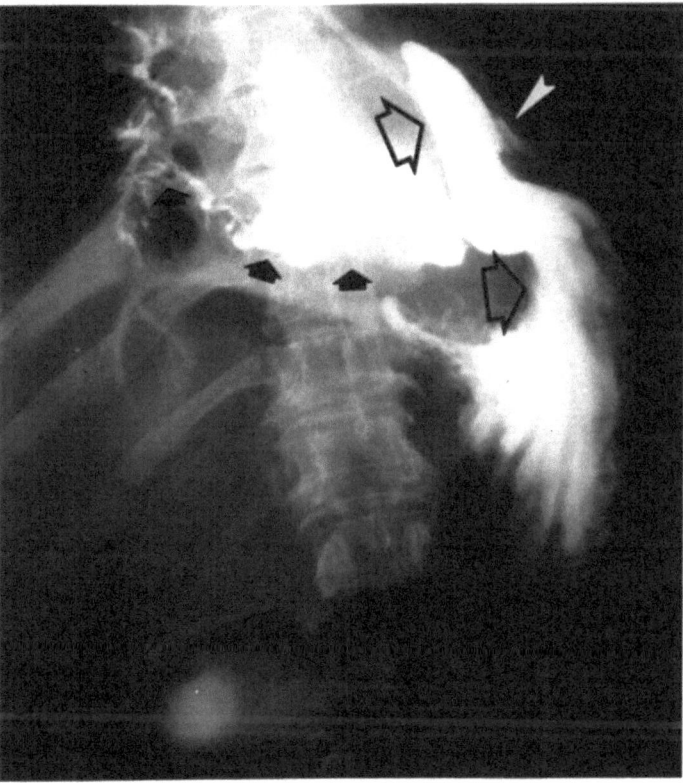

Fig. 5-32. Postoperative leakage and fistula. A Heimlich type of reversed gastric tube *(open arrows)* was constructed in a 56-year-old man whose esophagus was ruptured during resuscitation after cardiac arrest. Postoperative complications consist of leakage at the anastomosis *(arrowhead)* and esophagogastrobronchopericardial-cutaneous fistula *(black arrows)*.

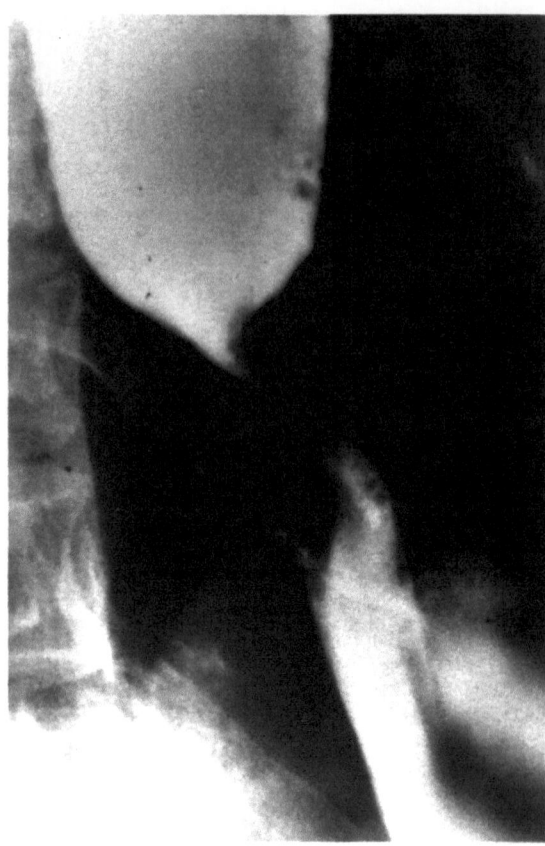

esophagus seen after gastrojejunostomy (44). In the different types of gastrojejunostomy and gastroduodenostomy (Fig. 5-34), all except the Roux-en-Y with a jejunal loop at least 6–7 cm long tend to eventually produce an alkaline stricture of the esophagus (Fig. 5-35).

Fundoplication

Complications attributed to fundoplication, either the Nissen or Belsey Mark IV type, include stenosis at the gastroesophageal junction, recurrent hiatus hernia, pouch deformity, deformity resembling a giant diverticulum (45), recurrent esophagitis, stricture, esophageal obstruction, trauma to the vagus, and gastric retention if pyloroplasty is not done (46) (Fig 5-36).

Hiatus Hernia Repair

Postoperative stricture following hiatal hernia repair can occur with the Allison type of operation (Fig. 5-37).

Vagotomy

Complications of vagotomy include esophageal fibrosis, esophagitis, intramural hematoma of the lower esophagus, perforation, and transient dysphagia (47).

Fig. 5-33. Postoperative narrowing. This occurred in a Beck type of reversed gastric tube at the distal end near passage through the diaphragm. It was due to bands of scar tissue. (Fetouh SA et al: Radiologic aspects of Beck gastric tube in esophageal reconstruction. Am J Roentgenol 129:425–431, 1977)

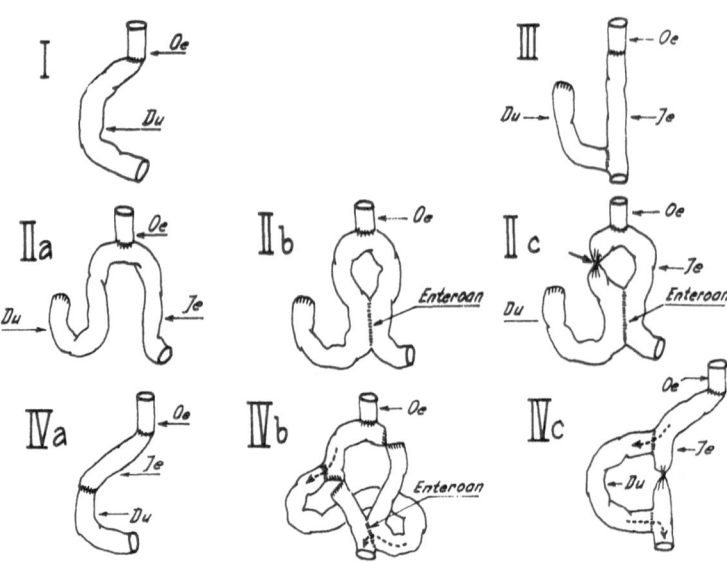

Fig. 5-34. Total gastrectomy with types of reconstruction affecting the esophagus. I Esophagoduodenostomy. **II** Esophagojejunostomies: **IIa** "simple"; **IIb** with enteroanastomosis (Braun). **IIc** With occlusion of the afferent jejunal limb (Efskind). **III** Roux-en-Y. **IV** Jejunal interpositions: **IVa** Henley-Longmire; **IVb** Tomoda; **IVc** Rosanov. All of these reconstructions, except the Roux-en-Y with a jejunal loop at least 6–7 cm, predispose to reflux of the duodenal contents into the esophagus with resulting stricture. *Oe*, esophagus; *Du*, duodenum; *Je*, jejunum; Enteroan, enteroanastomosis. (Helsingen N Jr: Oesophagitis following total gastrectomy. A clinical and experimental study. Acta Chir Scand 273:1–19, 1961)

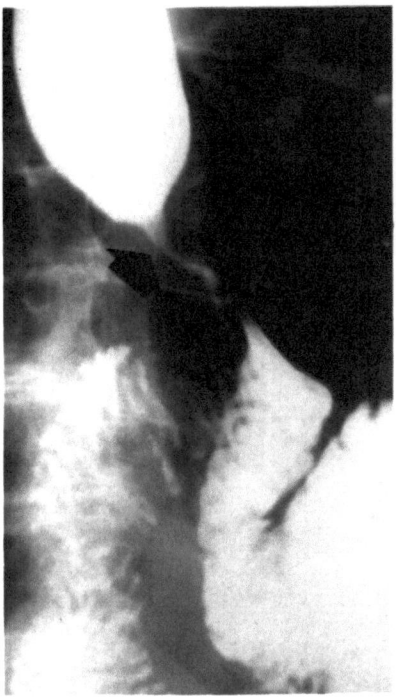

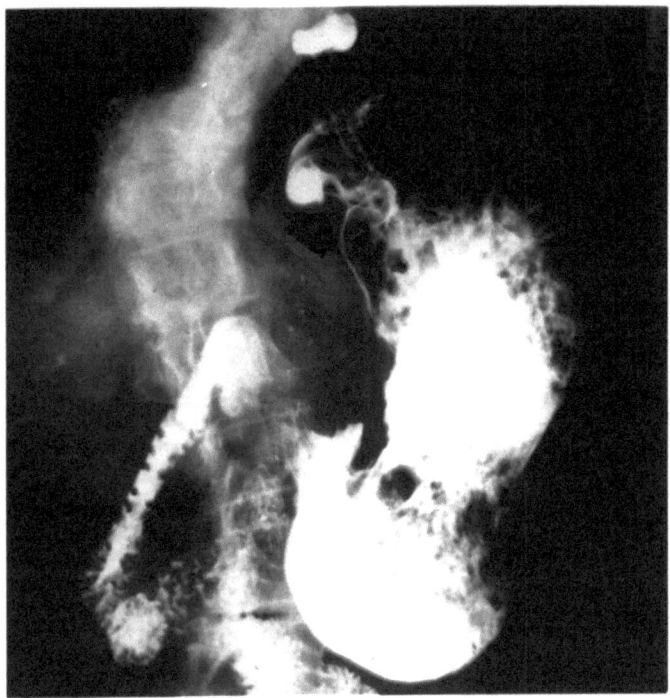

Fig. 5-35. Postoperative alkaline stric-ture of the lower esophagus. Sticture *(arrows)* developed 3 months after esophagojejunostomy. Reconstruction in this 65-year-old man with carcinoma of the lower esophagus was as in IVa in Fig. 5-34.

Fig. 5-36. Postoperative gastric retention. This eventually occurred because pyloroplasty was not performed in Belsey Mark IV fun-doplication *(arrow)* in a 75-year-old man.

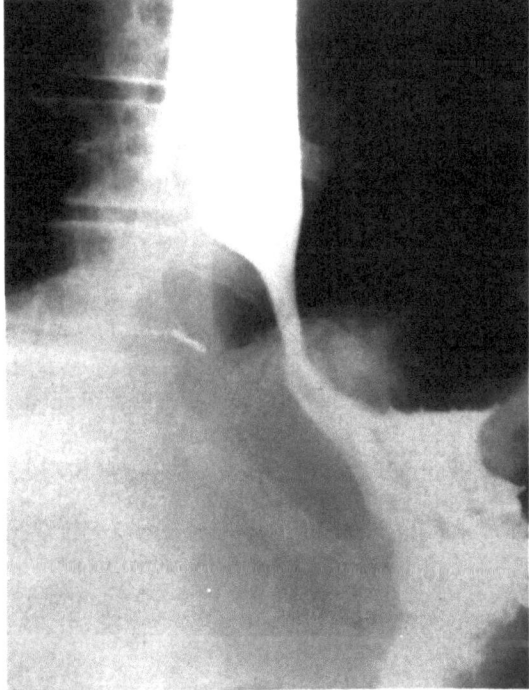

Transient dysphagia is the most common, although infrequent, complication of vagotomy in the immediate postoperative period. Treat-ment consists only of temporary exclusion of solid food. The diagnosis is readily made from the clinical history and the characteristic radio-graphic findings (Fig. 5-38). The onset of dys-phagia occurs with the first ingestion of solid food on the 7th to 14th postoperative day. A bar-ium swallow reveals persistent tapered narrow-ing of the terminal 3–4 cm of the esophagus. The symptoms usually disappear in 2–6 weeks with-out clinical or radiographic residua. The condi-tion results from denervation of the lower esoph-ageal segment during the operation (47).

◀ Fig. 5-37. Postoperative stricture. One year earlier the 77-year-old man had a massive hiatus hernia repaired (Allison type). (Calenoff L, Rogers LF: Radiologic manifestations of iatrogenic changes of the esophagus. Gastrointest Radiol 2:229–237, 1977)

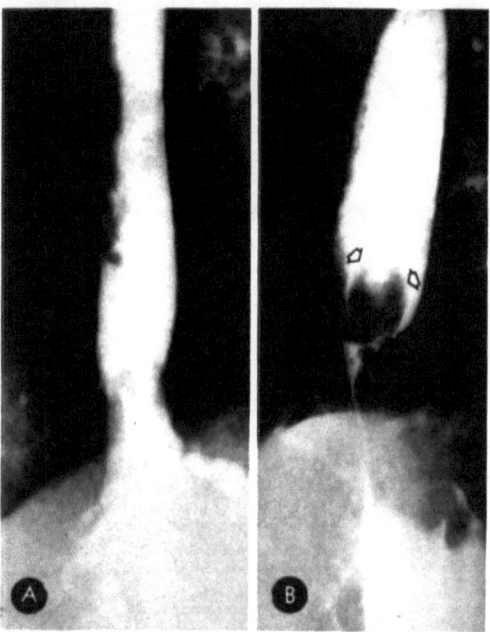
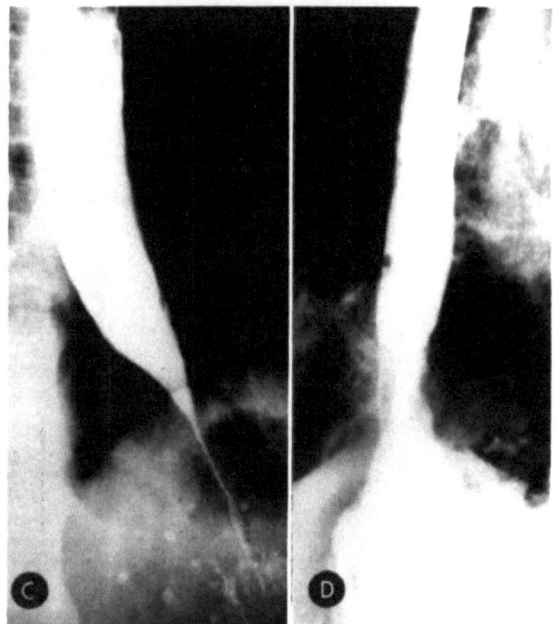

Fig. 5-38, a–d. Esophagograms in transient postvagotomy dysphagia. a Esophagogram 4 weeks prior to surgery in a 38-year-old woman. **b** On the 15th postoperative day she experienced dysphagia. A meat bolus is identified *(arrows)*. The lower esophageal segment is narrowed with tapered proximal margins. **c** The bolus has been dislodged, and the narrowed segment is seen better. The dysphagia was relieved in 20 days. **d** A normal esophagogram was obtained months later. (Rogers LF: Transient post-vagotomy dysphagia: A distinct clinical and roentgenographic entity. Am J Roentgenol 125:956–960, 1975)

Cervical Reconstruction

Hairy Esophagus

In extensive reconstruction of the cervical esophagus with skin flaps rotated to fashion a cervical esophagus, the outer surface of skin becomes the inner layer of the esophagus and forms the lumen. There are instances when hair follicles are present on the inner surface of the reconstructed tube. Hair may grow and cause dysphagia (48). In barium contrast studies of the esophagus, particularly double-contrast, the hair follicles are seen as small filling defects (Fig. 5-39). Occasionally if hair has grown and cannot be removed it has the appearance of a bezoar.

Heller Myotomy

Mucosal Herniation

Reflux esophagitis occurs occasionally after myotomy for achalasia. Peptic strictures can develop. Another complication is mucosal herniation at the site of the myotomy (Fig. 5-40). When the mucosal herniation becomes significant in size, symptoms occur (49).

Other Organs Affected by Esophageal Surgery

Neighboring organs can be easily affected by esophageal surgery or any iatrogenic complications involving the esophagus. Included are subcutaneous structures, the mediastinum, the abdomen, the diaphragm, trachea, bronchi, lungs, pleural space, and pericardium. Most of these can be identified by radiographic examination.

Mediastinum and Soft Tissue

A rent in the esophageal wall will permit air to escape from the esophagus and penetrate into the mediastinum. From there, it may extend to the subcutaneous structures of the neck, chest, and abdominal wall (Fig. 5-41). Air can dissect from the mediastinum into the retroperitoneal space and be the only manifestation of an injury to the esophagus. Although no direct communications exist between the retroperitoneal and intraperitoneal spaces, a large amount of retro-

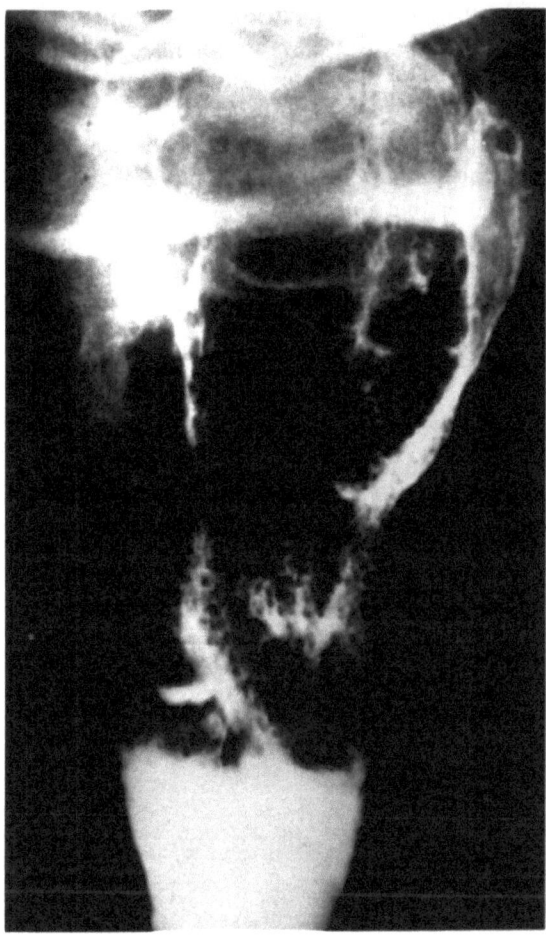

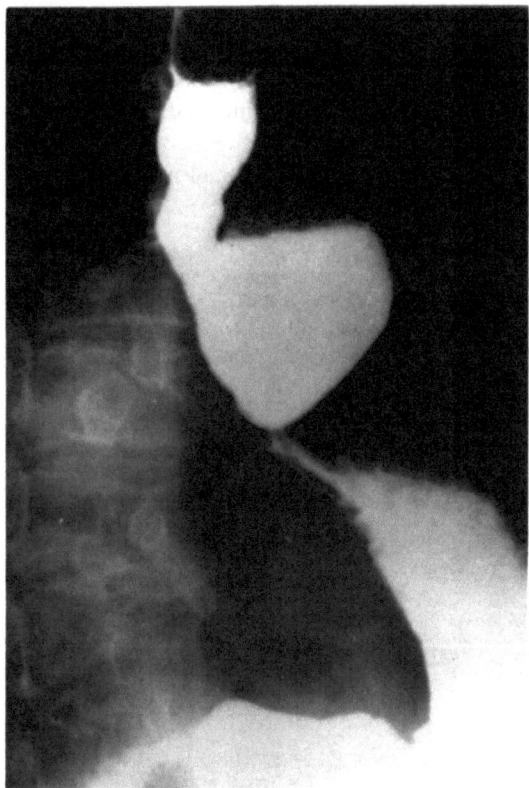

Fig. 5-40. Large postoperative mucosal hernia. After Heller's procedure the hernia developed at the site of the cardiomyotomy. (Menzies-Gow N et al: Results of Heller's operation for achalasia of the cardia. Br J Surg 65:483, 1978)

Fig. 5-39. Hairy esophagus. Endopharyngeal hair follicles growing on the skin flaps used to reconstruct the pharynx produce multiple filling defects. The growth of hair may cause dysphagia. (McLean GK, Laufer I: Hairy esophagus: A complication of pharyngoesophageal reconstructive surgery in two cases. Am J Roentgenol 132:269–270, 1979)

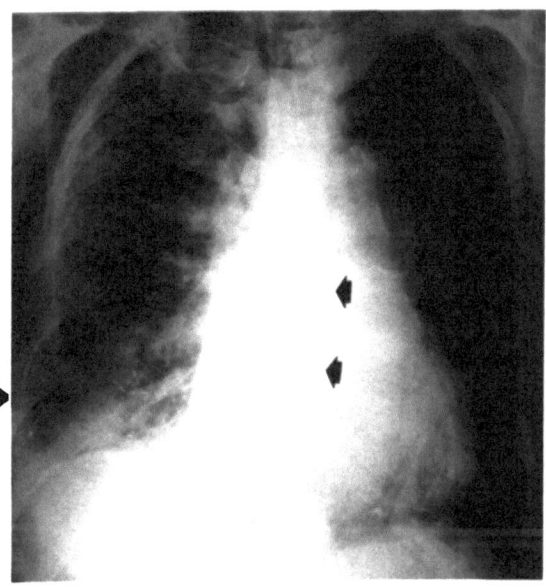

Fig. 5-41. Postoperative subcutaneous and mediastinal ▶ emphysema. A polyethylene tube *(arrows)* was inserted across the lesion to establish a lumen in a 64-year-old woman treated for obstructed carcinoma of the esophagus. (Calenoff L, Rogers LF: Radiologic manifestations of iatrogenic changes of the esophagus. Gastrointest Radiol 2:229–237, 1977)

peritoneal air can find its way to the intraperitoneal space.

Spillage of esophageal contents into the mediastinum can result in mediastinitis or mediastinal abscess. The abscess can, spontaneously or by surgical incision, extend to the outside, resulting in an esophagocutaneous fistula (Fig 5-42).

Trachea, Bronchus, Lung

The intimate relationship between the trachea and the esophagus accounts for tracheal injury during operation. The posterior wall of the trachea in the neck can be easily torn during dissection for gastric pull-up operations (20). Even

without injury the trachea becomes involved in postoperative aspiration problems, which can result in aspiration pneumonia, lung abscess, and death.

Esophagobronchial fistula can be caused by surgical trauma or instrumentation. It has been estimated that one-third of acquired nonmalignant esophagobronchial fistulas are of traumatic origin, including surgical (50). A fistula can be tenacious and sometimes require multiple surgical repairs (Fig. 5-43).

Pleura

A rent in the lower esophagus can easily find its way to the pleural space, usually on the right side (Fig. 5-44). Postsurgical esophagopleural fistula can be related to hiatal hernia repair (51) or occur as a consequence of perforation of the esophageal transplant (52).

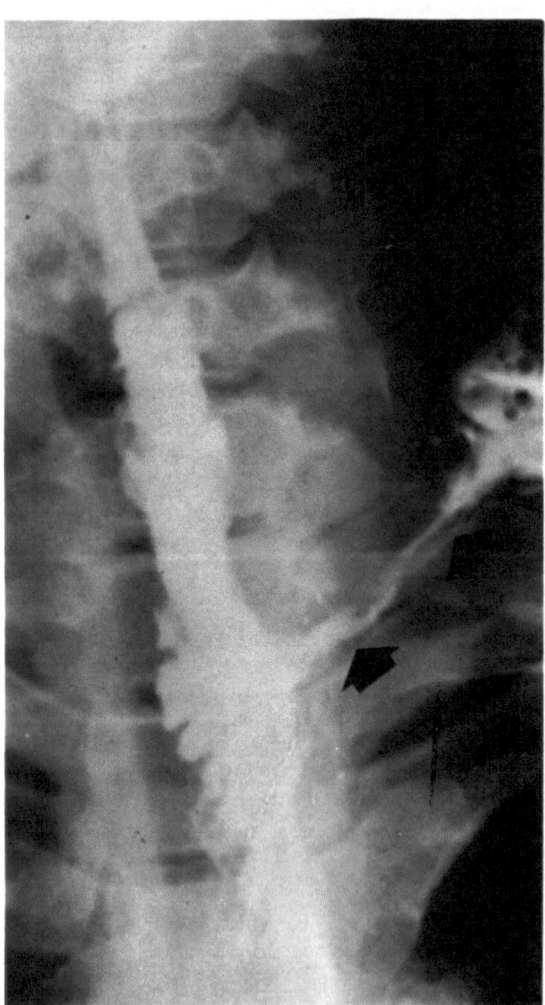

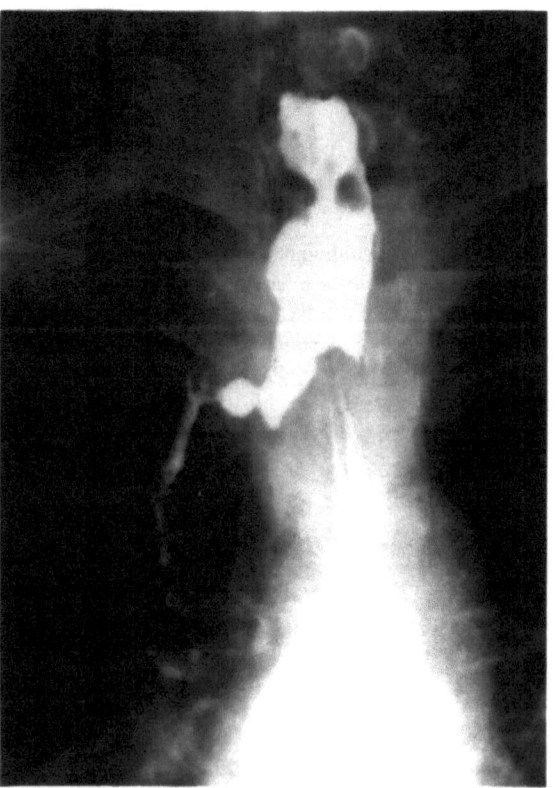

Fig. 5-42. Esophagocutaneous fistula. The fistula *(arrows)* developed after surgical drainage of a mediastinal abscess in a 40-year-old woman. (Courtesy of G. G. Ghahremani, MD, Evanston, Illinois)

Fig. 5-43. Esophagobronchial fistula. It resulted in a 64-year-old woman from prior perforation of an esophageal diverticulum by passage of a nasogastric tube.

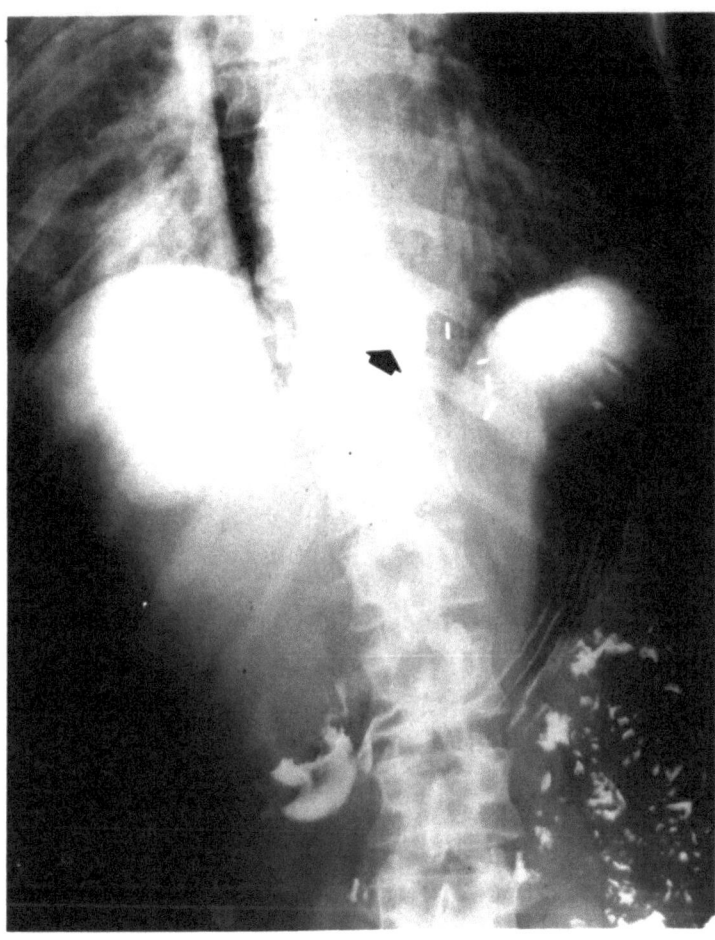

Fig. 5-44. Esophageal tear. Radiograph obtained in a 43-year-old woman after swallow of Gastrografin following attempt to remove meat lodged in the lower esophagus shows contrast medium around the foreign body *(arrow)*, stomach, and right pleural space. (Calenoff L, Rogers LF: Radiologic manifestations of iatrogenic changes of the esophagus. Gastrointest Radiol 2:229–237, 1977)

Pericardium

Tearing of the esophagus due to the trauma of surgery or instrumentation can create a communication with the pericardial sac (Fig. 5-45). An unusual case of gastric ulcer perforation into the pericardium was reported by Pellegrini and Cenni (53). The ulcer developed in the gastric segment used to patch the lower esophagus in a Thal operation. Ikard and Jacobs reported gastropericardial fistula and pericardial abscess as complications of subphrenic abscess following Nissen fundoplication (54).

Diaphragm

The diaphragm is affected by lower esophageal operations such as hiatal hernia repair, Heller's procedure, fundoplication, and the Thal procedure. Postsurgical herniation may occur following hiatal hernia repair and fixation of the gastroesophageal junction below the diaphragm.

Such herniation may be esophageal or paraesophageal or separated from the hiatus by a segment of intervening diaphragm. This last type of hernia, through an opening in the left hemidiaphragm, has been reported by Hoyt and Kyaw (55); this "disparaesophageal" hernia is the result of the small incision created in the diaphragm to admit the surgeon's fingers when the thoracic approach is used for hiatal hernia repair.

Stomach

The stomach is the recipient of the lower end of the intestinal transplant used to reconstruct the esophagus. It is generally accepted that the lower esophageal anastomosis should be placed high at the lesser curvature of the stomach. It is also common practice to provide for good gastric drainage by performing vagotomy and pyloroplasty. This is disputed by Lortat-Jacob and Giuli, however, who performed the lower anas-

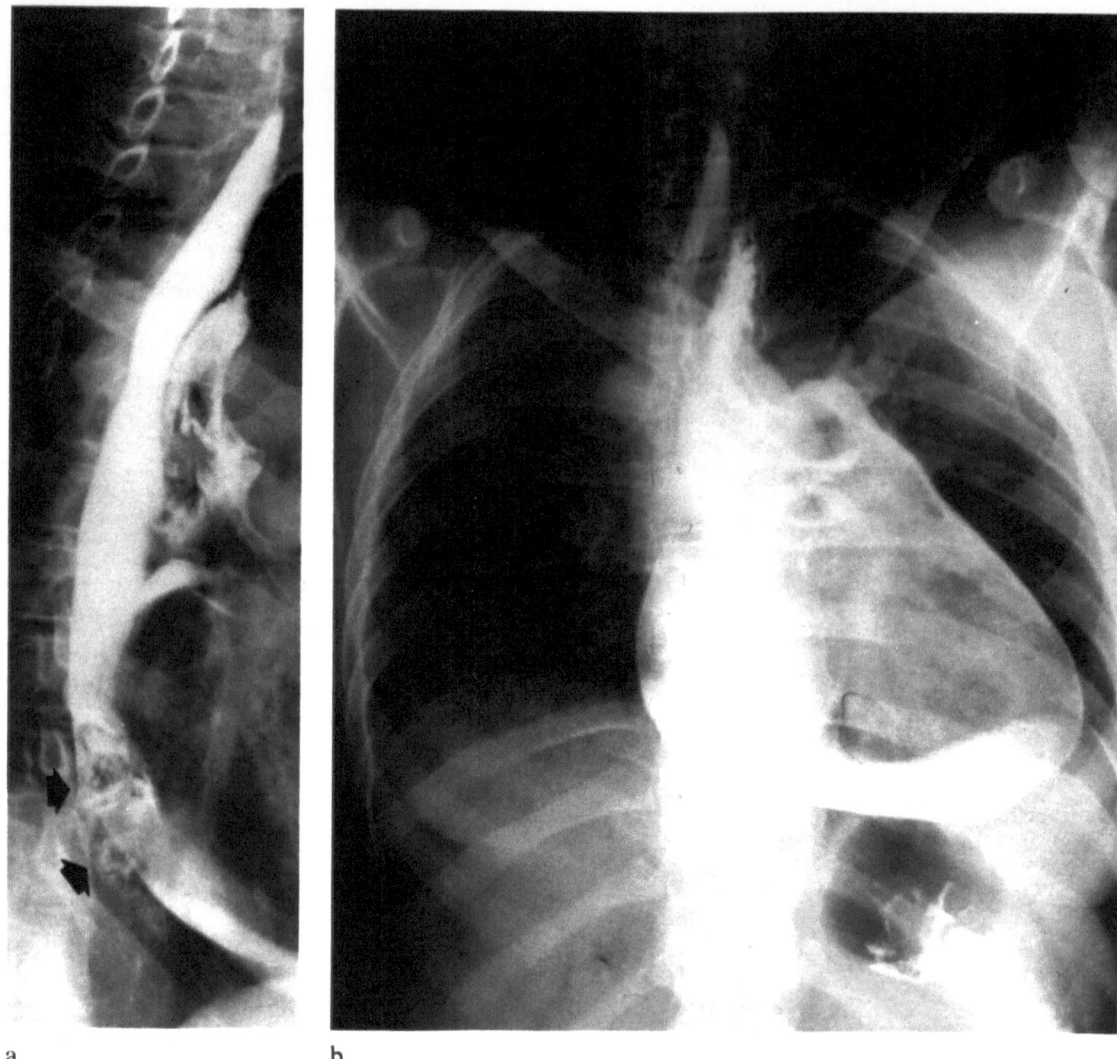

a   b

Fig. 5-45, a and b. Esophageal tear communicating with the pericardium. This occurred in a 43-year-old woman during an endoscopic attempt to remove meat lodged in the lower esophagus (*arrows* in **a**). At sur-gery, esophageal content and Gastrografin were aspir-ated from the pericardial sac. (Calenoff L, Rogers LF: Radiologic manifestations of iatrogenic changes of the esophagus. Gastrointest Radiol 2:229–237, 1977)

tomosis at the level of the gastric antrum with good tolerance in 80% of their patients (38). Only 15% of the patients eventually required pyloro-plasty. When the distal anastomosis is at the gas-tric antrum and pyloroplasty has not been per-formed, gastric retention is a common complaint (Fig 5-46).

A rent in the lower esophagus can create a fis-tula, which may extend to the lesser sac and present as an abscess projected behind the stom-ach (Fig 5-47).

Surgery on Other Organs Affecting the Esophagus

Surgery on neighboring organs does affect the esophagus. Sometimes there is only simple dis-placement, but in other instances, such as tho-racic surgery and surgery on the aorta, the cer-vical spine, and particularly the larynx, the esophagus can be profoundly affected.

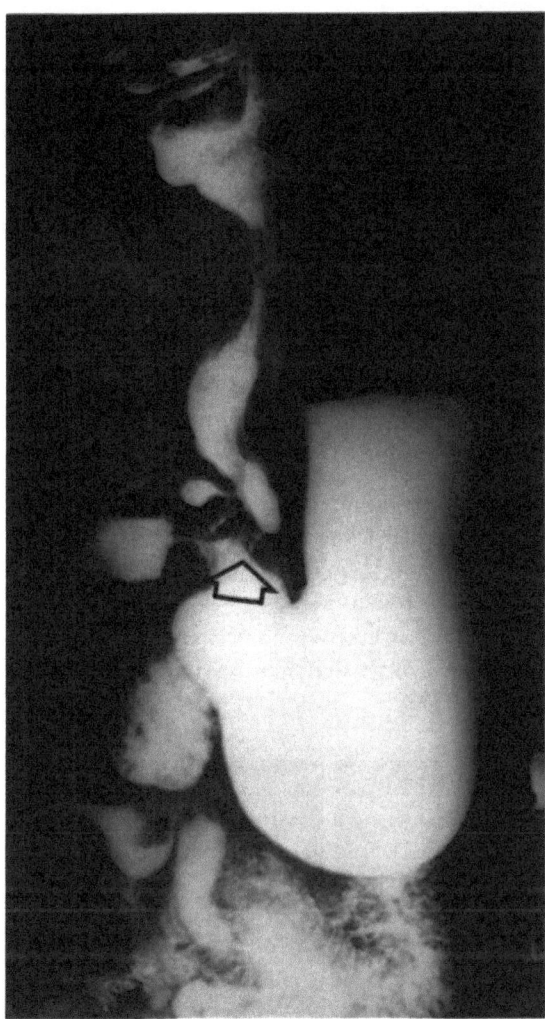

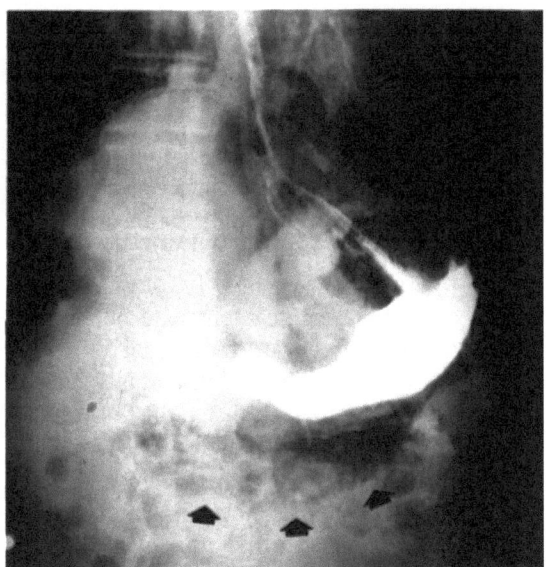

Fig. 5-47. Lesser-sac abscess. The abscess *(arrows)* in a 43-year-old man followed perforation of the esophagus during dilatation of a lower esophageal stricture.

Fig. 5-46. Gastric retention. Esophageal reconstruction was for lye stricture in a 36-year-old man. The distal colonic anastomosis *(arrow)* is nonphysiologic, and pyloroplasty was not performed. (Calenoff L, Norfray J: The reconstructed esophagus. Am J Roentgenol 125:864–876)

Aortic Prosthesis

Although complications of aortic prosthetic surgery rarely affect the esophagus, in a case reported by Seymour, an aortoesophageal fistula was secondary to infection of the graft and led to active bleeding (56). A barium swallow demonstrated the coil-spring appearance of the graft (Fig. 5-48).

Pneumonectomy

Pneumonectomy will often result in a shift of the mediastinal structures, the esophagus included,

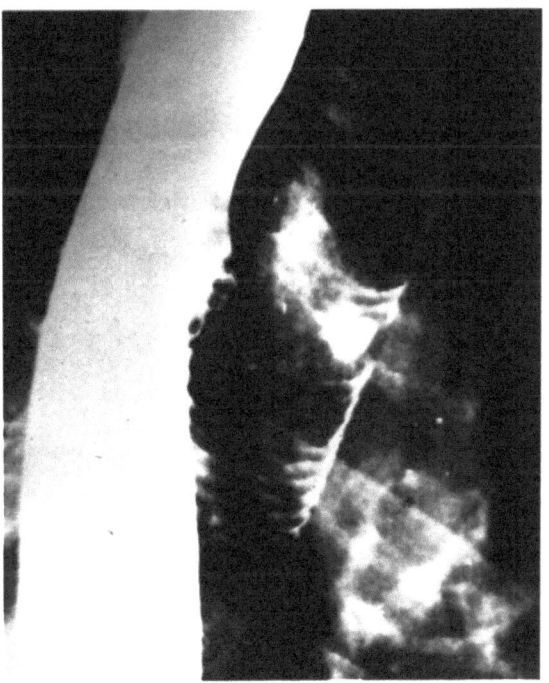

Fig. 5-48. Aortoesophageal fistula. This developed as a complication of aortic prosthetic grafting in a 22-year-old man in whom the thoracic aorta had been transected in a motorcycle accident. Barium outlines the Dacron graft (coil-spring effect). (Seymour EQ: Aortoesophageal fistula as a complication of aortic prosthetic graft. Am J Roentgenol 131:160–161, 1978)

toward the operated side. This can create dysphagia. The position of the esophagus can be identified by the nasogastric tube on a postoperative chest radiograph or by a barium swallow (Fig. 5-49). Esophageal-pleural fistulas related to pneumonectomy are divided into two categories (57). Early esophageal-pleural fistula occurs in the immediate postoperative period and is attributed to operative injury, namely, devascularization of an esophageal segment; late occurrence of fistula is usually due to recurrence of a neoplastic process. The majority of fistulas occur in the midportion of the esophagus at the level of the carina. Tecaro et al. noted 33 esophagopleural fistulas after 934 pulmonary resections for tuberculosis (58). Fistulas that appeared within 3 months of the operation were considered to be due to surgical trauma, while the others were attributed to chronic infection; 75% of the fistulas involved the right pleural space, which is more intimately associated with the esophagus.

Cervical Fusion

There has been an increase in the number of surgical procedures on the cervical spine, primarily spinal fusion for traumatic fracture-dislocations or for degenerative osteoarthritis. In half of the cases the approach to the cervical spine is anterior. This makes the cervical esophagus prone to surgical injury. In addition, postsurgical infection of bone graft can result in an esophagocutaneous fistula (Fig. 5-50).

Laryngectomy

Total laryngectomy, with or without reconstruction of the cervical esophagus, can leave a residual sinus tract (Fig 5-5l). Laryngectomy, usually performed for a neoplastic process, in most cases is followed by reconstructive surgery, the extent of which depends on the nature of the laryngectomy.

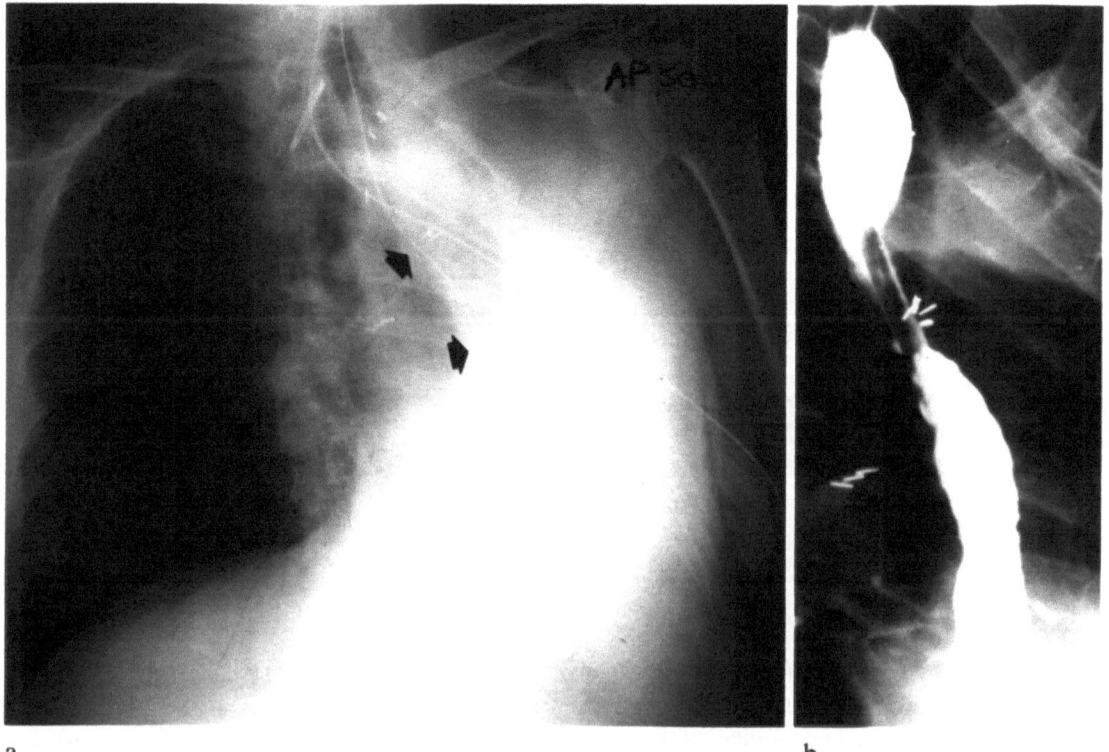

a

b

Fig. 5-49, a and b. Esophageal shifting. This was due to left pneumonectomy in a 71-year-old man with bronchogenic carcinoma. **a** The nasogastric tube *(arrows)* shows the marked shift of the esophagus to the left. **b** This is confirmed by a radiograph obtained after a barium swallow. (Courtesy of G. G. Ghahremani, MD, Evanston, Illinois)

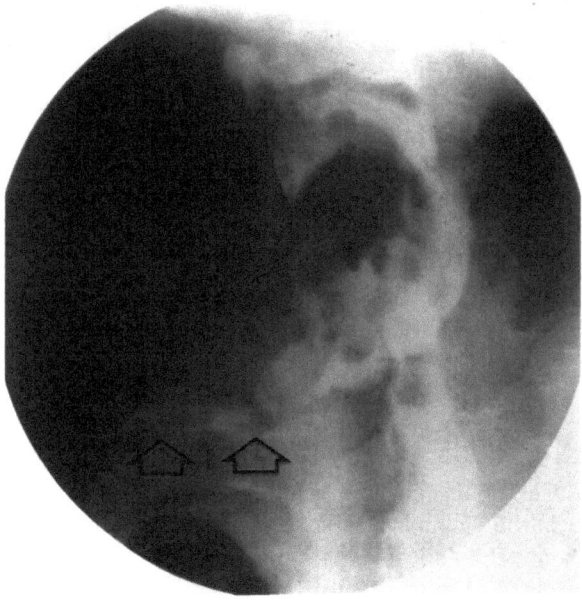

a

Fig. 5-50, a and **b. Esophagocutaneous fistula. a** The site of anterior spinal fusion in a 46-year-old man with ankylosing spondylitis and quadriplegia, due to injury at C-6 in a car accident, had become infected and resulted in a tenacious esophagocutaneous fistula *(arrows)*.

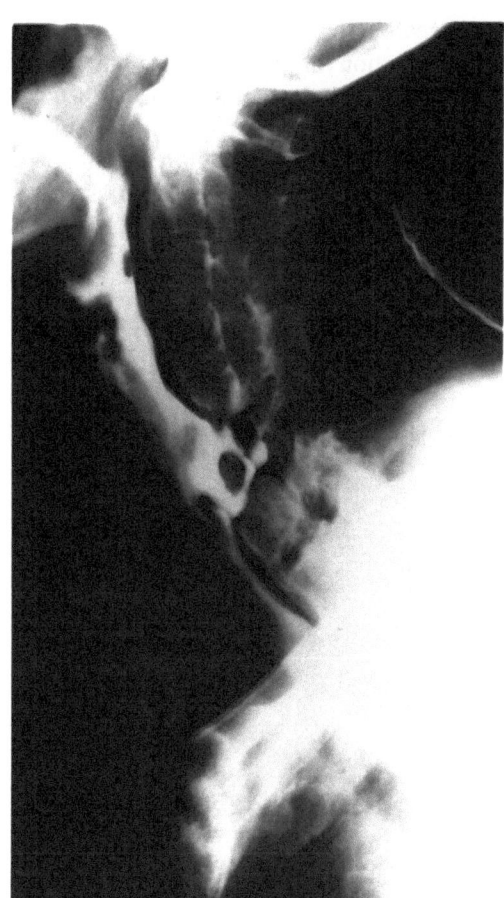

b

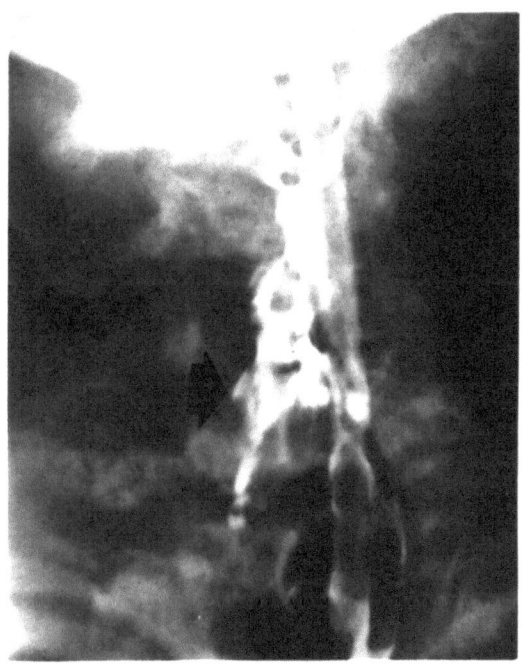

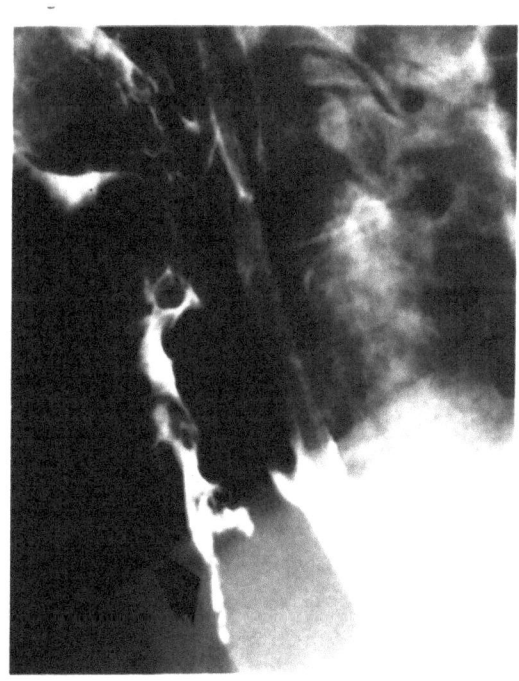

a   b

Fig. 5-51, a and **b. Postlaryngectomy sinus tract.** The sinus tract *(arrows)* originated in the hypopharynx in an 80-year-old woman who had total laryngectomy for carcinoma. (Courtesy of G. G. Ghahremani, MD, Evanston, Illinois)

Esophageal Speech

In rehabilitation of postlaryngectomy patients they are taught the use of alaryngeal speech. In most cases the esophagus is used for this purpose, and the swallowed air stored in the esophagus is expelled to make sound. As a result of air accumulation the esophagus dilates, and occasionally a diverticulum forms (Fig. 5-52). It has been established that the wider the dilated esophagus the better the alaryngeal speech (59).

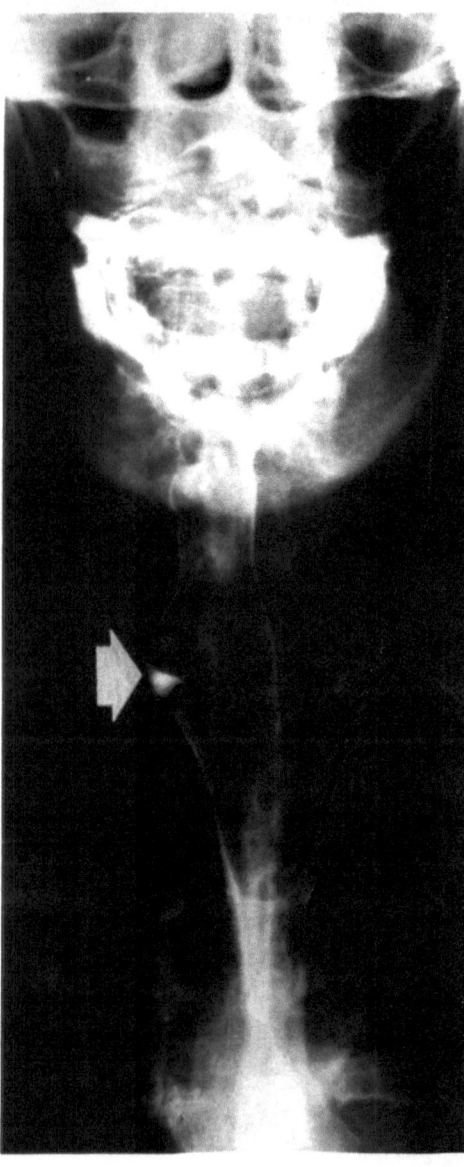

Fig. 5-52. Dilatation of the cervical esophagus and diverticulum *(arrow).* This is seen in a 56-year-old woman 9 years after total laryngectomy for carcinoma. Air stored in the esophagus and used for alaryngeal speech may result in this appearance.

Neoglottis

In uncomplicated larygectomy without radical dissection the hypopharynx is closed, and the only communication of the trachea with the outside is the tracheostoma. Since this is not satisfactory for adequate speech, an operation has been devised for construction of a neoglottis. Also known as pseudoglottis or neolarynx construction, two techniques are available, the Staffieri and the Serafini (60–62). A tracheopharyngeal shunt, small enough to simulate a vocal cord area, is created. Speech originates in the trachea, is clear, and differs from alaryngeal speech in which air stored in the esophagus is used to make sound, which is difficult to understand. The pharyngostoma is connected to the trachea in the vicinity of the tracheostoma. In the Serafini technique the pharyngostoma is sutured to the posterior edge of the tracheostoma, and in the Staffieri technique the hypopharyngeal mucosa is rotated over the tracheal opening and sutured to the anterior half of the tracheostoma (Fig. 5-53). The procedure is not without complications; pharyngocutaneous fistula and aspiration are the two main problems encountered.

To eliminate aspiration through the neoglottis Saito et al. change the direction of the shunt (63). The neoglottis is constructed from a midline full-thickness esophageal flap approximately 2–4 cm long and directed on a sharp angle to a lower point in the esophagus (Fig. 5-54). Ghosh, on the other hand, advocates transverse tracheoesophagoplasty to form the neoglottis, which is 2 cm long and 6 mm wide and constructed at the posterior wall of the trachea (64). The slit in the esophagus is made slightly below the slit in the trachea. To prevent early closure of the neoglottis, Silastic sheets are kept inside the neoglottis for 5 weeks.

Diverting Tracheoesophageal Anastomosis

For patients with intractable aspiration, a diverting tracheoesophageal anastomosis has been advocated by Lindeman (65). This type of anastomosis is created between the upper trachea and the esophagus above the level of the tracheostoma. Barium swallow in these cases will show the contrast material passing into both the esophagus and larynx and then, via the tracheoesophageal fistula, reentering the esophagus rather than progressing down the trachea. This procedure is reversible if no longer needed.

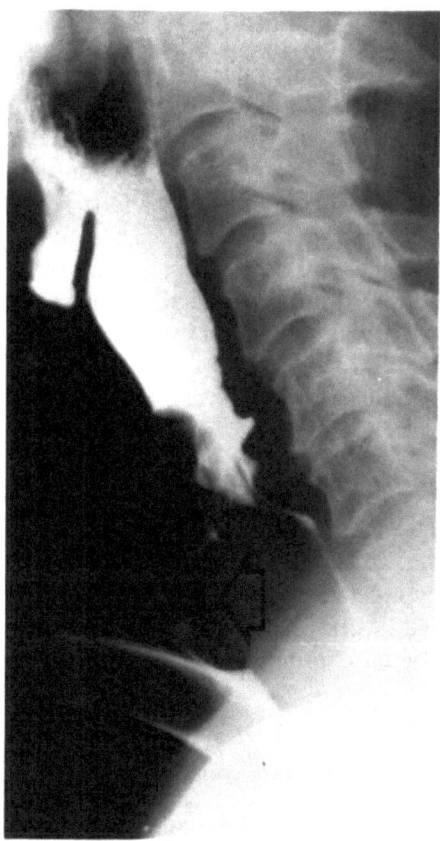

Fig. 5-53. Neoglottis, Staffieri type. In a 50-year-old man who had total laryngectomy for carcinoma, the neoglottis connects the anterior wall of the cervical esophagus to the trachea. Barium is running through the shunt into the trachea *(arrow)*.

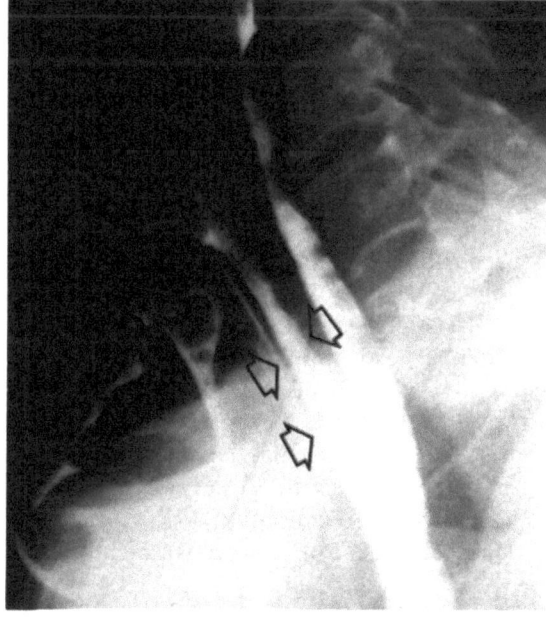

a

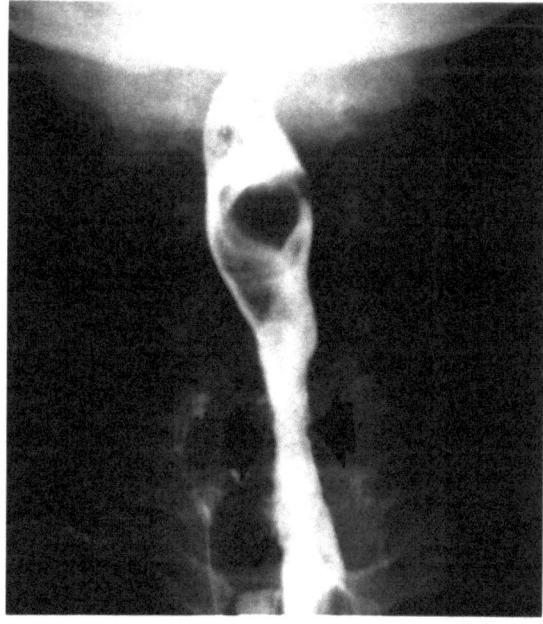

b

Fig. 5-54, a and b. Tracheoesophageal shunt for vocal rehabilitation following total laryngectomy for carcinoma. a The shunt *(arrows)* measures 4 cm in length and is at a sharp angle to the trachea and esophagus. **b** Anteroposterior appearance of esophagus after construction of the shunt. The slight stricture is the site of the flap *(arrows)*. (Saito H et al: Experiences with the tracheoesophageal shunt method for vocal rehabilitation after total laryngectomy. Arch Otorhinolaryngol 218:135–142, 1977)

Lifesaving Procedures Affecting the Esophagus

Lifesaving procedures used by physicians, hospital personnel, and paramedics at the scene of accidents may injure the esophagus. Esophageal trauma may be induced by lifesaving procedures in the neonate, the use of endotracheal intubation, the use of a cuffed tracheal tube, and the now widespread use of the esophageal obturator airway. Without use of any devices however, esophageal perforation can occur during resuscitation attempts after cardiac arrest (Fig. 5-55).

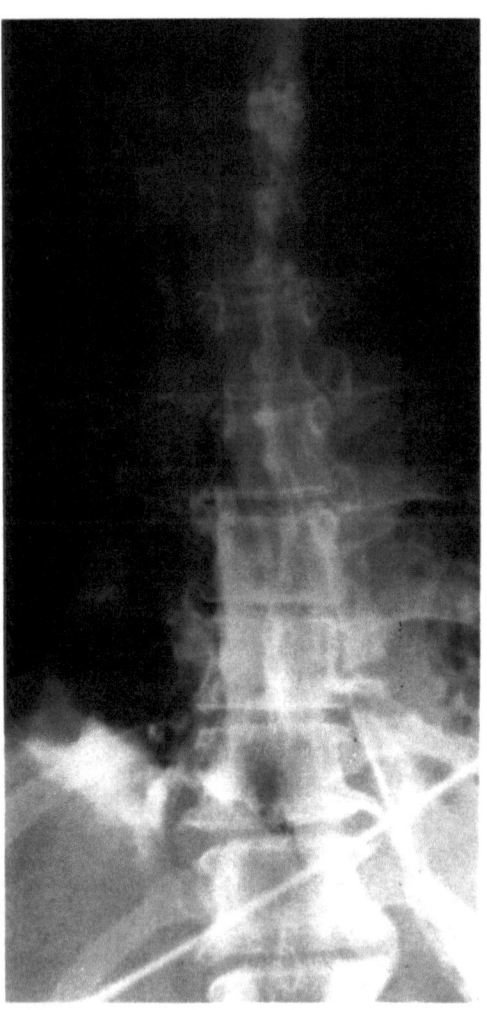

Fig. 5-55. Perforation of the esophagus during resuscitation following cardiac arrest. Gastrografin extravasated into the mediastinum.

Use of Esophageal Obturator Airway

The esophageal obturator airway (Fig. 5-56) is used by paramedics at the site of an accident. It is inserted more easily than an endotracheal tube. The esophageal airway has a balloon that is inflated after introduction. The balloon has a dual purpose: to prevent vomiting and to prevent the air blown into the esophageal airway from entering into the stomach. If the airway is properly positioned, the air is directed into the trachea through the appropriate air holes. When inflated the esophageal airway can be seen on a chest radiograph (66) (Fig. 5-57). Complications caused by an esophageal obturator airway include unrecognized endotracheal intubation, traumatic lacerations of the natural airway or hypopharynx, gastric dilatation if the balloon is not properly inflated, vomiting after removal of the tube and, worst of all, perforation of the esophagus by an overinflated balloon (67) (Fig. 5-58).

Endotracheal Intubation

When performed by skilled personnel, endotracheal intubation is usually harmless. Occasionally pharyngoesophageal perforation occurs, most often in the region of the cricopharyngeal sphincter or in the pyriform sinus (68,69). Such perforations result in pneumothorax, abscess formation, and mediastinal fistula.

Use of a Cuffed Tracheal Tube

Tracheostomy and intermittent positive pressure ventilation can result in tracheoesophageal fistula (70). Mechanical factors in the cuffed tracheal tube account for the occurrence of tracheoesophageal fistula (Fig. 5-59). It has been stressed that patients in whom a cuffed tracheal tube and nasogastric tube are utilized for long periods are more prone to develop fistula than patients without such tubes (71). A tracheoesophageal fistula can be demonstrated by a barium swallow (Fig. 5-60).

Neonatal Procedures

Lifesaving procedures in neonates include suctioning in the immediate postdelivery period and passage of nasogastric or nasojejunal feeding

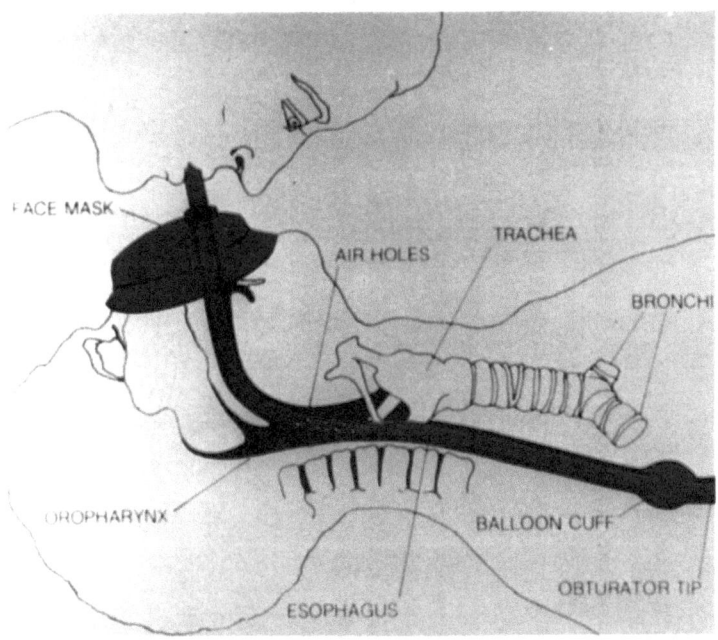

Fig. 5-56. Esophageal obturator airway. This is the airway used by paramedics at the site of an accident.

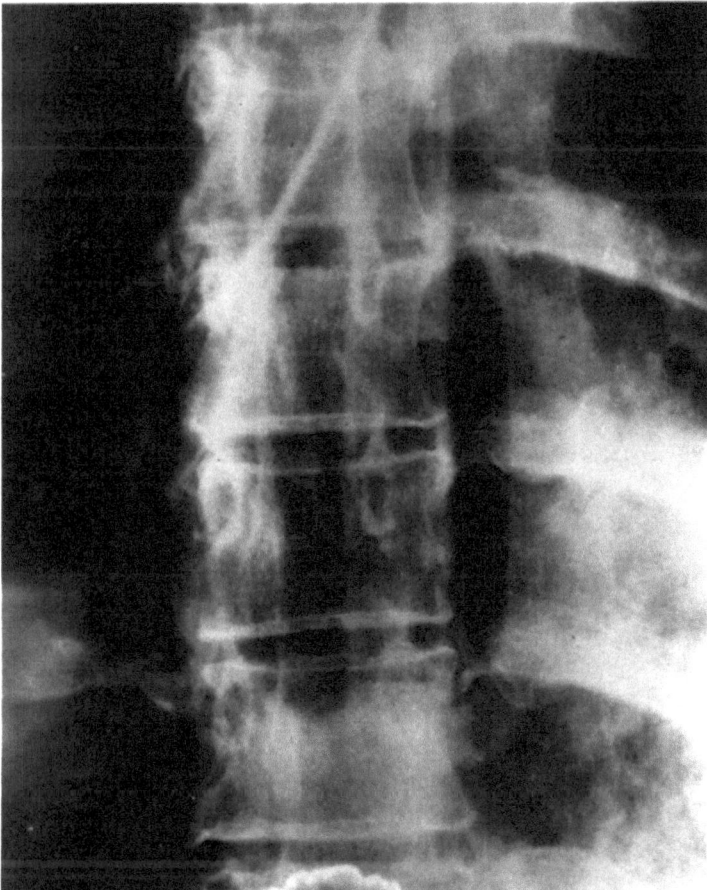

Fig. 5-57. Inflated obturator airway seen on a chest radiograph. Note that the endotracheal tube is in the right main-stem bronchus. (Pais MJ, Segal HB: Esophageal obturator airway: Radiographic appearance. Am J Roentgenol 132:267–268, 1979)

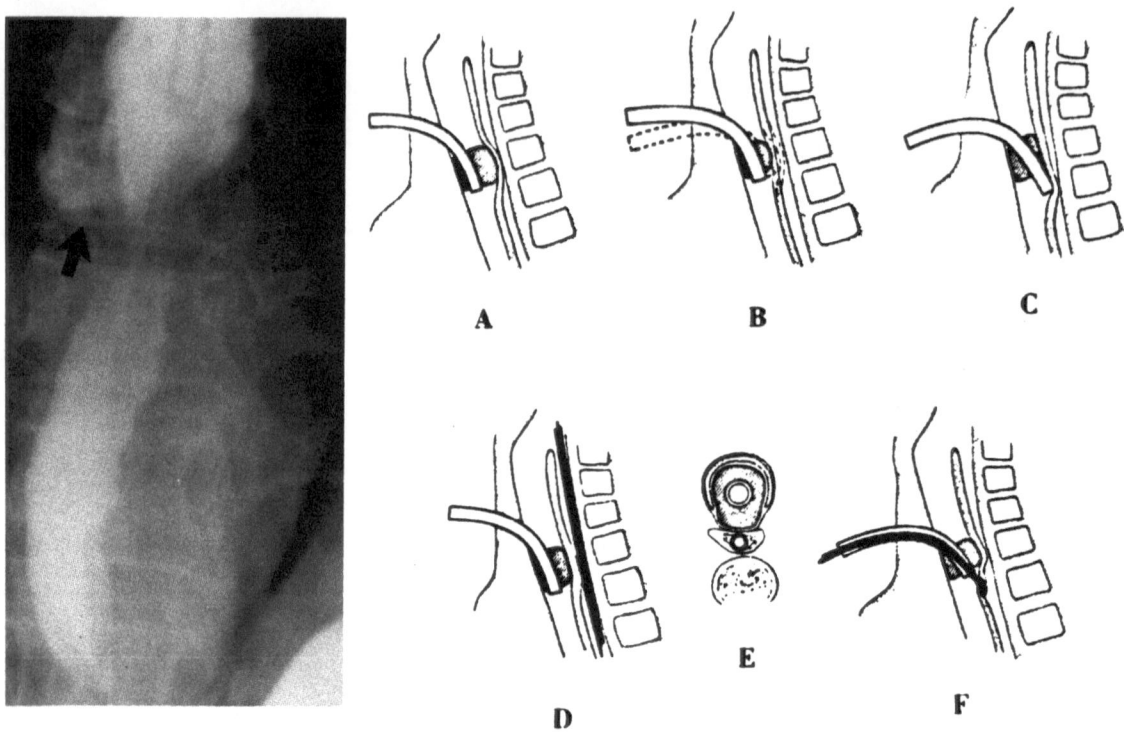

Fig. 5-58. Perforation of the esophagus by an overinflated balloon. The perforation *(arrow)* occurred in a 65-year-old woman who underwent resuscitation by paramedics using an esophageal obturator airway. (Scholl DG, Tsai SH: Esophageal perforation following the use of the esophageal obturator airway. Radiology 122:315–316, 1977)

Fig. 5-59, a–d. Mechanical factors in cuffed tracheal tube that can cause tracheoesophageal fistula. a Overinflation of tube cuff; b excessive mobility of cannula; c erosion by cannula tip between trachea and esophagus; d, e compression of wall of esophagus and trachea by nasogastric tube and cannula cuff; f penetration of esophagus by suction catheter. (Thomas AN: Management of tracheoesophageal fistula caused by cuffed tracheal tubes. Am J Surg 124:181–189, 1972)

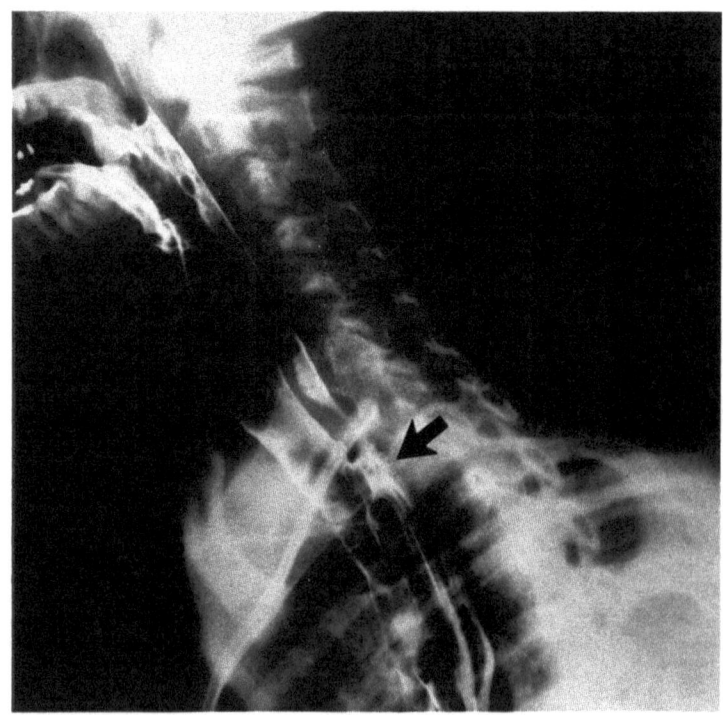

Fig. 5-60. Tracheoesophageal fistula due to prolonged use of a cuffed tracheal tube. The tube had been used in an 18-year-old quadriplegic for 1 year. The fistula *(arrow)* is 15 mm wide.

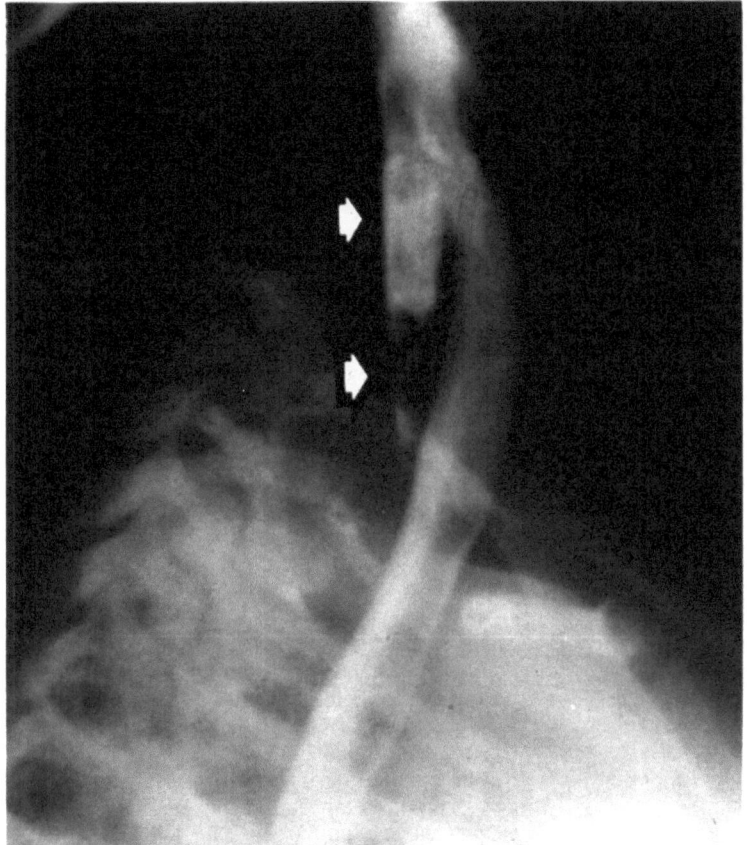

Fig. 5-61. Traumatic pseudodiverticulum. Perforation of the piriform sinus during suctioning in a 7-week-old infant resulted in the diverticulum *(arrows)*. (Calenoff L, Rogers LF: Radiologic manifestations of iatrogenic changes of the esophagus. Gastrointest Radiol 2:229–237, 1977)

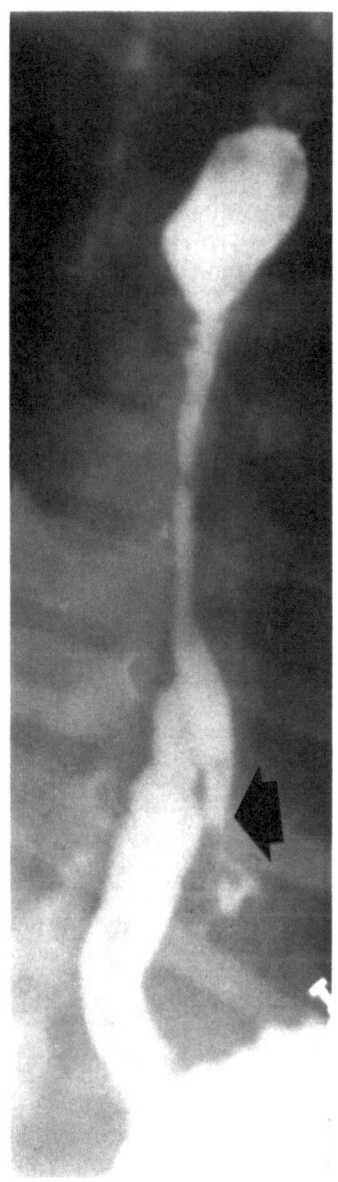

Fig. 5-62. False passage of a feeding tube. Evidence of false passage *(arrow)* is seen in the lower esophagus of a 3-month-old infant in whom passage had been difficult. (Calenoff L, Rogers LF: Radiologic manifestations of iatrogenic changes of the esophagus. Gastrointest Radiol 2:229–237, 1977)

tubes. Perforation from such procedures usually occurs in the hypopharynx or cervical esophagus. The perforation can be a catastrophic event (72), or it can be self-contained and result in a traumatic pseudodiverticulum (Fig. 5-61) or in false passage unexpectedly found during an upper gastrointestinal examination (Fig. 5-62).

References

1. Tuszewski FK: The radiologic appearance of the reconstructed esophagus. Acta Radiol 12:193–216, 1972
2. James AE, Montali RJ, Chaffee V, et al: Barium or gastrografin: Which contrast media for diagnosis of esophageal tears? Gastroenterology 68:1103–1113, 1975
3. Dunbar JS, Skinner GB, Wortzman G, et al: An investigation of effects of opaque media on the lungs with comparison of barium sulfate, lipiodol and dionosil. Am J Roentgenol 82:902–926, 1959
4. Reich SB: Production of pulmonary edema by aspiration of water-soluble nonabsorbable contrast media. Radiology 92:367–370, 1969
5. Harris PD, Newhauser EBD, Gerth R: The osmotic effect of water soluble contrast media on circulating plasma volume Am J Roentgenol 91:694–698, 1964

6. Calenoff L, Rogers LF: Radiologic manifestations of iatrogenic changes of the esophagus. Gastroint Radiol 2:229–237, 1977

7. Calenoff L, Norfray J: The reconstructed esophagus. Am J Roentgenol 125:864–876, 1975

8. Carter R, Hinshaw DB: Use of the Celestin indwelling plastic tube for inoperable carcinoma of the esophagus and cardia. Surg Gynecol Obstet 117:641–644, 1963

9. Postlethwait RW, Sealy WC, Dillon ML, et al: Colon interposition for esophageal substitution. Ann Thorac Surg 12:89–109, 1971

10. Vincent RG, Webster JH: Total esophagectomy and descending colon bypass for squamous cell carcinoma of the esophagus. Am J Surg 121:527–530, 1971

11. Orringer MB, Kirsh MM, Sloan H: New trends in esophageal replacement for benign disease. Ann Thorac Surg 23:409–416, 1977

12. Turney SZ: Lye stricture of the esophagus in children: The role of colon interposition. Am Surg 40:105–109, 1974

13. Schiller M, Frye TR, Boles ET Jr: Evaluation of colonic replacement of the esophagus in children. J Pediatr Surg 6:753–760, 1971

14. Baerg RD, Butler ML: Colon transplant for esophageal carcinoma. Manometric study of a case. Am J Gastroenterol 58:156–161, 1972

15. Jones EL, Skinner DB, Demeester TR, et al: Response of the interposed human colonic segment to an acid challenge. Ann Surg 177:75–78, 1973

16. Heimlich HJ: Esophagoplasty with reversed gastric tube. Review of fifty-three cases. Am J Surg 123:80–92, 1972

17. Heimlich HJ: Reversed gastric tube (RGT) esophagoplasty for failure of colon, jejunum and prosthetic interpositions. Ann Surg 182:154–160, 1975

18. Fetouh SA, Daffner RH, Postlethwait RW, et al: Radiologic aspects of Beck gastric tube in esophageal reconstruction. Am J Roentgenol 129:425–431, 1977

19. Dave KS, Wooter GH, Holden MP, et al: Esophageal replacement with jejunum for nonmalignant lesions: 26 years experience. Surgery: 72:466–473, 1972

20. Silver CE: Gastric pull-up operation for replacement of the cervical portion of the esophagus. Surg Gynecol Obstet 142:243–245, 1976

21. Okada N, Tagami Y, Morishita H, Reconstruction of the esophagus by posterior invagination esophagogastostomy. World J Surg 1:361–370, 1977

22. Mullens JE, Pezacki ZJ: Reconstruction of the cervical esophagus by revascularized autografts of intestine. An experimental study using the Inokuchi stapler and reporting the use of revasularized intestine to construct an artificial human larynx. Int Surg 55:157–171, 1971

23. Silver CE: Reconstruction after pharyngolaryngectomy-esophagectomy. Am J Surg 132:428–434, 1976

24. Petty CT, Theogaraj SD, Cohen IK: Secondary reconstruction of the cervical esophagus. Plast Reconstr Surg 56:70–76, 1975

25. West EM Jr, Baker HW: Esophageal dysphagia treated by cricopharyngeal myotomy. Am Surg 43:703–708, 1977

26. Sariyannis C, Mullard KS: Oesophagomyotomy for achalasia of the cardia. Thorax 30:539–542, 1975

27. Effler DB, Barr D, Groves LK: Epiphrenic diverticulum of the esophagus. Arch Surg 79:459–467, 1959

28. Takasaki T, Kobayashi S, Muto H, et al: Transabdominal esophageal transection by using a suture device in case of esophageal varices. Int Surg 62:426–428, 1977

29. Teixidor HS, Evans JA: Roentgenographic appearance of the distal esophagus and the stomach after hiatal hernia repair. Am J Roentgenol 119:245–258, 1973

30. Skucas J, Mangla JC, Adams JT, et al: An evaluation of the Nissen fundoplication. Radiology 118:539–543, 1976

31. Maulsby GO, Fontenelle LJ, Dalinka MK, Radiographic appearance of the chest following the Thal procedure. Radiology 100:293–294, 1971

32. Love L, Berkow AE: Trauma to the esophagus. Gastrointest Radiol 2:305–321, 1978

33. Rosenkrantz JC, Cozzetto FJ: Distal esophageal perforation: Complication of staged repair of esophageal atresia. Surgery 54:678–680, 1963

34. Huguier M, Gordin F, Maillard JN, et al: Results of 117 esophageal replacements. Surg Gynecol Obstet 130: 1054–1058, 1970

35. Ong GB: Resection and reconstruction of the esophagus. Curr Probl Surg 8:3–56, 1971

36. Hermreck AS, Crawford DG: The esophageal anastomotic leak. Am J Surg 132:794–798, 1976

37. Guidicelli R, Fuentes P, Reboud E: Surgical complications of esophageal surgery. Ann Anesthesiol Fr 18:373–376, 1977

38. Lortat-Jacob JL, Giuli R: Esophageal replacement. Prog Surg 12:77–95, 1973

39. Pradhan DJ, Ikins PM: Ischemic colitis in esophageal substitution: An unusual and lethal complication of colon interposition. Am Surg 41:427–428, 1975

40. Schiller M, Frye TR, Boles ET Jr: Evaluation of colonic replacement of the esophagus in children. J Pediatr Surg 6:753–760, 1971

41. Malcolm JA: Occurrence of peptic ulcer in colon used for esophageal replacement. J Thorac Cardiovas Surg 55:763–772, 1968

42. Raia A, Gama AH, Pinotti HW, et al: Diverticular disease in the transposed colon used for esophagoplasty: Report of two cases. Ann Surg 177:70–74, 1973

43. Hivet M, Blanchon P: Ischemic gastric ulcer in stomach transposed in the chest. Treatment with aortohepatic graft. Sem Hop Paris 51:2719–2722, 1975

44. Helsingen N Jr: Oesophagitis following total gas-

trectomy. A clinical and experimental study. Acta Chir Scand 273:1–19, 1961

45. Thoeni RF, Moss AA: The radiographic appearance of complications following Nissen fundoplication. Radiology 131:17–21, 1979

46. Burnett HF, Read RC, Morris WD, Management of complications of fundoplication and Barrett's esophagus. Surgery 82:521–530, 1977

47. Rogers LF: Transient post-vagotomy dysphagia: A distinct clinical and roentgenographic entity. Am J Roentgenol 125: 956–960, 1975

48. McLean GK, Laufer I: Hairy esophagus: A complication of pharyngoesophageal reconstructive surgery in two cases. Am J Roentgenol 132:269–270, 1979

49. Menzies-Gow N, Gummer JWP, Edwards DAW: Results of Heller's operation for achalasia of the cardia. Br J Surg 65:483–485, 1978

50. Sacks RP, DuBois JJ, Geiger JP, et al: The esophagobronchial fistula. Case report and review of the literature. Am J Roentgenol 99:204–209, 1967

51. Melamed M, Barker WL, Langston HT: Unusual pleural fistulas. Am J Roentgenol 120:876–882, 1974

52. Kovarik JL, Gipson BF: Spontaneous perforation of intrathoracic colon following total esophagectomy. Rocky Mt Med J 70:27–29, 1973

53. Pelligrini AN, Cenni LJ: Gastric ulcer perforated into pericardium. A unique complication of Thal's esophagogastroplasty. J Kans Med Soc 73:363–365, 1972

54. Ikard RW, Jacobs JK: Gastropericardial fistula and pericardial abscess: Unusual complications of subphrenic abscess following Nissen fundoplication. South Med J 67:17–19, 1974

55. Hoyt T, Kyaw MM: Acquired paraesophageal and disparaesophageal hernias. Complications of hiatal hernia repair. Am J Roentgenol 121:248–255, 1974

56. Seymour EQ: Aortoesophageal fistula as a complication of aortic prosthetic graft. Am J Roentgenol 131:160–161, 1978

57. Symes JM, Page AJF, Flavell G: Esophagopleural fistula: A late complication after pneumonectomy. J Thorac Cardiovasc Surg 63:783–786, 1972

58. Takaro T, Walkup HE, Okano T: Esophagopleural fistula as a complication of thoracic surgery. A collective review. J Thorac Cardiovasc Surg 40:179–193, 1960

59. Diedrich WM, Youngstrom KA: Alaryngeal Speech. pp 33–34, Springfield, Ill, Thomas, 1966

60. Staffieri M: Functional total laryngectomy. Surgical technique indication and results of an own technique for glottis-plasty with reconstruction of the voice. Monatsschr Ohrenheilkd Laryngorkinol 107:77–89, 1973

61. Griffiths CM, Love JT Jr: Neoglottic reconstruction after total laryngectomy. A preliminary report. Ann Otol 87:180–189, 1978

62. Sisson GA, Bytell DE, Becker SP, Total laryngectomy and reconstruction of a pseudoglottis: Problems and complications. Laryngoscope 88:639–650, 1978

63. Saito H, Matsui T, Tachibana M, et al: Experiences with the tracheoesophageal shunt method for vocal rehabilitation after total laryngectomy. Arch Otorhinolaryngol 218:135–142, 1977

64. Ghosh P: Transverse tracheo-esophagoplasty. A new one-stage operation for construction of a "neo-larynx." J Laryngol Otol 91:1077-1083, 1977

65. Lindeman RC: Diverting the paralyzed larynx: A reversible procedure for intractable aspiration. Laryngoscope 85: 157–180, 1975

66. Pais MJ, Segal HB: Esophageal obturator airway: Radiographic appearance. Am J Roentgenol 132:267–268, 1979

67. Scholl DG, Tsai SH: Esophageal perforation following the use of the esophageal obturator airway. Radiology: 122:315–316, 1977

68. Hirsch M, Abramowitz HB, Shapira S, et al: Hypopharyngeal injury as a result of attempted endotracheal intubation. Radiology 128:37-39, 1978

69. Wolff AP, Kuhn FA, Ogura JA: Pharyngeal-esophageal perforations associated with rapid oral endotracheal intubation. Ann Otol 81:258–261, 1972

70. Harley HRS: Ulcerative tracheo-oesophageal fistula during treatment by tracheostomy and intermittent positive pressure ventilation. Thorax 27:338–352, 1972

71. Thomas AN: Management of tracheoesophageal fistula caused by cuffed tracheal tubes. Am J Surg 124:181–189, 1972

72. Lee SB, Kuhn JP: Esophageal perforation in the neonate. A review of the literature. Am J Dis Child 130:325–329, 1976

6 Complications of Gastric and Duodenal Surgery

Morton Burrell and Bernard S. Jay

Many patients suffer complications, concurrent illness, recurrent disease, and generalized debilitation following major gastroduodenal surgery. Some of these problems represent the inherent risk of operation to relieve the original symptoms. It is difficult, however, to clearly define the iatrogenic complications because surgical procedures are initiated by physicians, and thus any subsequently encountered problem may be technically considered iatrogenic in nature. In this chapter we will review those complications that may be created by and related to specific surgical procedures but that do not necessarily imply error in technique. Problems directly due to surgical oversights will also be discussed and the postsurgical radiographic anatomy of the upper gastrointestinal tract presented with emphasis on findings that may simulate other diseases.

General Considerations

In several long-term studies comparing surgical and medical treatment of peptic ulcer disease the results in terms of hospitalization time, physical fitness, and ability to work seem to have favored the operative approach. This has led to earlier surgical intervention, especially in peptic ulcer disease (1). The availability of cimetidine and development of other H_2-receptor antagonists, however, may alter this outlook in the future.

Three major operations are currently in vogue for treatment of peptic ulcer disease: partial gas-trectomy, vagotomy with a drainage procedure, and vagotomy with hemigastrectomy (2–4). The associated mortality is generally between 1% and 2%, particularly after vagotomy and partial gastric resection (5–7). In a 25-year review of truncal vagotomy and partial gastric resection by Herrington et al. a mortality of 1.6% was found among 3500 patients (6). In comparison, in a series of 1000 patients who underwent truncal vagotomy and drainage procedure the mortality was only 0.5%.

The recurrence rate of ulcer is another important consideration. Dodsworth and Fischer noted a recurrence rate of less than 2% after vagotomy-hemigastrectomy as compared to a 6%–8% following vagotomy-drainage procedures (5). Other reviews confirm this reduced incidence of recurrent ulceration after vagotomy and partial resection, although this is offset by slightly increased morbidity (7–8).

Three types of vagotomy are available: truncal (most widely used), selective (total gastric), and the highly selective proximal vagotomy (9). It appears that the last operation has the least postvagotomy sequelae of all. Severe dumping and diarrhea occur rarely. According to Johnston et al. there is a decreased incidence of diarrhea with selective vagotomy (10). The incidence of recurrent ulcers after this procedure has been reported from ten centers, but follow-up is only a few years and further observation is needed for statistical accuracy. However, one may infer from several available studies that the incidence of recurrent ulceration is probably as low as or lower than that of other types of vagotomy (11,12).

In addition to the surgical morbidity and recurrence rate the immediate and long-term complications of surgery are important (Fig. 6-1). Dumping occurs in approximately 10% of patients. A 10%–25% incidence of diarrhea occurring with truncal vagotomy and hemigastrectomy is decreased with selective vagotomy without a drainage procedure. The associated weight loss may be related to decreased appetite and malabsorption. Anemia and metabolic bone disease are also frequent problems in patients who have undergone gastric surgery (5).

Presently in the United States the most popular operation for duodenal ulcer is antrectomy or limited distal gastrectomy (25%–40% of the stomach) combined with truncal vagotomy. Reconstitution is either via a Billroth I or II procedure (3).

Multiple operative methods directed toward reducing gastroesophageal reflux have been widely used. An excellent review by DeMeester, et al. strongly favors the Nissen repair over the Belsey mark IV and Hill repairs (13). It best controlled the gastroesophageal reflux and competency of the lower esophageal sphincter. All three procedures were limited by postoperative dysphagia and a high incidence (50%) of inability to vomit.

Radiographic Anatomy Following Gastroduodenal Surgery

Radiologic evaluation of the postoperative stomach represents a most challenging task because the established anatomic landmarks may be absent or so altered as to be unrecognizable and misleading. Surgically created plication deformities and contour irregularities of the gastric remnant often cause a diagnostic dilemma. Many of these difficulties can be avoided and recognition of subsequent complications made easier if a base-line postoperative upper gastrointestinal series is routinely obtained before the patient is discharged from the hospital.

Since numerous individual variations of common surgical procedures are in widespread use it is most helpful for the radiologist to be well acquainted with details of the operation prior to performance of the examination. In this context we will briefly describe only the surgical anatomy of common gastroduodenal operations and their associated radiographic findings. More comprehensive information about the subject is provided in several publications listed in the references.

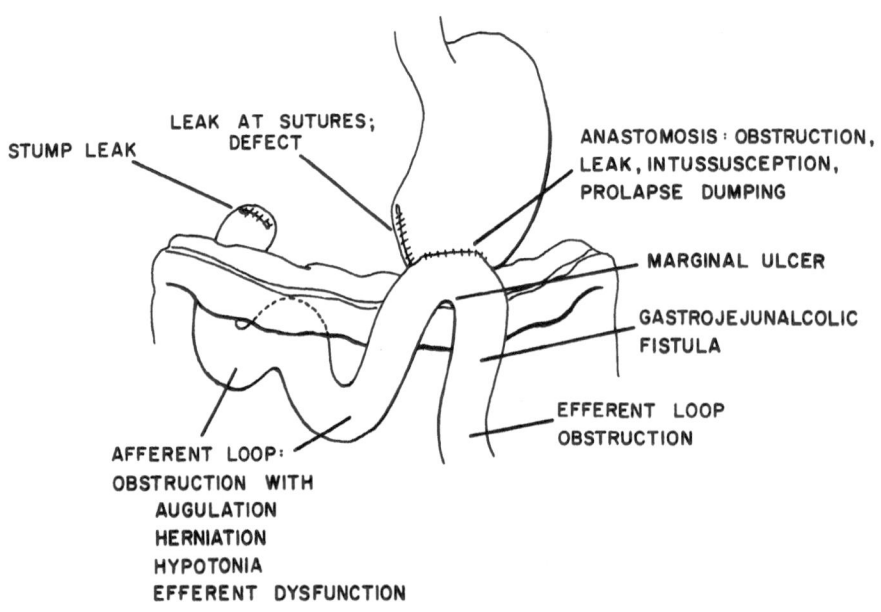

Fig. 6-1. Potential complications of gastric surgery.

The *Billroth I and II procedures* refer to a broad category of partial gastrectomy together with gastroduodenostomy and gastrojejunostomy, respectively (14–19). The original Billroth I operation consists of resecting the distal part of the stomach together with a very short cuff of duodenum and performing an end-to-end anastomosis between the gastric remnant and duodenal bulb. The Billroth II procedure also involves a partial gastrectomy. However, both the gastric and duodenal ends are tightly closed with multiple rows of sutures, and the continuity of the lumen is established through a gastrojejunostomy (Figs. 6-1, 6-2).

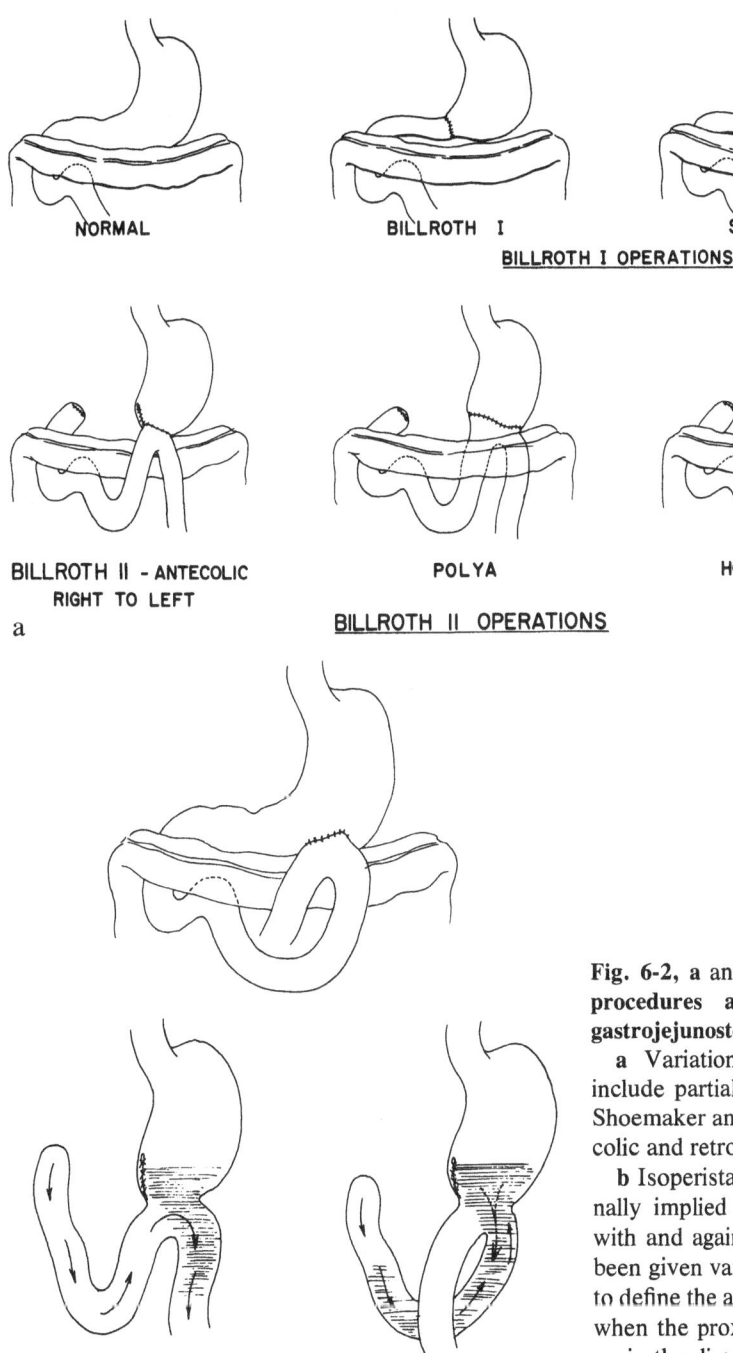

Fig. 6-2, a and b. Billroth I and Billroth II types of procedures and isoperistaltic and antiperistaltic gastrojejunostomy.

a Variations shown in the Billroth procedures include partial oversewing of the stoma, as with the Shoemaker and Hofmeister approaches, and the antecolic and retrocolic position of the anastomosis.

b Isoperistaltic and antiperistaltic, terms that originally implied emptying of the postsurgical stomach with and against peristaltic waves respectively, have been given varying interpretations. It is probably best to define the anatomic situation in terms of left to right when the proximal or afferent loop has been hooked up in the direction of greater to lesser curvature, and right to left in the direction of lesser to greater curvature.

In the *Polya operation* a retrocolic end-to-side anastomosis is performed between the open end of the gastric stump and the wall of jejunum. The same procedure may be performed by means of antecolic isoperistaltic gastrojejunostomy (Balfour operation) or antecolic antiperistaltic gastroenterostomy (Moynihan modification) (14,-18). A *retrocolic gastroenterostomy* involves upward mobilization of the jejunal loop through a rent in the transverse mesocolon and anastomosis with the posterior gastric wall close to the greater curvature. In contrast, the *antecolic gastroenterostomy* is made between a proximal jejunal loop and the anterior gastric wall just above and anterior to the transverse colon. The widely popular *Hofmeister technique* of gastrojejunostomy was developed to minimize the disadvantages of a very large stoma created during the Polya operation. This procedure involves closure of the open end of the gastric remnant by a line of sutures extending along the lesser curvature and performance of gastrojejunostomy using only the greater curvature side of the gastric lumen.

Pseudolesions Following Gastric Surgery

Several of the commonly performed operations on the upper gastrointestinal tract cause unusual radiographic findings that may be easily mistaken for more serious disorders. Insight into these potential problems can assist physicians in avoiding pitfalls in their recognition and subsequent management.

Simple closure or oversewing of a perforated ulcer may result in localized invagination of the wall, presenting as a small figure-3 type of deformity. This is usually seen on the early postoperative contrast studies but will later disappear.

Partial gastrectomy involving wedge or sleeve resection usually results in a recognizable radiographic deformity where the gastric wall is inverted and sutured (15,18).

Gastrostomy involves creation of an external opening in the anterior gastric wall near the greater curvature. This segment is also sutured to the anterior wall of the abdomen. After removal of the gastrostomy tube or draining catheter there is usually spontaneous closure of the gastric incision. However, the anterior walls of the stomach and abdomen remain attached by the sutures. Accordingly, persistent anterior deviation or localized tenting of the gastric wall may be visible on barium contrast examination (16). This and other problems associated with gastrostomy tubes will be described in more detail later in this chapter.

In the late 1950s Nissen and Rossetti developed a fundoplication for hiatal hernia repair (20). By means of an abdominal approach, the distal esophagus and upper portion of the stomach are mobilized and the gastric fundus is wrapped around the esophagus. The hiatus hernia itself is reduced, and the hiatus is closed posteriorly. In order to avoid excessive narrowing of the esophagus, the plication procedure is performed while a large-bore (no. 36 or no. 38 Ewald) nasogastric tube is within the esophagus. The postoperative radiographic appearance is characteristic (Fig. 6-3). A filling defect resembling a tumor is seen in the gastric cardia (21,22).

The Belsey mark IV hiatal hernia repair also distorts the radiographic appearance of the esophagogastric junction. The object of this operation is to use the fundus and diaphragm together to secure the formation of an intraabdominal segment of the esophagus. A left thoracotomy is done for this purpose, and a large nasogastric tube is inserted to avoid excessive narrowing of the esophagus. Because of the suture placement in this procedure an unusual appearance of the distal esophagus and fundus is seen on the subsequent barium contrast study. Radiographs may reveal the appearance of a stenosing lower esophageal lesion or a mass in the fundus (21,22).

A characteristic defect is noted radiographically in patients who have had gastroenterostomy with a Hofmeister type of anastomosis (Figs. 6-4, 6-5). As mentioned earlier, the procedure was developed to minimize the problems associated with a large stoma after partial gastrectomy (14,18). Here the open end of the gastric stump is closed with a line of sutures extending one-half to two-thirds of the distance from the lesser curvature to the greater curvature, and the anastomosis is then performed. In a study by Fisher of 100 patients who had a Hofmeister

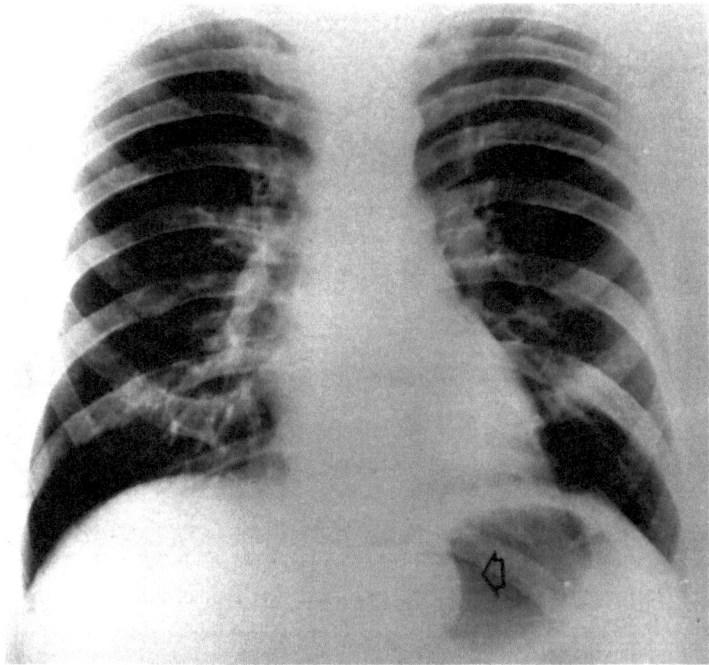

a

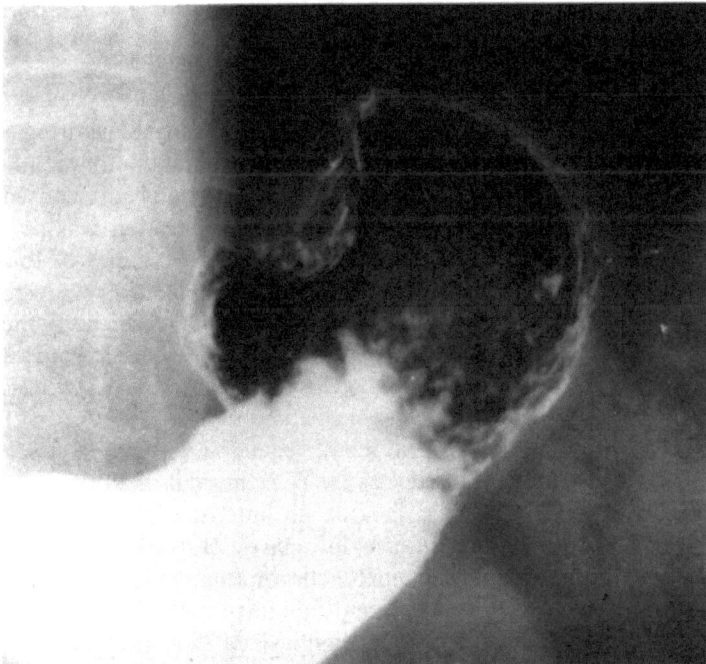

b

Fig. 6-3, a and **b. Nissen fundoplication. a** The characteristic mass *(arrow)* in the area of the gastric cardia is well seen in this posteroanterior radiograph of the chest. **b** Barium examination reveals a smoothly marginated mass distorting the gastric outline in the area of the esophagogastric junction. Despite the absence of surgical clips the possibility of surgery should always be considered when one is evaluating a stomach with this appearance.

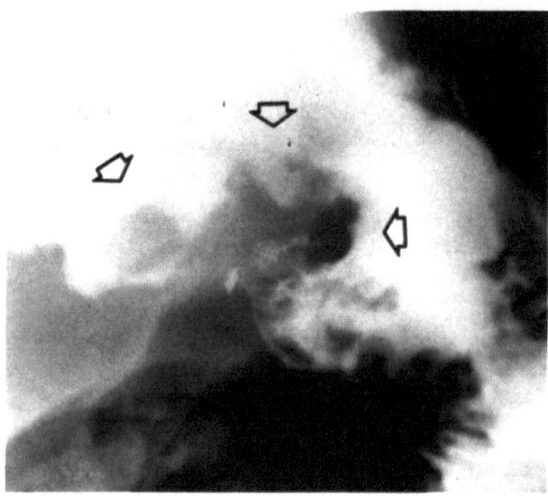

Fig. 6-4. Hofmeister defect. This is a characteristic deformity *(arrows)* seen on lesser curvature just proximal to Billroth II type anastomosis.

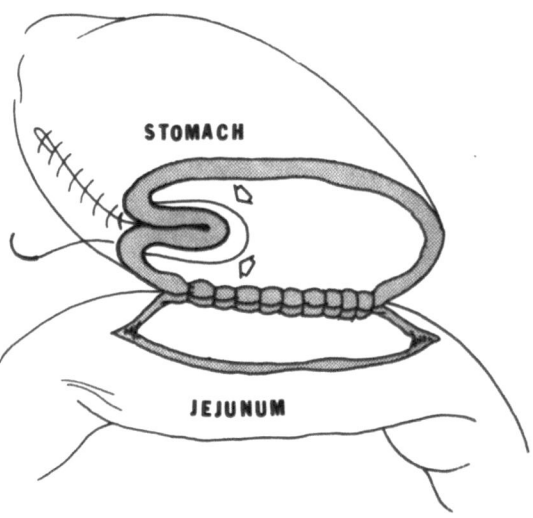

Fig. 6-5. Hofmeister defect. Diagrammatic representation of the surgical infolding *(arrows)* of stomach to reduce the size of anastomosis with jejunum that is responsible for the radiographic appearance of the defect.

operation, six showed this defect (23). The filling defect corresponds to the closure line of the invaginated cut surface of the stomach. It is more apparent on the initial postoperative study but may later decrease in size and become invisible. Similar changes are seen with other surgical procedures where there is plication proximal to the stoma (Fig. 6-6) or at the side of the gastroduodenal anastomosis in the Billroth I procedure (Fig. 6-7).

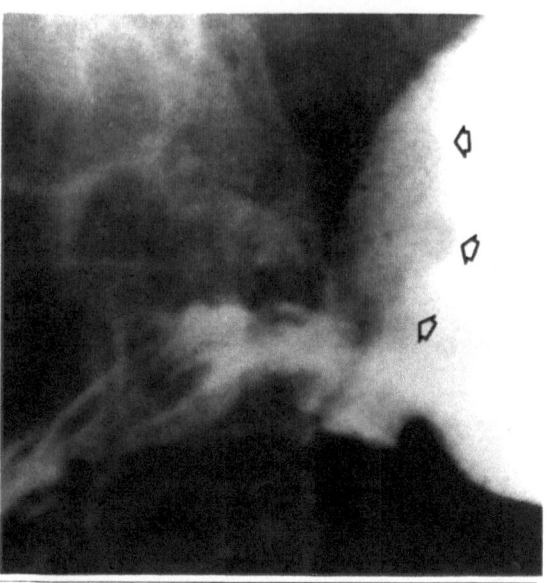

Fig. 6-6. Defect in Shoemaker type of Billroth I repair. The defect is seen on the lesser curve above the anastomosis *(arrows)*.

Following pyloroplasty of various types the vertical closure of the incision produces irregularity of the pyloric and duodenal contours, and to this is added the preexisting deformity caused by the lesion for which the operation was performed (24,25). Barium contrast studies of this area present typical and sometimes bizarre radiographic findings (Fig. 6-8). Occasionally the deformity does not fit into the classical mold (Fig. 6-9). This again emphasizes the value of a base-line study, particularly for differentiation of a commonly noted pseudodiverticulum from recurrent ulcer (15). The normal anatomic and physiologic landmarks are usually not clearly identified after pyloroplasty. Instead, a wide and irregular channel incorporating the lumina of the gastric antrum and duodenal bulb may be seen. Bloch and Wolf emphasized that the functional and anatomic evaluation of pyloroplasty is best achieved by cineradiography (25). They also noted that persistence of a radiographically normal and contractible pyloric channel together with evidence for gastric retention would indicate unsuccessful pyloroplasty.

Several authors have described postoperative plication deformity, sometimes with foreign-body granuloma simulating gastric tumor (26,-

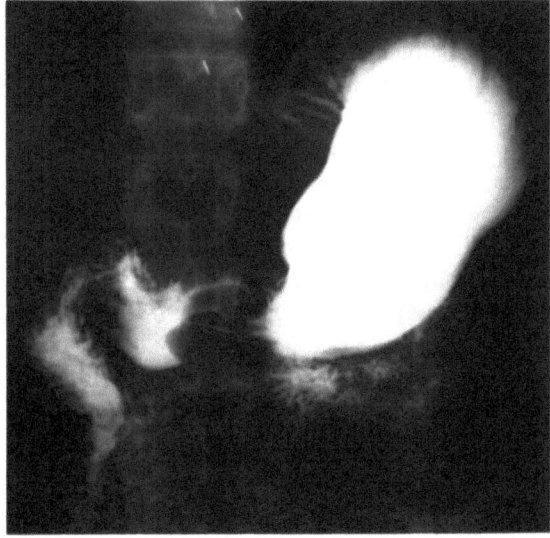

a

Fig. 6-7, a and b. Pseudotumor due to plication defect in gastroduodenostomy. a The patient had undergone vagotomy and Billroth I procedure because of a bleeding antral ulcer. **b** Close-up shows a lobulated mass projecting into the duodenal bulb.

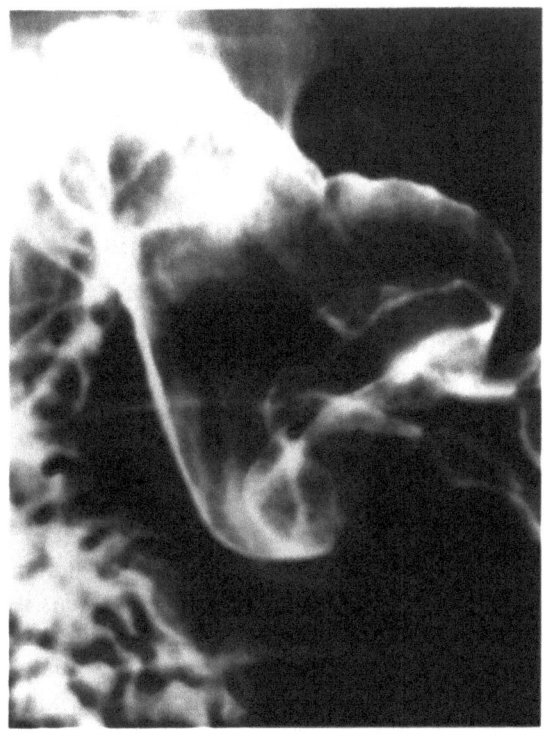

b

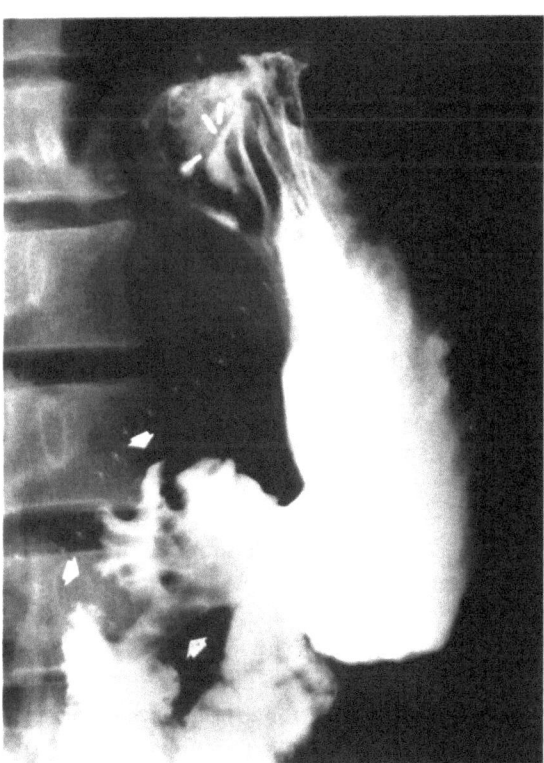

Fig. 6-8. Deformed duodenum and surgically created gastroduodenostomy channel *(arrows)*. These are characteristic features of a Jaboulay pyloroplasty.

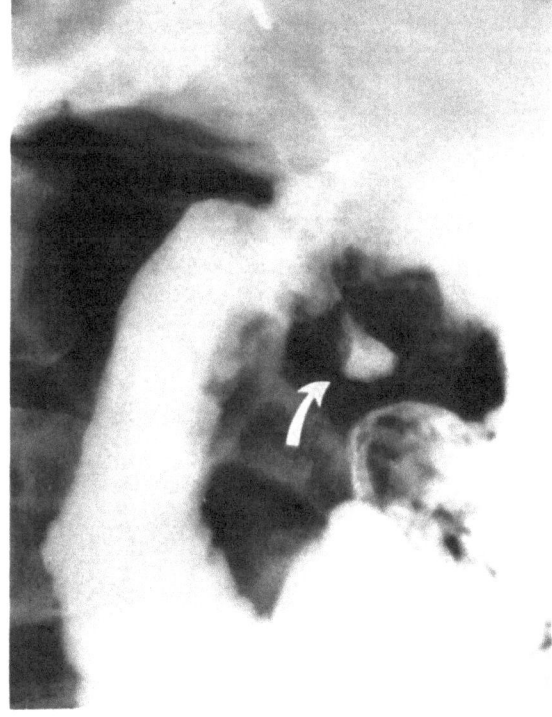

Fig. 6-9. Large outpouching after a Finney pyloroplasty. The outpouching *(arrow)* is somewhat unusual although the loss of a clear-cut pyloric canal and scalloping of the pyloroduodenal area are common.

27). These lesions, if large enough, may cause symptoms and actually ulcerate. Radiographically the findings consist of a well-defined filling defect appearing as a benign tumor (Fig. 6-10).

Postoperative Complications

Many of the complications of gastrointestinal surgery are related to the cardiopulmonary system and include atelectasis, pneumonitis, pulmonary embolism, shock lung, etc. These are not inherent to specific surgical procedures but are also seen in other types of abdominal surgery.

Postoperative ileus and acute gastric dilatation occur frequently (28–30). The degree of ileus is directly related to the extent of bowel manipulation during surgery. Although ileus is usually generalized the gastric atony may be a striking component. The proximal portion of the stomach does not display any significant motility. Therefore, evaluation of gastric emptying when the stoma is in the dependent position is necessary to distinguish atony from obstruction (28). It is not unusual for atony to persist for 2 or 3 days postoperatively (29). Acute gastric dilatation is another serious complication whereby the stomach becomes distended with fluid and gas, leading to nausea, vomiting, dehydration, and possibly shock. The causal mechanisms are unclear, but nasal administration of oxygen, use of respirators, and aerophagia have been implicated (30).

Pneumoperitoneum is extremely common after intraabdominal surgery and may not be dependent on the type of operation or the presence of peritonitis. It is stressed that pneumoperitoneum may increase when multiple abdominal drains are in place, and such observation should not be misinterpreted as perforation or stump blowout (31,32). The duration of pneumoperitoneum is variable and is affected by body habitus. It disappears fastest in children and thin individuals. However, persistence of free air for longer than 1 week or an increasing amount of free air should suggest the possibility of anastomotic leakage (28).

Tube-Related Problems

Nasogastric tubes and other devices are commonly used in postoperative patients. These occasionally have unusual clinical and radiographic findings, which are presented in Chapter 3.

Gastrostomy tubes are commonly used in the immediate postoperative period and for long-term feeding purposes. The feeding gastrostomy was introduced in 1896 (33). Complication rates associated with its use are reported to vary between 1 and 5% (34). These include hemorrhage, leakage, gastric prolapse through the ostia of the tube, and partial or complete obstruction (34,35). To avoid partial or complete obstruction from a gastrostomy tube, care must be taken in its proper positioning. The onset of severe vomiting and dehydration following recent placement of a gastrostomy tube, or in patients in whom a tube is being used for long-term feeding, should alert the physician to this potential complication (36). Without immediate diagnosis and treatment death may ensue quickly. Treatment is simple, consisting of repositioning the tube. Following removal of a gastrostomy tube, filling defects

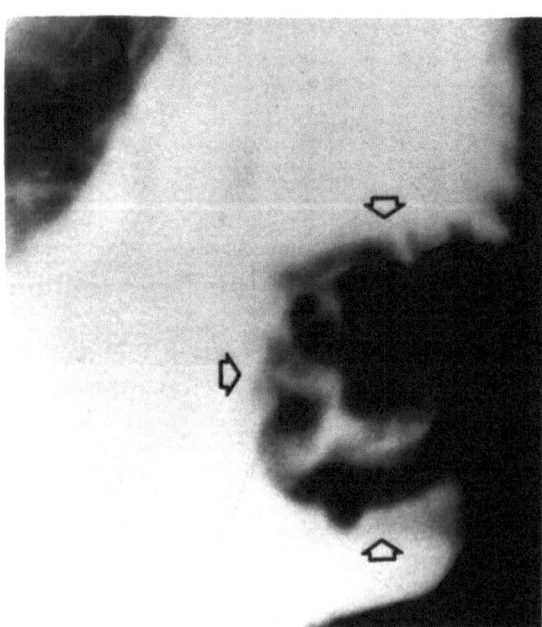

Fig. 6-10. Foreign-body granuloma simulating tumor. The greater-curvature mass *(arrows)* was due to a granuloma about retained suture material. The patient had had previous colon surgery, and a bleeding point in the gastrocolic ligament was ligated at that time.

and irregularity of the wall of the stomach may be observed on barium contrast studies. These defects are generally seen along the greater curvature of the stomach and may persist permanently (Figs. 6-11, 6-12). Anterior displacement of the gastric antrum with adherence to the ante-

rior abdominal wall or acute angulation of the gastric body in a medial direction may be noted (37) (Figs. 6-13, 6-14). Recognition of these defects will avoid unnecessary diagnostic studies or surgical intervention.

Prosthetic tubes are frequently used for palliative treatment of inoperable esophageal carcinoma (38). These tubes may be inserted surgically and sutured in place (Celestin tube), or simply positioned within the esophagus during endoscopy (Silastic tube) (38–40). A frequent complication is subsequent displacement of the

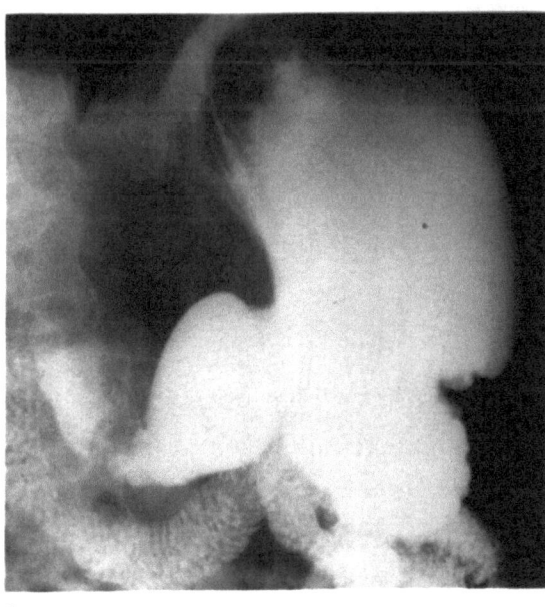

a

b

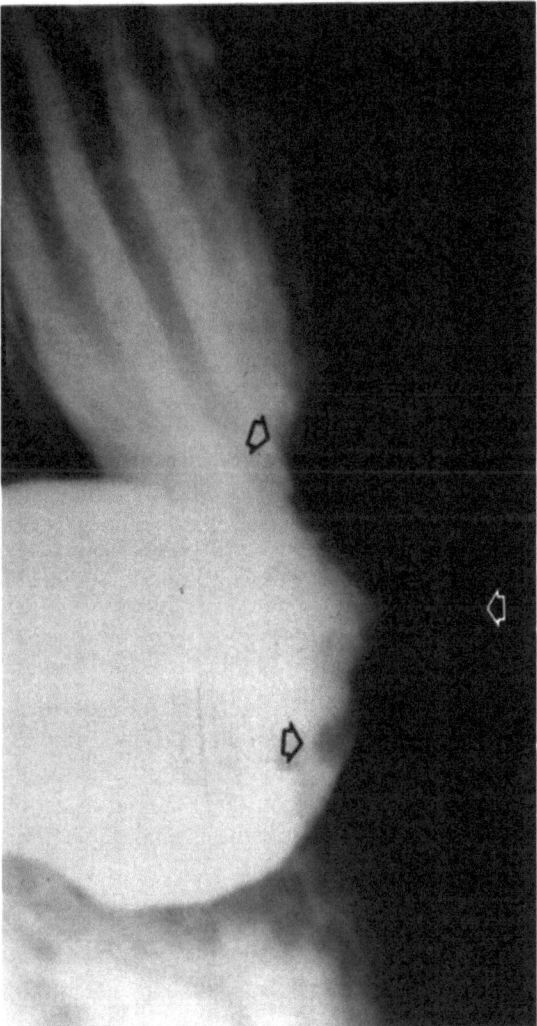

Fig. 6-11, a and b. Filling defect and irregularity of wall of stomach associated with use of gastrostomy tube. a The large defect about the gastrostomy tube is seen. b Years later a localized irregular scar is visible on the greater curvature.

Fig. 6-12. Filling defect and irregularity of wall of stomach associated with use of a gastrostomy tube. Several years after closure of gastrostomy in this patient the mucosal irregularity of the greater curvature *(black arrows)* and a pseudodiverticulum *(white arrow)* are noted.

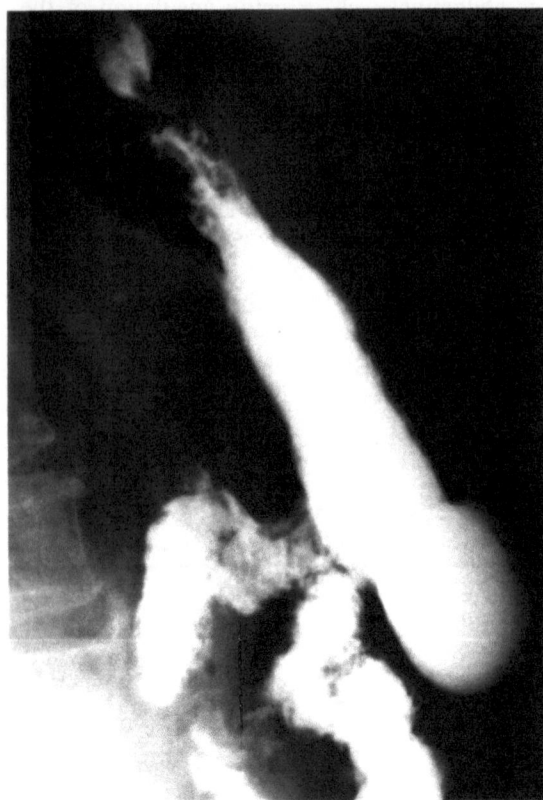

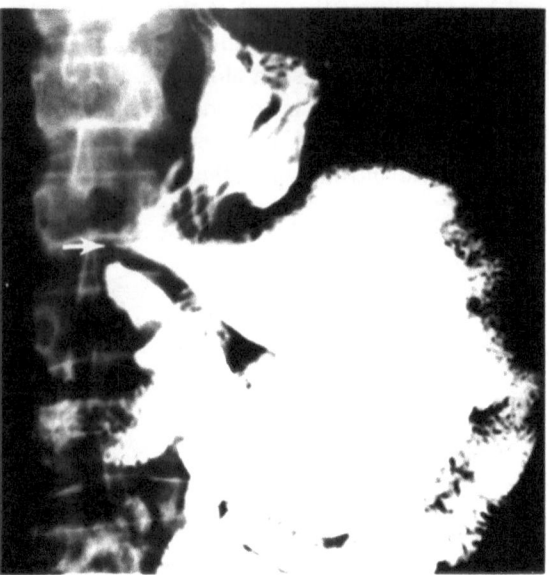

Fig. 6-14. Postgastrectomy deformity of stomach. Upper gastrointestinal series performed 2 years after splenectomy and tube gastrostomy. There is acute angulation of the body of the stomach toward the midline *(arrow)*. This configuration was not present on study performed prior to surgery. (Bryk D: Postgastrostomy deformity of the stomach. Gastrointest Radiol 2:259–261, 1977)

Fig. 6-13. Postgastrostomy deformity of stomach. Right lateral recumbent view reveals anterior position of the gastric antrum. This deformity is related to tube gastrostomy performed in conjunction with cholecystectomy 10 years previously. (Bryk D: Postgastrostomy deformity of stomach: Gastrointest Radiol 2:259–261, 1977)

prosthetic tube from the site of obstruction. Other potential complications include perforation, obstruction of the tube due to food impaction, and aspiration, Radiographs obtained with or without the use of contrast material assist in locating the slipped prosthesis and in further evaluation of complications (Figs. 6-15, 6-16).

Postsurgical Diverticula

Gastric diverticula are unusual in locations other than the cardia and juxtapyloric area, and their appearance following subtotal gastrectomy has

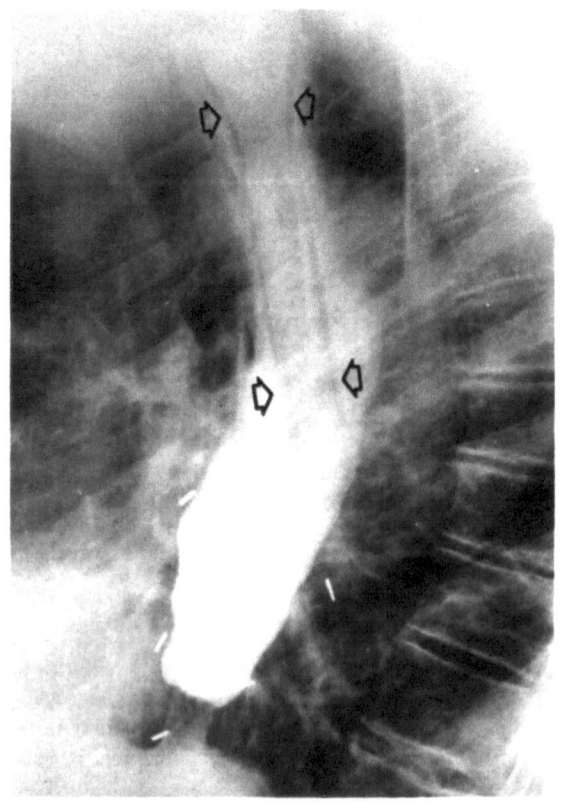

Fig. 6-15. Displacement of prosthetic tube. Celestin tube *(arrows)* used to maintain patency of the esophagus has become dislodged, and there is complete obstruction by distal esophageal carcinoma.

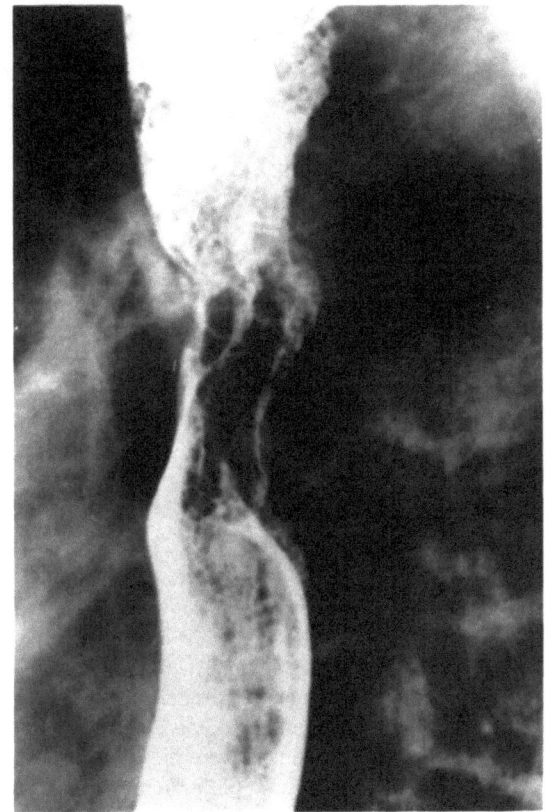

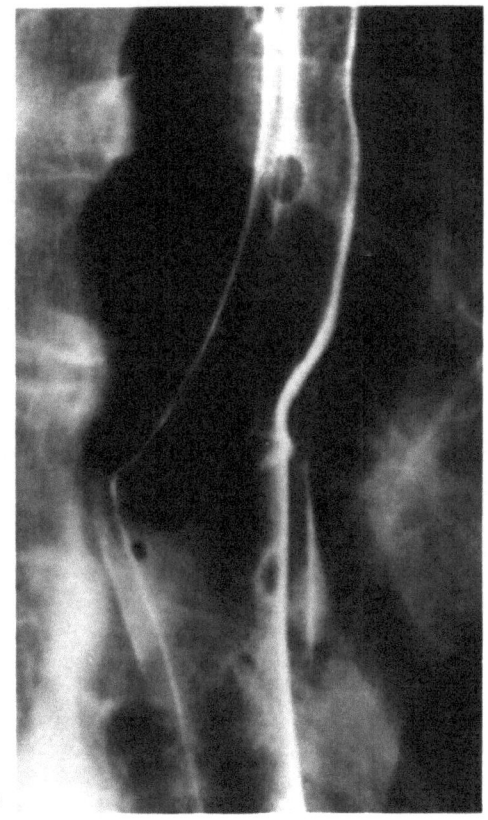

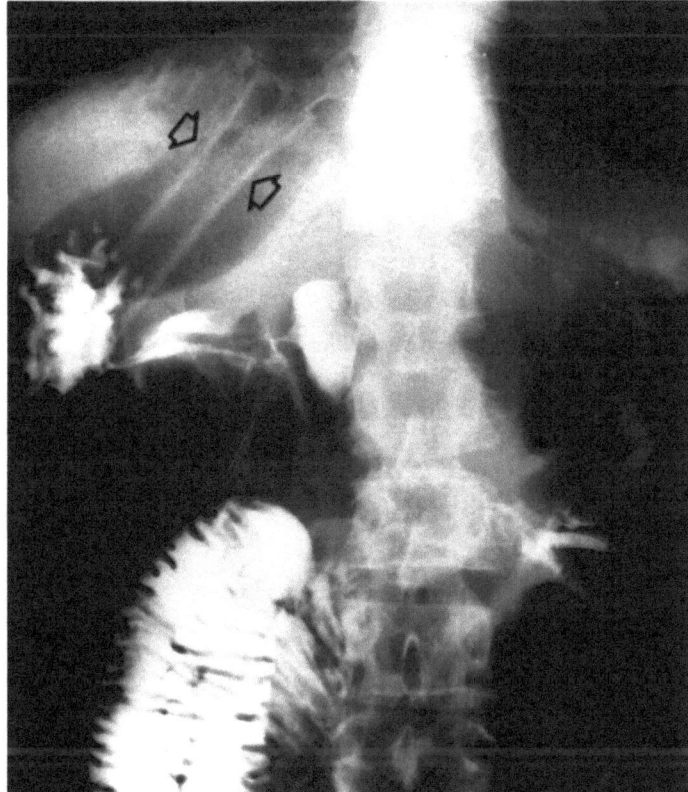

Fig. 6-16, a–c. Displacement of prosthetic tube. a Esophageal border is irregular and lumen narrowed secondary to carcinoma. b Silastic tube has been placed endoscopically to maintain patency of upper gastrointestinal tract. c After attempted endoscopic removal of a piece of steak impacted in the tube the tube was accidentally pushed into the stomach (arrows).

Another iatrogenic complication occurred when the surgeon in attempting to remove the tube from the stomach could not find it and created a feeding "gastrostomy" into the jejunum, failing to recall the presence of situs inversus and making too small an incision to appreciate true topography.

been generally ignored in the literature (41). These diverticula are probably true acquired pulsion diverticula and may be related to increased intragastric pressure (42). Adhesions secondary to perianastomotic inflammation also could produce traction diverticula. Three examples of gastric diverticula illustrated in Figs. 6-17 to 6-19 also show partial obstruction distal to the diverticulum, perhaps accounting for increased intragastric pressure and formation of a pulsion type of diverticulum.

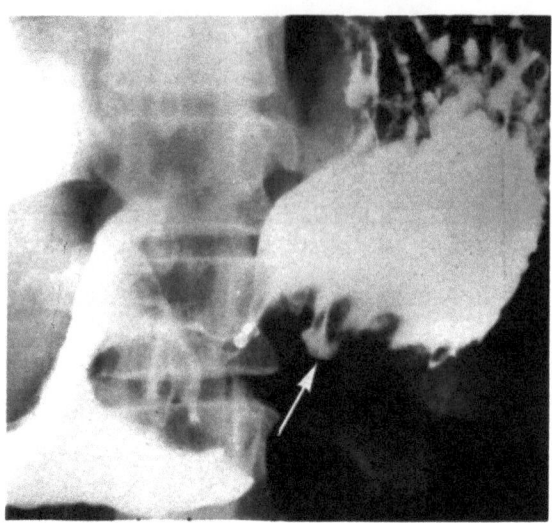

Fig. 6-18. Postsurgical diverticulum associated with gastric mucosal prolapse. A Billroth II procedure has been performed 17 years previously for bleeding duodenal ulcer in a 58-year-old man. During the year prior to admission to the hospital progressive obstructive symptoms developed, and on admission there was a 1-week history of vomiting after eating. There is prolapse of gastric mucosa into both afferent and efferent loops, and a small diverticulum is noted on the greater curvature of the stomach (arrow). (Mihas AA, Hans S: Gastric diverticula following subtotal gastrectomy. Gastrointest Radiol 2:263–265, 1977)

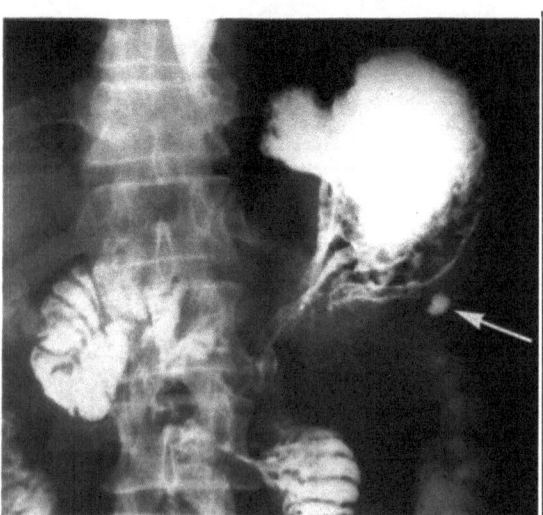

Fig. 6-17. Postsurgical diverticulum associated with gastric mucosal prolapse. A small diverticulum is seen on the greater curvature (arrow) proximal to obstructing prolapse of gastric mucosa into duodenum. Hyperplastic mucosa obstructing the pyloric stoma and a greatly dilated duodenum were confirmed endoscopically. The patient had repeated epigastric pain and vomiting. This obstructing mass of polypoid mucosa was excised surgically. (Mihas AA, Hans S: Gastric diverticula following subtotal gastrectomy. Gastrointest Radiol 2:263–265, 1977)

Fig. 6-19. Postsurgical diverticulum. Five years prior to admission with complaints of epigastric pain, nausea, and occasional vomiting, a 56-year-old man had undergone subtotal gastrectomy with Billroth II anastomosis for peptic ulcer disease. On upper gastrointestinal series a large greater-curvature diverticulum is noted proximal to the gastrojejunostomy (arrow). (Mihas AA, Hans S: Gastric diverticula following subtotal gastrectomy. Gastrointest Radiol 2:263–265, 1977)

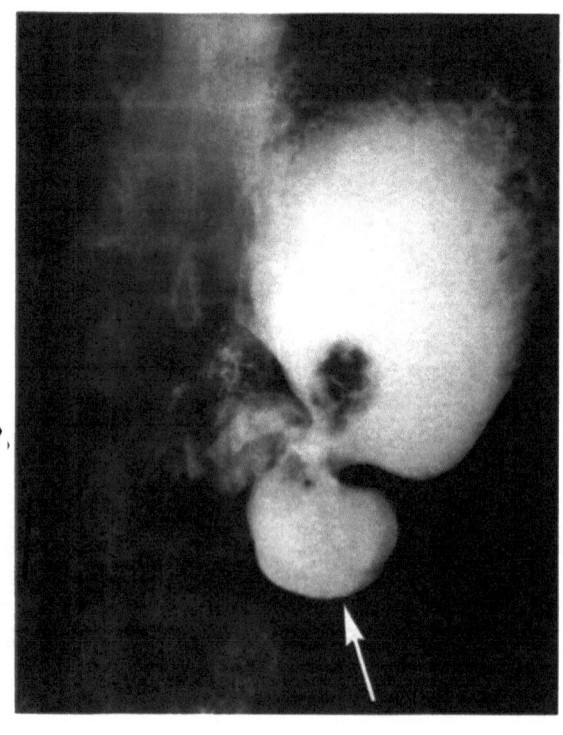

"Gas-Bloat Syndrome"

The "gas-bloat syndrome" generally occurs in patients who have undergone fundoplication procedures, but it also may be associated with other types of hiatal hernia repairs (43). The incidence is highest after the Nissen procedure. It varies from 10% to 25%, but one observer noted an incidence of 54% in a study of 68 patients (43–47).

The patient generally complains of inability to eructate or vomit. Air is trapped in the stomach, producing early satiety and epigastric fullness. As the patient attempts to relieve the discomfort by eructating or vomiting, air is swallowed. This vicious cycle leads to more entrapment of air, thus increasing symptoms of bloating and fullness. Radiographs show significant gastric distention and marked narrowing of the newly created intraabdominal esophagus (Fig. 6-20).

Goldstein and Butterfield evaluated the gas-bloat syndrome experimentally in animal models with complete and incomplete fundoplications (43). They noted that the extent of the fundoplication is not in itself important and contend that this syndrome is the result of a technically imperfect repair.

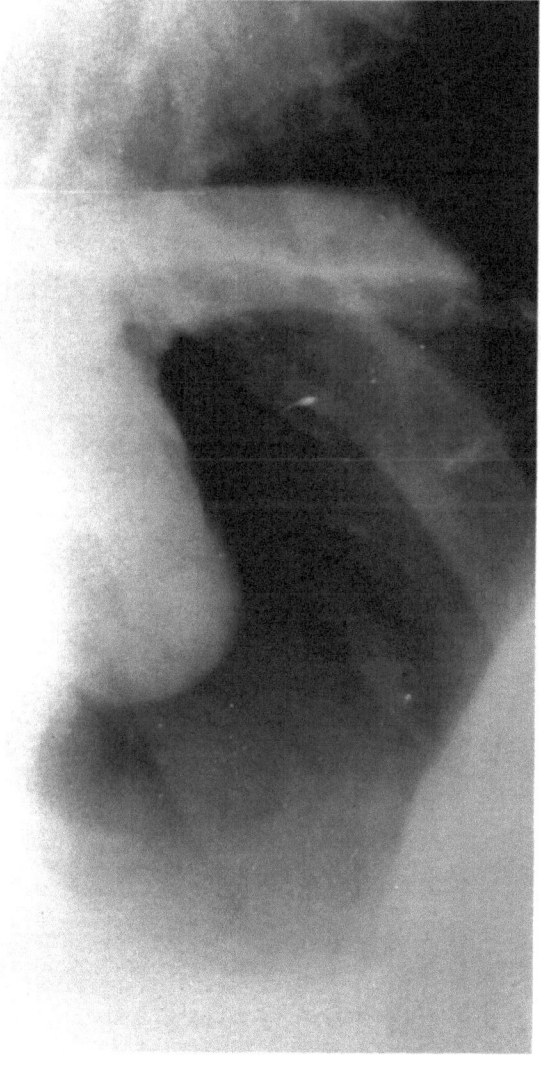
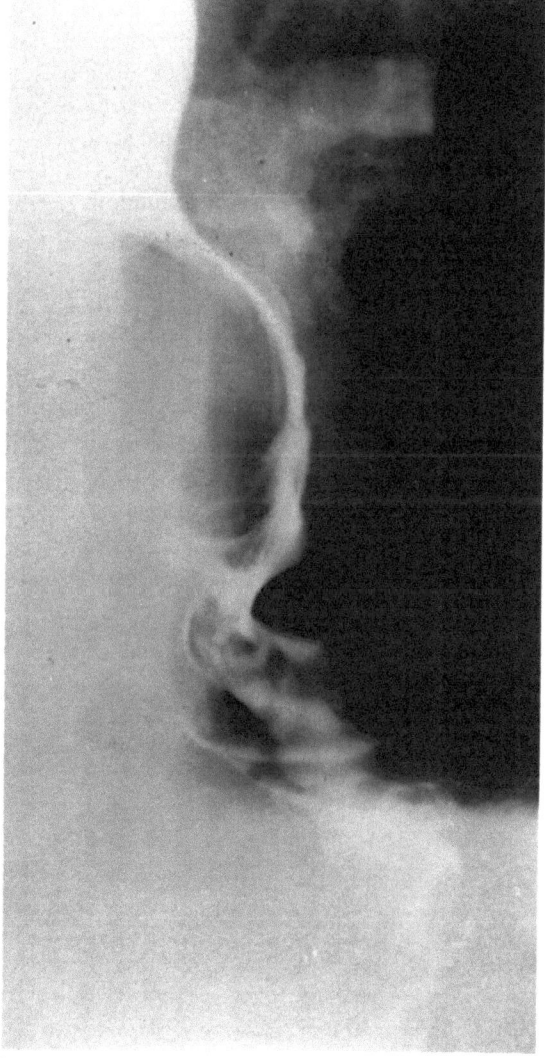

a   b

Fig. 6-20, a and **b. Gas-bloat syndrome. a** Gaseous distention of the stomach and a mass in the cardia are seen in a patient who has undergone a Belsey type of fundoplication and complained of bloating and inability to belch. **b** The narrowing of the newly created intraabdominal esophagus is desirable for preventing reflux, but it also produces gas-bloat type of symptoms.

As noted in the prior description of pseudolesions, current surgical technique for either the Nissen or Belsey repair includes placement of a large-bore nasogastric tube within the distal esophagus during the surgical procedure to allow for adequate patency of the esophagogastric surgical junction and, it is hoped, to minimize this problem (46).

Inadvertent Gastroileostomy

Another potential iatrogenic complication is inadvertent gastroileostomy. Clinical distinction from gastrojejunocolic fistula is readily made. Patients with a gastroileostomy have early onset of symptoms, which include inanition, marked diarrhea, and malabsorption. The diagnosis of inadvertent gastroileostomy is more readily made from an upper gastrointestinal series (Figs. 6-21, 6-22) while gastrocolic fistula is better demonstrated on barium enema examination.

Bezoars

One of the relatively frequent complications of gastric surgery is formation of bezoars (48–51). Over 80% of these are phytobezoars and consist of a conglomerate mass of undigested fruit and vegetable fibers coated with mucous secretions. Rarely the mass includes other material such as fungus balls and antacid concretions (49). In a series of 131 patients who underwent gastric surgery for ulcer, bezoars were subsequently diagnosed in 16, an incidence of over 12% (50). All these patients had vagotomy together with Billroth I (11) or Billroth II operation (3) and pyloroplasty (2). The majority of such bezoars form within the first postoperative year, but symptoms may develop several years later.

Bezoars within the gastric remnant are initially small and easily overlooked. Gradual enlargement leads to distention of the lumen, producing the sensation of epigastric fullness, early satiety,

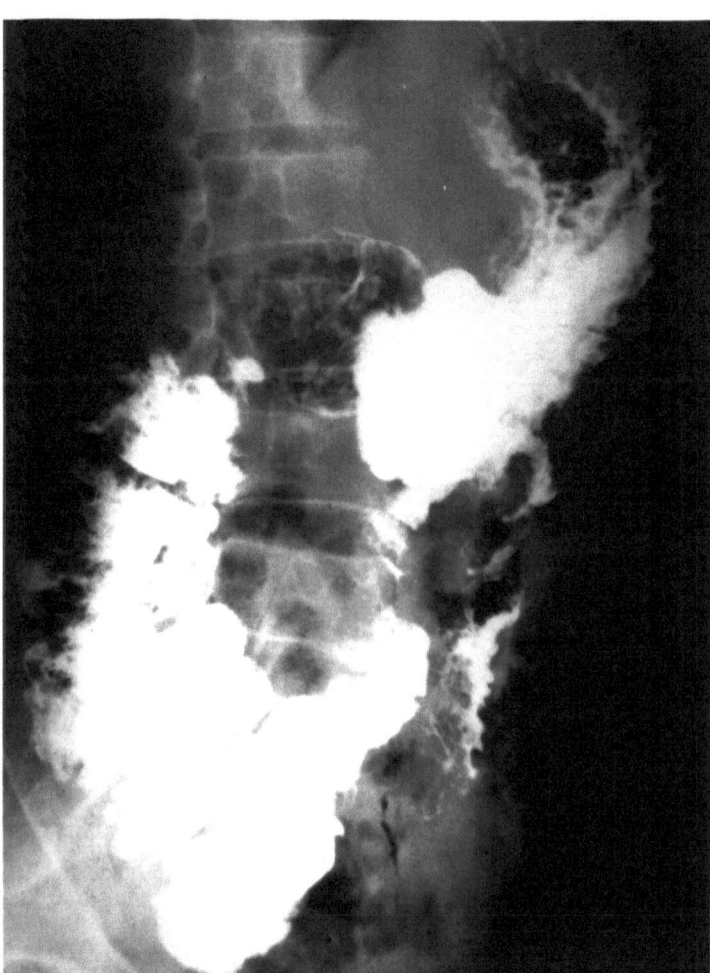

Fig. 6-21. Inadvertent gastroileostomy. The patient developed marked diarrhea within 2 weeks following surgery. Upper gastrointestinal series reveals short-circuiting of most of small bowel secondary to gastroileostomy. (Courtesy of R. Shapiro, MD, Connecticut)

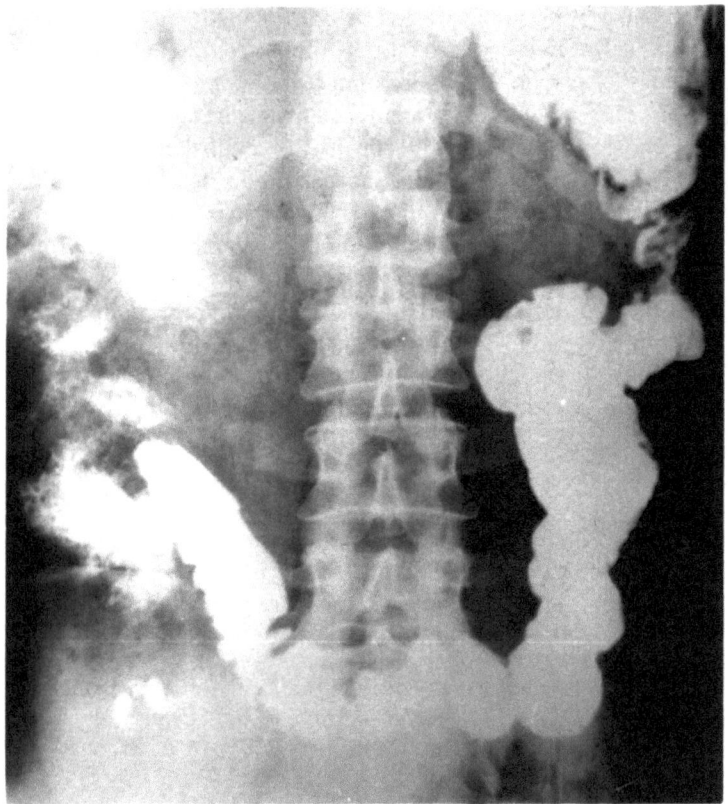

a

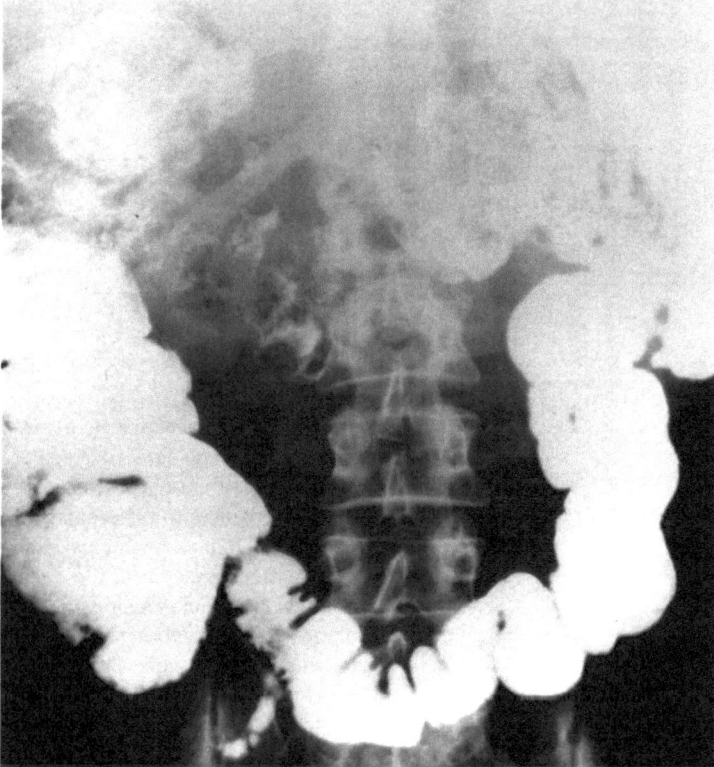

b

Fig. 6-22, a and **b. Inadvertent gastroileostomy.** Diagnosed by means of upper gastrointestinal study, it led to marked malabsorption in the postoperative period. **a** The anastomosis looks normal and only efferent segment is seen. The small bowel is slightly dilated. **b** The true location of the anastomosis is more clearly represented and lies approximately 12 in from ileocecal valve. (Courtesy of H. Bhatt, MD, Connecticut)

and nausea and vomiting. They may also cause pressure erosion of the gastric mucosa and bleeding, or retard gastric emptying because of intermittent occlusion of the stoma (49). The passage of bezoars beyond the anastomosis occurs more commonly after a Billroth II procedure and leads to acute obstruction of the terminal ileum (48,49) (Fig. 6-23).

Gastric bezoars may be visible on plain radiographs of the abdomen as a mottled soft-tissue mass that persists on repeated studies. Upper gastrointestinal series show a large filling defect that often conforms to the gastric outline and traps barium in its spongy matrix (50). In the upright position the mass tends to float and project partly above the level of barium. Differentiation from retained food particles is important although these usually divide and mix with barium when palpated at fluoroscopy. Administra-

tion of water or carbonated beverage and delayed radiographs often provide better visibility of the barium-impregnated bezoar.

The treatment of postgastrectomy phytobezoars usually consists of endoscopic breakage and removal. Successful dissolution has also been reported after oral administration of proteolytic enzymes and repeated gastric lavage (49–51). However, small bowel obstruction by an impacted bezoar requires surgical intervention. Because of the possibility of recurrence the patients must be instructed to avoid ingestion of citrus fruits and foods with considerable fiber content (50).

Postvagotomy Dysphagia

In the early postoperative period after vagotomy patients frequently experience dysphagia. Several mechanisms may explain this problem:

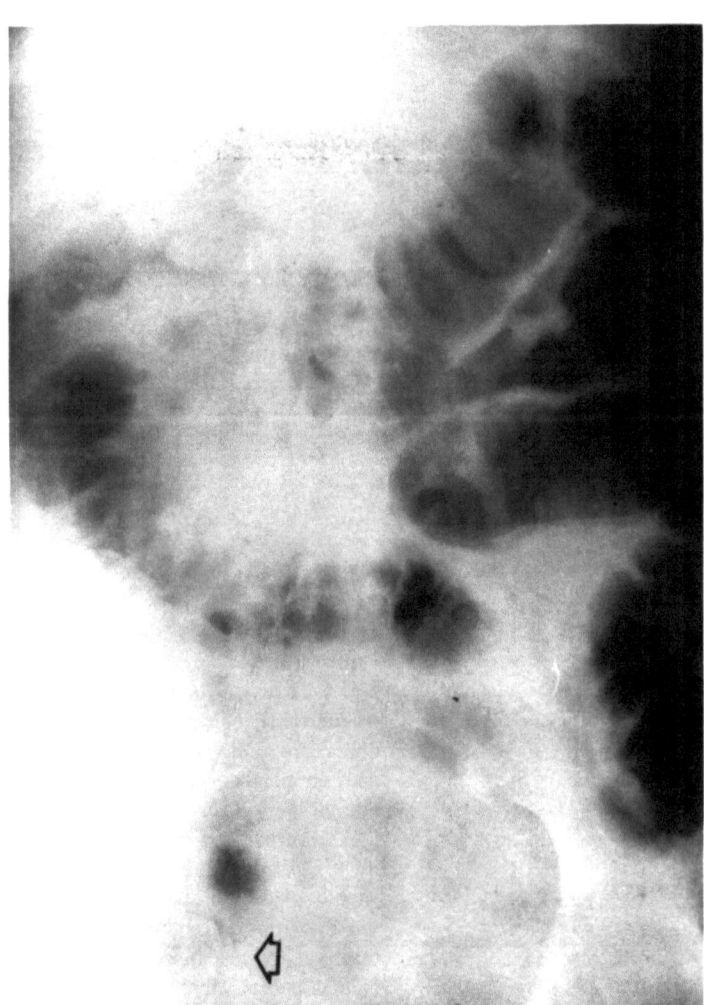

Fig. 6-23. Ileal obstruction by phytobezoar. Linear densities and irregular gas shadows in the right lower quadrant are secondary to a bezoar consisting of orange segments and fibrous matter impacted in the distal small bowel *(arrow)*. This resulted in small-bowel obstruction, which is also evident on the film. The patient was elderly and edentulous and had undergone gastric surgery for benign peptic ulcer disease 14 years earlier. (Courtesy of H. Moscowitz, MD, Connecticut)

vagal denervation of the esophagus, periesophageal edema, and postoperative esophagitis. A review of 1096 patients by Wirthlin and Malt showed a complication rate of 5% (52). Similar results are evident in a more recent study (11).

Study of esophageal motility in such patients demonstrates failure of the esophagogastric sphincter to relax. The radiographic appearance is similar to early changes in achalasia (Fig. 6-24). Generally the symptoms disappear with time and do not require further treatment.

Acute Obstruction of the Afferent Loop

Acute obstruction of the afferent loop is unusual and, if untreated, disastrous. Markowitz found no significant difference in incidence of acute afferent loop obstruction in antecolic and retrocolic anastomosis (53). However, 19 of 21 in his series were noted to be associated with right-to-left anastomosis. Appropriate placement of the anastomosis with closure of the potential retroanastomotic space may prevent this problem.

The incidence of this complication is 0.5%–1%; the mortality is about 50% (54,55). The onset may be during the immediate postoperative period or years after surgery. The syndrome consists of severe upper abdominal pain, nonbilious vomiting, and sometimes a tender, palpable mass in the left upper abdomen. Pancreatitis and jaundice may occur secondary to obstruction of the common bile duct (54). Herniation of the afferent loop through a surgical defect behind the gastroenteric anastomosis is the most common finding at surgery (Fig. 6-25). In clinically suspected cases the nonfilling of the afferent limb seen in upper gastrointestinal series and a palpable left upper quadrant mass would suggest the diagnosis. However, since failure of the afferent loop to fill with contrast material is commonly noted during fluoroscopy, this finding alone is not diagnostic in asymptomatic patients.

Chronic Obstruction of the Afferent Loop

Burhenne described an iatrogenic form of chronic afferent loop obstruction that is incomplete or functional in nature (56). In such cases there is apparent preferential gastric emptying into the afferent loop. These patients usually present with intermittent bilious vomiting,

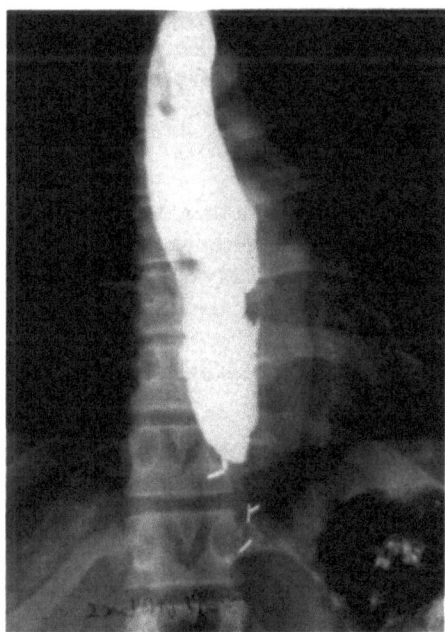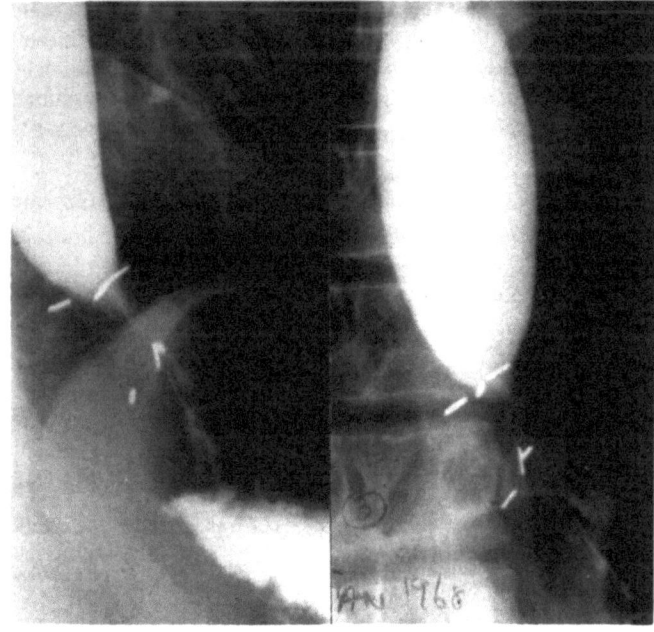

a   b

Fig. 6-24, a and **b. Postvagotomy dysphagia.** Solid food became stuck in the lower chest. **a** X-ray study reveals partial obstruction in the area of the esophagogastric junction. **b** The long smooth nature of this segment is demonstrated on the spot films. Symptoms abated in several months, and the appearance of the lower esophagus returned to normal.

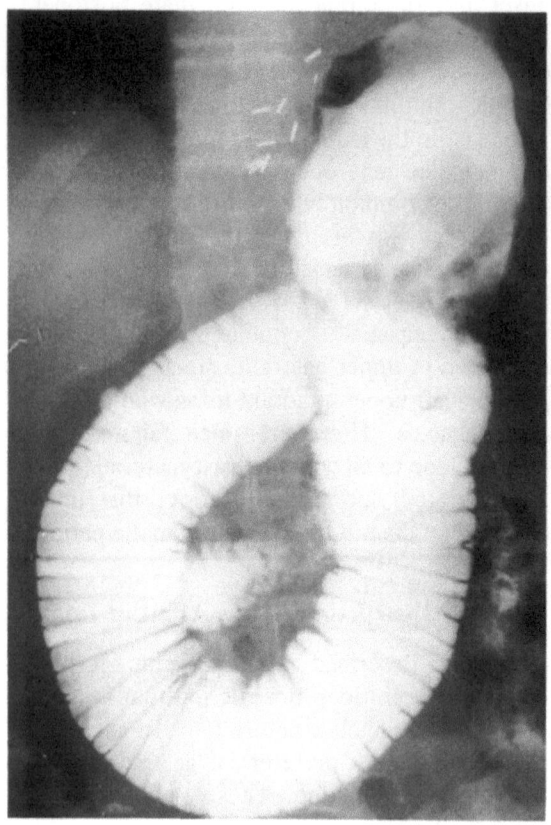 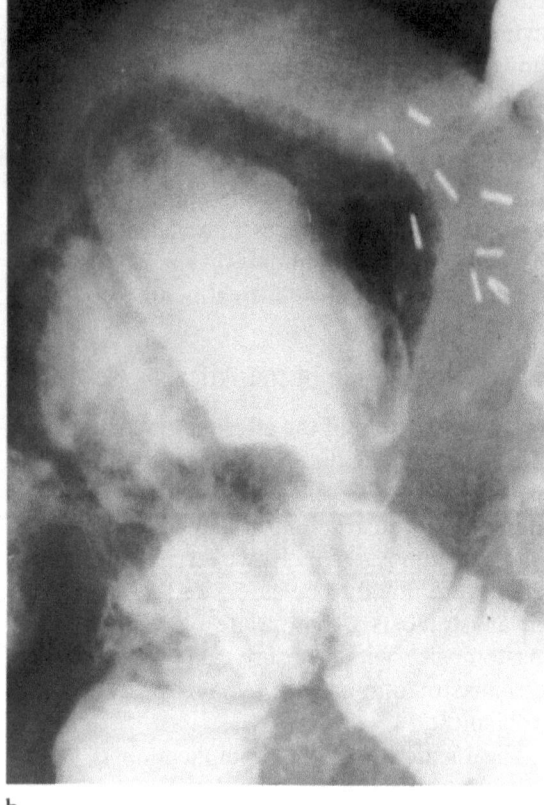

a   b

Fig. 6-25, a and b. Acute obstruction of the afferent loop. Acute abdominal pain was associated with marked distention of the afferent loop and a localized defect at the gastric stoma near the anastomosis. The defect was secondary to incarceration of a loop of bowel in this area. **a** There is massive distention of the afferent loop and no filling of the efferent loop. **b** The knuckle of bowel incarcerated near the anastomosis produces a scalloped defect in the gastric remnant above the anastomosis.

weight loss, anemia, malabsorption, and steatorrhea. The symptoms are believed to result from stasis in the afferent limb with accumulation of biliary and pancreatic secretions.

Radiographic findings include preferential filling of the distended afferent limb, retention of barium as seen on delayed films, and regurgitation of contrast material into the stomach (Figs. 6-26, 6-27). These findings are sometimes more obvious in the upright position (56).

It should be noted that preferential gastric emptying into the afferent limb or bidirectional flow of the contrast material is often noted during radiologic evaluation of asymptomatic patients who have had gastroenterostomy. However, persistent retention of contrast material or significant dilatation of the afferent loop is not normally seen. Furthermore, in patients with the clinical and radiographic diagnosis of chronic or

intermittent obstruction of the afferent loop, findings during surgical exploration may be completely normal. This is probably due to the effect of anesthesia, the fasting, and the recumbent position of the patient at the time of surgery. Nevertheless, revision of the anastomosis generally resolves the problem.

Dysfunction of the Efferent Loop

Efferent loop dysfunction is presumed to be due to localized, temporary disturbance in muscle function resulting from surgical trauma at the site of anastomosis. The onset is usually characterized by a lag of 8–10 days postoperatively. The condition may last from a few days to several weeks and often remits spontaneously. Therefore conservative management is appropriate, and surgical intervention for what appears to be obstruction is not indicated.

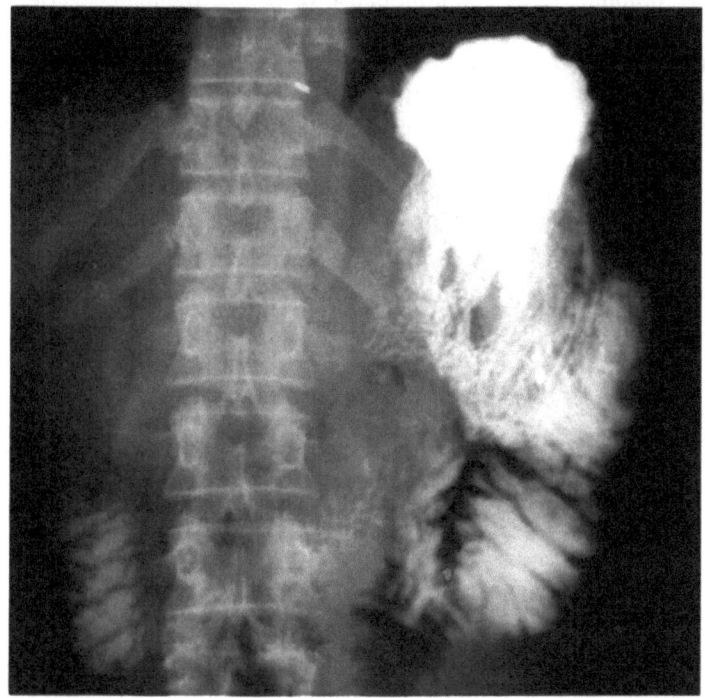

Fig. 6-26. Chronic obstruction of the afferent loop. The distended loop of bowel is the afferent loop, which is anastomosed in a left-to-right fashion, with obstruction secondary to knuckling of the efferent limb just distal to the anastomotic margin.

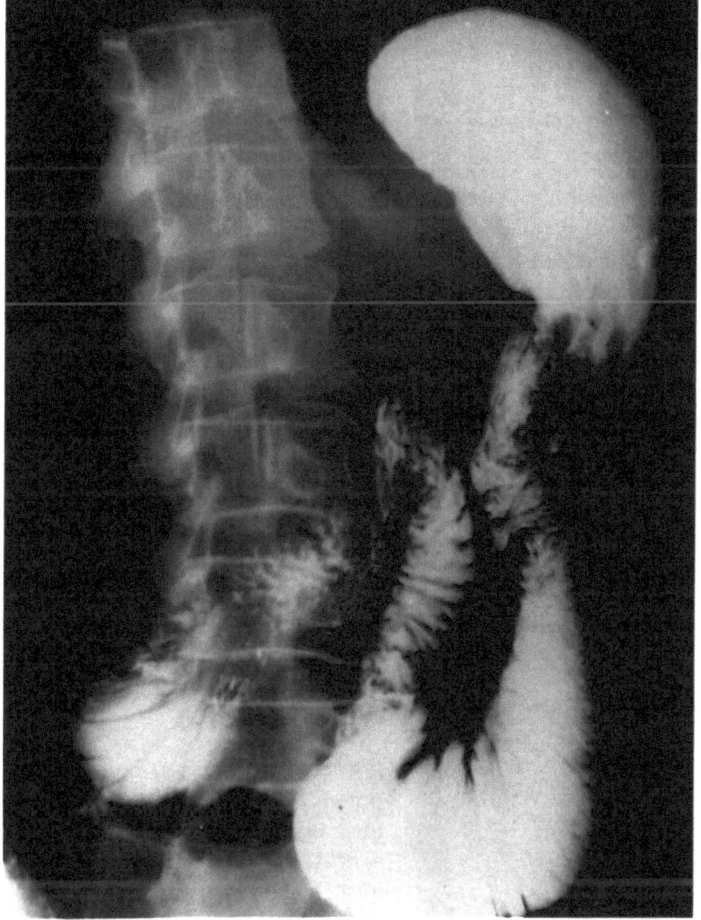

Fig. 6-27. Distended preferentially filled afferent loops due to relative obstruction at origin of efferent loop. The patient had an antecolic anastomosis and a relatively long and dependent afferent loop with essentially no filling of efferent loop. Intermittent obstructive symptoms with weight loss and vomiting were present.

The characteristic clinical feature is bilious vomiting (57,58). Radiographs reveal poor filling of the efferent loop 2–10 cm beyond the site of anastomosis. The mucosal pattern remains normal, but emptying is markedly delayed (Fig. 6-28).

Leakage

Postoperative leaks from the duodenal stump and gastroenteric anastomosis remain the single most common cause of death. Incidence varies from 1% to 5% with 40%–50% mortality (59–61). Leakage occurs more frequently at the stump closure site than at the gastroenteric anastomosis. This complication is thought to be secondary to devascularization around the duodenal stump or anastomotic site.

Duodenal stump leakage occurs within the first 2.5 weeks and most frequently during the third and fourth days following surgery. Clinically the patient has sudden onset of fever,

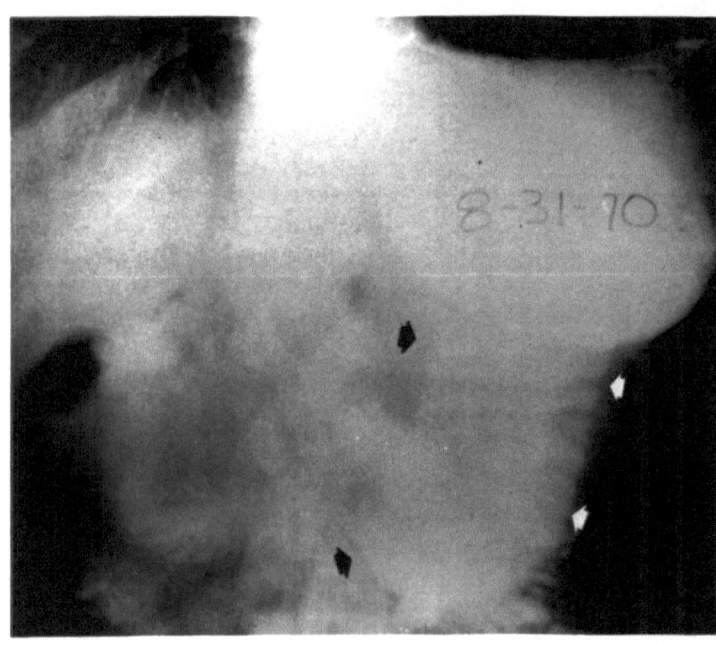

Fig. 6-28. Dysfunction of the efferent loop. There is dilution of contrast medium in the markedly dilated loop (arrows). This apparent obstruction resolved with conservative management.

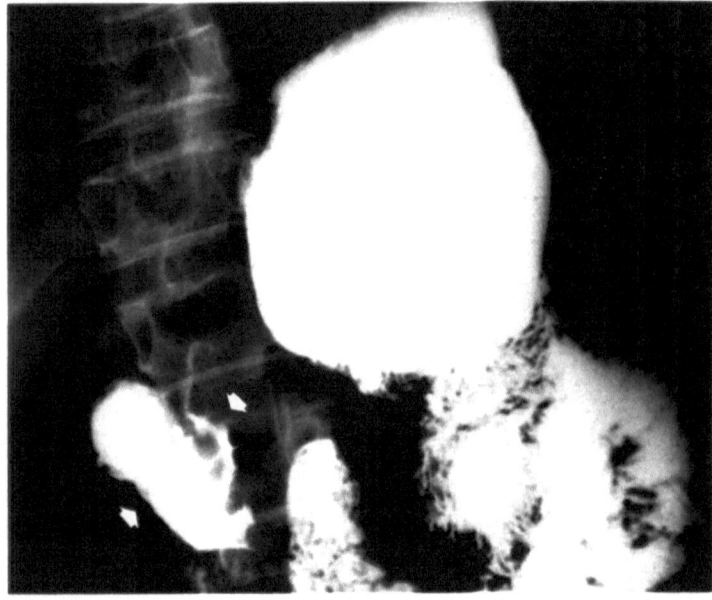

Fig. 6-29. Leakage from duodenal stump. Amorphous collection of contrast material is secondary to duodenal-stump perforation with contrast material pooling in abscess cavity (arrows).

abdominal pain, and tachycardia. Without surgery the mortality is almost 100% (60).

Radiographic findings indicating postoperative leakage include plain-film demonstration of pneumoperitoneum, abscesses, peritonitis, and obstruction. Upper gastrointestinal series using a water-soluble contrast medium can disclose the precise location of extravasation (Fig. 6-29). An anastomotic leak (Figs. 6-30, 6-31) may be generalized or localized to the left upper quadrant. With stump leakage, fixed radiolucent areas in the subhepatic space and deformity in the lesser curvature of the stomach may be seen (28). Elevation and restricted motion of the diaphragm and associated pleural effusion would further indicate the possibility of abscess complicating the anastomotic leakage (Fig. 6-32).

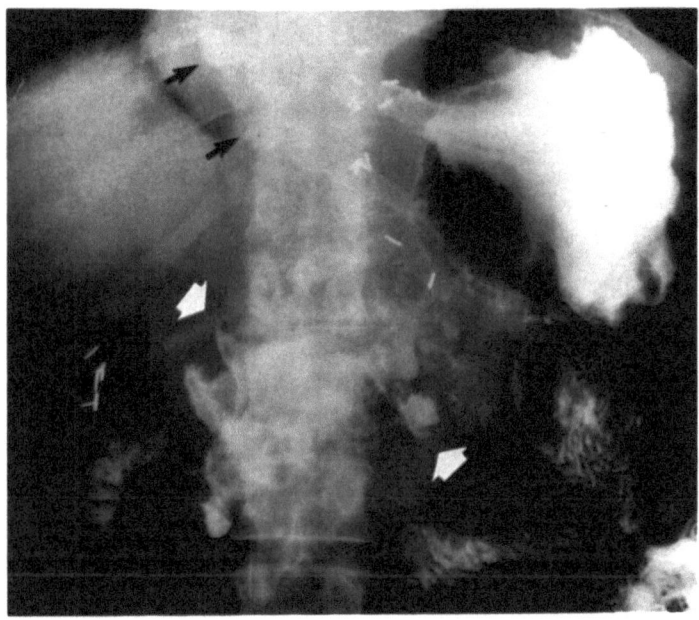

a

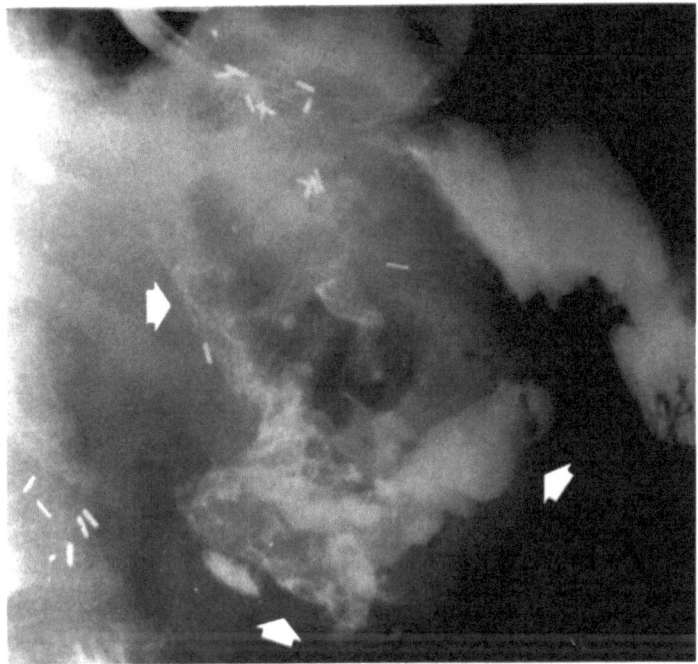

b

Fig. 6-30, a and b. Anastomotic leakage. Massive central collection of contrast agent and air is in large abscess related to leakage at gastroenteric suture line *(white arrows).* The defect in the area of gastric fundus is related to subdiaphragmatic abscess extending into the mediastinum *(black arrows).*

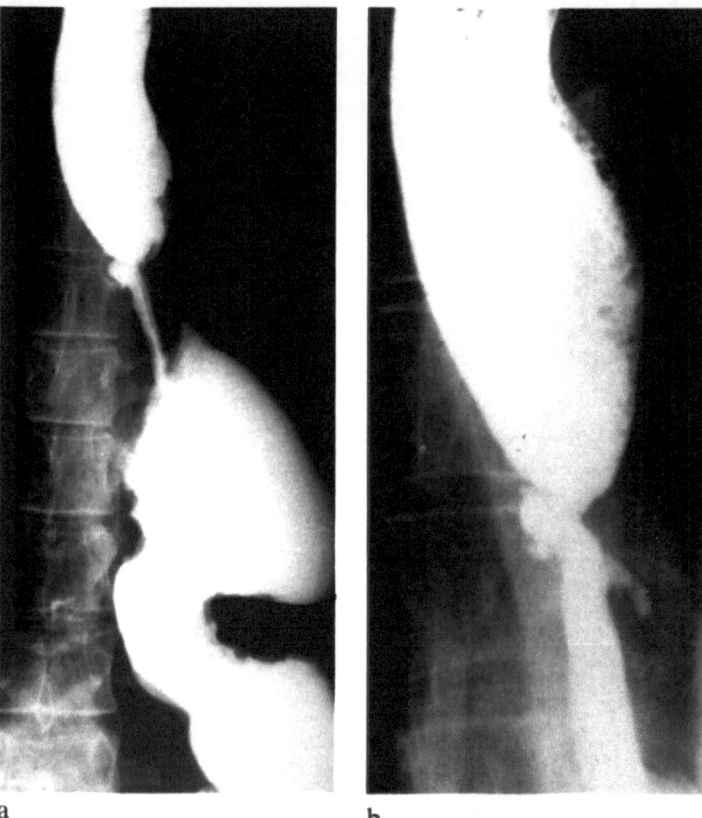

a

b

Fig. 6-31, a and b. Anastomotic leak following esophagogastrostomy for carcinoma of cardia. There is leakage at the site of anastomosis with partial obstruction of the proximal esophagus.

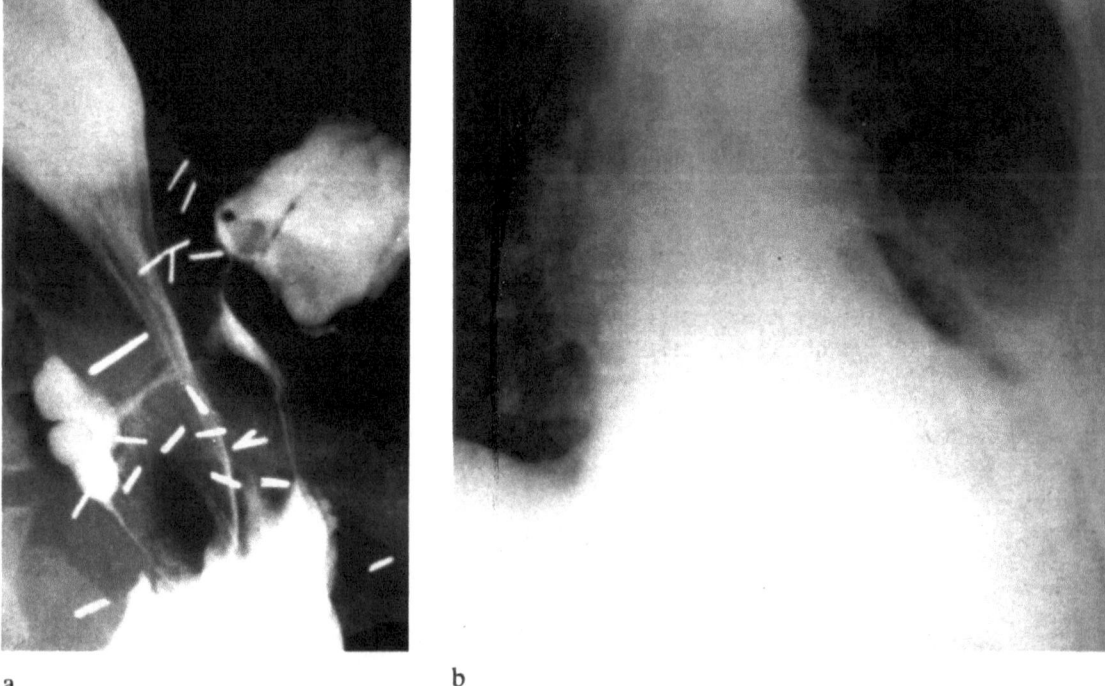

a   b

Fig. 6-32, a and b. Anastomotic leakage complicated by abscess. a Contrast material is extravasated after fundoplication, leading to mediastinal abscess. **b** Left pleural effusion is associated. (Courtesy of M. Koehane, MD, New Haven, Connecticut)

Obstruction

Failure of gastric emptying after recent gastric surgery is most commonly due to stomal edema (28,62). Other causes may be more iatrogenic: gastric atony as a result of vagal denervation, minor suture leak resulting in an abscess with surrounding edema, postischemic fibrosis of the duodenum, internal herniation (Fig. 6-33), and retrograde jejunogastric intussusception (63,64). Less frequent causes are volvulus about the gastrojejunostomy, perhaps due to excessive mobilization, and defective suturing of the transverse mesocolon, allowing slippage of both limbs of the anastomosis superiorly where they become entrapped within the opening of the transverse mesocolon.

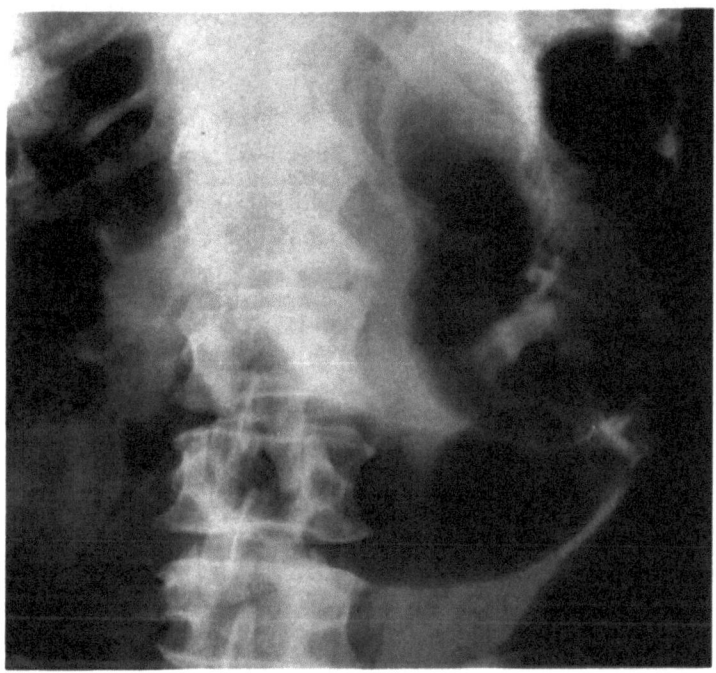

a

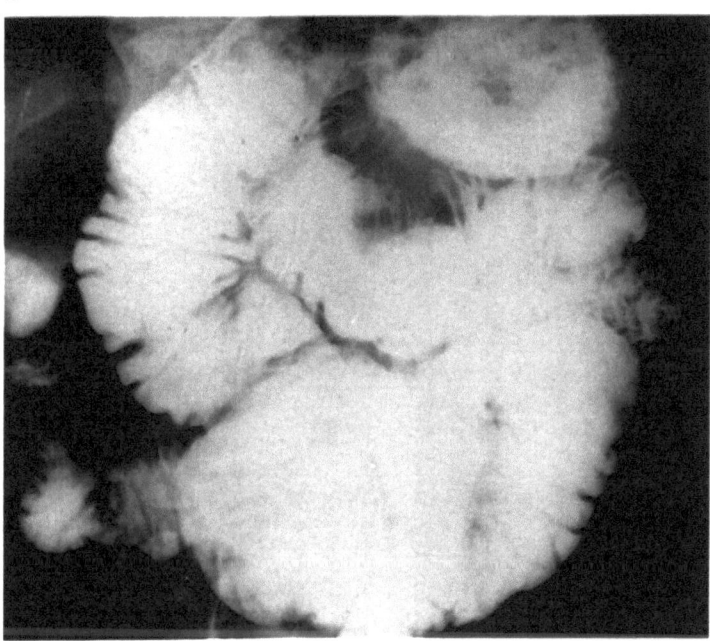

b

Fig. 6-33, a and b. Failure of gastric emptying due to internal herniation. a After Billroth II procedure a plain film demonstrates multiple dilated loops of small bowel in left upper abdomen. b Barium contrast study reveals these loops to be contained in a sac-like enclosure in the upper abdomen. At surgery these loops were entrapped in a large retroanastomotic hernia.

188   M. Burrell and B. S. Jay

Antral Stricture After Gastroenterostomy

The gastric antrum may become atrophic and
contracted long after the performance of gastroenterostomy. The radiologic appearance may
resemble infiltrating carcinoma, and knowledge
of this may prevent unnecessary surgery (65).

Hajdu et al. reviewed 132 patients with gastroenterostomy and found 13 (10%) patients with
hypertrophy of the pylorus and antrum (66). The
radiographic diagnosis rests on demonstration of
the relatively smooth, concentric narrowing of
the pyloric antrum (Fig. 6-34). The incidence in
this group of patients was higher than in a ran-
dom group of upper gastrointestinal studies (21
out of 6456 patients or 0.32%).

Another type of stricture occurs in the proximal efferent loop, presumably secondary to scarring after marginal ulceration.

Fistula

Stomal ulcers, if unrecognized or inadequately
treated, may pursue an aggressive course, having a well-known tendency to perforate into the
peritoneal cavity or transverse colon and resulting in gastrojejunocolic fistula (Fig. 6-35). The
most common site for fistulization is at the
suture line of anastomosis (gastroenteric) or in
the Hofmeister suture line of the gastric remnant. Diarrhea and weight loss are present in
80% of the cases. Fecal vomiting and fecal
breath occur in less than 30% of cases. It may
occur immediately or up to 25 years after surgery
(67). The malabsorption that may occur with
such fistulas is due to bacterial overgrowth of
regurgitated fecal material into the small bowel.
The result is severe diarrhea (68).

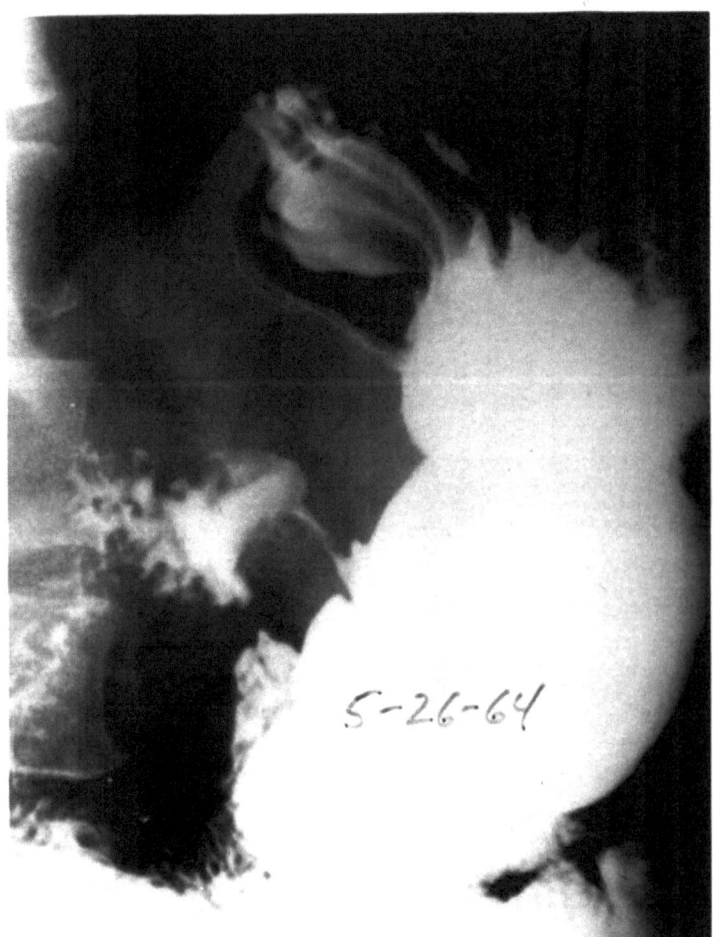

**Fig. 6-34. Benign hairline stricture of
antrum after gastroenterostomy.**
This stricture eventually became
completely fibrotic, and emptying
occurred only via gastroenterostomy.

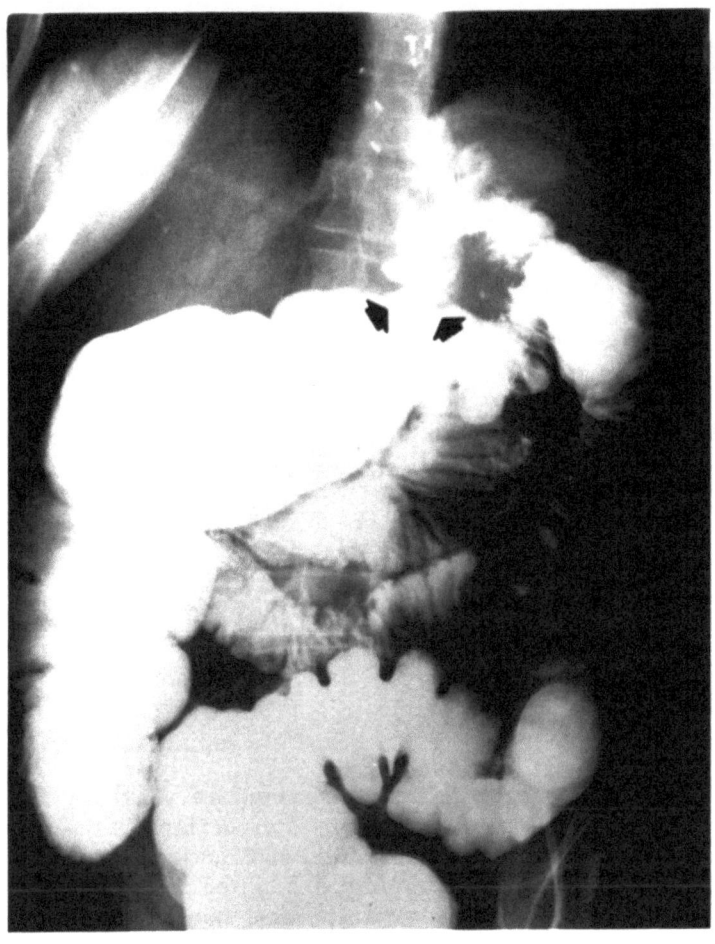

Fig. 6-35. Gastrojejunocolic fistula. Barium enema study reveals reflux of contrast material into the stomach and afferent loop due to gastrojejunocolic fistula complicating Billroth II procedure *(arrows)*.

Radiographically the best way to demonstrate a gastrocolic or gastrojejunocolic fistula is with barium enema (Fig. 6-35). In one study, barium enema examinations provided the diagnosis in 100% of cases and upper gastrointestinal studies in only 11% of cases (69). Another type of fistula, enterocutaneous, is secondary to leakage from the duodenal stump, gastroenteric anastomosis, or Hofmeister suture line.

Marginal Ulcer (Anastomotic Ulcer, Stomal Ulcer)

The two most common causes of marginal ulcers are inadequate vagotomy and simple gastroenterostomy without vagotomy. This latter procedure diverts secretions from the stomach but does not disrupt the gastrin-producing mechanism. Other potential factors are inadequate gastric resection, increased gastrin secretion from a retained distal antrum in the duodenal stump, or unrecognized Zollinger-Ellison syndrome (70).

It is estimated that a marginal ulcer will subsequently develop in 3%–10% of patients operated on for duodenal ulcer. It is much more common in men than women, with a ratio of 6:1. Of the current operative procedures, vagotomy with partial gastric resection consistently has the lowest reported ulcer recurrence rate:0–2% (71).

The radiographic appearance of marginal ulcers is sometimes very difficult to appreciate. Many authors report a positive diagnostic rate of 50% for these ulcers and a suspicion rate of approximately 80%. The site of ulceration is generally within the first 2 cm of the anastomosis on the jejunal side (Fig. 6-36). Secondary findings to assist in making the diagnosis consist of rigidity and lack of peristalsis in the proximal jejunum and spasm of the transverse colon adjacent to the anastomosis (72). As mentioned earlier, approximately 17% of stomal ulcers will lead to formation of gastrojejunocolic fistula if untreated (18).

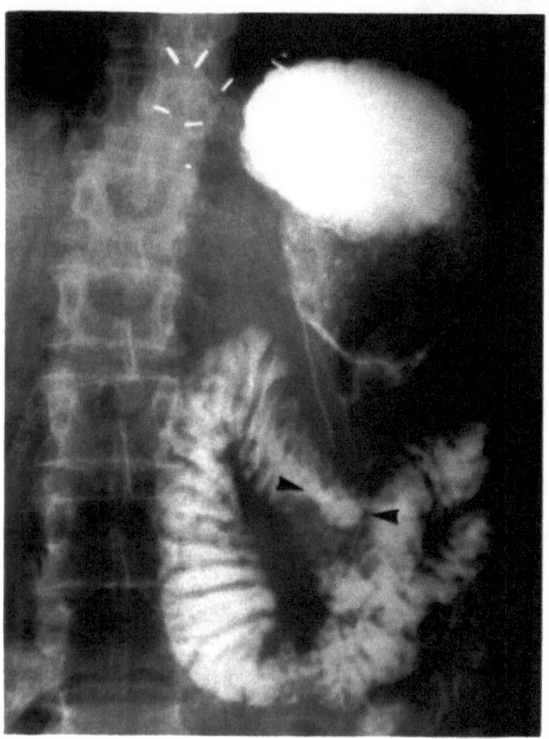
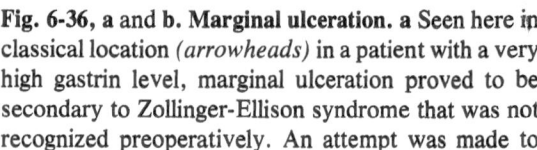
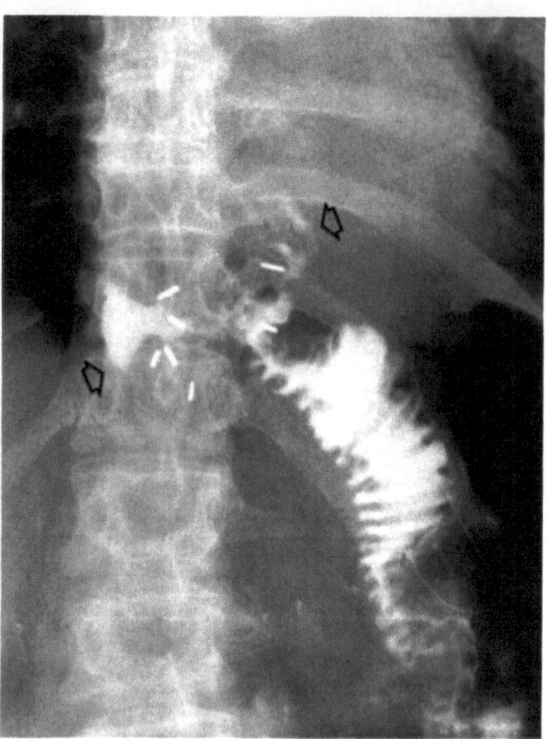

Fig. 6-36, a and b. Marginal ulceration. a Seen here in classical location *(arrowheads)* in a patient with a very high gastrin level, marginal ulceration proved to be secondary to Zollinger-Ellison syndrome that was not recognized preoperatively. An attempt was made to manage the patient with cimetidine, and although the ulcer decreased in size at first the lack of any further resolution necessitated complete gastrectomy. b The additional complication of anastomotic leak and mediastinal abscess was also noted subsequently *(arrows)*.

Zollinger-Ellison Syndrome

The presence of a gastrin-secreting tumor, although rare, is an important cause of recurrent ulcers. This can be ruled out with gastric acid secretory tests and determination of gastrin levels. The radiographic picture consists of evidence of hypersecretion on the upper gastrointestinal series associated with the occurrence of multiple ulcers in unusual locations (71,73,74). If this diagnosis is not recognized the usual partial gastrectomy for ulcer disease will invariably lead to problems, i.e., recurrent ulceration (Fig. 6-36).

Once the diagnosis is confirmed the surgery of choice is total gastrectomy with reconstitution of a gastric pouch from the remaining small bowel (Hunt-Lawrence pouch).

Retained Gastric Antrum

Although a rare occurrence, retained gastric antrum produces symptoms similar to those found in Zollinger-Ellison syndrome. The normal inhibitory factors of acid and distention cannot act upon the antrum, which is no longer in continuity. Thus gastrin production proceeds continuously, acting on the fundus and parietal cells to cause hypersecretion, hyperacidity, and predisposition to ulcer (75).

Radiographic demonstration is extremely difficult. The afferent loop must be seen, as well as the duodenum and duodenal stump. A search is then made for residual antrum and pylorus (76,-77)(Fig. 6-37).

Technetium Tc 99m may be helpful in locating residual antral tissue (78). It is well known that gastric mucosa actively secretes pertechnetate ion (79) and that this secretion is so efficient that sodium pertechnetate Tc 99m scintigraphy has been utilized in the diagnosis of Barrett's esophagus and Meckel's diverticulum with ectopic gastric mucosa. It has been suggested that his technique can be utilized to differentiate retained

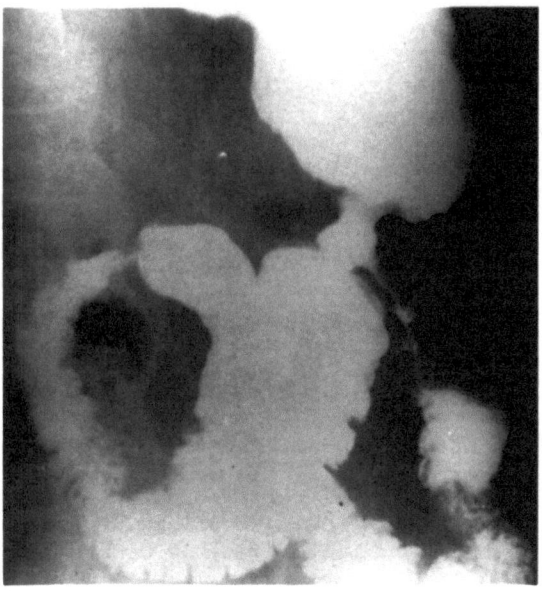

a

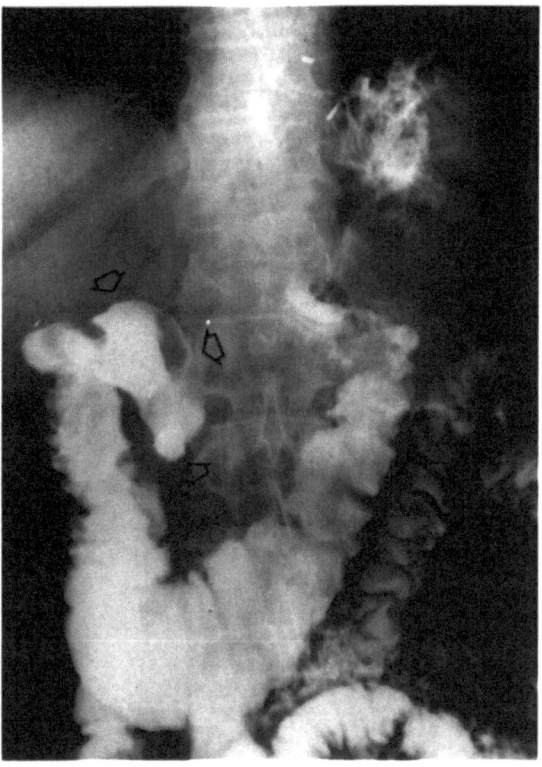

b

Fig. 6-37, a and **b. Marginal ulceration. a** The film demonstrates ulceration associated with marked edema and narrowing of the efferent loop adjacent to the anastomosis. These changes are secondary to excessive gastrin secretion from retained antral tissue that is not in continuity and thus cannot be inhibited by acid or distention. **b** Further filling of afferent loop allows reflux into duodenal stump and through pylorus, demonstrating antral folds *(arrows)*. (Courtesy of A. Clemett, MD, New York, New York)

antrum from Zollinger-Ellison syndrome (80,81). Its visualization is time related, and its accuracy is limited by varying blood concentrations and time of maximum concentration of the isotope within the retained antral tissue.

Prolapse

Mucosal prolapse into the stoma may be iatrogenic in the sense that the predisposition for this problem is thought by some to be related to the type of surgical closure (82). It may be related to mucosal redundancy about a Hofmeister closure (83). It also has been described with the Polya procedure.

Patients with this condition may present with bleeding. However, it is difficult to relate the radiologic picture to the clinical problem.

Roentgenograms are characteristic; a smooth, sharply demarcated filling defect, resulting from the prolapsed mucosa, is seen in the postanasto-

motic small bowel (82,83). The size of the prolapse varies; it may originate symmetrically from either anterior or posterior margin of the stoma, producing the appearance of two separate masses (Fig. 6-38).

Treatment is generally symptomatic since prolapse is usually self-reducing. However, it must be differentiated from more serious conditions such as actual intussusception or recurrent tumor in the juxtastomal segment, both of which may require surgery.

Dumping Syndrome

The dumping syndrome is due to disruption or bypass of the pyloric sphincter mechanism and can occur after any type of gastric surgery. The stomal size may also be directly related to the development of the dumping syndrome; however, this has not been definitely proven to be a major cause. The symptoms are both vasomotor (flushing, sweating, tachycardia) and intestinal (cramps, diarrhea) (84). Because of the great fluctuation in blood glucose levels, some patients may faint or actually have hypoglycemic seizures. Generally the symptoms start 15–30 min after eating and may last for an hour. Fortu-

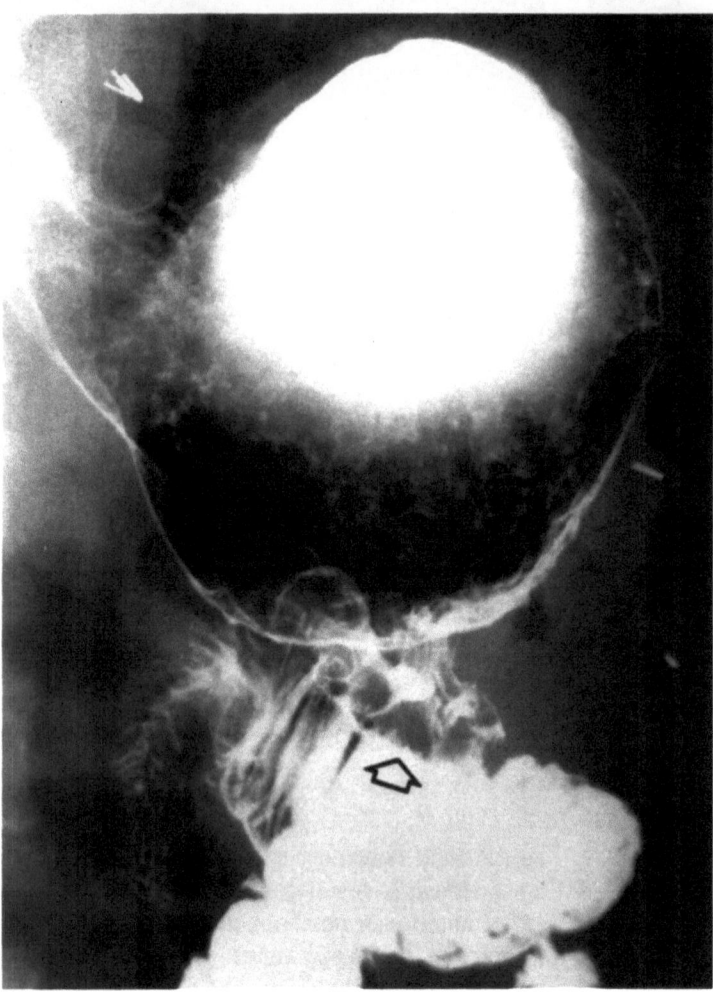

Fig. 6-38. Mucosal prolapse. The sharply marginated defects at the anastomotic site in this patient with Billroth II procedure are characteristic of gastrojejunal mucosal prolapse *(arrows)*.

nately the symptoms tend to decrease in severity with the passage of time. Statistics as to the frequency of occurrence of this syndrome vary. However, in a study of 604 patients by Hardy, 29 (4.8%) developed the dumping syndrome (85).

Radiographic correlation is not very accurate when compared with the physiologic problems associated with this syndrome. An upper gastrointestinal study may reveal extremely rapid transit, with simultaneous visualization of the stomach and distal colon after a barium meal (Fig. 6-39).

Treatment is generally symptomatic and aimed at control of the diet. In severe cases, surgical intervention is needed (86).

Miscellaneous

Carcinoma of the gastric stump is very rare, accounting for approximately 1% of all forms of gastric carcinoma. There is a definite increase in the frequency of this entity in postgastrectomy patients in comparison with the general population (87). The radiographic picture reveals an irregular polypoid mass at the anastomotic margin or within the stomach (88). There may also be diffuse shrinkage of the stomach and possibly findings of gastric outlet obstruction (89).

Esophagitis, gastritis, and jejunitis occur postoperatively. Esophagitis may occur secondary to nasogastric intubation or bile reflux, or it may occur with esophageal vestibular spasm after vagotomy (90–93). Strictures may further complicate prolonged retention of a nasogastric tube and its associated reflux. Reflux gastritis is recognized as another complication after surgery to remove, alter, or bypass the pyloric sphincter mechanism (93). Another uncommon complication of gastroduodenal surgery is development of acute pancreatitis during the immediate postoperative period, probably as a result of surgical trauma (Fig. 6-40).

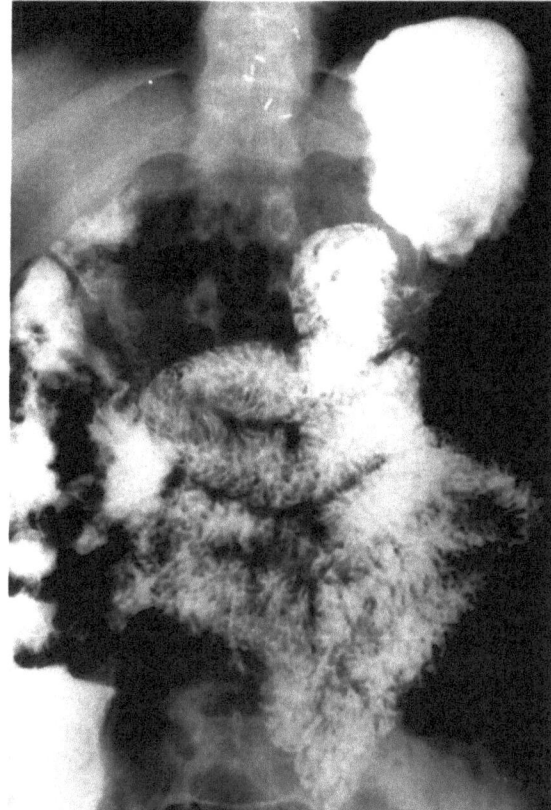

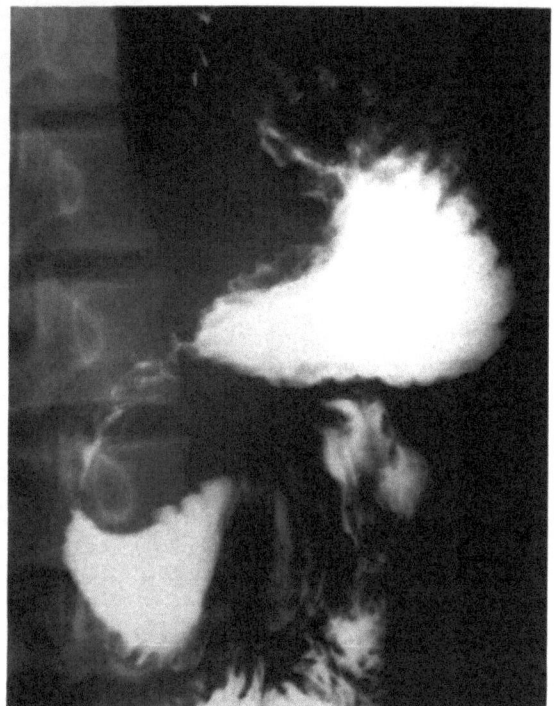

a

b

Fig. 6-39. Dumping syndrome. Contrast material is already in the colon on this film taken 15 min after a barium meal in a patient with clinical symptoms of dumping. In general, we have not found good correlation between the radiographic transit time of contrast material and clinical symptoms.

Fig. 6-40, a and b. Acute pancreatitis complicating gastroduodenal surgery. a Eight days after vagotomy and Billroth I procedure abnormalities are seen along the lesser curvature and in the duodenal loop. b Air-contrast view of the duodenum clearly shows the edematous folds and extrinsic pressure caused by pancreatitis.

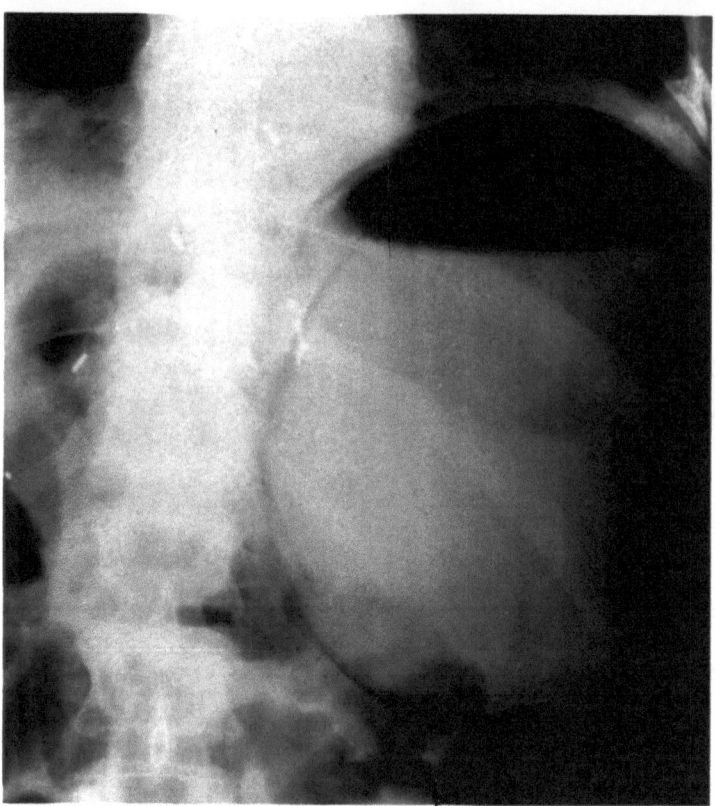

Fig. 6-41. Pneumatosis of wall of stomach. Linear gas collection is seen in the wall of the stomach of a patient who had received respiratory assistance after gastric surgery. The patient was managed conservatively, and pneumatosis resolved without consequence.

Unusual cases of stomach rupture have been reported in association with oxygen therapy by nasal catheter (94). Furthermore, pneumatosis of the wall of the stomach can occur following respiratory therapy, intermittent positive pressure breathing therapy, and nasal administration of oxygen (Fig. 6-41).

References

1. Macleod JB: The surgery of peptic ulcer. Scott Med J 16:141–145, 1971
2. Tanner NC: The surgical treatment of peptic ulcer. Br J Surg 51:5–23, 1964
3. Hoerr SO: A review and evaluation of operative procedures used for chronic duodenal ulcer. Surg Clin North Am 56:1289–1296, 1976
4. Hardy JD: Problems associated with gastric surgery—A review of 604 consecutive patients with annotation. Am J Surg 108: 699–716, 1964
5. Dodsworth JM, Fischer JE; Surgical therapy of chronic peptic ulcer—Preoperative assessment, choice of operations and consequences. Surg Clin North Am 54:529–547, 1974
6. Herrington JL, Sawyers JL, Scott HW: A 25-year experience with vagotomy—antrectomy. Arch Surg 106:469–474, 1973
7. Johnston D: A therapeutic index (scoring system) for the evaluation of operations for peptic ulcer. Gastroenterology 70:433–438, 1976
8. Johnston D: Operative mortality and postoperative morbidity of highly selective vagotomy. Br J Surg 62:160–161, 1975
9. Dozois R, Kelly KA: Gastric secretion and motility in duodenal ulcer: Effect of current vagotomies. Surg Clin North Am 56:1267–1296, 1976
10. Johnston D, Humphrey CS, Walker BE, et al: Vagotomy without diarrhea. Br Med J 3:788–790, 1972
11. Baron JH, Spencer J: Facts and heresies about vagotomy. Surg Clin North Am 56:1297–1312, 1976
12. Johnston D, Goligher JC: Selective, highly selective, or truncal vagotomy in 1976—A clinical appraisal. Surg Clin North Am 56:1313–1334, 1976
13. DeMeester TR, Johnson LF, Kent AH: Evaluation of current operations for prevention of gastroesophageal reflux. Ann Surg 180:511–525, 1974
14. Maingot R: Abdominal Operations, 6th ed, vol 1, New York: Appleton-Century-Crofts 1974
15. Burhenne HJ: Roentgen anatomy and terminology of gastric surgery. Am J Roentgenol 91:731–743, 1964
16. Burhenne HJ: Postoperative defects of the stomach. Semin Roentgenol 6:182–192, 1971
17. Burrell M, Curtis AM: Sequelae of stomach surgery. CRC Crit Rev Diagn Imaging 10:17–97, 1977
18. Zatzkin HR, Riera A: Upper gastrointestinal examination after gastric surgery. Radiology 55:193–206, 1950
19. Gold RP, Seaman WB: The primary double-con-

trast examination of the postoperative stomach. Radiology 124:297–305, 1977

20. Nissen R, Rossetti M: Surgery of hiatal and other diaphragmatic hernias. J Int Coll Surg 43:663–674, 1965

21. Feigin DS, James AE Jr, Stitik FP, et al: The radiological appearance of hiatal hernia repairs. Radiology 110:71–77, 1974

22. Skucas J, Mangla JC, Adams JT, Cutcliff W: An evaluation of the Nissen fundoplication. Radiology 118:539–543, 1976

23. Fisher MS: The Hofmeister defect—A normal change in the postoperative stomach. Am J Roentgenol 84:1082–1086, 1960

24. Burhenne HJ: The postoperative stomach. In Margolis AR, Burhenne HJ (eds): Alimentary Tract Roentgenology, vol 1. St. Louis: Mosby 1973, pp 740–783

25. Bloch C, Wolf BS: The gastroduodenal channel after pyloroplasty and vagotomy: A cineradiographic study. Radiology 84:43–51, 1965

26. Eklof O, Ohlsson S: Postoperative plication deformity with foreign-body granuloma simulating tumor of the stomach. Report of 3 cases. Acta Chir Scand 123:125–130, 1962

27. Sasson L: Tumor-simulating deformities after subtotal gastrectomy. JAMA 174:280–283, 1960

28. Ochsner SF, Watson JD: Radiologic evaluation of early postoperative abdominal complaints. South Med J 58:1439–1446, 1965

29. Kraft RO, Fry WJ, DeWeese MS: Postvagotomy gastric atony. Arch Surg 88:865–874, 1964

30. Rimer DG: Gastric retention without mechanical obstruction: A review. Arch Intern Med 117:287–299, 1966

31. Bryant LR, Woit JF, Kloecker RJ: A study of the factors affecting the incidence and duration of postoperative pneumoperitoneum. Surg Gynecol Obstet 117:145–150, 1963

32. Heslin DJ, Malt RA: Progressive postoperative pneumoperitoneum: Air entering through drain sites. Am J Roentgenol 92:1166–1168, 1964

33. Engel S: Gastrostomy. Surg Clin North Am 49:1289–1295, 1969

34. Connar RG, Sealy WC: Gastrostomy and its complications. Ann Surg 143:245–250, 1956

35. Goodman LR, Wittenberg J, Messer R: Duodenal obstruction—An unusual complication of a gastrostomy feeding catheter. Br J Radiol 44:883–885, 1971

36. Haws EB, Sieber WK, Kiesewetter WB: Complications of tube gastrostomy in infants and children. Ann Surg 164:284–290, 1966

37. Bryk D: Postgastrostomy deformity of the stomach. Gastrointest Radiol 2:259–261, 1977

38. Manfredi D, Campioni N, LaFerla G, et al: Tube prosthesis in the palliative treatment of cancer of the esophagus and cardia. Ann Ital Chir 48:215–225, 1976

39. Anscombe AR, Pearson K, Taylor TV: A simple method for the introduction of an oesophageal tube in advanced carcinoma of the esophagus. Br J Surg 63:947–948, 1976

40. Atkinson M, Ferguson R: Fibroptic endoscopic palliative intubation of inoperable oesophagogastric neoplasms. Br Med J 1:266–267, 1977

41. Mihas AA, Han S: Gastric diverticula following subtotal gastrectomy. Gastrointest Radiol 2:263–265, 1977

42. Brown CH, Disconnectte RP, Albee RD: Diverticula of the stomach. Gastroenterology 12:10–23, 1949

43. Goldstein R, Butterfield W: Modified Nissen fundoplication and the "gas-bloat" syndrome as measured by the inability to vomit—An experimental study. Am J Surg 126:89–92, 1973

44. Woodward ER, Thomas HF, McAlhany JC: Comparison of crural repair and Nissen fundoplication in the treatment of esophageal hiatus hernia with peptic esophagitis. Ann Surg 173:782–792, 1971

45. Polk HC Jr, Zeppa R: Hiatal hernia and esophagitis: A survey of indications for operation and technic and results of fundoplication. Ann Surg 173:775–781, 1971

46. Bushkin FL, Neustein CL, Parker TH, et al: Nissen fundoplication for reflux peptic esophagitis. Ann Surg 185: 672–677, 1977

47. Nicholson DA, Nohl-Oser HC: Hiatus hernia: A comparison between two methods of fundoplication by evaluation of the long-term results. J Thorac Cardiovasc Surg 72:938–943, 1976

48. Cain GD, Moore P Jr, Patterson M: Bezoars—A complication of the postgastrectomy state. Am J Dig Dis 13:801–809, 1968

49. Rogers LF, Davis EK, Harle TS: Phytobezoar-formation and food boli following gastric surgery. Am J Roentgenol 119:280–290, 1973

50. Goldstein HM, Cohen LE, Hagen RO, et al: Gastric bezoars: A frequent complication in the postoperative ulcer patient. Radiology 107:341–344, 1973

51. Pollard H, Block G: Rapid dissolution of phytobezoar by cellulase enzyme. Am J Surg 116:933–936, 1968

52. Wirthlin LS, Malt RA: Accidents of vagotomy. Surg Gynecol Obstet 135:913–916, 1972

53. Markowitz AM: Internal hernia after gastrojejunostomy. Surgery 49:185–194, 1961

54. Buckberg GD: Acute obstruction of the afferent loop after gastrectomy. Am J Surg 113:682–687, 1967

55. Quinn WF, Gifford JH: The syndrome of proximal jejunal loop obstruction following anterior gastric resection. Calif Med 72:18–25, 1950

56. Burhenne HJ: The iatrogenic afferent-loop syndrome. Radiology 91:942–947, 1968

57. Golden R: Functional obstruction of efferent loop of jejunum following partial gastrectomy. JAMA 148:721–724, 1952

58. Bodon GR, Ramanath HK: The gastrojejunostomy efferent loop syndrome. Surg Gynec Obstet 134:777–780, 1972

59. Petterson S, Wallensten S: Leakage at suture lines after partial gastrectomy for peptic ulcer. Acta Chir Scand 135:229–234, 1969

60. Rudko M, Price WE: Duodenal stump perforation. J Okla State Med Assoc 58:337–340, 1965
61. Howlett SA: Perforation of duodenal stump ten years after partial gastrectomy. South Med J 68:639–640, 1975
62. Samuel E, Duncan JG, Philip T, et al: Radiology of the postoperative abdomen. Clin Radiol 14:133–142, 1963
63. Jordan GL Jr, Walker LL: Severe problems with gastric emptying after gastric surgery. Ann Surg 177:660–668, 1973
64. Donovan I, Alexander-Williams J: Postoperative gastric retention and delayed gastric emptying. Surg Clin North Am 56:1413–1419, 1976
65. Carter TL, Martel W: Contraction of the gastric antrum following a long-term gastrojejunostomy—Report of 2 cases. Radiology 91:514–516, 1968
66. Hajdu N, Hyde I, Riddell V: Antro-pyloric hypertrophy in patients with long-standing gastroenterostomies—A study of 13 cases. Br J Radiol 41:49–55, 1968
67. Marshal SF, Knud-Hansen J: Gastrojejunocolic and gastrocolic fistulas. Ann Surg 145:770–782, 1957
68. Schwartz SI, Lillehei RC, Shires GT, et al: Principles of Surgery, 2nd ed. New York: McGraw-Hill 1969
69. Thoeny RH, Hodgson JR, Scudamore HH: The roentgenologic diagnosis of gastrocolic and gastrojejunocolic fistulas. Am J Roentgenol 83:876–881, 1960
70. Wychulis AR, Priestley JT, Foulk WT: A study of 360 patients with gastrojejunal ulceration. Surg Gynecol Obstet 122:89–99, 1966
71. Passaro E Jr, Gordon HE. Stabile BE: Marginal ulcer: A guide to management. Surg Clin North Am 56:1435–1444, 1976
72. Schatzki R: The significance of rigidity of the jejunum in the diagnosis of postoperative jejunal ulcers. Am J Roentgenol 103:330–338, 1968
73. Christoforidis AJ, Nelson SW: Radiological manifestations of ulcerogenic tumors of the pancreas: The Zollinger-Ellison syndrome. JAMA 198:511–516, 1966
74. Isenberg JI, Walsh JH, Grossman MI: Zollinger-Ellison syndrome. Gastroenterology 65:140–165, 1973
75. van Heerden JA, Bernatz PE, Rovelstad RA: The retained gastric antrum—Clinical considerations. Mayo Clin Proc 46:25–30, 1971
76. Burhenne JH: The retained gastric antrum. Preoperative roentgenologic diagnosis of an iatrogenic syndrome. Am J Roentgenol 101:459–466, 1967
77. Beneventano TC, Glotzen P, Messinger NH: Retained gastric antrum. Am J Gastroenterol 59:361–365, 1973
78. Safaie-Shirazi S, Chaudhuri TK, Chauduri TK, et al: Visualization of isolated retained antrum by using technetium 99-m. Surgery 73:278–283, 1973
79. Irvine WJ, Stewart AG, McLoughlin GP: Appraisal of application of technetium 99-m in the assessment of gastric function. Lancet 2:644–653, 1967
80. Dunlap JA Jr, McLane RC, Roper TJ: The retained gastric antrum—A case report. Radiology 117:371–372, 1975
81. Chaudhuri TK, Chaudhuri TK, Shirazi SS, et al: Radioisotope scan—A possible aid in differentiating retained gastric antrum from Zollinger-Ellison syndrome in patients with recurrent peptic ulcer. Gastroenterology 65:697–698, 1973
82. Seaman WB: Prolapsed gastric mucosa through a gastrojejunostomy. Am J Roentgenol 110:304–314, 1970
83. Levine M, Boley SJ, Mellins HZ, et al: Gastrojejunal mucosal prolapse. Radiology 80:30–38, 1963
84. Tanner NC: Personal observations and experiences in the diagnosis and management of ulcer disease and disabilities that follow peptic ulcer operations. Surg Clin North Am 56:1349–1363, 1976
85. Hardy JD: Problems associated with gastric surgery—A review of 604 consecutive patients with annotation. Am J Surg 108: 699–716, 1964
86. Jordan GL, Angel RT, McIlhaney JS, et al: Treatment of the postgastrectomy dumping syndrome with a reversed jejunal segment interposed between the gastric remnant and the jejunum. Am J Surg 106:451–459, 1963
87. Stalsberg H, Taksdal S: Stomach cancer following gastric surgery for benign conditions. Lancet 2:1175–1177, 1971
88. Burrell, M, Tovloukian JS, and Curtis, AM, Roentgen manifestations of carcinoma in the gastric remnant. Gastrointest Radiol In Press
89. Feldman F, Seaman WB: P,rimary gastric stump cancer. Am J Roentgenol 115:257–267, 1972
90. Moffat RC, Berkas EM: Bile esophagitis. Arch Surg 91:963–966, 1965
91. Clarke SD, Penry JB, Ward P: Oesophageal reflux after abdominal vagotomy. Lancet 2:824–826, 1965
92. Dagradi AE, Stempien SJ, Seifer HW, et al: Terminal esophageal (vestibular) spasm after vagotomy. Arch Surg 85:955–968, 1962
93. Herrington JL, Sawyers JL, Whitehead WA: Surgical management of reflux gastritis. Ann Surg 180:526–537, 1974
94. Barichello AW, Pimblett T, Dyck FJ, et al: Rupture of the stomach following oxygen therapy by nasal catheter. Can Med Assoc J 98:855–858, 1968

7 Complications of Biliary Tract Surgery

H. Joachim Burhenne and Peter Cooperberg

Operations on the biliary tract are the most frequent intraabdominal surgical procedures, about 500,000 being performed annually in the United States (1). Included in this figure are cholecystectomies, choledochotomies, bypass procedures, and reoperations for complications.

Although the incidence of cholelithiasis appears to be increasing, the surgical treatment of gallstones is one of the most satisfactory of modern therapeutic measures. The morbidity and mortality associated with biliary tract surgery have gradually been reduced over the past several decades. The mortality of cholecystectomy is about 1.5%, but it increases with associated common duct exploration. Even when cholecystectomy was originally described in 1882 there had been only one death among the first nine patients who underwent cholecystectomy (2).

In a large series of 1614 patients undergoing a variety of biliary tract procedures, including reoperation, the overall mortality was slightly less than 4% (3). In cholecystectomy the mortality was about 1% and in reoperation it was up to 8%. Among the 64 fatalities 19 were due to local complications, 5 to pulmonary complications, 16 to cardiovascular complications, 21 to metabolic disturbances, and 3 to miscellaneous causes.

It has been pointed out in the surgical literature that many of these complications could have been prevented (4). Accuracy in preoperative diagnostic assessment helps to reduce morbidity and mortality materially. Judicious application of radiographic procedures before, during, and after operation is an important part of biliary tract surgery, particularly in prevention of iatrogenic injuries. Demonstration of bile duct anomalies by routine operative cholangiography, for instance, is important in prevention of surgical bile duct injury.

Radiologic study is often crucial in preoperative diagnostic evaluation and in differentiation of the postoperative status from iatrogenic injuries.

Postoperative Fluid Collections

Some degree of subhepatic accumulation of blood, bile, lymph, and peritoneal fluid occurs in the majority of patients undergoing operations on the biliary tract (Fig. 7-1). Fluid collects in the operative bed surrounding the gallbladder and is usually controlled by drainage tubes. Unusual amounts of fluid usually indicate slippage of a cystic duct ligature (Fig. 7-2) or indicate extravasation from a cut or torn artery or bile duct.

The signs and symptoms of postoperative subhepatic fluid collections depend on the amount of fluid and on the presence of infection. There may be severe pain in the right upper quadrant associated with an increase in both temperature and white blood cell count.

Meticulous surgical technique and drainage of the right upper quadrant should prevent subhepatic collections. Large accumulations of fluid usually necessitate surgical intervention.

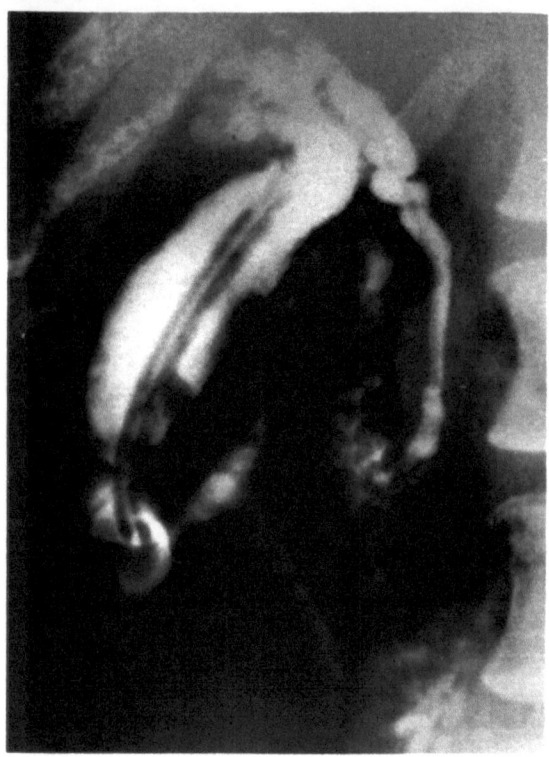

Fig. 7-1. Subhepatic leakage from cholecystostomy site. Note retained stones in the gallbladder.

Hemorrhage

Operations upon the biliary tract are not excepted from hemorrhage, one of the great hazards of surgery. Potential sources include laceration of the liver; avulsion or tear in the cystic or right hepatic arteries, accessory arteries, or vessels in the gallbladder bed; and a large bleeding surface of the gallbladder bed after cholecystectomy for acute cholecystitis. Hemorrhage due to injury to the inferior vena cava has occurred rarely.

Postoperative hemorrhage results from failure to control bleeding in the above areas at operation as well as slippage of sutures. In a significant number of patients postoperative bleeding also occurs from the lateral stab wound for T-tube insertion and from the incision.

The hepatic artery and its branches may be injured during biliary tract surgery, particularly because of variations in anatomy. Because of its anatomic location the right hepatic artery is injured or ligated more commonly (5), and this iatrogenic complication may be associated with injury to the common duct (Fig. 7-3).

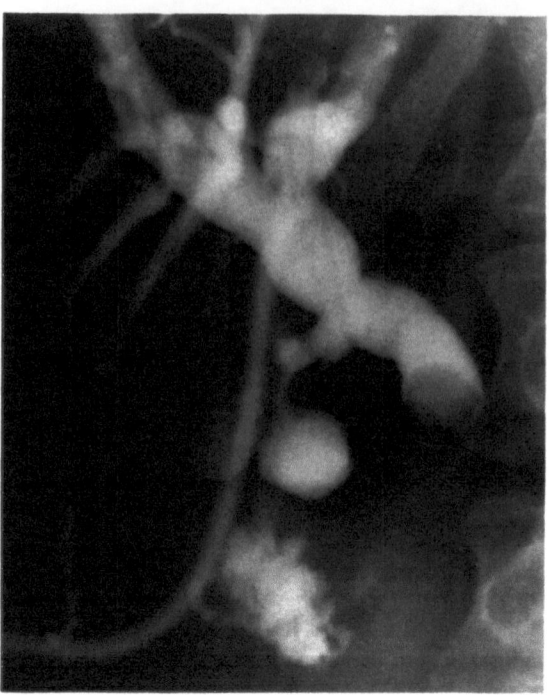

Fig. 7-2. Collection of subhepatic bile and contrast agent from leaking cystic duct stump. Note that the common duct is obstructed by a single retained common duct stone. The T-tube has been placed into the common hepatic duct and not the common bile duct. One short arm lies in the left hepatic radicle; the tip of the other short arm lies in the cystic duct.

Nonoperative stone extraction resulted in free duodenal drainage. The bile leak from the cystic duct ceased.

Bleeding at or after operation may occur in patients with liver disease and slow prothrombin time not corrected with vitamin K therapy prior to surgery.

Upper gastrointestinal hemorrhage following biliary tract surgery is less common. If duodenotomy has been performed for exploration of the distal common duct, this area is the most probable source of upper gastrointestinal bleeding. Bleeding from varices in coexistent portal hypertension must also be considered.

Bile Collections and Bile Peritonitis

Bile collections derive usually from the extrahepatic ductal system. Little or no problem arises if the rate of bile escape is slow. Free escape of bile in large amounts within the peritoneal cavity, however, may cause a fall in blood pressure

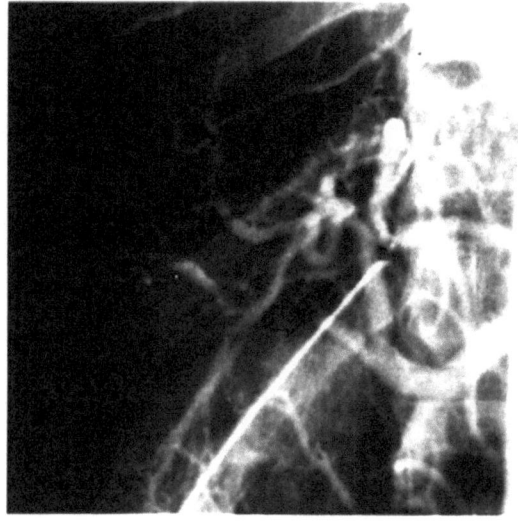
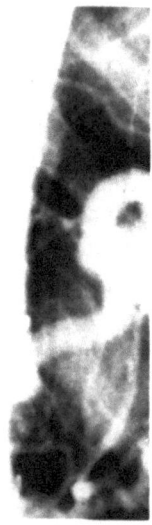

Fig. 7-3. Cutoff of right hepatic artery *(arrow)* due to inadvertent ligation. (Love L et al.: Radiology of cholecystectomy complications. Gastrointest Radiol 4:33–40, 1979)

and clinical manifestations of shock. It may be fatal. This complication is particularly feared, since large quantities of bile in the peritoneal cavity may give little evidence of peritoneal irritation. Loculated fluid collections occur if the bile leak results in chemical peritonitis. These patients then have generalized abdominal pain. Associated infections accelerate the course of events.

Abscess

Abscesses may be subhepatic or subdiaphragmatic.

Encapsulated collections of pus in the subphrenic region between the convexity of the liver and the diaphragm are less common than subhepatic abscess formation. They develop either as an extension of a subhepatic abscess (Fig. 7-4, 7-5 and 7-6) or by extension of infectious material into the subphrenic space, or rarely by rupture of a liver abscess.

Subhepatic abscesses may also extend to the lesser sac. Persistent infection of the subhepatic space can develop in a patient with an infected bile leak from a choledochotomy or from a cystic duct stump.

Combinations of blood and bile favor the formation of abscesses, particularly if postoperative drains have not been placed. Subhepatic drains are therefore good prophylaxis against subdiaphragmatic abscesses.

Drainage of subphrenic abscesses may be accomplished under ultrasonic guidance.

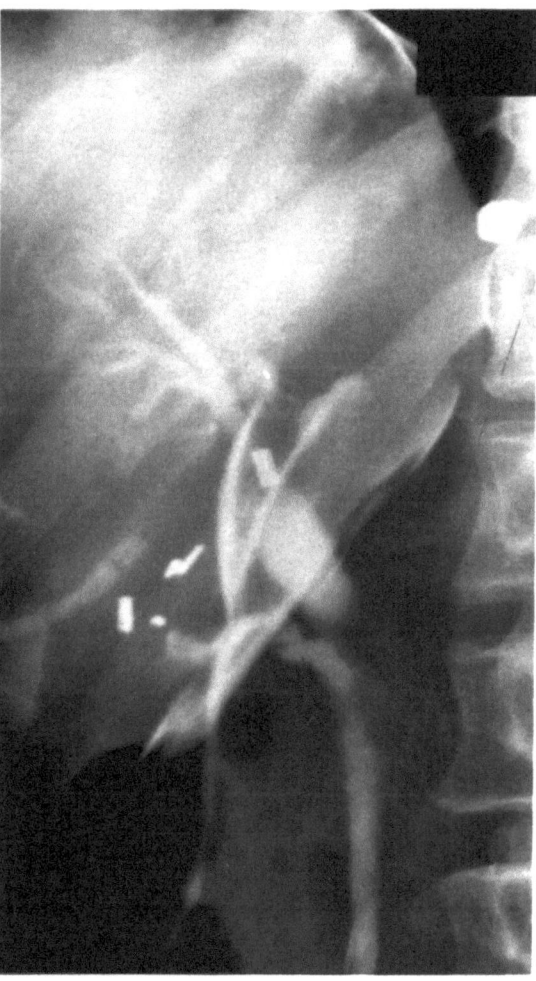

Fig. 7-4. Subhepatic extravasation from cystic duct leak. It has extended into subphrenic space over the liver.

Diagnosis

Radiographic signs of subphrenic abscess include elevation or limitation of motion of the right hemidiaphragm, right pleural effusion, and visualization of subdiaphragmatic air-fluid levels. Modern methods of ultrasound and computed tomography are more accurate in identification of subphrenic abscesses (Fig. 7-5).

Radiographic differentiation of blood, bile, serous fluid, and abscess is often difficult. Plain abdominal radiographs are obtained first. Films in multiple projections, particularly the left lateral decubitus view, help to identify air-fluid levels in abscesses. The appearance of multiple soft-tissue masses without air-fluid levels is often due to multiple localized bile collections associated with peritonitis. Right pleural effusion is associated more commonly with right upper-quadrant abscesses.

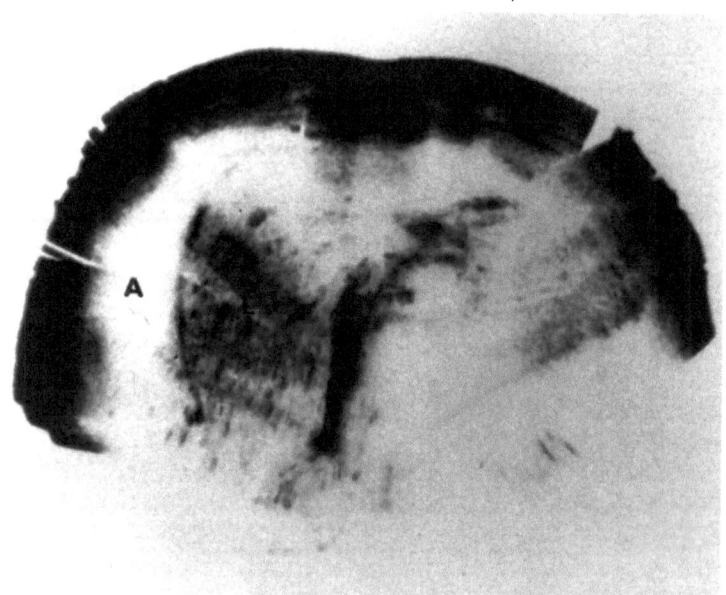

a

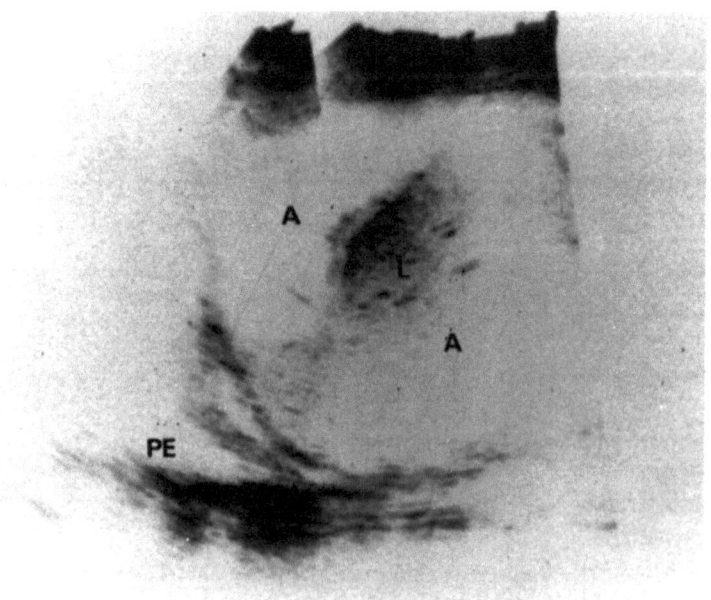

b

Fig. 7-5, a and b. Subhepatic and subphrenic abscess. Transverse (a) and longitudinal (b) ultrasonograms demonstrate a large abscess (A) of the subhepatic space surrounding the liver (L) and extending into the subphrenic space. Note associated pleural effusion (PE), usually present with subdiaphragmatic abscess.

Ultrasonography is an effective method for investigating suspected fluid collections after biliary tract surgery (6). Diagnostic investigation with ultrasound or computed tomography may lead to earlier diagnosis, and aspiration of the bile collection under ultrasonic guidance represents a safe therapeutic approach (Fig. 7-6). It should be the first step in the approach to suspected localized bile collections and abscesses. Bile collections or "bilomas" must be differentiated from abscesses and pseudocysts of the pancreas (7).

Imaging procedures such as ultrasonography and computed tomography are usually not helpful in differentiating between blood and bile, however. If hemorrhage is suspected clinically, selective arteriography may be required for identification of the bleeding vessel.

External and Internal Biliary Fistulas

In addition to localized bile collections, external biliary fistulas through the drain tract or incision and internal biliary fistulas to the intestinal tract may occur.

External biliary fistula is seen more frequently in patients with acute cholecystitis and in those who have undergone choledochostomy. It may result from slippage of cystic duct ligatures, severance of accessory ducts, or incomplete cholecystectomy. It occurs more frequently if the gallbladder fossa extends partially into the liver. It has been described following cholecystostomy, particularly after premature removal of drainage tubes or obstruction of T-tubes.

T-tubes should be removed only after good bile drainage has been shown by T-tube cholangiography because bile seepage from the drain site may continue, particularly with obstruction of the common bile duct. Radiographic interventional procedures are then indicated to relieve possible obstruction and diagnose other causes of external biliary fistula. Complications of biliary fistula are particularly difficult to diagnose if the fistula is internal, and transhepatic cholangiography may then be necessary. When the gallbladder is not entirely removed a mucous discharge from the remaining mucosal lining may develop.

Internal fistula may result from dehiscence of a duodenostomy after surgery on the distal common duct at the ampulla of Vater. This duodenal fistula may discharge bile as well as other intestinal juices. Fortunately this complication is less

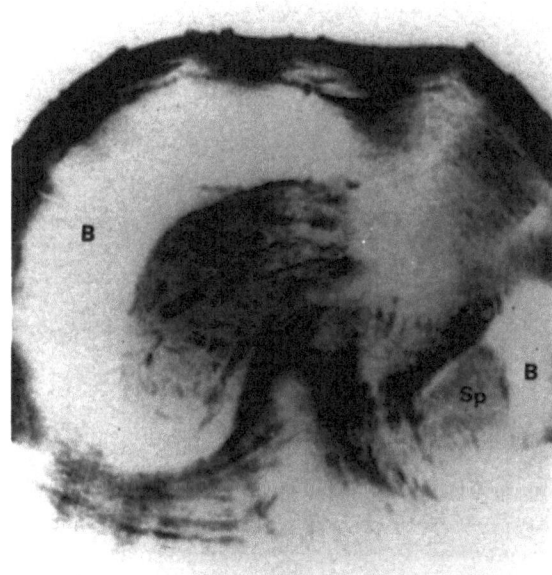

Fig. 7-6. Bile collection. Huge sonolucent collection (B) surrounding the liver (L) from a bile duct leak is shown by transverse ultrasonography. Note second localized bile collection adjacent to spleen (Sp).

frequent. Upper gastrointestinal studies with water-soluble contrast material will demonstrate the site of leakage. In the absence of jaundice, postoperative intravenous cholangiography is often of help. Optimal radiographic visualization is obtained by direct cholangiography if the T tube remains in place.

The surgical procedure for correction of biliary fistula depends on its cause. If the fistula is due to common duct obstruction by calculus (Fig. 7-7), percutaneous stone removal through the T-tube tract will correct the underlying problem. The fistula, however, may persist. If the duct system has been injured, reoperation and repair are indicated. However, since the second operation has at least twice the mortality of the initial surgical procedure, every effort must be made to avoid it. Attempts to dissect out the fistulous tract are usually of no help.

The exact etiology of postoperative pancreatitis remains controversial. Although it is often attributed to reflux of contrast material during cholangiography, there is no scientific evidence to support this theory. In fact, pancreatitis is seen particularly after surgical instrumentation of the ampulla of Vater, sphincterotomy, biopsy, impaction of distal common duct stones, and damage to pancreatic ducts. Specific attention has been focused on the possible association of acute hemorrhagic pancreatitis with choledochal sphincterotomy, indicating that direct trauma to the pancreas is the most likely cause (9).

Regurgitation of bile into pancreatic ducts may be indirectly diagnosed during cholangiography in a patient with pancreatitis. Adequate external drainage must be provided if spasm or other temporary obstruction is present at the distal end of the common duct.

Postoperative Pancreatitis

Postoperative pancreatitis occurs characteristically within the first 48 hours following surgery. Pancreatitis is one of the most dreaded complications of biliary tract surgery. Its incidence and mortality are high, particularly if common duct exploration is added to cholecystectomy (8).

Drainage Tube Problems

Cholecystostomy tubes are placed for drainage in acute cholecystitis, and T-tubes are placed routinely after exploration of the common duct. These drainage tubes may become dislocated or obstructed, or they may disintegrate.

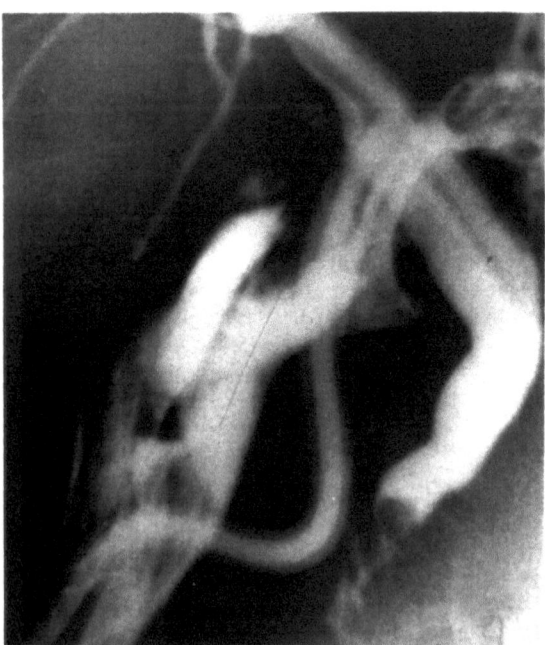

Fig. 7-7. External biliary fistula from choledochotomy site. This is secondary to partial obstruction of the distal common bile duct due to a retained stone.

Faulty placement of a T-tube is sometimes evident. One short arm of the drainage tube may be outside the duct system (Fig. 7-8). A long proximal arm of the T-tube can obstruct bile drainage from part of the liver or prevent passage of intrahepatic retained stones. Improper bile drainage is readily diagnosed during T-tube cholangiography after surgery. Replacement of a T-tube over a guide wire or replacement with a

straight catheter can be accomplished by the radiologist.

A T-tube is usually secured to the skin by sutures. A T-tube inadvertently extracted by a patient or medical personnel can almost always be replaced by the radiologist if replacement is accomplished within 24 hours after extraction.

Formation of a tract along the course of such a drain tends to allow the bile that escapes from the common duct to pass to the exterior rather than to accumulate in the periductal and subhepatic areas (10). The shorter the time between operation and inadvertent extraction of the tube, the more serious the accident is likely to be.

A drainage tube may become obstructed in the early postoperative period by a blood clot, calculus, gravel, or kinking. The longer the tube remains within the ductal system the more likely it is to become obstructed by encrusted material. The radiologist may be called upon to reestablish drainage. This can be done by reopening the obstructed tube with a guide wire. It is usually best, however, to exchange the tube over a guide wire (11).

Disintegration of a rubber T-tube occurs only if it is left in place for a prolonged period. The tube may become brittle and fragile and may come apart near the site of exit in the skin. Retained segments of a drainage tube must be removed.

Operative placement of a T-tube into the common duct must be accomplished with at least a 14 F drainage catheter. This permits radiologic interventional procedures for retained stones and other postoperative complications. Use of a T-tube smaller than 14 F must be considered poor operative technique. Proper placement also involves exit through a lateral anterior stab wound. This permits easy access for the radiologist. A T-tube should not be placed through a midline incision. Bivalving of a T-tube permits placement of an even larger T-tube into a small common duct.

A bile-tight closure about the point of entrance of the T-tube is advocated to keep periductal accumulation of bile to a minimum. Placement of a small V segment in the T-tube wall opposite the limb of the tube leading to the exterior makes extraction easiest. Again, it is good practice to cut away half of the circumference of the short arms of the tube before it is placed into the common duct. This also facilitates later removal.

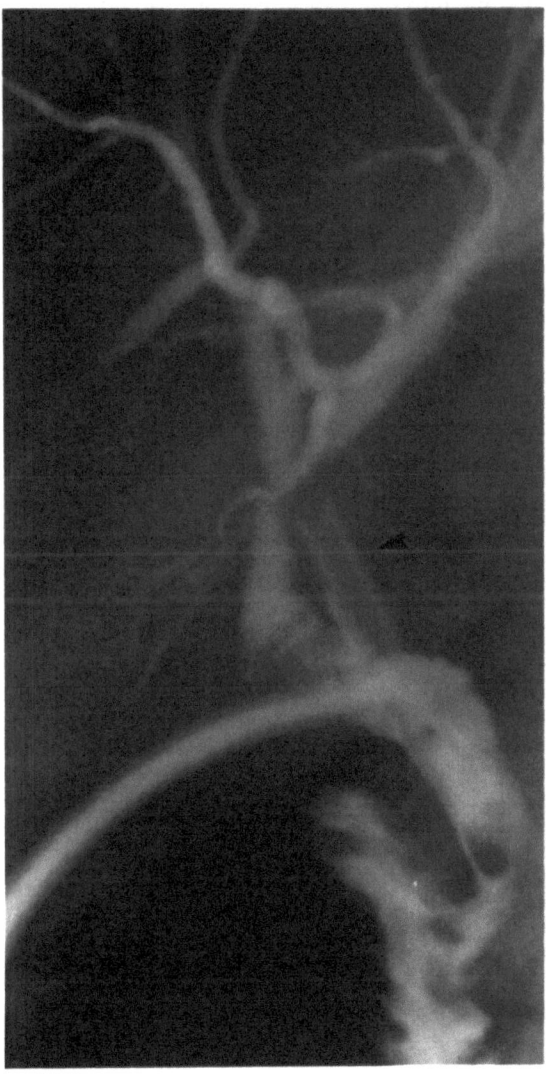

Fig. 7-8. Superior short arm of T-tube lying outside the common duct *(arrow)*. The T-tube was exchanged over a guide wire for a straight tube inserted for drainage into the common hepatic duct. The retained common duct stone was removed 4 weeks later.

Bile Duct Severance and Stricture

Common bile duct injury during operation on the biliary tract has a high fatality rate. The injury may result in stricture. Perhaps less than half of those with stricture due to operative injury survive for 10 years (10). Postoperative stricture of the bile duct most commonly is secondary to cholecystectomy, but it may follow gastrectomy, choledochostomy, or radical operations on the pancreas (12). Stricture usually results because the common duct has been injured (Fig. 7-9). The incidence of bile duct injury may be as high as 1% in patients undergoing cholecystectomy (13). Familiarity with anatomic variations of the biliary tract is mandatory if this dreaded complication is to be avoided (Fig. 7-10).

If the cystic duct is not properly dissected at operation the common or right hepatic bile duct may be mistaken for it and divided. The true junction of the cystic and common duct must be demonstrated. This is best accomplished by means of routine operative cholangiography with direct injection of contrast material into the cystic duct before common duct exploration.

Blind clamping of bleeding vessels may also injure the common duct, particularly when hemorrhage from the cystic artery obscures the operative field. This situation can also result in inadvertent placement of a ligature around the common duct.

Nonoperative spontaneous stricture of the bile ducts is rare but may result from erosion of a gallstone into the biliary tract or from infection.

The diagnosis of bile duct injury (Fig. 7-11) must be entertained when either a biliary fistula or jaundice occurs after biliary tract surgery. In jaundiced patients, bile duct enlargement may be first demonstrated by a noninvasive imaging procedure (Fig. 7-12) and then confirmed by transhepatic cholangiography (Fig. 7-13) or endoscopic retrograde cholangiography (Fig. 7-14). If sphincterotomy or choledochoenterostomy has

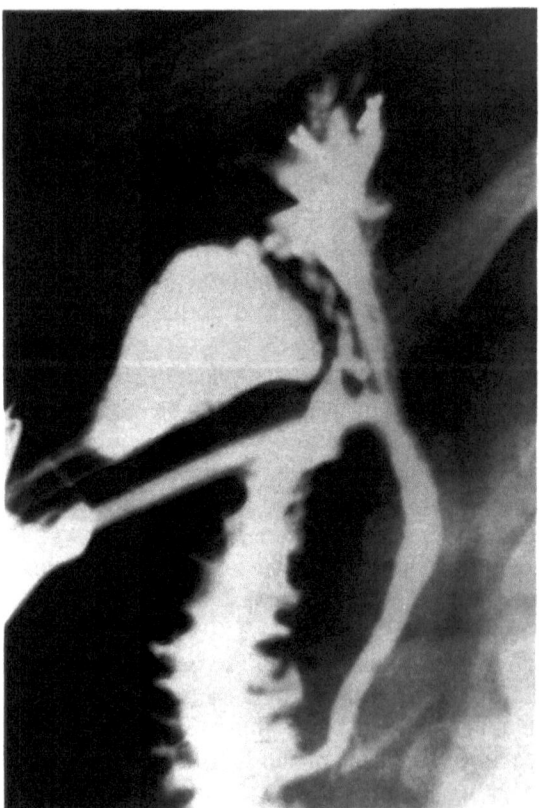

Fig. 7-9. Common hepatic duct injury. Extravasation has resulted from unsuccessfully repaired common hepatic duct injury.

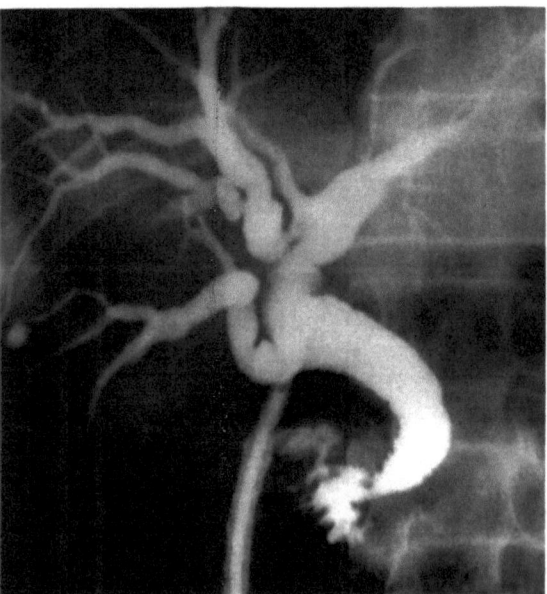

Fig. 7-10. Low insertion of right hepatic radicle. This is not a rare occurrence. Familiarity with this anatomic variation and identification by cholangiography before common duct exploration may prevent bile duct injury, particularly as the cystic duct lies in proximity to the low right hepatic radicle. The cystic duct may also enter into the right radicle.

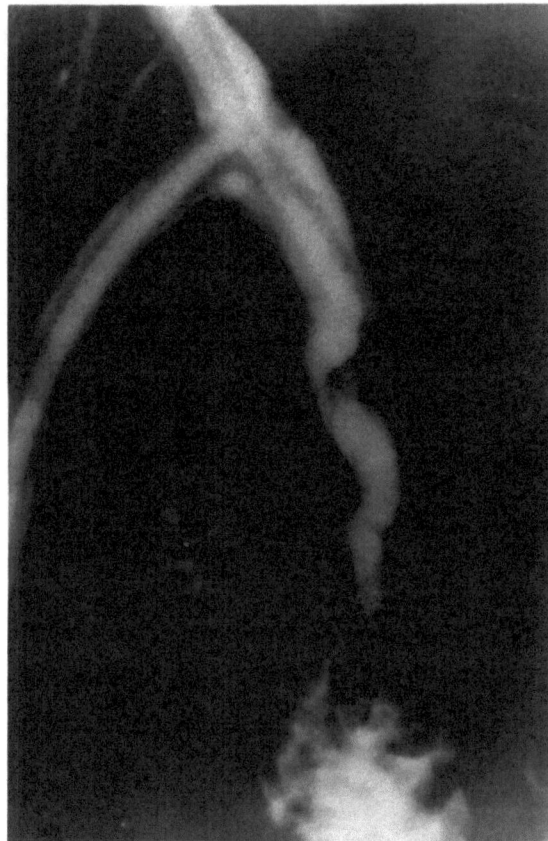

Fig. 7-11. **Early stricture formation.** T-tube cholangiography shows this 10 days after repair of common duct injury.

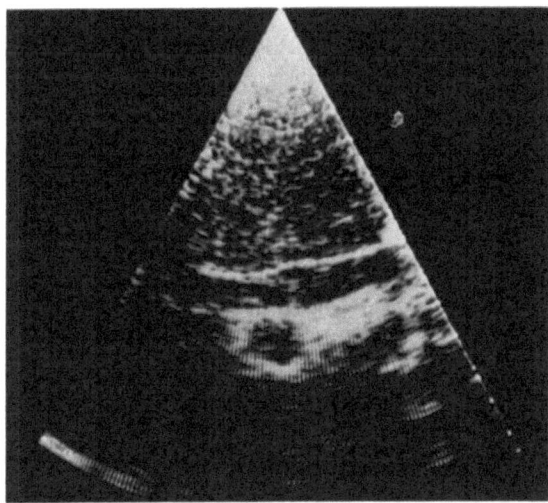

Fig. 7-12. **Ultrasonic demonstration of distended common hepatic duct.** This identifies obstruction in this jaundiced patient. The distended duct is seen in longitudinal fashion above the portal vein, which is seen in cross-section.

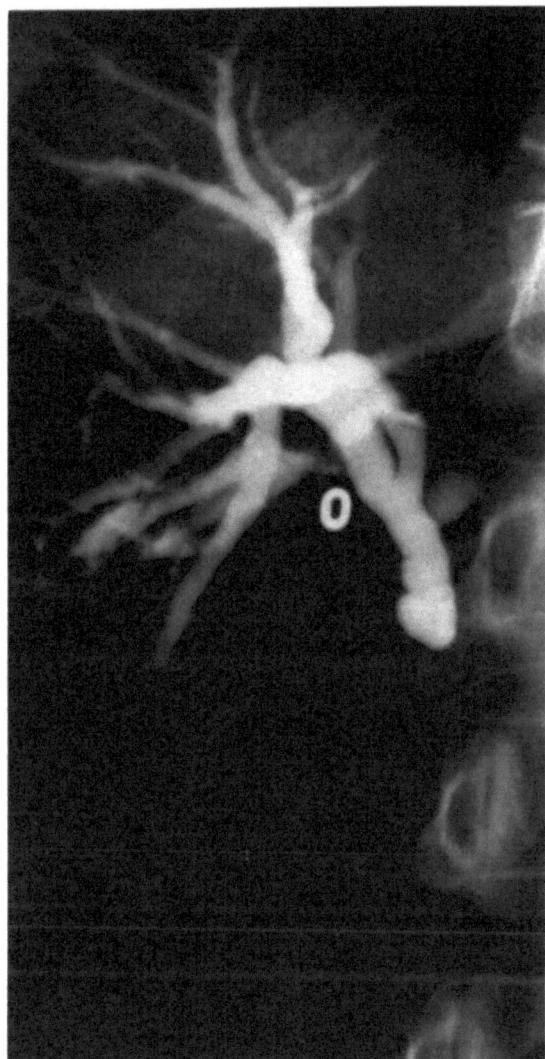

Fig. 7-13. **Inadvertent ligature of the common hepatic duct.** Transhepatic cholangiography identifies almost complete obstruction.

been performed, reflux of barium into the common duct from an upper gastrointestinal study can also identify the stricture. This approach is often useful in stricture at the site of hepatojejunostomy.

Reoperation has usually been undertaken to repair stricture. However, with the advent of interventional radiology of the biliary tract, dilatation and management of previous strictures can now be accomplished without operation (Figs. 7-15, 7-16). This is usually a palliative procedure, because stricture may recur after splint removal.

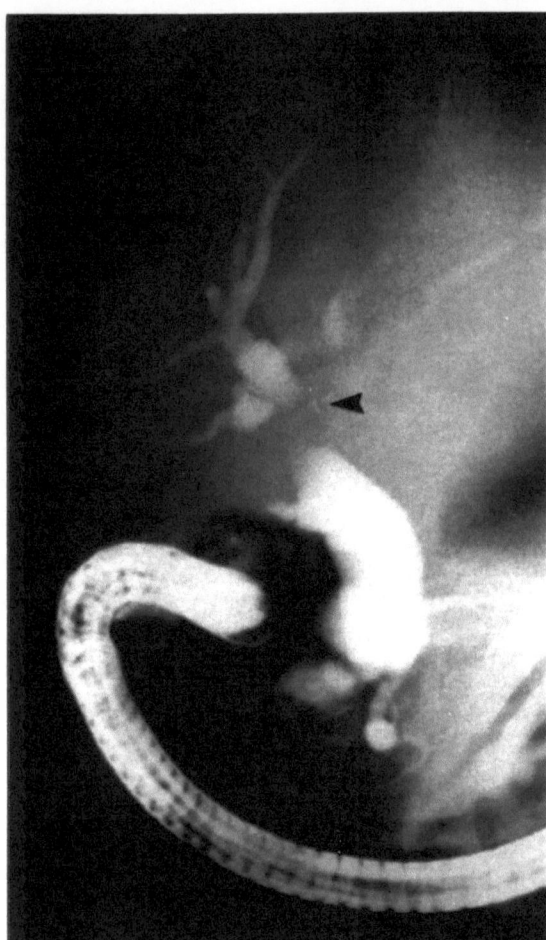

Fig. 7-14. Common hepatic duct stricture *(arrow).*
This is visualized by retrograde endoscopic cholangiography in jaundiced patient 6 weeks after repair of
iatrogenic duct injury.

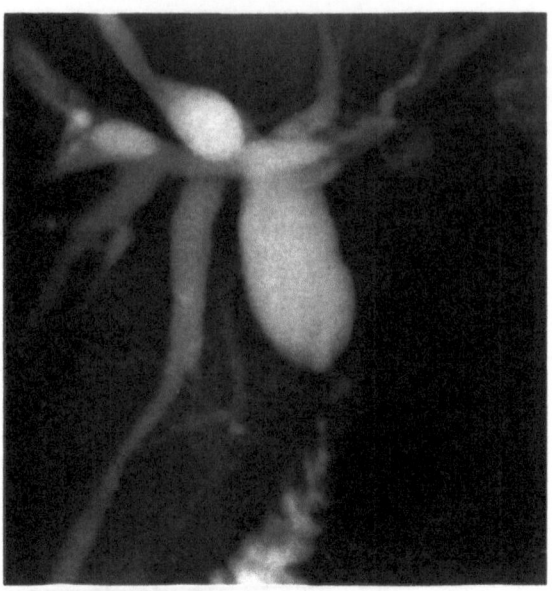

a

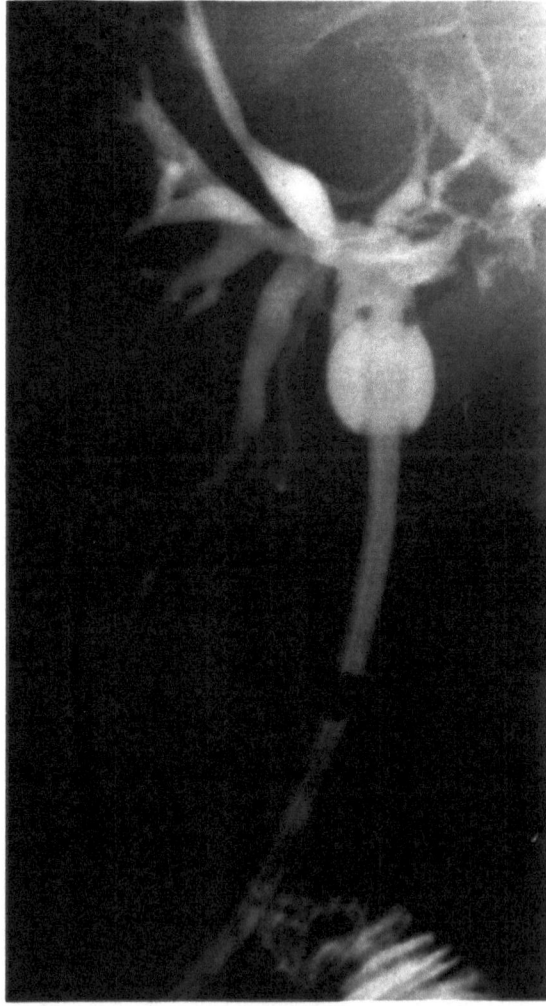

b

**Fig. 7-15, a and b. Stricture at hepatojejunostomy
anastomosis. a** This is seen in jaundiced patient 3
months after operation. **b** A retention balloon catheter
was inserted after stricture dilatation by a radiologic
interventional procedure. Side hole in the catheter
permits internal drainage.

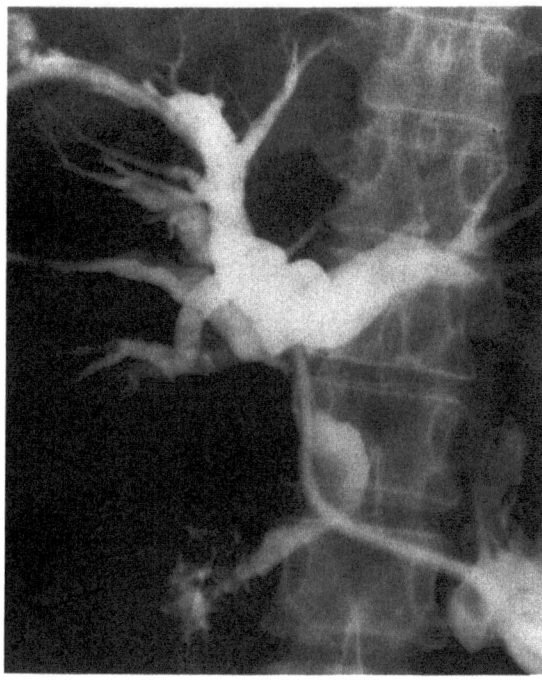

Fig. 7-16. Recurrent common duct stricture after stent fell out. By use of the catheter drainage tract and addition of a second opening via a percutaneous transhepatic approach, a U tube was placed after stricture dilatation.

Intraoperative Instrumentation

Instrumentation of the common duct may lead to iatrogenic injuries. Mucosal flaps may be lifted by metallic probes and dilators used in the distal common duct (Fig. 7-17). The same instruments may perforate the common duct (Fig. 7-18).

Intrahepatic injury with the Fogarty balloon catheter is not uncommon (14) (Fig. 7-19). This balloon catheter is not infrequently used to attempt extraction of intrahepatic stones, which is a difficult surgical maneuver as the operator is usually not sure into which second-division hepatic duct the catheter passed and if it is in fact distal to the retained stone. The surgeon cannot visualize the balloon without fluoroscopy and thus is not aware if it has been overdistended.

Postcholecystectomy Syndrome

The postcholecystectomy syndrome is not one particular complication. Rather the term applies to a variety of abnormalities after biliary tract surgery that cause right upper-quadrant pain, including retained stone; cystic duct remnant;

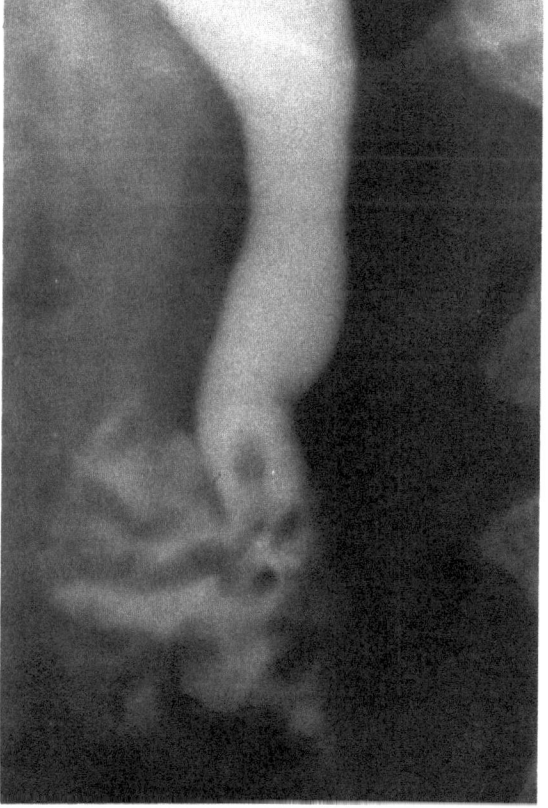

Fig. 7-17. Elevated mucosal flap. This is seen in distal common duct 6 days after operative instrumentation.

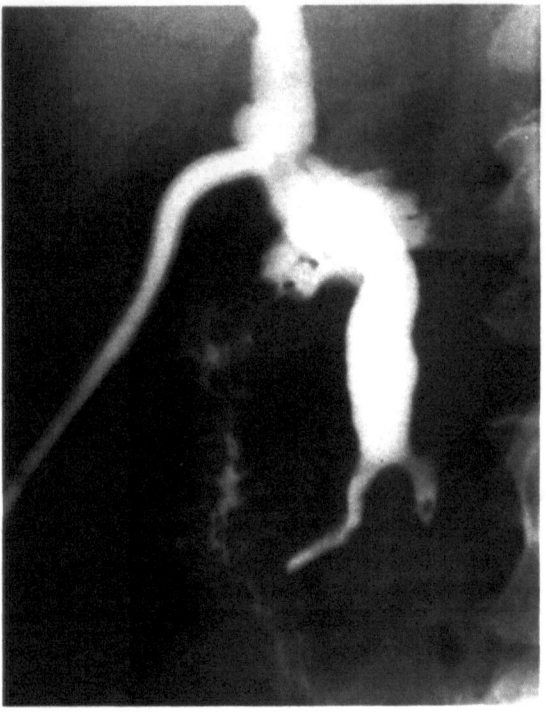 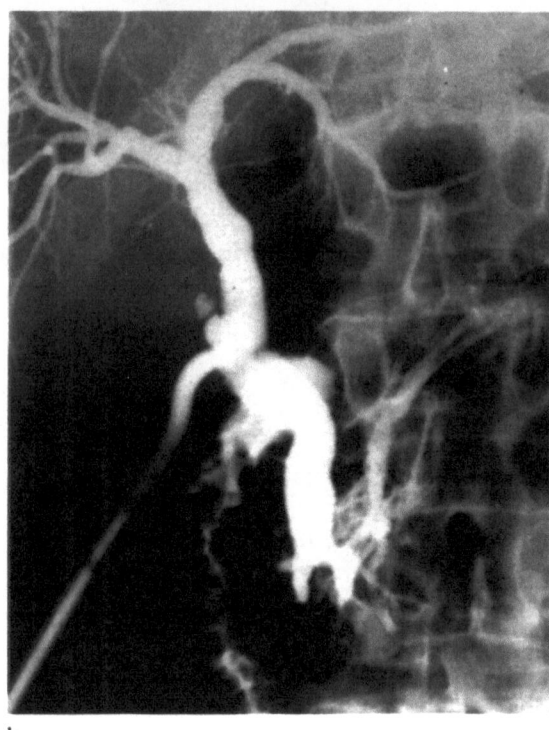

a   b

Fig. 7-18, a and b. Common duct perforation due to surgical instrumentation with metallic dilator. a A false channel was created. **b** Perforation resulted in internal fistula with pancreatic duct communication. (Courtesy M. Smart, MD)

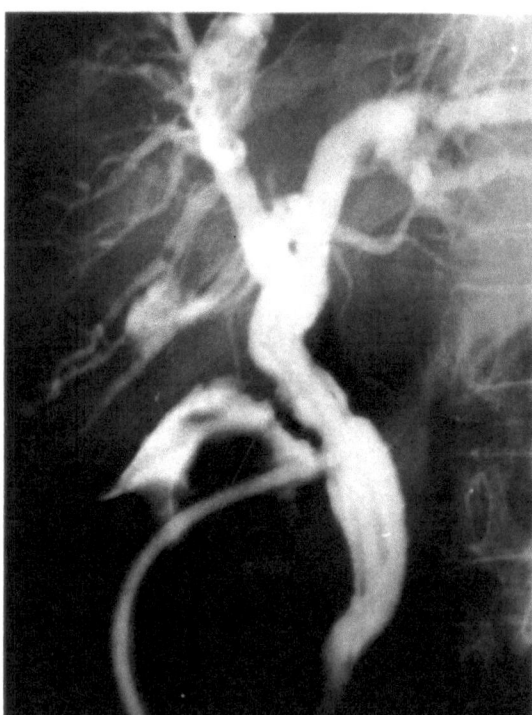

Fig. 7-19. Injury by Fogarty balloon catheter. Two areas of intrahepatic bile duct extravasation are evident.

amputation neuroma; periductal adhesions; abnormality at the sphincter of Oddi such as hypertrophy, fibrosis, and spasm; stricture; carcinoma; and erroneous preoperative diagnosis.

Retention of stones occurs almost always after common duct exploration and rarely after cholecystectomy alone (Fig. 7-20). Overlooked, forgotten, or retained stones are usually found in the distal common duct but may be anywhere in the biliary duct system. They are detected usually on postoperative T-tube cholangiography. Nonoperative extraction through the sinus tract of the T-tube is the treatment of choice. The radiologist places a steerable catheter through the sinus tract of the T tube, inserts a stone basket, and extracts the retained stones (15). The success rate for the procedure is 95% and complication rate is less than 5%; we have had no fatalities (16).

Retention of stones represents probably the most common complication after biliary tract surgery. The incidence is variously reported as 2%–15%. The use of routine operative cholangiography and intraoperative choledochoscopy contributes to a low incidence of stone retention, but retained stones do not always represent an iatrogenic complication. Intrahepatic stones may

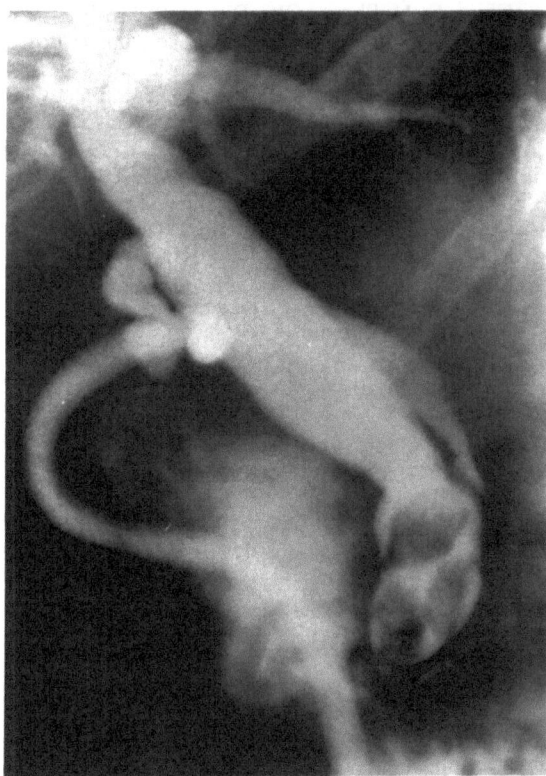

Fig. 7-20. Multiple retained common duct stones. Note the long cystic duct remnant. The common duct measures only 3 cm in length.

not be visible at the time of operative cholangiography and subsequently move into distal ducts postoperatively. Furthermore, it may be impossible to differentiate stones from blood clots or gas at the time of operation.

Cystic ducts or gallbladder remnants are detected on postoperative T-tube cholangiography. Assertions that cystic duct stumps are responsible for postoperative symptoms have not been substantiated. Cystic duct remnants are probably the cause of postoperative complaints only if they harbor retained stones (Fig. 7-21). Moreover, it is no longer accepted that the postoperative biliary tract and the cystic duct or gallbladder remnant dilate after cholecystectomy. If, in comparison to preoperative and intraoperative cholangiographic studies there is enlargement of the duct system on postoperative studies, partial distal common duct obstruction must be suspected.

Cystic duct remnants have been reported in 13%–21% of patients after cholecystectomy (17). It is our experience that careful cholangiography after cholecystectomy reveals the presence of

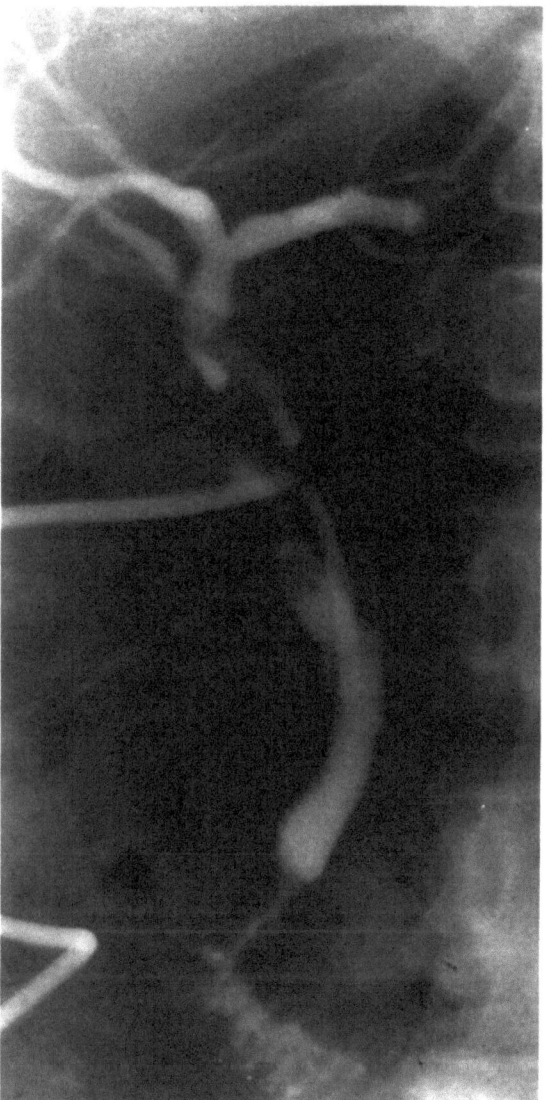

Fig. 7-21. Retained stone in cystic duct remnant (*arrow*). T-tube has been placed into the common hepatic duct.

cystic duct remnants in about 40% of patients. However, in a series of 661 patients with cystic duct remnants detected by postoperative cholangiography, we have not seen any symptoms unless there were also retained cystic duct stones.

Partial obstruction at the sphincter of Oddi due to fibrotic narrowing, spasm, or hypertrophy may be associated with common duct dilatation. Fibrosis of the sphincter of Oddi, however, is unusual and difficult to diagnose. Cholangiographic evidence of pronounced narrowing of the sphincteric portion is of greater diagnostic significance than manometric studies. These strictures are usually quite short and limited to the sphincteric portion. Longer strictures are more likely caused by pancreatic disease.

Erroneous Preoperative Diagnosis

Many patients with stone-bearing gallbladders have no symptoms. In those with symptoms, careful preoperative investigation is needed to rule out other causes unless actual biliary colic is noted. Hiatus hernia and gastroesophageal reflux, peptic ulcer disease, aerophagia, irritable colon, diverticulitis, urinary tract disease, coronary artery disease, and appendicitis may simulate cholelithiasis. Another complicating factor is the frequent association of biliary and pancreatic disorders. If symptoms persist after cholecystectomy, then hepatitis, cholelithiasis, tumor of the bile ducts or pancreas, and pancreatitis must be considered.

References

1. PAS Data. Hospital Record Study by CPHA. Ann Arbor, Mich. 1972, p 23
2. Langenbuch CJA: A case of extirpation of the gallbladder because of chronic cholelithiasis. Berl Klin Wochenschr 19:725–730, 1882
3. Hess W: Surgery of the Biliary Passages and the Pancreas. Princeton, N.J.: Van Nostrand, 1965
4. Glenn F, McSherry CK, Dineen P: Morbidity of surgical treatment for nonmalignant biliary tract disease. Surg Gynecol Obstet 126:15–26, 1968
5. Love L, Kucharski P, Pickleman J: Radiology of cholecystectomy complications. Gastrointest Radiol 4:33–40, 1979
6. Hillman BJ, Smith EH, Holm HH: Ultrasound diagnosis and treatment of gallbladder fossa collections following biliary tract surgery. Br J Radiol 52:390–392, 1979
7. Gould L, Patel A: Ultrasound detection of extrahepatic encapsulated bile: "Biloma." AJR 132:1014–1016, 1979
8. Bartlett MK, Carter EL: Special complications of gallbladder surgery. Surg Clin North Am 43:741–754, 1963
9. Warren KW, Cattrell RB: Pancreatic surgery. N Engl J Med 261:333–340. 1959
10. Artz CP, Hardy JD: Management of Surgical Complications. Philadelphia: Saunders, 1975
11. Burhenne HJ: Non-operative instrumentation of post-operative biliary tract. In Najarian JS, Delaney JP (eds): Surgery of the Liver, Pancreas and Biliary Tract. Miami: Symposia Specialists 1975, pp 177–207
12. Warren KW, Braasch JW: Repair of benign strictures of the bile ducts. Surg Clin North Am 45:617–619, 1965
13. Rosenquist H, Myrin SO: Operative injuries to the bile ducts. Acta Chir Scand 119:92–107, 1960
14. Eaton SB Jr, Wirtz RD, Ten Eyck JR, et al: Iatrogenic liver injury resulting from ductal instrumentation with the Fogarty biliary balloon catheter. Radiology 100:581–584, 1971
15. Burhenne HJ: The technique of biliary stone extraction. Radiology 113:567–572, 1974
16. Burhenne HJ: Complications of non-operative extraction of retained common duct stones. Am J Surg 131:260–262, 1976
17. Raymer JB, Tarpinian DA, Myers SG: Symptoms following cholecystectomy. Am J Dig Dis 5:55–62, 1960

8 Complications of Intestinal Surgery

James L. Clements, Jr., James V. Rogers, Jr.,
and William E. Torres

Radiologic examination of the abdomen plays an important role in the diagnosis and management of postoperative complications of surgery of the small bowel and colon. Plain films of the abdomen in supine and erect positions are usually the first examination, often followed by barium contrast studies of the small intestine and colon, in a patient with suspected intraabdominal disease occurring as the result of recent or remote surgical procedure on the small bowel and colon. Recently,the more sophisticated methods of imaging such as abdominal ultrasound and abdominal computed tomography have added a new dimension to the evaluation of intraabdominal diseases.

Postoperative Ileus and Mechanical Obstruction

Postoperatively the motility of the gastrointestinal tract is temporarily impaired. Small bowel activity returns to normal within a few hours, but gastric inertia persists for 24–72 hours. After extraabdominal operations or blunt trauma, colonic activity is absent for an average of 16 hours and after abdominal surgery for an average of 40–48 hours.

In uncomplicated cases, colonic decompression is usually seen radiographically in 3 days after extraabdominal surgery, in 4 days after laparotomy without gastrointestinal resection, in about 5 days after gastric surgery, and in about 7 days after partial colon resection. The extent

of surgery and administration of postoperative analgesics apparently have little effect on resumption of colonic activity (1,2).

Since gaseous distention of the small bowel is not a feature of uncomplicated postoperative cases, plain abdominal films (supine and upright or decubitus if feasible) are quite helpful in distinguishing uncomplicated ileus from mechanical obstruction and nonobstructive complications associated with small and large bowel distention (3,4). If only colonic or colonic and gastric distention is present, uncomplicated ileus is likely (Fig. 8-1). If small bowel distention is also present, some complication such as peritonitis, bowel leak, ischemia, abscess, retroperitoneal hemorrhage, or electrolyte disturbance should be suspected (Fig. 8-2). It may be quite difficult to distinguish these cases radiographically from partial small bowel obstruction, but administration orally or by nasogastric tube of 30–40 cc Gastrografin with follow-up films at hourly intervals for 3–5 hours frequently resolves this problem (Fig. 8-3, 8-4). The small bowel transit time is normally 30–90 min, but postoperatively it is usually 1.5–4 hours. A delay in small bowel passage of more than 3–5 hours is strongly suggestive of small bowel obstruction. This is further confirmed by a gasless bowel more distally. Demonstration of dilated proximal small bowel loops and normal-diameter distal loops indicates partial obstruction.

Barium enema study may be helpful in evaluating the cause of delayed postoperative distention, particularly if the distal small bowel can be filled by reflux through the ileocecal valve (Fig. 8-4). Demonstration of a normal diameter of the

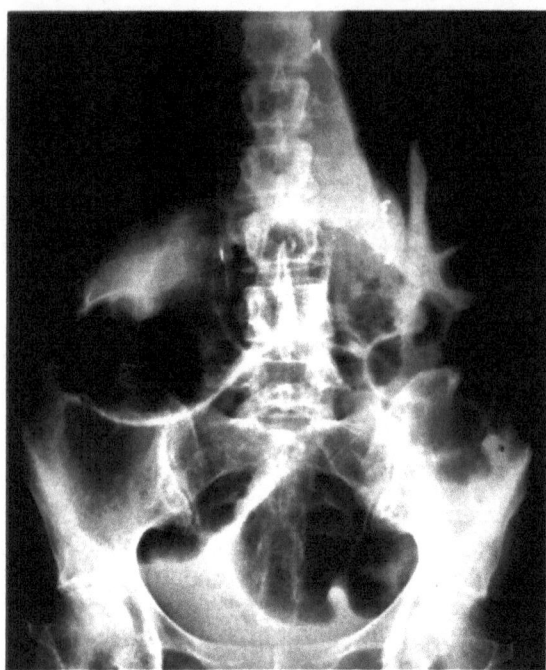

Fig. 8-1. Adynamic ileus 3 days after Whipple operation. Supine film of abdomen of a 56-year-old white female shows moderate gastric and colonic distention without small bowel distention.

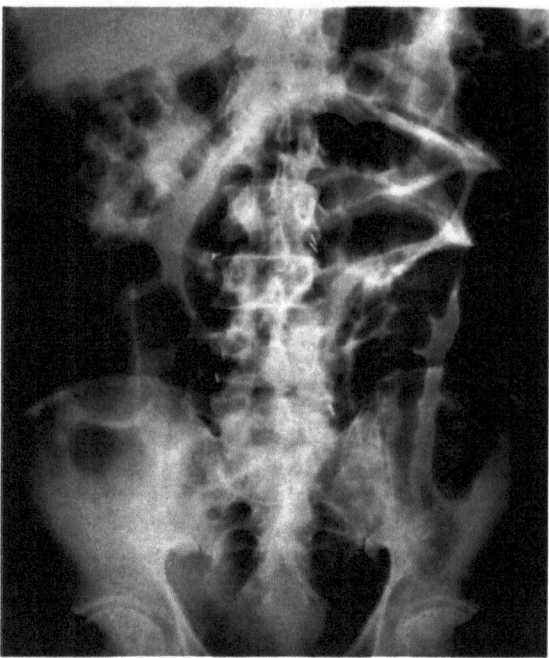

Fig. 8-2. Postoperative ileus accompanying retroperitoneal hematoma. This 66-year-old white male recently had a femoral-tibial artery bypass. Previously he had had an aorta-femoral bypass. Supine film shows extensive small and large bowel distention suggesting nonobstructive ileus.

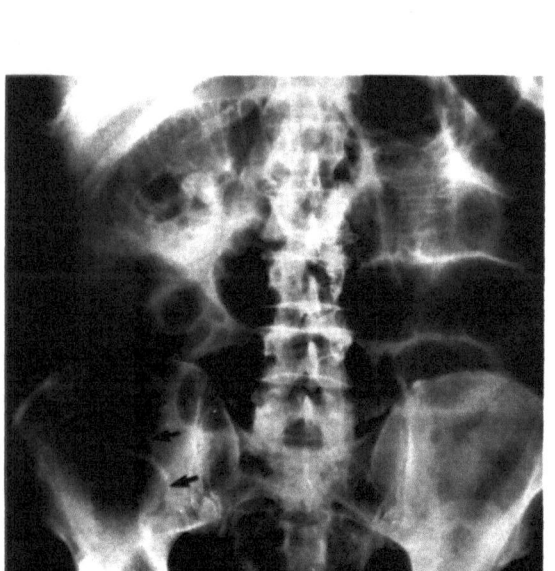

a

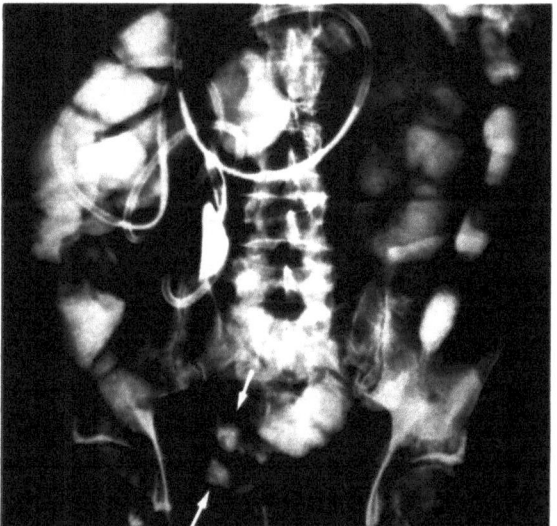

b

Fig. 8-3, a and b. Postoperative partial small bowel obstruction. This 72-year-old patient had recently undergone peristomal hernia repair. Left lower-quadrant colostomy had been done previously after abdominoperineal resection for carcinoma. Extensive abdominal adhesions were noted at operation. a Supine film of the abdomen 11 days postoperatively shows extensive small bowel distention. Gas is apparent in cecum and right colon (arrows). b Three days later a diatrizoate meglumine (Gastrografin) study through a Cantor tube confirms partial small bowel obstruction (3-hour film). There are dilated proximal small bowel loops and nondistended distal loops (arrows) with contrast material throughout the colon. The patient was treated successfully by bowel decompression with the Cantor tube and discharged 3 days later.

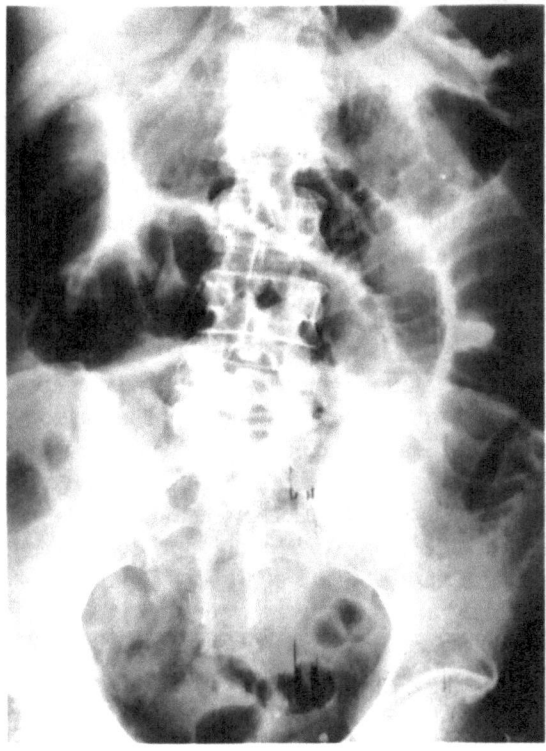

a

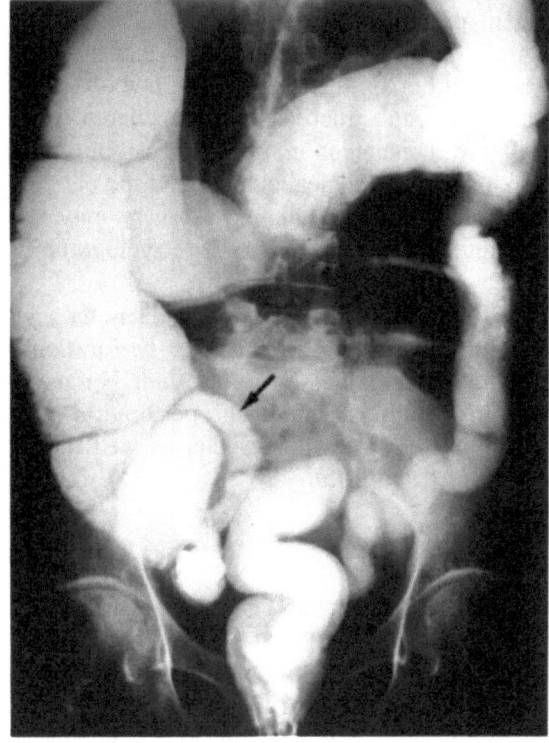

b

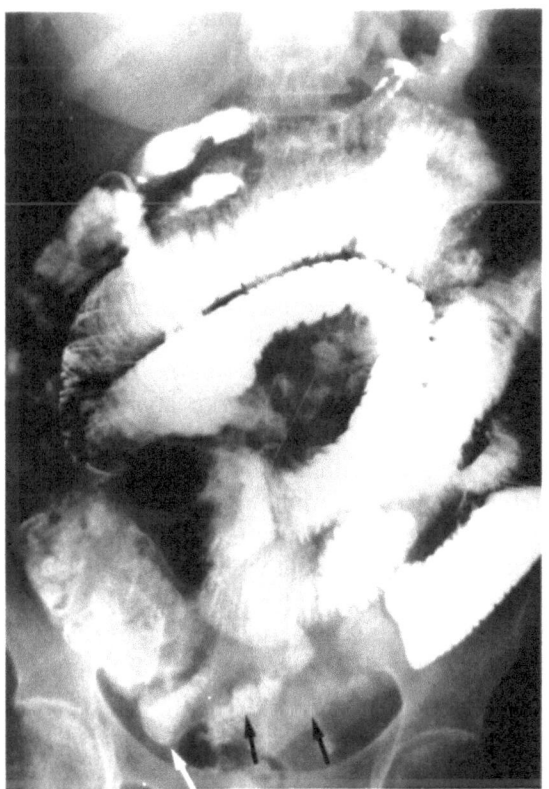

c

Fig. 8-4, a–c. Partial small bowel obstruction. This occurred in a 58-year-old white female following vaginal and rectocele repair. a Supine film of abdomen 11 days postoperatively shows continued gastric and small bowel distention with some gas throughout the colon. b After a barium enema there is reflux into nondistended terminal ileum (arrow). Proximal gas-distended small bowel indicates partial small bowel obstruction. c A 3-hour film after oral administration of diatrizoate meglumine (Gastrografin) confirms partial obstruction by demonstration of distended proximal small bowel loops and distal loops of normal diameter (arrows). The patient responded to conservative treatment (intubation and constant suction).

terminal ileum by reflux in the presence of distended proximal bowel is an indication of obstruction. It must be emphasized that there is a significant error rate in distinguishing obstruction from nonobstructive ileus in patients with small bowel distention in the early postoperative period, and if the clinical condition of the patient does not improve or worsens, surgery may be indicated, regardless of the radiographic findings.

Cecal distention of over 10 cm in diameter signals the possibility of impending perforation. Intraluminal pressures of 20–55 mm Hg may result in rupture. Spontaneous perforation has been reported in adynamic ileus as well as in colonic obstruction (5).

Short-Bowel Syndrome

This clinical syndrome results from functional deprivation of an extensive portion of the small bowel. This may be secondary to surgical resection, surgical exclusion, or extensive enteropathy. Resection of 50%–60% of the small bowel is compatible with normal existence, and more extensive resection of up to 75% may have a good result. It is doubtful if an individual can survive on oral intake alone with less than 60 cm of mesenteric small bowel (6). However, with parenteral support, a person can probably survive with as little as 20–45 cm of mesenteric small bowel.

The anatomic portion of small intestine remaining has an influence on the symptoms and deficiencies since there tends to be selective absorption of certain nutrients and chemicals. For instance, iron is absorbed predominantly in the duodenum; lipids, amino acids, and glucose in the upper small bowel; and vitamin B_{12} and bile salts in the distal ileum (7).

Manifestations of the short-bowel syndrome include severe diarrhea, steatorrhea, fat and protein malabsorption, megaloblastic anemia, hypovolemia, metabolic acidosis, tetany due to calcium loss, hypomagnesemia, impaired glucose absorption, hypoalbuminemia and edema, lactose deficiency, and gastric hypersecretion (8,9).

Although there is a likelihood of increased gallstone formation secondary to a decreased bile acid pool, this has not been substantiated clinically. There is an increased incidence of urinary tract calculi, including oxalate stones as well as uric acid stones (Fig. 8-5a).

Radiographically the shortened bowel and rapid transit time may be demonstrated by a barium meal. The adaptation of the small intestine by dilatation, elongation, villous hypertrophy, and cellular hyperplasia of the mucosa is demonstrable as dilatation with a coarse mucosal pattern (7) (Fig. 8-5b, c).

Medical treatment includes intravenous hyperalimentation (10), elemental and other special diets, vitamin and mineral supplementation, antidiarrheal and antiperistaltic drugs, and cimetidine therapy to counteract gastric hypersecretion (11,12). Surgical therapy includes a reverse (antiperistaltic) loop or recirculating loop to slow intestinal transit time (13), artificial sphincters or ileocecal valve substitutes when the right colon has also been resected, vagotomy and pyloroplasty for gastric hypersecretion, and as-yet unsuccessful attempts at small bowel transplantation.

The bowel proximal to a reversed loop tends to be even more dilated. If the reverse loop is too short it is ineffective, and if too long a complete functional obstruction will result.

Continent Ileostomy (Kock Pouch)

In 1969 Kock reported his initial efforts at construction of an ileal reservoir in patients who had undergone proctocolectomy (14). These first pouches were constructed with approximately 40 cm of terminal ileum; about 30 cm were used to create an aperistaltic pouch, and 10 cm, an efferent isoperistaltic limb. Although the reservoir functioned it was incontinent. Kock subsequently modified the efferent limb to an intussuscepted isoperistaltic nipple valve (15,16) (Fig. 8-6), thereby creating a continent ileostomy requiring catheter drainage. The capacity of the pouch was designed to be about 400 cc, requiring drainage two or more times each day. The design is such that opposing contractile forces prevent an effective stripping (peristaltic) wave.

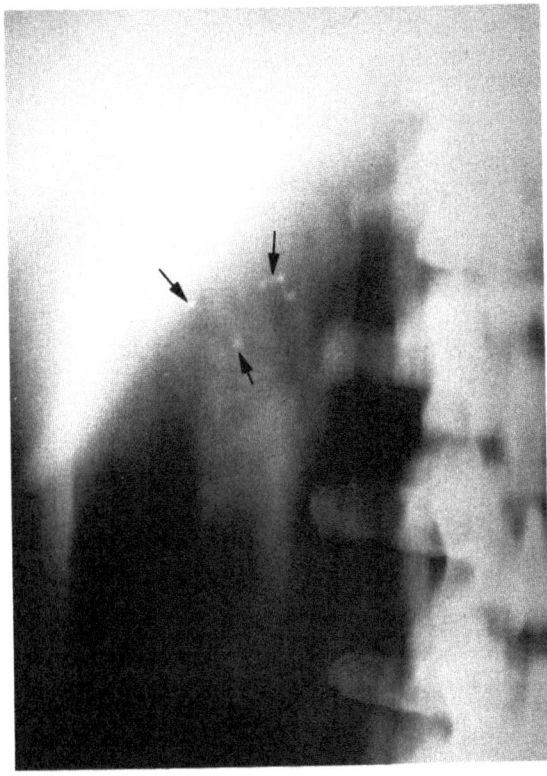

a

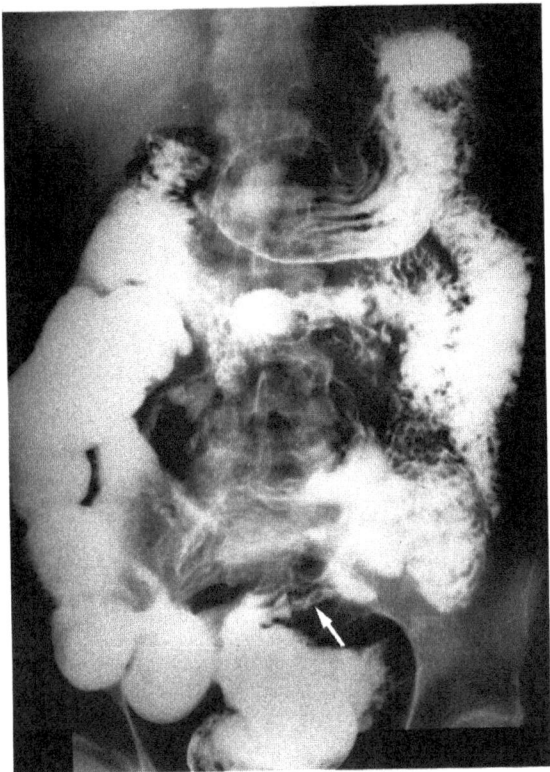

b

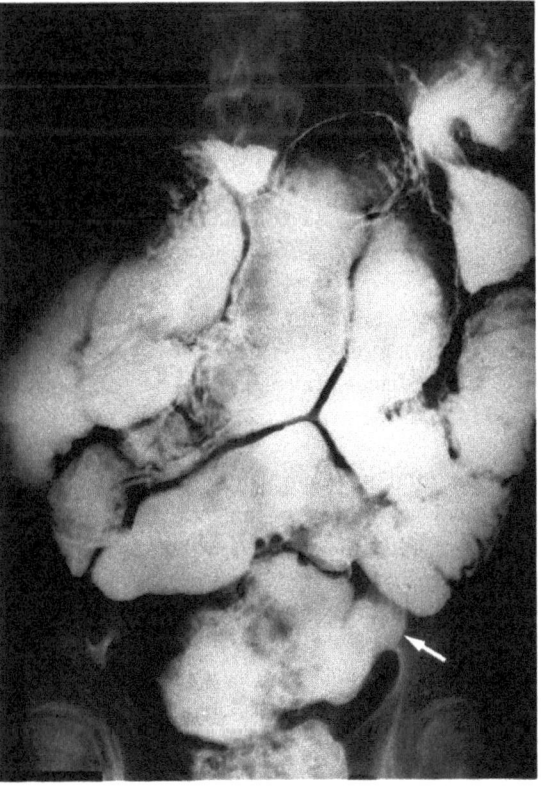

c

Fig. 8-5, a–c. Short-bowel syndrome. A 45-year-old male had approximately 5 ft of small intestine and rectum remaining after multiple resections for regional enteritis. **a** *Arrows* on the tomogram indicate renal calcium oxalate calculi. **b** On antegrade barium study at 45 min slight dilation and coarsened mucosal pattern are noted. *Arrow* indicates site of enterosigmoidostomy. **c** Seven years later, antegrade study at 60 min shows further dilation and elongation of the bowel. *Arrow* indicates site of enterosigmoidostomy.

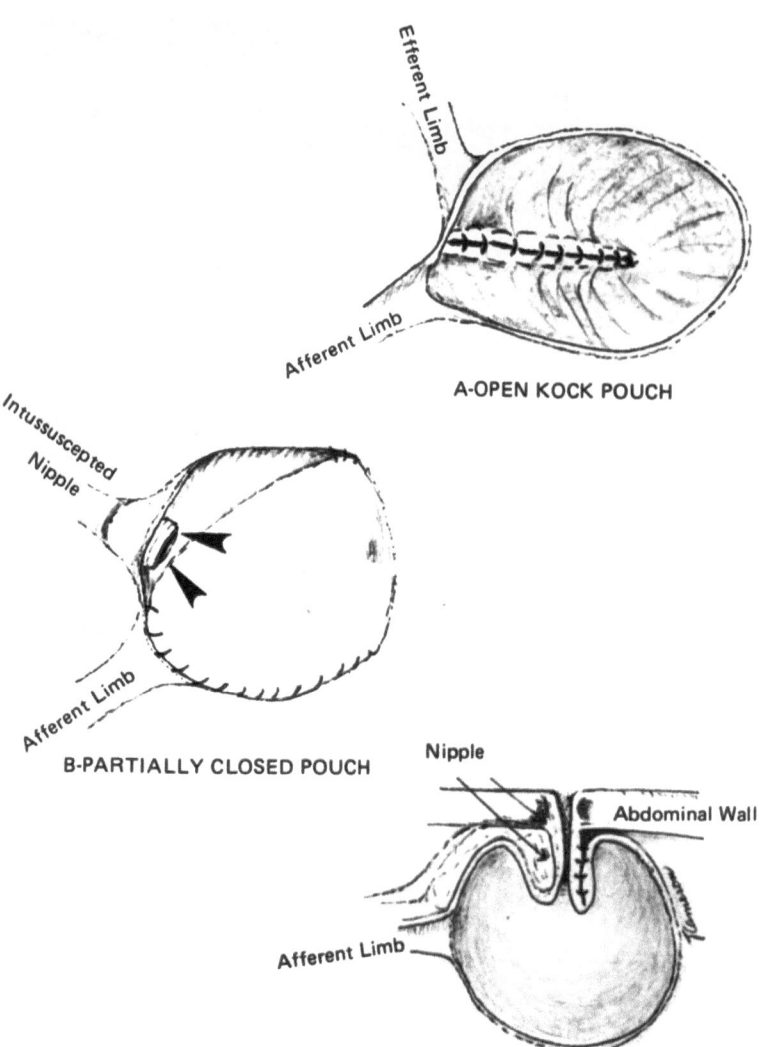

A-OPEN KOCK POUCH

B-PARTIALLY CLOSED POUCH

C-FINAL POSITION OF POUCH

Fig. 8-6, A–C. Kock pouch. A The initial step in formation of an aperistaltic ileal reservoir is shown. **B** Transformation of efferent limb of reservoir into a reverse intussuscepted segment creates a "nipple valve" *(arrows).* **C** In the representation of the final position of the Kock pouch in relation to the anterior abdominal wall, the proximal end of the nipple valve projects into the reservoir and the distal end forms the ileal stoma.

The advantages of a properly functioning continent ileostomy are all related to the absence of the constant efflux of ileal content. These include absence of the necessity for an ileostomy bag, absence of skin irritation, and absence of unpleasant odor.

The indications for continent ileostomy are primarily to permit a more nearly normal functional state in patients (particularly young patients) who have undergone proctocolectomy and to avoid the skin irritation that commonly occurs with an incontinent ileostomy. Patients undergoing proctocolectomy for idiopathic ulcerative colitis or familial polyposis of the colon are usually good candidates for this procedure.

A Kock pouch is generally contraindicated in patients who have undergone proctocolectomy for Crohn's disease because of the likelihood of recurrence in the pouch or afferent loop or both (Fig. 8-7).

The immediate postoperative complications are those common to small bowel resection, including obstructive and nonobstructive ileus, suture-line leakage or disruption, peritonitis, abscess, bowel necrosis, wound dehiscence, and wound infection. Delayed complications include abscess, fecal fistula from the pouch or around the intussuscepted nipple (Fig. 8-8), nonspecific ileitis in the pouch, recurrent regional enteritis (Fig. 8-7), and mechanical obstruction from adhesions, internal hernia, or volvulus (Fig. 8-9).

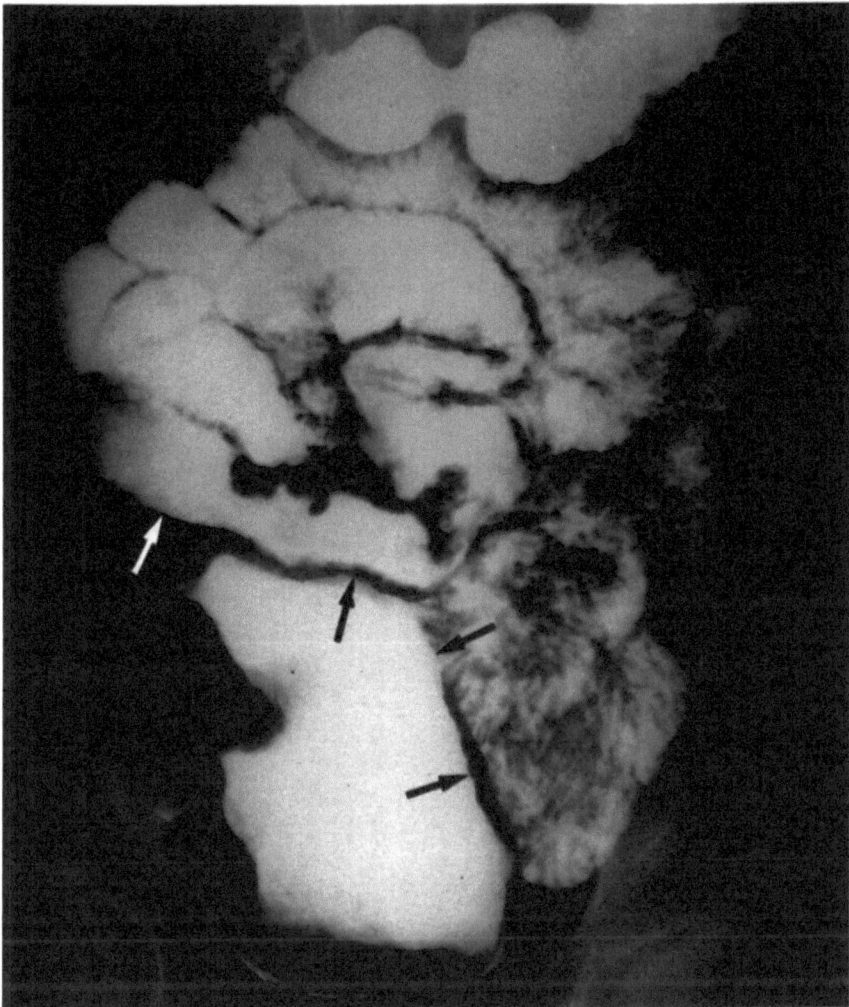

a

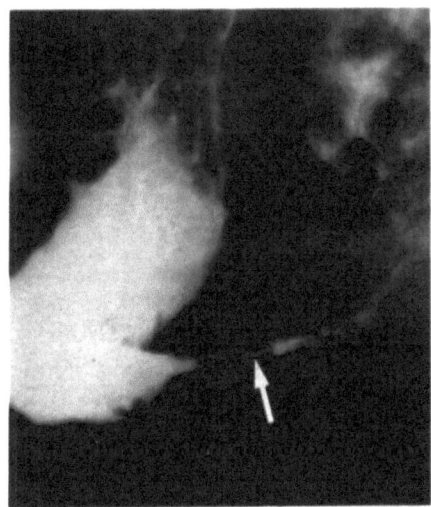

b

Fig. 8-7, a and **b. Recurrent regional enteritis in afferent limb and Kock pouch.** This occurred after proctocolectomy for supposed idiopathic ulcerative colitis. **a** Antegrade barium study demonstrates serrated appearance of ulcerations in pouch and afferent limb *(arrows)*. **b** Antegrade study 4 months later shows marked stenosis of afferent limb proximal to reservoir and changes of Crohn's disease in afferent limb *(arrow)*.

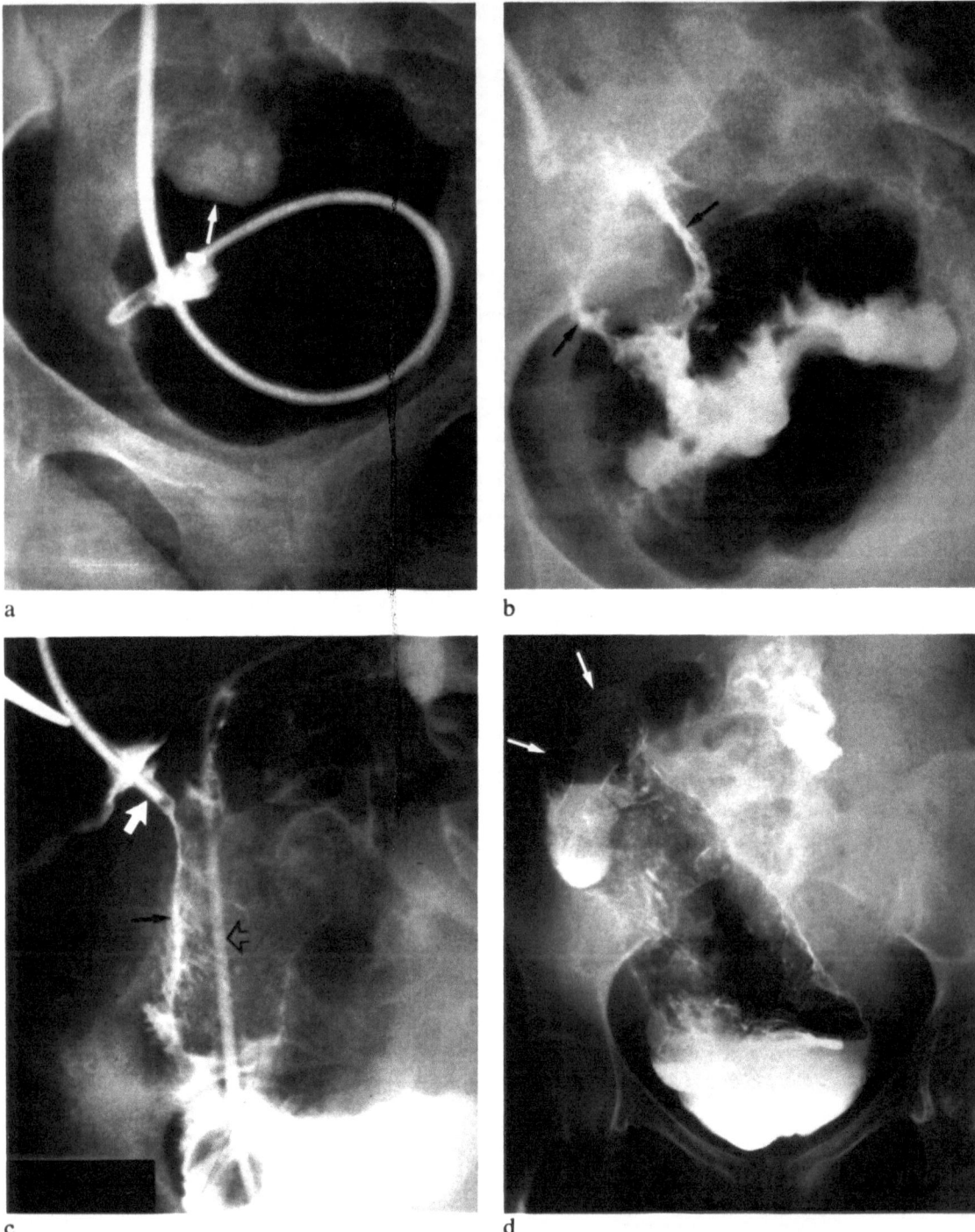

Fig. 8-8, a–d. Fecal fistula between intussusceptum and intussuscipiens of nipple valve of Kock pouch. This developed in a 26-year-old white female following proctocolectomy for idiopathic ulcerative colitis. **a** In catheterization of the fistula the catheter enters the air-filled Kock pouch beside the nipple *(arrow)*. **b** On injection of the fistulous tract, contrast material surrounds the nipple *(arrows)* between the intussusceptum and intussuscipiens before entering the reservoir.

c During simultaneous catheterization of the nipple valve and fistula injection the catheter entering the pouch is properly centered in the nipple valve *(open arrow)*. The other catheter is in the fistulous tract, and contrast medium outlines the fistula and Kock pouch *(closed arrows)*. A normal mucosal pattern is demonstrated in the pouch. **d** The anteroposterior projection shows the Kock pouch filled with contrast material and reflux into the afferent loop *(arrows)*.

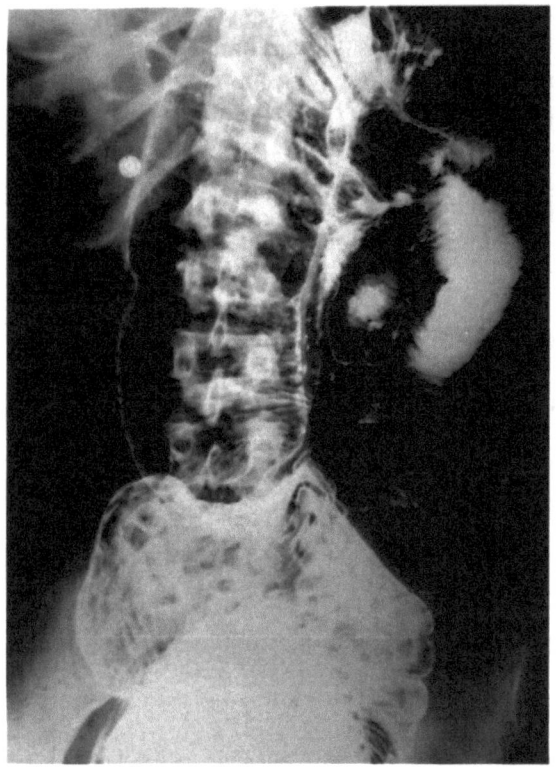

a

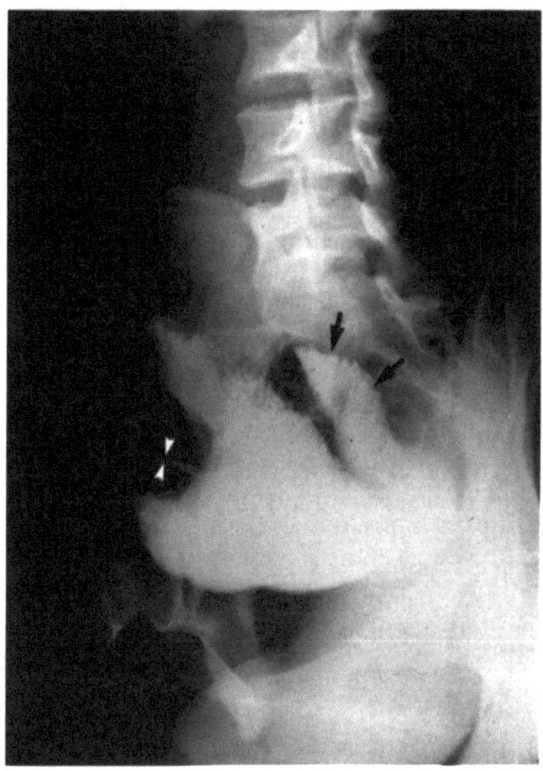

b

Fig. 8-9, a and b. Recurrent small bowel distention associated with Kock pouch. a Antegrade barium study shows marked small bowel distention without complete obstruction proximal to the pouch. Distention abated without surgery but recurred episodically, and a provisional diagnosis of recurrent volvulus was made. **b** In a later retrograde study during an asymptomatic period the catheter is properly centered in nipple valve *(arrowheads)*, and mucosal pattern of pouch and afferent limb *(arrows)* is normal. There is no distention of small bowel.

The most common complication is incontinence due to partial or complete deintussusception of the nipple. This may also lead to difficulty in intubation of the nipple because of kinking of the efferent limb. Cauterization of the serosa of the intussuscepted segment and fixation with nonabsorbable sutures have markedly reduced this complication.

The pouch can be studied radiologically by retrograde injection of barium through the nipple valve (Fig. 8-9b). This can be by either single- or double-contrast technique. Usually 200–300 cc's of barium suspension will satisfactorily outline the pouch and afferent limb (17).

Ulcerations in nonspecific ileitis and recurrent regional enteritis may be demonstrated in this manner (Fig. 8-7). Retrograde injection of the nipple may also reveal tortuosity or kinks associated with partial deintussusception (18). Retrograde endoscopy is also very useful in assessing the status of the mucosa of the pouch and of the afferent and efferent limbs. Antegrade barium studies are indicated particularly when disease is suspected in the small bowel proximal to the Kock pouch (Figs. 8-7, 8-9). Injection of contrast material into a fistulous tract should demonstrate the site of communication with the bowel (Fig. 8-8).

Jejunoileal Bypass Procedure

Massive obesity is a disabling and life-threatening condition that responds very poorly to long-term medical therapy. Surgical management offers a method for control or cure in those patients in whom medical treatment is ineffective (19–21). Surgical bypass of a major portion of the small intestine has definite value in the control of obesity. This technique is associated with considerable morbidity, however, and is still considered to be experimental by many observers.

The indications for the procedure are generally (1) body weight of more than 150% of normal; (2) massive obesity of more than 5 years' duration with failure of long-term medical management; (3) associated complications of obesity, such as hypertension, diabetes mellitus, and hypercholesterolemia; (4) absence of endocrine and other somatic disorders such as Cushing's disease and severe liver disease (19–21). Evidence of patient willingness to cooperate in preoperative and postoperative management and the absence of severe psychiatric aberration are further considerations.

Cirrhosis is a contraindication to the procedure, although impaired liver function without evidence of cirrhosis is not considered a contraindication. Mental retardation and alcoholism are considered relative contraindications. It is preferred that the procedure be carried out at any early age. Patients past the age of 50–55 years are more prone to develop complications following this procedure.

There are currently two types of surgical procedures utilized to bypass the majority of the absorptive surface of the intestinal tract (19-21) (Fig. 8-10): the end-to-side jejunoileostomy (Payne-DeWind) and the end-to-end jejunoileostomy (Scott).

Most weight loss, up to 40%, occurs in the first 40–80 weeks (19,20). The end-to-side jejunoileal shunt produces less weight loss than the end-to-end jejunoileal shunt (21). The latter, however, is accompanied by a higher rate of complications. There may be variable degrees of weight gain occurring 2–4 years after the proce-

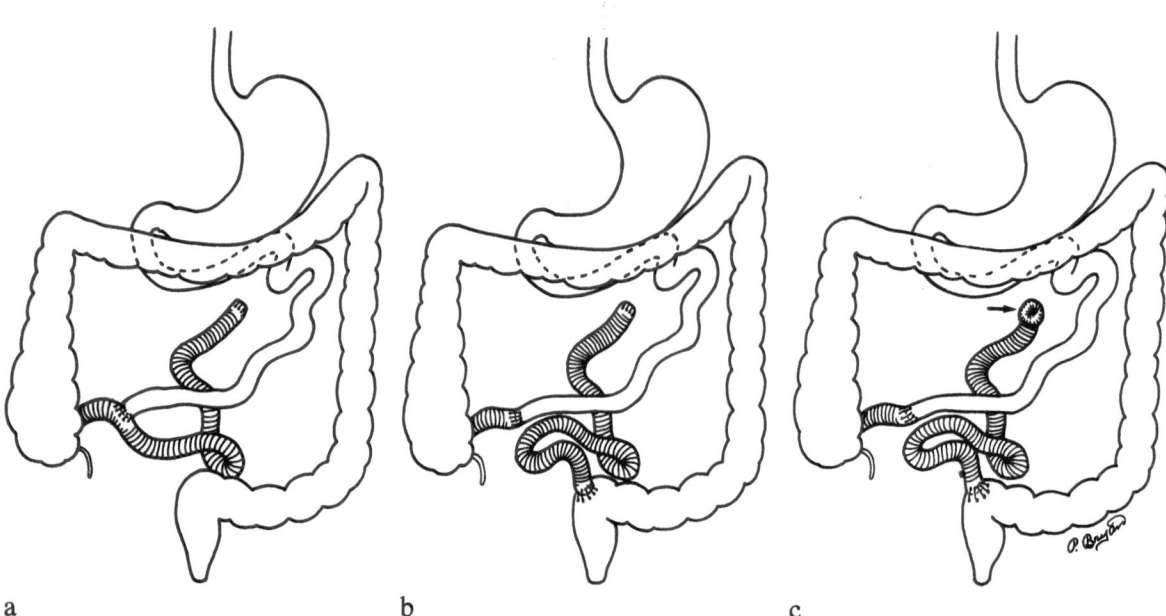

a   b   c

Fig. 8-10, a–c. Jejunoileal bypass procedures. a In the end-to-side jejunoileostomy (Payne-DeWind) the jejunum is divided approximately 40 cm distal to the ligament of Treitz and anastomosed end-to-side to the ileum approximately 15 cm proximal to the ileocecal valve. The proximal end of the bypassed small intestine is closed blindly and left within the abdominal cavity. **b** In the end-to-end jejunoileostomy (Scott) the jejunum is divided approximately 30 cm distal to the ligament of Treitz and anastomosed end-to-end to the ileum, approximately 15–30 cm from the ileocecal valve. The proximal end of the bypassed small intes- tine is closed blindly and left within the abdomen. The distal end of the bypassed small bowel is anastomosed end-to-side to the sigmoid, transverse, or right colon for drainage. **c** In a modification of the end-to-end jejunoileostomy (Scott) the proximal end of the bypassed small bowel is brought out as a jejunostomy to the abdominal wall *(arrow)*. This modification provides an entrance for alimentation in the event of severe nitrogen imbalance, impaired liver function, or electrolyte imbalance. The jejunostomy also provides a route for the radiologist to investigate the bypassed small bowel by injecting contrast material into the jejunostomy.

dure (19). This may be attributed to hypertrophy of the functioning intestine.

There is probably no elective surgical procedure performed on the intestinal tract that is associated with as many and varied complications as the jejunoileal bypass procedure. The overall mortality from the procedure has been reported as 6%, including postoperative complications and late death (22).

Diarrhea is a constant sequela of the procedure as a result of osmotic effect of unabsorbed bile and fatty acids (20). Usually the degree of diarrhea gradually decreases, and after 1 year only a few patients complain of diarrhea (19). In one series the bypass procedure had to be partially refunctionalized in 8% because of intractable diarrhea (23). Electrolyte disturbances occur as the result of rapid intestinal transit and diarrhea. The most serious late complication of the procedure is liver disease. In a review of the literature Hallberg et al. reported 13 deaths due to liver injury in 1165 cases (19). Possible explanations for the liver injury include protein malnutrition, altered biliary metabolism, and formation of toxic materials within the bypassed intestinal tract secondary to bacterial action (20,24). Arthritis and arthralgias similar to those associated with inflammatory bowel disease may occur. The only radiographic change that has been described is juxtaarticular demineralization (25,26).

Radiologic examination plays an important part in diagnosis and management of many complications of the jejunoileal bypass procedure. Reflux into the bypassed ileum may normally occur from the small intestine following the end-to-side procedure and from the colon following the end-to-end procedure (23,27). Filling of an 8–12-cm segment is not considered to be of significance, but if reflux occurs into a longer segment it may be of significance and account for poor weight loss.

The size and length of the functioning segment of the intestine frequently increase (23,26,28) (Fig. 8-11). The mucosal pattern of the bypassed segment thickens, secondary to villous hypertrophy (27,28). The most impressive changes are seen in the terminal ileum with so-called jejunization (Fig. 8-12). These changes may account for stabilization of the weight following the procedure.

Mechanical small intestinal obstruction is the most common complication of the jejunoileal bypass procedure. In a retrospective analysis of

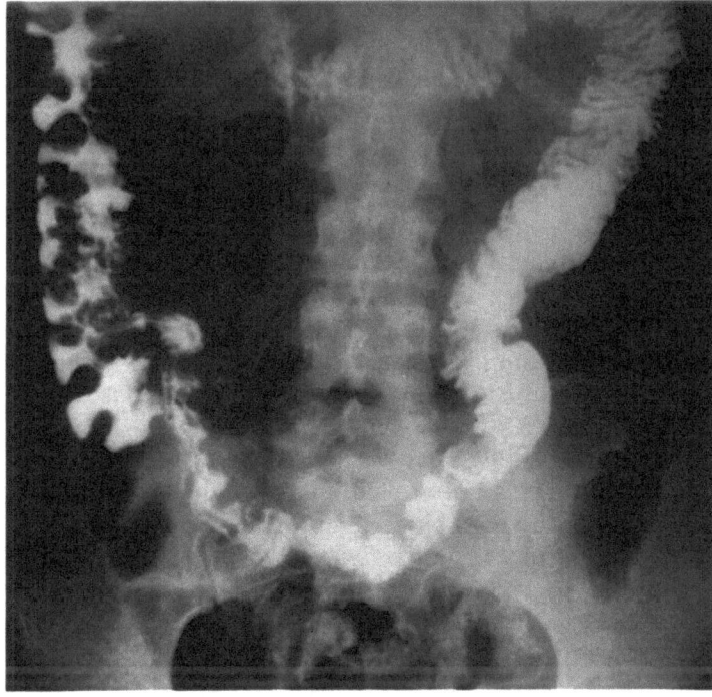

Fig. 8-11. End-to-end jejunoileostomy. Small bowel study 2 years after operation demonstrates dilatation and elongation of the functioning small bowel with hypertrophy of the mucosal folds of the jejunum and ileum.

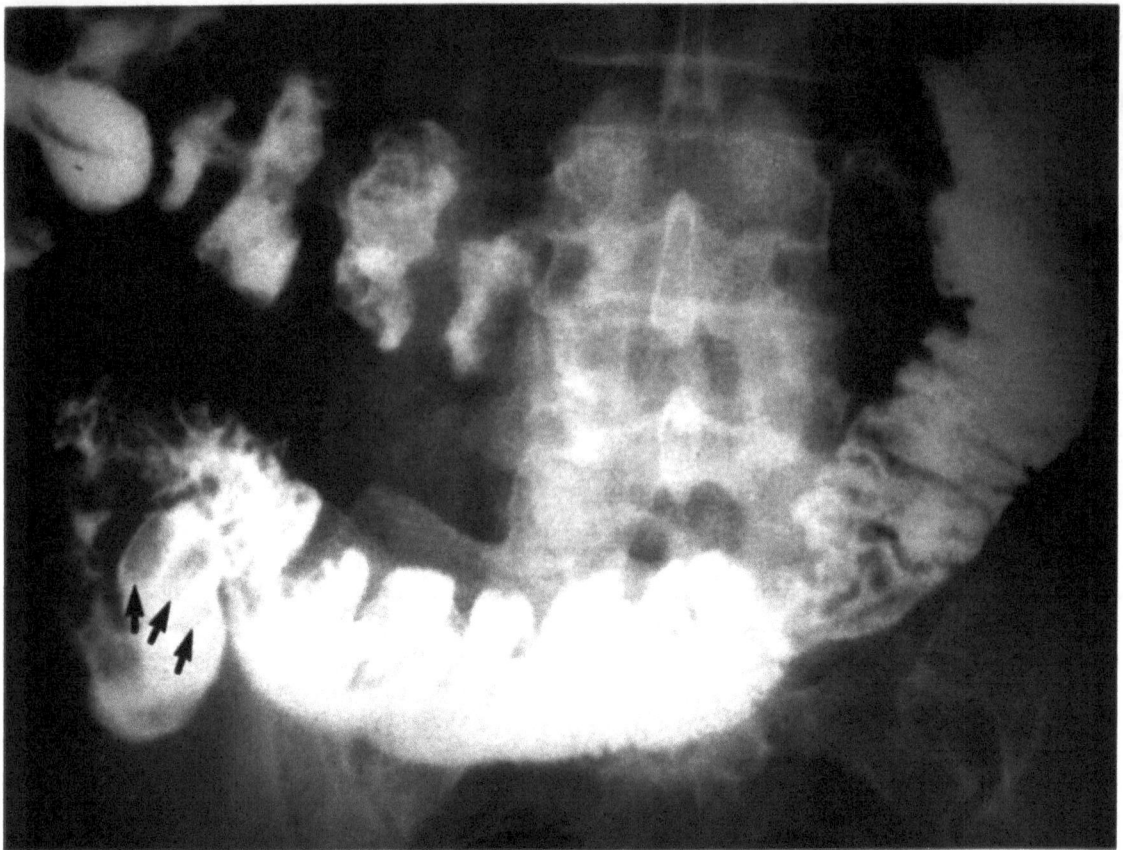

Fig. 8-12. End-to-end jejunoileostomy. The ileum distal to the anastomosis demonstrates "jejunization" of the mucosa. The *arrows* indicate unabsorbed medication in the colon.

89 patients, Moss et al. found the incidence of obstruction to be 10.1% (28). Jejunoileal intussusception, volvulus (Figs. 8-13, 8-14), and incarcerated hernia accounted for most. Half of the obstructions occurred within 2 weeks of surgery, and all were diagnosed by barium contrast examination of the small bowel or by plain films. Sanders (29) and Menguy (30) have reported three cases of volvulus of the sigmoid colon or ileosigmoid junction following the end-to-end (Scott) procedure in patients with symptoms suggestive of "bypass enteritis" or paralytic ileus. Both authors point out that the end-to-side ileosigmoidostomy with a mobile sigmoid loop and mobile ileum predisposes to rotation and volvulus. Sanders suggested that an ileotransverse colostomy be employed rather than ileosigmoidostomy in patients undergoing the end-to-end procedure to avoid this complication.

Dilatation of the colon and of small intestinal loops with air-fluid levels but without evidence of organic obstruction is encountered not uncommonly following the jejunoileal bypass procedure. Wade et al. observed dilatation of the colon to a diameter of more than 7 cm in 50% of 38 patients (23). The colon may be dilated to the point that mechanical obstruction is strongly suggested from plain films (22,31). Barium contrast studies are indicated before a diagnosis of mechanical obstruction of the colon can be made. In a review of 47 patients at the Emory University affiliated hospitals who had follow-up examinations after the jejunoileal bypass procedure, plain films were strongly suggestive in six cases of colonic or small intestinal obstruction (Figs. 8-15, 8-16).

Bypass enteritis has been suggested as a cause of the megacolon and pseudo-obstruction (25, 26,31). This enteropathy is attributed to an inflammatory process with invasion by intestinal bacteria within the bypassed small bowel rather than the sequelae of surgically produced short-bowel syndrome. This enteropathy may mimic a surgical intraabdominal emergency (25).

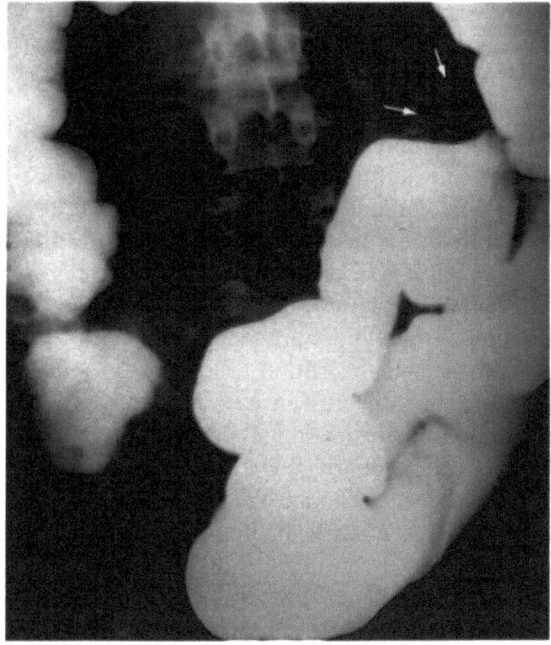

a

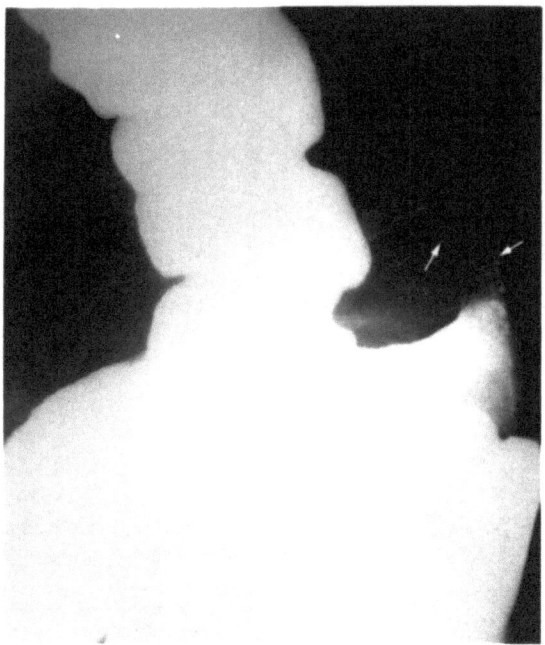

b

Fig. 8-13, a and b. Mechanical obstruction of bypassed small bowel after end-to-end jejunoileostomy. This was secondary to volvulus at the ileosigmoid anastomosis. a Barium enema examination demonstrates complete filling of the colon. The *arrows* indicate a small channel at the site of ileosigmoidostomy. b Oblique film demonstrates the typical beaked appearance of volvulus of the ileum at the ileosigmoid anastomosis *(arrows)*.

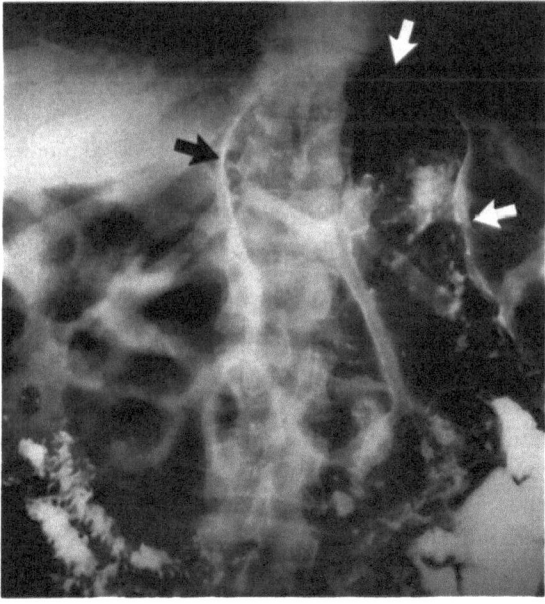

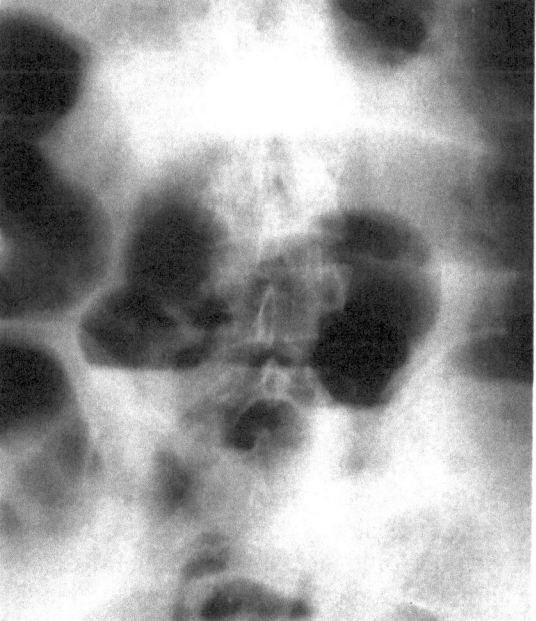

Fig. 8-14. Volvulus and partial obstruction of a segment of bypassed small intestine after modified end-to-end jejunoileostomy. This was demonstrated on small bowel study by way of the feeding jejunostomy. The *arrows* indicate a dilated segment of the bypassed small bowel.

Fig. 8-15. Intestinal pseudo-obstruction following end-to-end jejunoileostomy. Erect film of abdomen indicates distention of both large and small intestinal loops in a patient with no clinical evidence of mechanical obstruction.

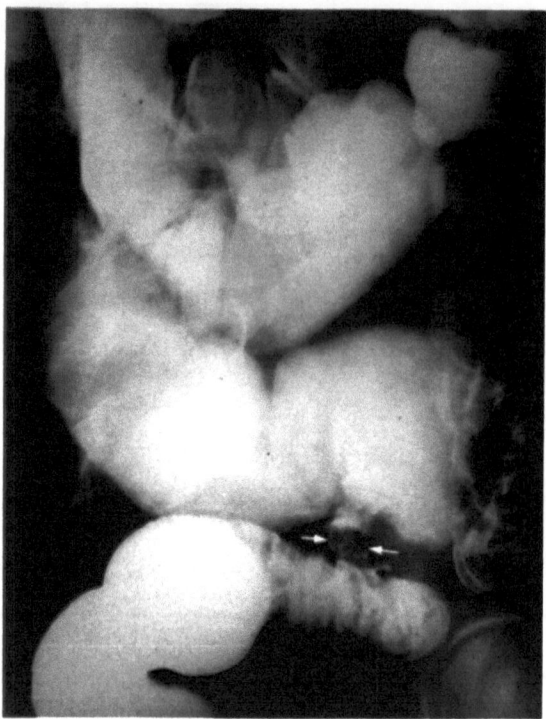

Fig. 8-16. Filling of markedly dilated bypassed small bowel after end-to-end jejunoileostomy. Barium enema study shows that there is filling by way of the ileosigmoidostomy *(arrows).* The dilated loops of small bowel were seen to empty completely on a postevacuation film, ruling out organic obstruction at the anastomosis.

There is an increased incidence (10%–14%) of renal calculi postoperatively (22,28,32,33). Most are composed of calcium oxalate (32). Hyperoxaluria is almost always present following the jejunoileal bypass procedure; the mechanism is still uncertain and has been attributed to bacterial degradation of the glycine-conjugated bile salts in the colon with production of large amounts of glyoxalate, which is then reabsorbed from the intestine and metabolized in the liver to form oxalate (32). A more important source of increased urinary oxalate appears to be the absorption of oxalate directly from the intestinal tract due to binding of calcium ions with the fecal fats, reducing the amount of calcium available for forming a complex with the oxalate to render a more insoluble form of oxalate (32). There is also an increased incidence of uric acid calculi attributable to the patient's anabolic state and dehydration (32,33). It is postulated that the increased clearance of uric acid following the bypass procedure may form a potential nidus for subsequent growth of oxalate calculi (32).

An increased incidence of acute cholecystitis also develops after the jejunoileal bypass procedure (28). It has been observed to occur in patients having normal gallbladders as well as those with cholelithiasis with no evidence of cholecystitis at the time of the bypass procedure. Radiologic evaluation of the gallbladder is recommended preoperatively; if it is found to contain calculi or demonstrate any evidence of disease, cholecystectomy should be performed at the time of the bypass procedure (28).

With the malabsorption following the jejunoileal bypass procedure, it is to be expected that absorption of medication is also decreased (Fig. 8-12). This is true for medications used in treatment of electrolyte disturbances, psychiatric difficulties, birth control medication, and the oral gallbladder contrast media. Little reliance can be placed upon nonvisualization of the gallbladder by oral cholecystography in this group of patients (23). All patients with nonvisualization of the gallbladder following 2 days of medication should undergo intravenous cholangiography before gallbladder disease is diagnosed.

Another striking complication of the procedure is the development of intestinal pneumatosis (34–38). Feinberg et al. observed pneumatosis intestinalis in 24 of 148 patients (36). Symptoms varied from none to nausea and vomiting and abdominal distress. None were considered for abdominal surgery on the basis of their clinical findings. Clements has observed pneumatosis in six patients, in all of whom the course was benign (35). The pneumatosis was observed to develop from 10 days to 30 months following the procedure. Involvement is most commonly confined to the colon (Figs. 8-17, 8-18), primarily the right colon, but, the pneumatosis may involve the bypassed small intestine (Fig. 8-19) or rarely both (34) (Fig. 8-20). The occurrence of pneumatosis appears to be more common in patients undergoing the end-to-end (Scott) procedure than the end-to-side (Payne-DeWind) procedure.

The pattern of the pneumatosis is similar to that of mechanical or infectious origin rather than the benign idiopathic form (pneumatosis cystoides intestinalis) in which large cyst-like collections of gas accumulate in the bowel wall. Since the pattern may thus suggest changes secondary to intestinal ischemia or necrotizing enterocolitis, the radiologist should avoid the pitfall of suggesting a catastrophic event, which

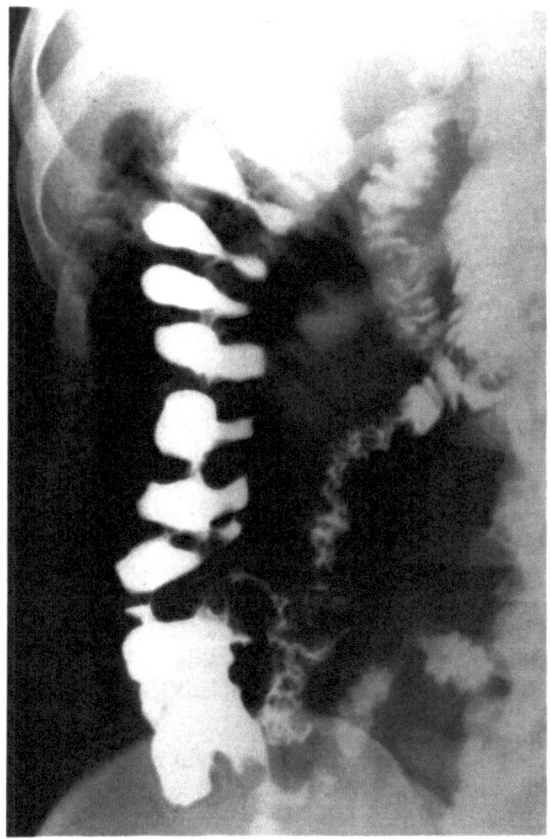

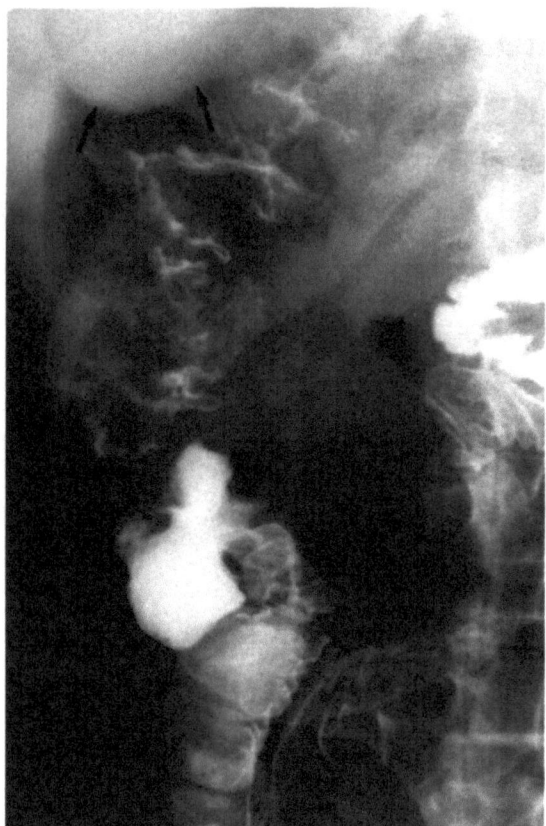

Fig. 8-17. Extensive pneumatosis involving the ascending colon after jejunoileal bypass. The patient had no symptoms referable to the intestinal tract. (Clements JL Jr: Intestinal pneumatosis—A complication of the jejuno-ileal bypass procedure. Gastrointest Radiol 2:267–271, 1977)

Fig. 8-18. Pneumatosis involving the ascending colon after jejunoileal bypass. The patient had intractable diarrhea, requiring takedown of the bypass. Free air within the peritoneal cavity is localized to the subhepatic area on this recumbent film. *Arrows* indicate the inferior margin of the gallbladder outlined by the free intraperitoneal air. (Clements JL Jr: Intestinal pneumatosis—A complication of the jejuno-ileal bypass procedure. Gastrointest Radiol 2:267–271, 1977)

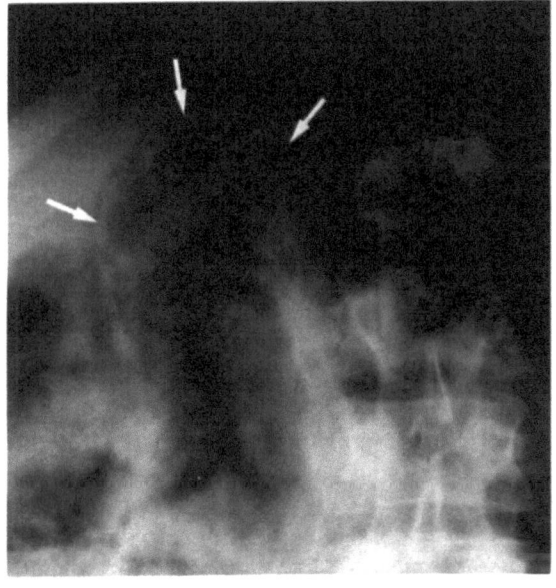

Fig. 8-19. Intestinal pneumatosis involving the bypassed small bowel *(arrows)*. The patient was asymptomatic and was admitted for elective cholecystectomy. Free air was in the peritoneal cavity. At surgery pneumatosis was documented, and there was no evidence of peritonitis. (Clements JL Jr: Intestinal pneumatosis—A complication of the jejuno-ileal bypass procedure. Gastrointest Radiol 2:267–271, 1977)

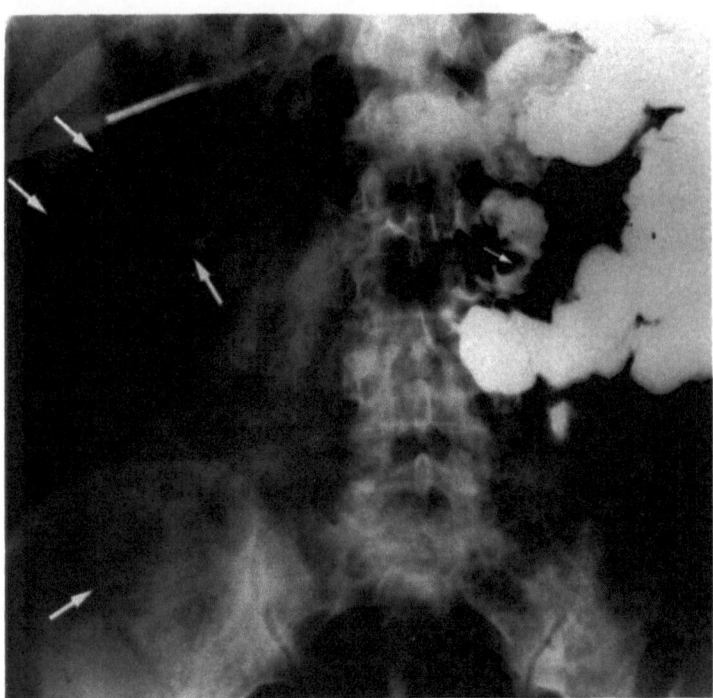

Fig. 8-20. Intestinal pneumatosis involving the bypassed small intestine and right colon. Pneumatosis of the right colon is indicated by the *larger arrows*. The small bowel study by way of the feeding jejunostomy demonstrates nodularity of the small bowel wall produced by intramural gas cysts *(small arrow)*. (Clements JL Jr: Intestinal pneumatosis—A complication of the jejuno-ileal bypass procedure. Gastrointest Radiol 2:267–271, 1977)

may lead to unnecessary surgery. Sterile pneumoperitoneum may accompany the process (Fig. 8-18). Clements observed free air in the peritoneal cavity in three of six cases of intestinal pneumatosis following jejunoileal bypass (35). None had evidence of peritonitis.

The origin of the intestinal pneumatosis is obscure. Mechanical and infectious origins have been suggested. Martyak and Curtis have pointed out that colonic intraluminal pressure is higher than the ileal intraluminal pressure and suggested dissection of gas from the intestinal lumen at the ileosigmoid anastomotic line in patients undergoing the end-to-end procedure with ileosigmoidostomy (38). Menguy has reported intestinal pneumatosis secondary to obstruction due to sigmoid volvulus in a patient with ileosigmoidostomy (30). Drenick et al. have suggested an inflammatory basis for pneumatosis, after observing pneumatosis in two patients with bypass enteritis (32).

The treatment of pneumatosis intestinalis in a patient who has had bypass is conservative. This condition appears to be asymptomatic and self-limited in most patients. It has been documented to respond to oxygen inhalation, 70%–75% by mask (35,39). However, Ganel et al. have reported a case of chronic pneumatosis intestinalis involving the bypassed small intestine that resulted in irreversible segmental mucosal atrophy and mural fibrosis, which was treated by resection (40).

Blind Loop Syndrome

The blind (stagnant) loop syndrome is a clinical syndrome of diarrhea-steatorrhea, weight loss, and macrocytic anemia secondary to intestinal stasis and small bowel bacterial overgrowth.

The surgical causes include (1) intestinal anastomosis resulting in a "blind pouch" formation or recirculation of small intestinal contents; (2) afferent loop dysfunction following gastrojejunostomy; (3) gastrojejuno-colic fistula; and (4) partial obstruction secondary to adhesions or strictures (41).

In infants and children the syndrome occurs most often as a result of surgical treatment of ileal atresia, jejunal stenosis or atresia, and duodenal atresia (42,43).

Some authors differentiate between the blind loop syndrome and the blind pouch syndrome (44,45). The blind pouch syndrome occurs as a result of a side-to-side intestinal anastomosis with subsequent dilatation of the proximal intestinal segment secondary to the motility disturbances from division of the circular muscles during the surgical procedure (44). The classic blind loop syndrome occurs as a result of bypassing a segment of small intestine by an enteroanastomosis. In addition to malabsorption, the conditions may be associated with abdominal cramps, intestinal hemorrhage, and perforation. Many months or years may lapse between the time of intestinal surgery and the onset of symptoms attributable to the blind pouch or blind loop syndrome (41).

The mechanism whereby bacterial proliferation within the small intestine produces the syndrome is attributed to bacterial hydrolysis of conjugated bile salts, leading to a deficiency of bile salts and resultant steatorrhea. Direct bacterial uptake of vitamin B_{12} results in macrocytic anemia. The involved intestinal pouch may ulcerate and bleed and result in iron deficiency anemia (41).

Radiographic examination plays an important part in diagnostic evaluation. Plain films of the abdomen may be of value in demonstrating an intestinal gas pattern of partial mechanical obstruction or abnormal gas accumulations or air-fluid levels in the dilated blind pouch (45). Barium-contrast small intestinal study usually indicates the dilated blind pouch (44,45) (Fig. 8-21), afferent-loop dysfunction following gastrojejunostomy, enteric fistula, or evidence of partial obstruction. Barium enema study may be of value when the previous surgical procedure had been performed in the ileocecal area, where the terminal ileum may be refluxed with demonstration of a blind pouch, and in cases of suspected gastrojejunocolic fistula.

Surgical revision of a localized abnormality causing small bowel stasis is the treatment of choice (41). This is particularly true in blind loops produced by side-to-side anastomosis, afferent-loop syndrome, enteric fistula and partial obstruction secondary to peritoneal adhesions or stricture. In patients in whom surgery is not feasible, or when the underlying cause is extensive, long-term antibiotic therapy to suppress intraluminal bacterial proliferation is utilized along with appropriate administration of nutrients and vitamins (41).

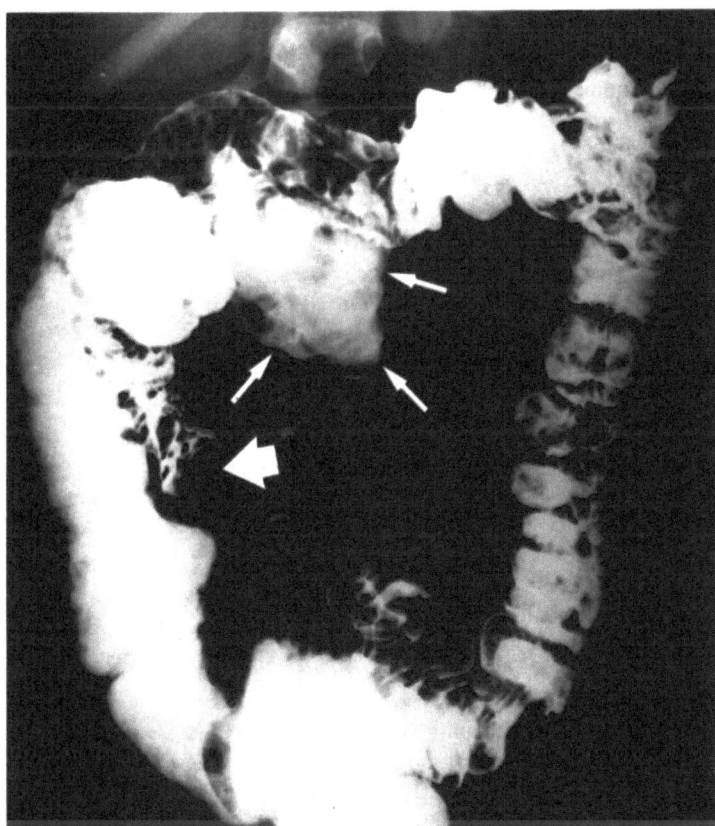

Fig. 8-21. Blind loop syndrome. A small bowel follow-through in a 10-year-old male who as a neonate had undergone a 25-cm terminal ileum resection for ileal atresia with a side-to-side ileal-transverse colostomy. Since the age of 1 year he had chronic malabsorption and anemia, which responded to treatment with iron and parenterally administered vitamin B_{12}. The *small arrows* indicate a 10-cm blind pouch of ileum in the region of the ileocolostomy with dilatation of the ileum proximal to this pouch. The *large arrow* indicates the blind-ending cecum.

Complications of Colostomy

Colostomy is a surgical procedure frequently employed to divert the fecal stream from a distal process such as perforation or colonic anastomosis and to decompress the colon proximal to an obstructing lesion. Colostomies are also produced as permanent structures when the distal colon, rectum, and anus have been removed.

There are three basic types of colostomy procedures (46):

1) *Loop colostomy*, including exteriorizing colostomy, resectional colostomy, and Mikulicz colostomy: In this procedure both the proximal and distal segments of the colon are brought through the same abdominal wall defect.

2) *End colostomy:* Only a single stoma is produced with the proximal colonic segment. The distal segment is left blindly closed within the abdominal cavity. Restoration of continuity in this type of colostomy is difficult.

3) *Divided-stoma colostomy:* In this procedure the proximal and distal segments of the colostomy are brought through separate abdominal wall defects. This type is most effective in diverting the fecal stream from the colon distal to the colostomy.

The complications of temporary and permanent colostomies include obstruction and abscess formation. Local complications at the colostomy site may be diagnosed clinically, including strictures, retraction, and prolapse. Hernias of both colon and small bowel (47), and rarely of the stomach (48), may develop at the colostomy site. Radiographic examination plays a minor role in the management of these complications.

Before closure of a temporary colostomy it is customary to evaluate its proximal and distal segments radiographically. The radiologist bears the responsibility of ruling out obstruction, persistent perforation, or inflammatory disease of the distal segment, which would preclude closure.

Anorectal Complications

Complications following surgery and instrumentation of the rectosigmoid can occur despite good technique. They are usually due to destruction of anatomic structures and barriers that are necessary for normal function. Several of the complications are common to all colonic operations, including wound infection, wound disruption and fistula formation, sepsis, and ileus. Frequently these complications coexist. Anastomotic dehiscence can lead to all simultaneously (49–51).

Postoperative wound infections vary from superficial to irreversible with subsequent death. Organisms found in the gastrointestinal tract account for one-half of the wound infections (51).

Anastomotic dehiscence and fistula are more frequent in sigmoid and anterior resections than in right or transverse colonic surgery. Fistula on the right usually requires reoperation, while fistula formation on the left with a drainage tract does not require reoperation if obstruction is not present (49). If the patient is having bowel movements the rectal fistula will usually close spontaneously. Obstruction at the anastomotic site is infrequent and is usually temporary, secondary to either edema or inflammation (49).

Rectosigmoid abscess produces, besides the usual signs of infection, diarrhea or increased mucus per rectum or both. A palpable soft, tender boggy mass is felt anterior to the rectum. The abscess usually drains into the rectum (52).

Postoperative ileus is usually shortlived. Peristalsis is present usually within 48–72 hours (49).

Plain films and barium contrast examinations play a minor role in the diagnosis of anorectal surgical complications. However, abdominal and pelvic computed tomography (Fig. 8-22) and ultrasonography (Fig. 8-23) are making increasingly important contributions in the diagnosis of these complications.

Arteriovenous Fistula

An arteriovenous fistula can be either congenital or acquired (traumatic or iatrogenic) and becomes pathologic when significant hemodynamic changes occur because of its location or size (53).

The majority of iatrogenic arteriovenous fistulas result from intestinal and gynecologic surgery (54,55) (Fig. 8-24). Aorto-inferior vena caval fistulas are rare and are always acquired

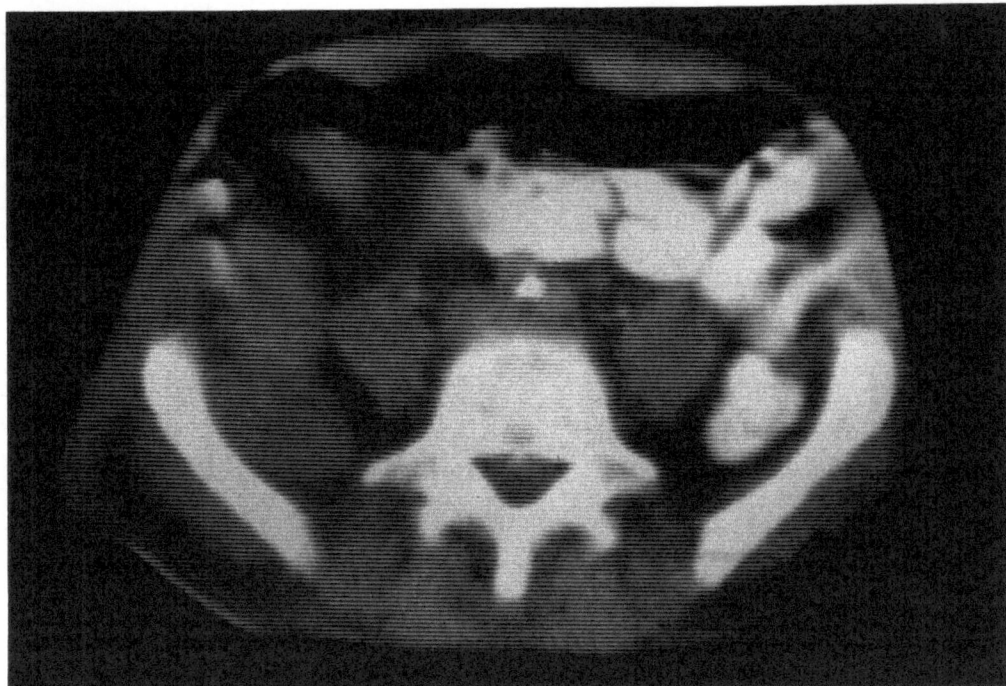

a

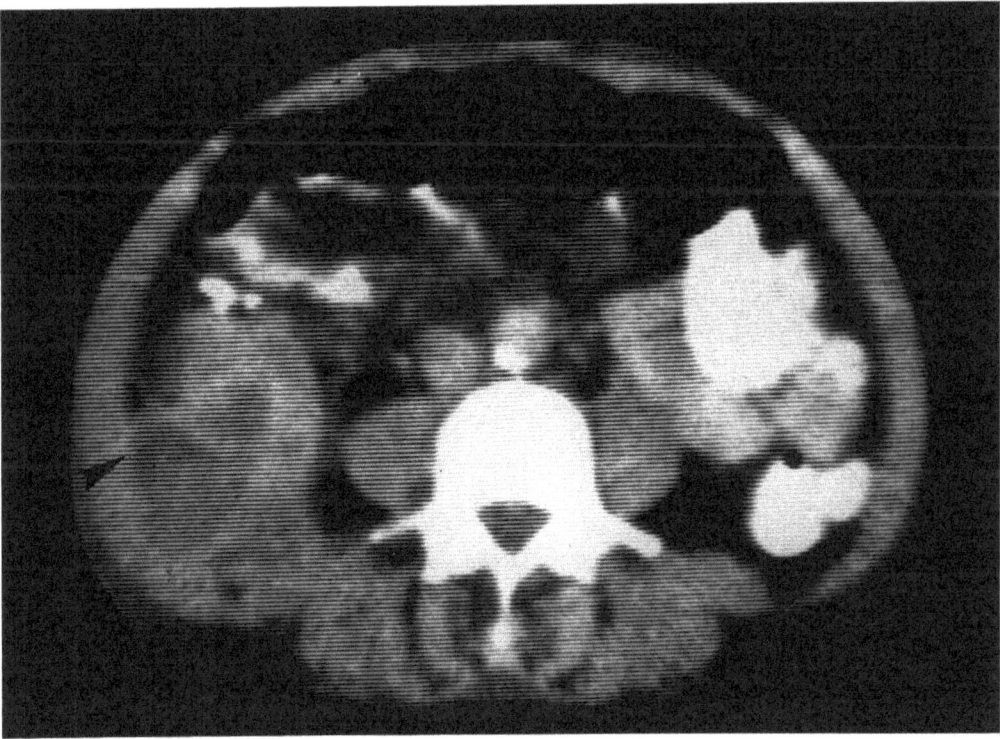

b

Fig. 8-22, a and **b. Retroperitoneal cellulitis and abscess.** Extending from pelvis into the mid-abdominal region, they are secondary to recent anorectal sur-gery. **a** CT scan at level of iliac crest demonstrates mass in right iliac fossa. **b** Scan at midabdominal level reveals upward extension of abscess *(arrowhead).*

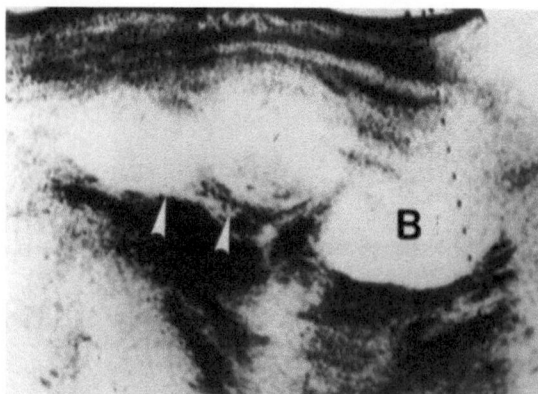

Fig. 8-23. Pelvic abscess. Abscess *(arrowheads)* superior to urinary bladder (*B*) demonstrated by ultrasound midline longitudinal scan.

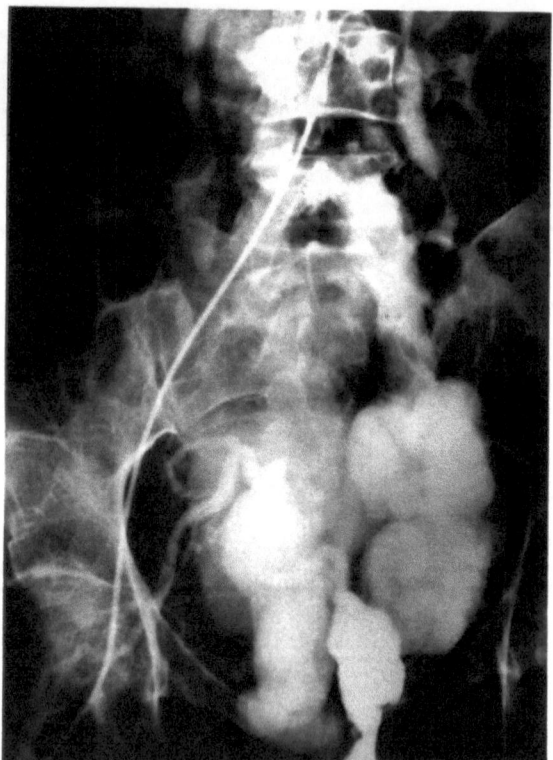

b

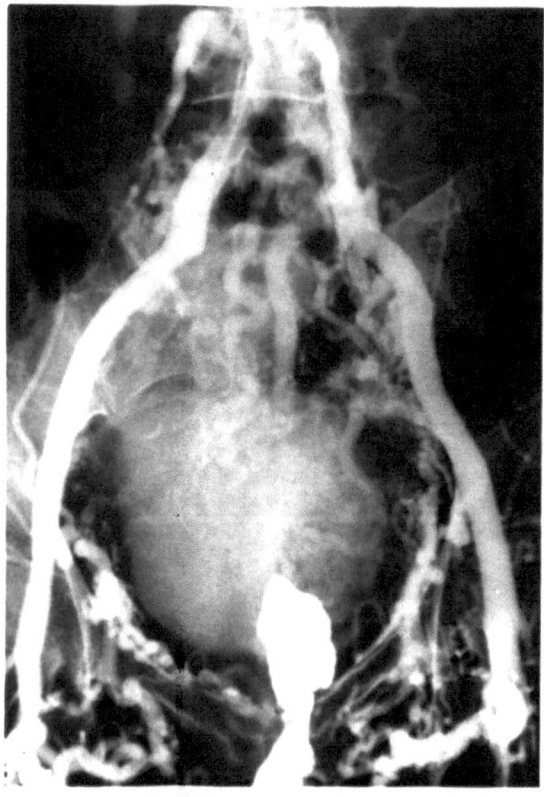

a

Fig. 8-24, a–c. Arteriovenous fistula secondary to pelvic surgery. This type can result from both gynecologic and intestinal surgery. **a** Abdominal aortogram shows multiple arterial feeders. **b** Venous phase demonstrates multiple dilated and tortuous pelvic veins. **c** Midline longitudinal ultrasound scan of pelvis displays multiple cystic areas *(arrowheads)* posterior to urinary bladder (*B*) representing dilated tortuous pelvic vessels.

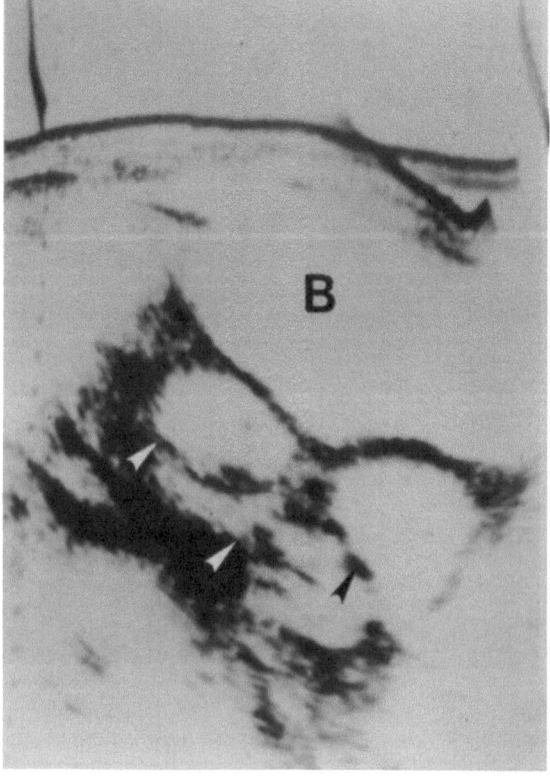

c

(53). They can be iatrogenic—secondary to lumbar disk surgery; traumatic—due to penetrating injury; or spontaneous—as in rupture of an aortic aneurysm into the inferior vena cava. The aorta and inferior vena cava can also be injured inadvertently at the time of intestinal surgery.

Several etiologic factors have been proposed in the occurrence of arteriovenous fistula following surgery. There may be direct injury to the artery and vein during the procedure. One of the most common causes is accidental passage of the surgical needle through the two vessels during suture-ligation of the vascular pedicle; this, of course, creates a direct communication (54, 55). Infection and necrosis of the vessel wall with pseudoaneurysm formation and subsequent communication between an artery and vein have also been described.

Clinical manifestations can be systemic or local (56). Systemic manifestations are those associated with circulatory overload and may present as easy fatigability, dyspnea on exertion, or overt congestive heart failure. Malabsorption may result from large intestinal arteriovenous fistulas. Local manifestations are pain or a pulsatile mass in the area of the lesion. Physical findings usually are a thrill and continuous bruit at the site of the lesion.

A considerable time may elapse between the original operation and presentation of the arteriovenous fistula. Intervals have varied from 2 months to 25 years (57). The diagnosis may not be obvious and is related to systemic blood pressure, the size of the aneurysm, and the size of the shunt. Many cases are diagnosed by physical examination, but arteriography is extensively used for confirmation. Newer methods such as ultrasound (Fig. 8-24) and abdominal computed tomography are also proving valuable (55).

Suture and Starch Granuloma

The development of suture and starch granuloma is secondary to a foreign-body reaction as the result of a surgical procedure (58).

Suture granuloma can simulate a localized benign neoplasm and can appear as an adherent extrinsic mass or an intramural mass. Erosion of granuloma through the peritoneum and into the mesentery has been reported (58).

Starch granuloma results from a hypersensitivity reaction to the cornstarch used as a lubricating agent for surgical gloves (59). Numerous reports have cited the complications caused when talcum powder was used for glove lubrication, but recently, there has been an increase in the number of reported cases attributed to cornstarch for glove lubrication (59–61). Symptoms, which are usually manifest 2–5 weeks postoperatively, characteristically include abdominal pain, paralytic ileus, ascites, a palpable abdominal mass, and low-grade fever. The disease is said to be self-limiting, with most patients recovering after 2–6 weeks. Many patients have nonspecific findings that may disappear without diagnosis. Pathologically the process is similar to granulomatous disease from any foreign body (59). Contrast examination of the small bowel with demonstration of a mass may suggest the possibility of a suture or starch granuloma in the proximity of recent surgery (58,59) (Fig. 8-25).

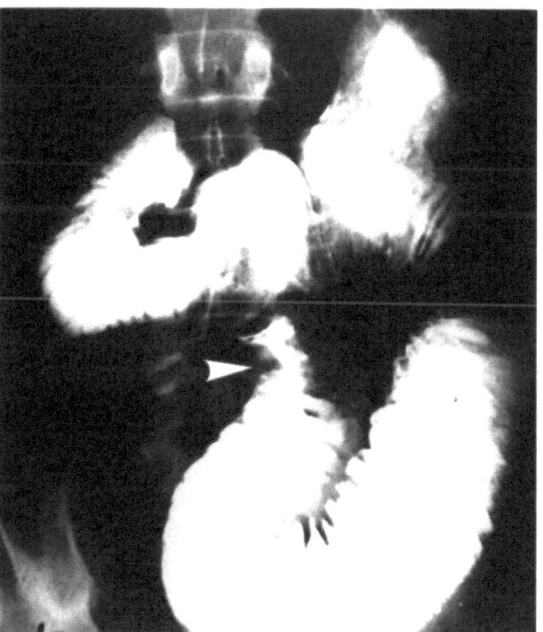

Fig. 8-25. Recurrent starch granulomatous peritonitis. It presented as longstanding paralytic ileus. Small bowel examination demonstrates obstruction of the jejunum (arrowhead). At surgery this was proved to be secondary to a thick adhesion, with multiple peritoneal starch granulomas. (Han SY, Whitten DM: Starch granulomatous peritonitis. Gastrointest Radiol 1:281–283, 1976.)

References

1. Wilson JP: Post-operative motility of the large intestine in man. Gut 16:689–692, 1972
2. Post-operative ileus. (editorial). Lancet 2:1186–1187, 1978
3. Sykes PA, Shofield PF: Early post-operative small bowel obstruction. Br J Surg 61:594–600, 1974
4. Vest B, Margulis AR: The roentgen diagnosis of postoperative Ileus-Obstruction. Surg Gynecol Obstet 115:421–427, 1962
5. Fromm SH: Spontaneous perforation of the cecum due to adynamic ileus. Bol Asoc Med PR 70:217–218, 1978
6. Stuart JR: Short bowel syndrome. RI Med J 56:66–71, 1973
7. MacKenzie GW, Boileau GR, St. Clair WR: Short gut syndrome: A review with case report. Can J Surg 16:3–11, 1973
8. Buxton B: Progress report—Small bowel resection and gastric acid hypersecretion. Gut 15:229–238, 1934
9. Hislop IG, Grant AK: The sequelae of small intestinal resection and homeostatic role of the terminal ileum. Med J Aust 2:963–965, 1970
10. Heizer WD, Orringer EP: Parenteral nutrition at home for 5 years via arteriovenous fistula. Supplemental feedings for a patient with severe short bowel syndrome. Gastroenterology 72:527–532, 1977
11. Cortot A, Fleming RC, Malagelada JR: Improved nutrient absorption after cimetidine in short-bowel syndrome with gastric hypersecretion. N Engl J Med 300:79–80, 1979
12. Murphy JP Jr, King DR, Dubois A: Treatment of gastric hypersecretion with cimetidine in the short-bowel syndrome. N Engl J Med 300:80–81, 1979
13. Perlman MM, Stein A, Shamroth L: Reversal of an intestinal segment in the long-term management of the short-bowel syndrome. S Afr Med J 46:1730–1733, 1972
14. Kock NG: Intra-abdominal "reservoir" in patients with permanent ileostomy. Arch Surg 99:223–231, 1969
15. Kock NG: Continent ileostomy. Prog Surg 12:180–201, 1973
16. Kock NG: Present status of the continent ileostomy. Dis Colon Rectum 19:200–212, 1976
17. Diner WC, Cockrill HH: The continent ileostomy (Kock pouch): Roentgenologic features. Gastrointest Radiol 4:65–73, 1979
18. Montagne JP, Kressel HY, Moss AA, et al: Radiologic evaluation of the continent (Kock) ileostomy. Radiology 127:325–329, 1978
19. Hallberg D, Backman L, Espmark S: Surgical treatment of obesity. Prog Surg 14:46–83, 1975
20. Current status of jejuno-ileal bypass for obesity. Nutr Rev 32:333–336, 1974
21. Scott WH Jr, Dean RH, Shull HJ, et al: Surgical management of morbid obesity; current consider-

ations in the use of extensive jejuno-ileal bypass. S Med J 69:789–798, 1976
22. Fikri E, Cassella RR: Jejuno-ileal bypass for massive obesity: Results and complications in 52 patients. Ann Surg 179:460–464, 1974
23. Wade DH, Richards V, Burhenne HJ: Radiographic changes after small bowel bypass for morbid obesity. Radiol Clin North Am 14:493–498, 1976
24. Galambos JT: Jejuno-ileal bypass and nutritional liver injury. Arch Pathol Lab Med 100:229–232, 1976
25. Drenick EJ, Ament ME, Finegold SM, et al: Bypass enteropathy, intestinal and systemic manifestations following small bowel bypass. JAMA 236:269–272, 1976
26. Drenick EJ, Ament ME, Finegold SM, et al: Bypass enteropathy: An inflammatory process in the excluded segment with systemic complications. Am J Clin Nutr 30:76–89, 1977
27. Balthazar EJ, Goldfine S: Jejuno-ileal bypass: Roentgenographic observations. Am J Roentgenol 125:138–142, 1975
28. Moss AA, Goldberg HI, Koehler RE: Radiographic evaluation of complications after jejuno-ileal bypass surgery. Am J Roentgenol 127:737–741, 1976
29. Sanders GB: Bypass enteritis or obstructive volvulus? Arch Surg 112:668, 1977
30. Menguy R: Pneumatosis intestinalis after jejunoileal bypass: Etiological mechanism in one case. JAMA 236:1721–1724, 1976
31. Barry RE, Benfield JR, Nicell P, et al: Colonic pseudo-obstruction: A new complication of jejuno-ileal bypass. Gut 16:903–908, 1975
32. Thomas MH, Madura JA: Urolithiasis after intestinal bypass for morbid obesity. Urology 9:170–172, 1977
33. O'Leary JP, Thomas WC Jr., Woodward ER: Urinary tract stone after small bowel bypass for morbid obesity. Am J Surg 127:142–147, 1974
34. Meyers MA, Ghahremani GG, Clements JL Jr., et al: Pneumatosis intestinalis. Gastrointest Radiol 2:91–105, 1977
35. Clements JL Jr: Intestinal pneumatosis—A complication of the jejuno-ileal bypass procedure. Gastrointest Radiol 2:267–271, 1977
36. Feinberg SB, Schwartz MZ, Clifford S, et al: Significance of pneumatosis cystoides intestinalis after jejuno-ileal bypass. Am J Surg 133:149–152, 1977
37. Wandtke J, Skucas J, Spataro R, et al: Pneumatosis intestinalis as a complication of jejuno-ileal bypass. Am J Roentgenol 129:601–604, 1977
38. Martyak SN, Curtis LE: Pneumatosis intestinalis—A complication of jejuno-ileal bypass. JAMA 235:1038–1039, 1976
39. Forgacs P, Wright PH, Wyatt AP: Treatment of intestinal gas cysts by oxygen breathing. Lancet 1:579–581, 1973
40. Ganel A, Haspel Y, Ben-Ari G, et al: Surgical treatment for pneumatosis cystoides intestinalis

complicating jejuno-ileal bypass. Am J Gastroenterol 71:306–310, 1979

41. Donaldson RM Jr.: The blind loop syndrome. In Gastrointestinal Disease, volume II Sleisenger MH, Fordtran JS (eds): 2nd edn. Philadelphia: Saunders 1978, pp 1094-1095, 1101-1102

42. Schreiner RL, Ternberg JL, Shackelford GD, et al: The stagnant loop syndrome in childhood; review and report of four patients. Am J Dig Dis 20:23–30, 1975

43. Challacombe DN, Richardson JM, Edkins S, et al: Ileal blind loop in childhood. Am J Dis Child 128:719–723, 1974

44. Maglinte DT: "Blind pouch" syndrome—A cause of gastrointestinal bleeding. Radiology 132:314, 1979

45. Levine M, Katz I, Lampros PJ: Blind pouch formation secondary to side-to-side intestinal anastomosis. Am J. Roentgenol 89:706–719, 1963

46. Colin I Jr, Nance FC: The colon and rectum. In Sabiston DC Jr (ed): Davis-Christopher Textbook of Surgery, 11th edn. Philadelphia: Saunders 1977, pp 1080–1083

47. Welch CE, Hedberg SE: Complications in surgery of the colon and rectum. In Artz CP, Hardy JD (eds): Complications in Surgery and Their Management, 2nd edn. Philadelphia: Saunders 1967, pp 600–603

48. Cohn HE, Deardoff CL Jr.: Volvulus of the stomach—Complications of colostomy. Arch Surg 88:1013–1015, 1964

49. Rousselot LM, Slattery JR; Immediate complications of surgery of the large intestines. Surg Clin North Am 44:397–410, 1964

50. Hedberg SE, Welch CE: Complications following surgery of the colon. Surg Clin North Am 43:775–788, 1963

51. Smith EB: Complications of colon and rectal surgery. JAMA 60:386–390, 1968

52. Heidenreich A: Anorecto-colonic iatrogenic wounds. Prensa Med Argent 57:436–439, 1970

53. Gomes MM, Bernatz PE: Arteriovenous fistula: A review and ten year experience at the Mayo Clinic. Mayo Clin Proc 45:81-102, 1970

54. Rossi PA, Carillo FG, Alfidi RJ, et al: Iatrogenic arteriovenous fistulas. Radiology 111:47, 1974

55. Torres WE, Sones PJ, Thames FM: Ultrasound appearance of a pelvic arteriovenous malformation: Case report. J Clin Ultrasound 7:383–385, 1979

56. Ellis R, Saunders WG: Acquired pelvic arteriovenous fistulae: Case report and literature review. Milit Med 137:308–310, 1972

57. Colvin GL: Pelvic arteriovenous fistula: Report of a case and review of literature. J Am Osteopath Assoc 74:325–330, 1974

58. Golden R, Cimmino CV: Digestive tract. Golden's Diagnostic Roentgenology, Sect 5 (Robbins, LL, ed.). Baltimore: Williams & Wilkins 1969, pp 5.681–5.682

59. Han SY, Whitten DM: Starch granulomatous peritonitis. Gastrointest Radiol 1:281–283, 1976

60. Sneierson H, Woo ZP: Starch powder granuloma: A report of two cases. Ann Surg 142:1045–1050, 1955

61. Ignatus JA, Hartman WH: The glove starch peritonitis syndrome. Ann Surg 175:398–402, 1972

9 Hemorrhage Complicating Gastrointestinal Surgery

Gary G. Ghahremani, Morton A. Meyers, Sven-Ola Hietala, and William H. Brewer

Even in the era of modern medicine the occurrence of internal bleeding after operation on the digestive organs frequently presents a formidable diagnostic and therapeutic challenge. Conventional radiographic techniques often fail to indicate the source of hemorrhage. Postoperative examination of the gastrointestinal tract with barium or an iodinated contrast medium may reveal multiple abnormalities, each capable of being the potential bleeding point. The task is made further difficult by the presence of postsurgical plication defects and distortion of anatomic landmarks (1–4). Fortunately the widespread application of arteriography and fiberoptic endoscopy has significantly reduced the number of cases of unexplained postoperative bleeding, often eliminating the necessity for reexploration of the patient (5–8).

Etiology of Postoperative Bleeding

Among various gastrointestinal operations, partial gastrectomy is commonly complicated by subsequent hemorrhage. The incidence has been reported to be 3% (2). However, in patients who are initially operated upon because of gastric bleeding the incidence of postoperative rebleeding is markedly higher (30%–50%) (2,9).

Many different causes of bleeding after gastrointestinal surgery have been described in the literature (11–16). Some of these are considered iatrogenic while others are more clearly defined as the inherent risk of operative procedure. The possible causes include the following:

Misplaced or slipped sutures
Bleeding sites overlooked during initial operation
Recurrent or marginal ulcer
Postoperative coagulation problems
Hemorrhagic gastritis
Mucosal erosions over plication defects
Arteriovenous fistula created by surgical trauma
Inadvertent laceration of adjacent organs
Hematoma of rectus sheath or abdominal wall
Mucosal prolapse, intussusception, etc.

In many instances minimal and self-limiting hemorrhage from the site of incision occurs during the immediate postoperative period. If the bleeding does not stop with conservative measures, radiologic or endoscopic diagnosis of its precise source may be crucial prior to surgical intervention (5,7,10,12–14). It is also important to distinguish bleeding into the bowel lumen from intramural, intraperitoneal, and abdominal-wall hematomas. In this chapter we shall emphasize the major causes of postoperative bleeding that are detectable by radiologic studies.

Intraluminal Hemorrhage

Postoperative bleeding into the lumen of the gastrointestinal tract occurs frequently despite exercise of the highest degree of surgical skill and care. The complication is generally clinically suspected or diagnosed from the appearance of blood either in the aspirates from indwelling nasogastric tubes or in the stool specimens.

The *anastomotic site* is the most common source of bleeding within the first postoperative day (2–5). Bleeding is usually minimal and subsides spontaneously. The incidence of significant hemorrhage from the suture line is approximately 1% after gastrectomy and is slightly higher among patients operated upon because of duodenal ulcer disease (2,4,5). However, if surgery was performed because of bleeding, the rate of its recurrence might be as high as 30% (2,9).

Slipped ligature is the usual cause of bleeding from the suture line on the first day after surgery. Delayed bleeding episodes may occur between the seventh and tenth postoperative days and are probably due to mucosal sloughing at the suture line (4,5).

Several authors have emphasized the value of selective visceral arteriography in the diagnostic and therapeutic management of this postoperative complication (5–8,10–14) (Figs. 9-1, 9-2).

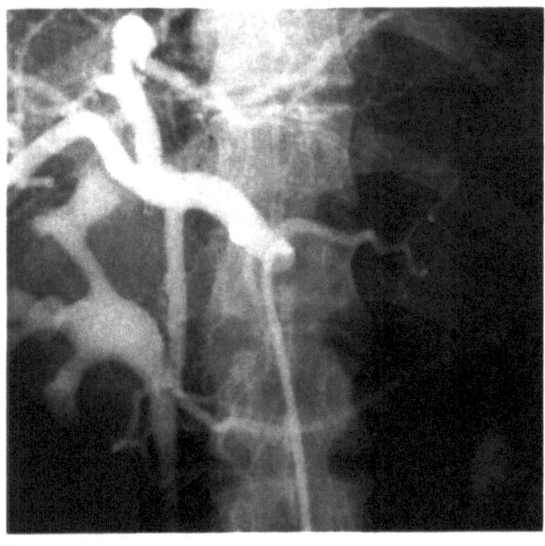

a

Fig. 9-1, a–c. Bleeding from suture line after partial gastrectomy. Massive hematemesis occurred in a 45-year-old man after splenectomy and partial gastrectomy done because of stab wounds. **a** and **b** Films obtained during arterial phase of celiac angiography show beginning extravasation of contrast material (*arrow* in **b**) from the left gastric artery. **c** Late venous phase shows the gastric pouch outlined with contrast material (*arrows*).

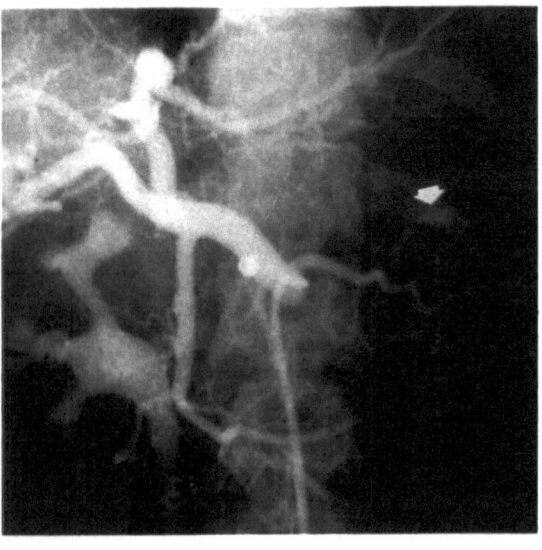

b

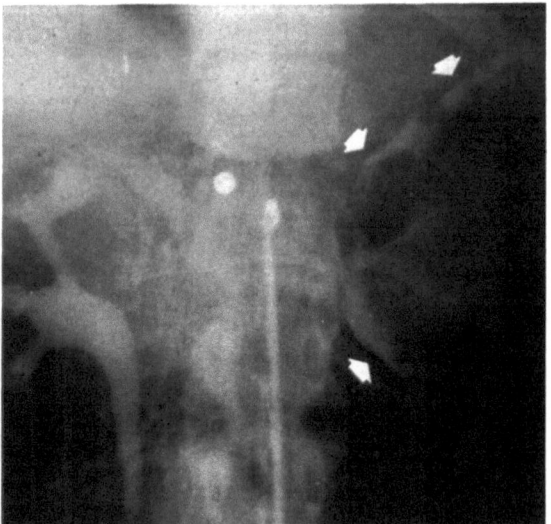

c

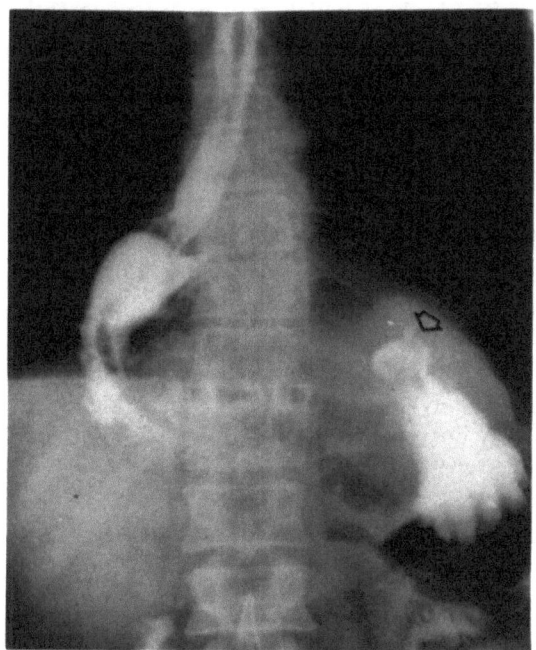

a

Fig. 9-2, a–c. Bleeding from the suture line of an interposed ileal loop. Bleeding developed in this 67-year-old man 8 days after resection of an adenocarcinoma of gastroesophageal junction. **a** Upper gastrointestinal series with iodinated contrast material shows an ileal loop interposed between the esophagus and stomach. The collection of contrast material in the superior aspect of the gastric pouch *(arrow)* was initially considered to represent a bleeding ulcer. **b** and **c** Superior mesenteric arteriograms demonstrate progressive extravasation from branches supplying the distal margin of the ileal loop at the anastomotic site *(arrow)*.

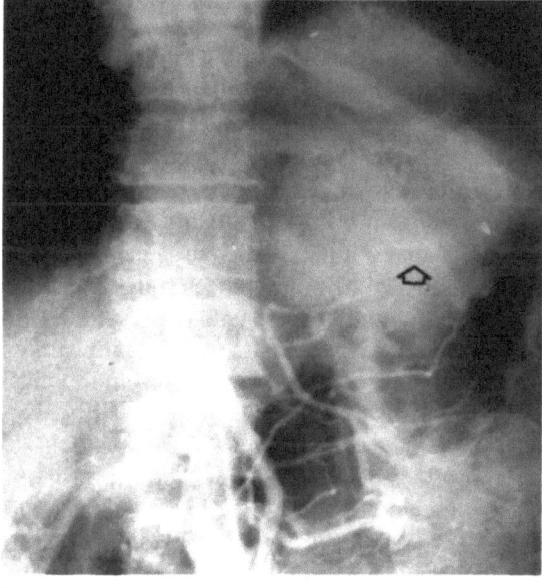

b

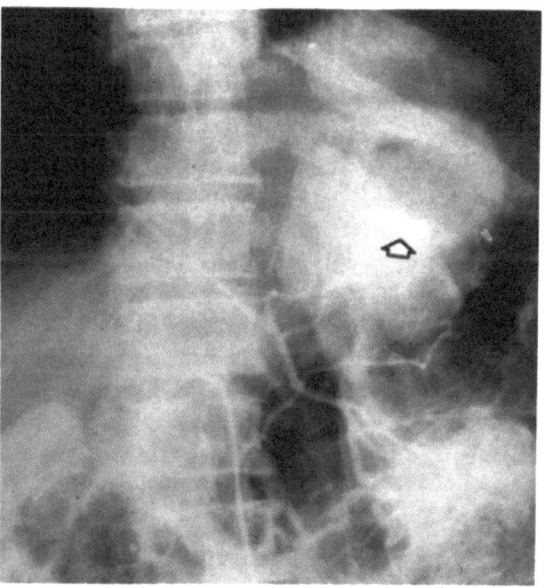

c

Among 11 cases reported by Athanasoulis et al., bleeding from the suture line occurred on the first day after surgery in 5 and during the eighth to tenth days in another 4 patients. In all 9 cases the bleeding point was correctly identified by angiographic evidence of contrast extravasation and successfully controlled with selective intraarterial infusion of posterior pituitary extract. Arteriography demonstrated fully unexpected bleeding sites distant from the suture line in only 2 of 11 patients in their series. Surgical reexploration was necessary in both patients because infusion therapy failed to arrest the hemorrhage (5).

Hemorrhagic gastritis is estimated to account for 16.8% of all upper gastrointestinal bleeding (9). Its existence may occasionally go unrecognized at the time of initial operation, or it can develop later as the result of postoperative bile reflux into the gastric remnant (17–19). The usual surgical therapy for this condition is often unsatisfactory. Even after subtotal gastrectomy the incidence of rebleeding may be as high as 50% (20). Several authors advocate total gastrectomy or 85% subtotal resection with vagotomy as the procedure of choice (9,21). Vagotomy is shown to diminish gastric blood flow and thus control the hemorrhage, but its vasoconstrictor effect may be temporary (9). With the advent of selective angiography for diagnosis and pharmacologic control of bleeding, the radiologist can play an important role in the management of this complication, often eliminating the need for further surgical intervention (5,6,8,22). As an alternative method LeVeen et al. believe that intraperitoneal or intragastric administration of norepinephrine may be sufficient to produce hemostasis even in patients with relatively massive upper gastrointestinal bleeding (9).

Alkaline reflux gastritis is a well-recognized complication of several types of gastroduodenal operations. It occurs most commonly after partial gastrectomy and the Billroth II procedure because the bile and pancreatic juice from the afferent loop can readily enter the gastric pouch (2,17–19). However, Billroth I gastroduodenostomy and even pyloroplasty can lead to reflux gastritis (18). The symptoms consist of epigastric pain unrelieved by food intake, nausea, bile-stained vomitus, anemia, and bleeding from superficial mucosal ulcerations within the gastric pouch (17). Endoscopic evaluation shows diffusely inflamed and friable gastric mucosa, usually with multiple bleeding erosions and scattered bile lakes. Administration of antacids and cholestyramine, a bile-acid absorbent, often relieves the symptoms (19). Some patients do not respond to conservative therapy and require surgical diversion of duodenal content away from the gastric pouch (18,19). In one of our patients with clinical and endoscopic features of alkaline gastritis, arteriography showed evidence of bleeding into the afferent loop from a large, inflamed duodenal diverticulum (23) (Fig. 9-3). In another patient, selective superior mesenteric arteriography permitted diagnosis and accurate localization of a clinically unsuspected retrogastric hematoma (Fig. 9-4). These observations emphasize the need for careful search for multiple or unrelated sources of postoperative bleeding. It should also be noted that the reflux of bile and pancreatic juice can induce esophagitis and

jejunitis, both of which may be other potential sources of postsurgical hemorrhage (2).

Marginal ulcers occur usually within the first 2 cm distal to a gastroenterostomy. They often produce more pain, bleeding, and perforation than the initial peptic ulcer for which the operation had been performed. The average incidence of marginal ulcer is 0.5% after gastric ulcer surgery and 8% when the operation is done because of duodenal ulcer disease (2). A significantly higher incidence (up to 25%) has been reported after pancreaticoduodenal surgery (2). Unfortunately only about half of marginal ulcers are clearly documented on postoperative upper gastrointestinal series because many are small and superficial. Air-contrast studies and endoscopy represent better methods for their detection.

Although marginal ulcers can develop within a few weeks after surgery, most become symptomatic several years later (2,24). Bleeding occurs in approximately 50% of the cases (24,-25). It can be localized (Fig. 9-5) and controlled by selective arteriography (5,22). More recently, technetium Tc 99m sulfur colloid scanning has been introduced for detection of the source of gastrointestinal bleeding (26). The method has the advantage of being simple and noninvasive yet detects intestinal hemorrhage at rates much slower than can be visible by arteriography.

Stress bleeding from the midduodenum is seldom considered a potential source of postoperative hemorrhage. Baum et al. first described the radiologic features of the entity in 1970 (27). In their series of 8 patients, 5 were demonstrated by arteriography to have bleeding from the junction of the second and third portions of the duodenum. This segment appears susceptible to ischemia because it is in the periphery of the celiac and superior mesenteric arterial systems. Diminished blood flow caused by stress of surgery or other ailments can induce the midduodenal bleeding (28,29). These ulcers are usually shallow and lack an indurated margin, often escaping recognition during routine radiographic or endoscopic evaluation (27–29). However, extravasation of contrast material during arteriography can correctly localize the site of bleeding (Fig. 9-6) and permit its nonoperative control.

Arteriovenous fistula occurring within the abdomen is usually congenital, arteriosclerotic, or posttraumatic. During the past two decades

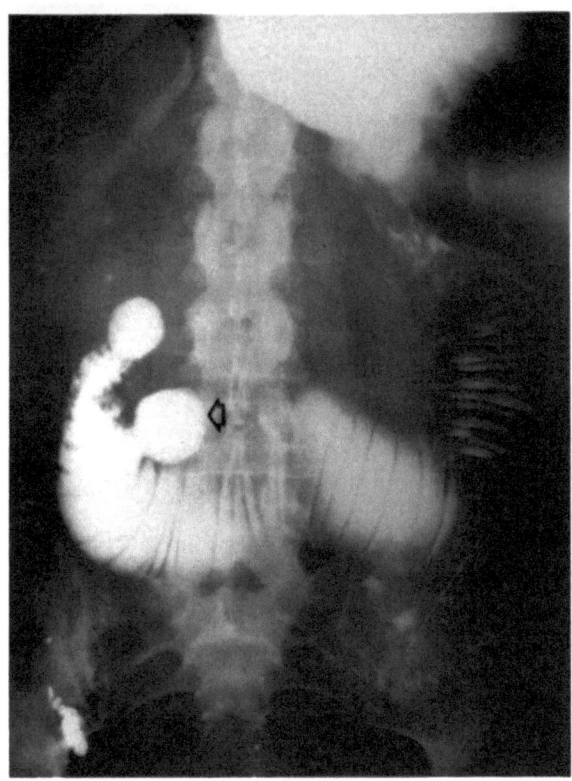

a

Fig. 9-3, a–c. Postoperative bleeding from an inflamed duodenal diverticulum. The patient had alkaline reflux gastritis following Billroth II procedure. a Upper gastrointestinal series demonstrates prominent gastric rugae and marked dilatation of afferent loop harboring a duodenal diverticulum (arrow). There is obstruction of the efferent jejunal limb. b and c Common hepatic arteriogram reveals evidence for hypervascularity and contrast extravasation (arrows) in the region of the duodenal diverticulum. (Ghahremani GG, Hietala SO: Arteriography of a bleeding duodenal diverticulum. Am J Dig Dis 22:445–448, 1977)

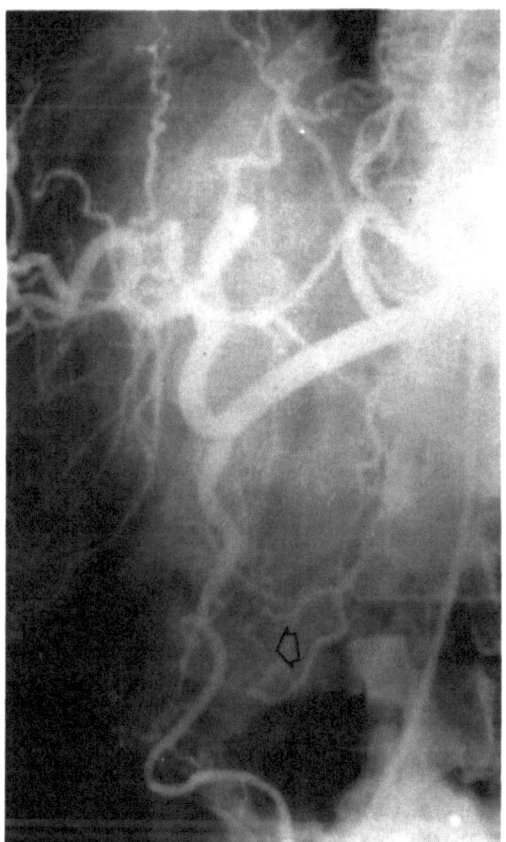

b

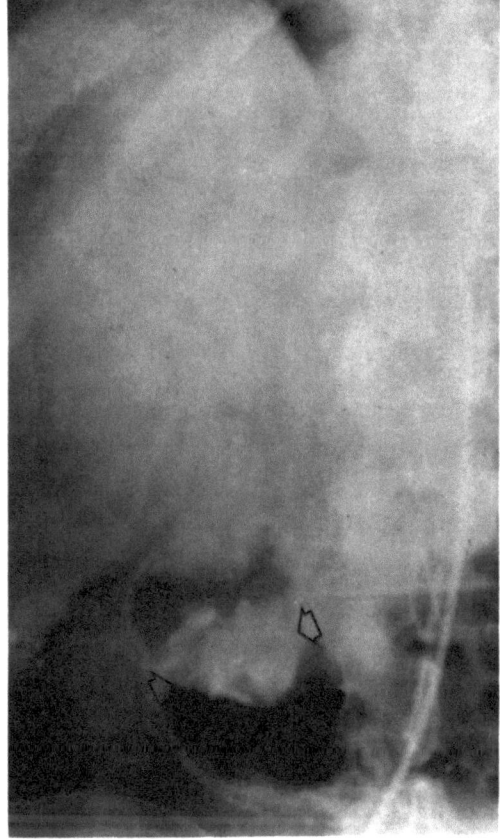

c

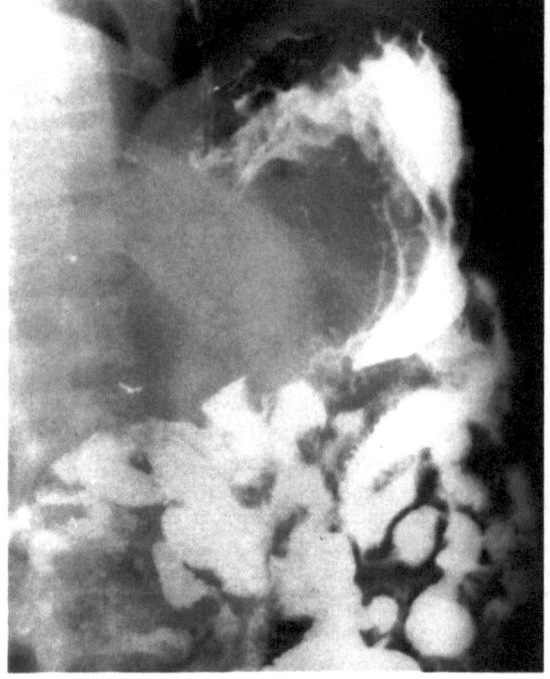

a

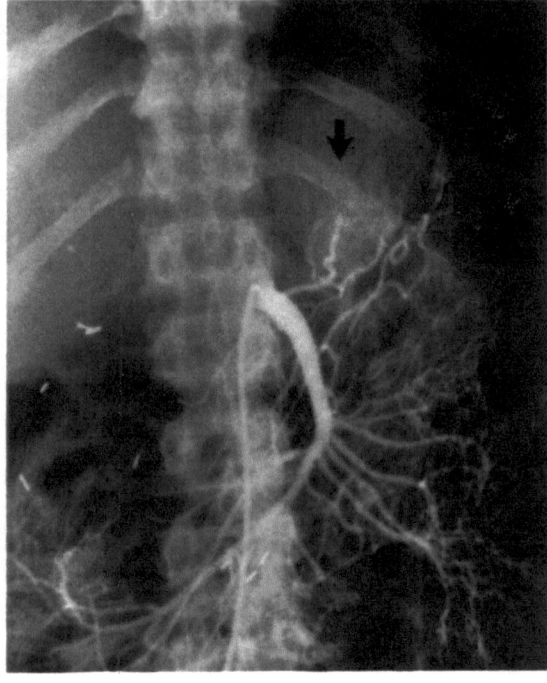

b

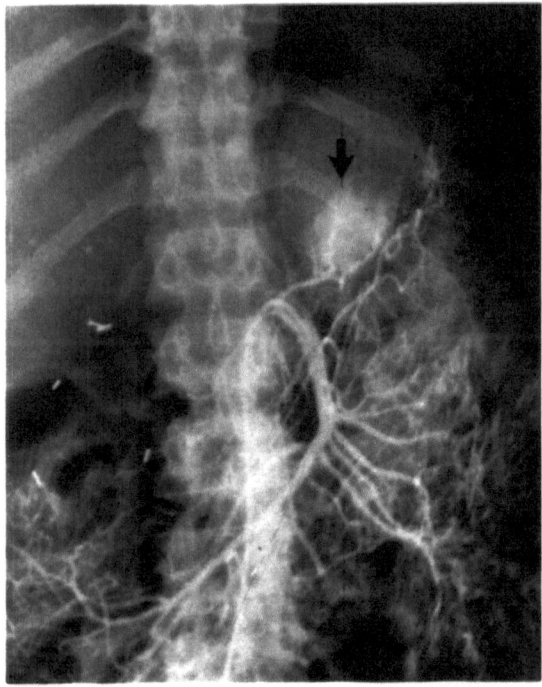

c

Fig. 9-4, a–c. Postsurgical retrogastric hematoma. This 48-year-old man had had multiple abdominal operations, including Billroth I gastroduodenostomy. **a** Examination with Gastrografin shows enlarged gastric rugae and evidence of extrinsic compression on the posteromedial aspect of the stomach. **b** and **c** Selective superior mesenteric arteriograms demonstrate progressive opacification with contrast material *(arrow)* derived from an artery supplying proximal jejunum. Laparotomy revealed a partially organized hematoma in the region of the ligament of Treitz and tail of the pancreas.

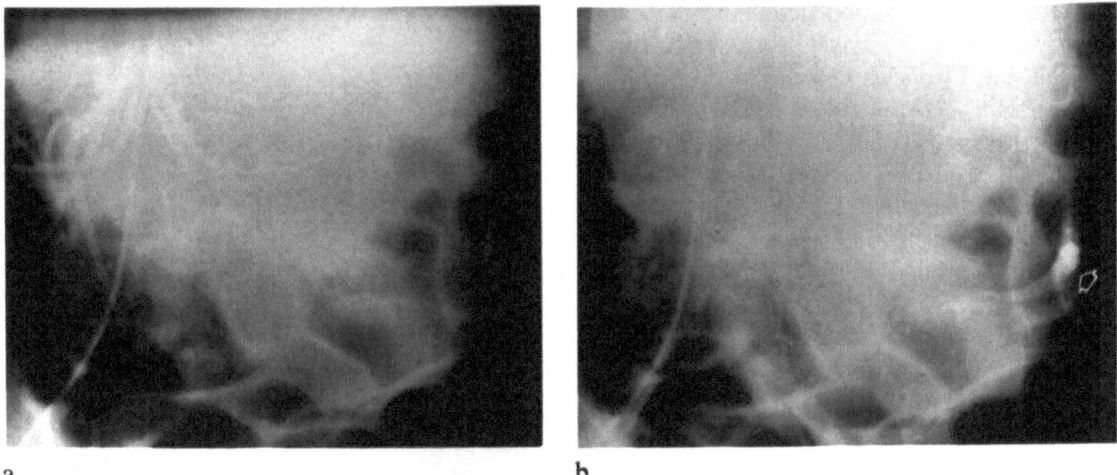

a   b

Fig. 9-5, a and **b. Bleeding marginal ulcer.** This is seen 2 years after partial gastrectomy and Billroth II procedure. **a** Early phase of superior mesenteric arteriography is shown. **b** Venous phase shows extravasation of the contrast material *(arrow)* from a marginal ulcer in the efferent jejunal limb.

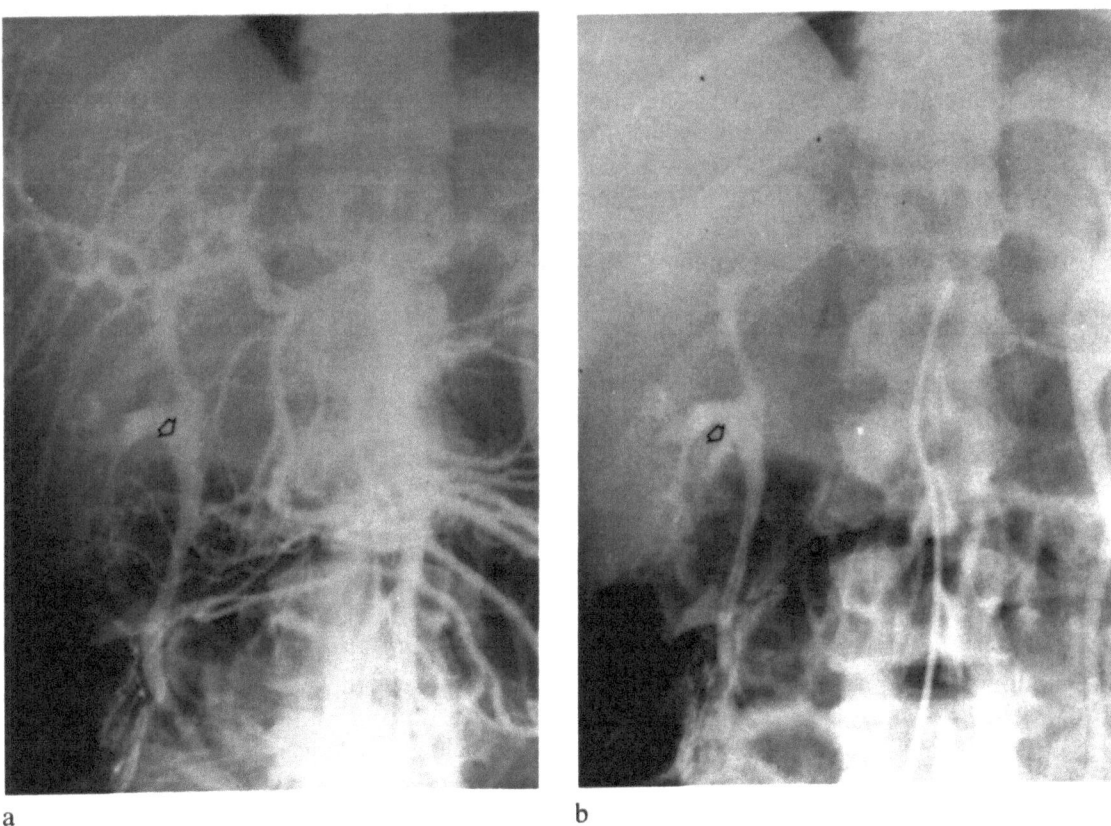

a   b

Fig. 9-6, a and **b Postoperative stress bleeding from midduodenum.** This occurred in a 52-year-old man who was recovering from vagotomy and pyloroplasty. **a** and **b** Celiac angiograms show extravasation from a branch of gastroduodenal artery supplying midduodenum *(arrow)*.

operative procedures and percutaneous biopsy of abdominal organs have been clearly recognized as causes of this lesion (7,8,10–14,30–36) (Fig. 9-7). It is generally believed that a postsurgical arteriovenous fistula develops as a result of placement of mass ligatures around vascular pedicles or direct injury of an adjoining artery and vein by transfixation sutures. Postoperative inflammation around the site of incision or anastomosis may also damage the wall of adjacent vessels, causing formation of a mycotic aneurysm or pseudoaneurysm that erodes into a neighboring vessel.

Korobkin et al. reported three cases and reviewed five other examples of arteriovenous fistula between the mesenteric and portal circulation, all complicating previous partial gastrectomy (10). The interval between surgery and discovery of the lesion was 4–20 years (7,10,12).

Arteriovenous fistula has also occurred after operations on the duodenum (7), small bowel (33), colon (11), and other abdominal organs (14,30). In most instances the lesion remained clinically silent until its perforation into the gastrointestinal lumen or the peritoneal cavity led to massive hemorrhage. The possibility of an arteriovenous fistula may be considered when a bruit or a pulsatile mass develops after abdominal surgery (10). A unique feature of fistula between the portal vein and visceral branches of the abdominal aorta is the tendency to produce portal hypertension and its associated symptoms. This was present in 17 of 22 reported cases in which the portal pressure was measured (34). The classic findings of other large and systemic arteriovenous fistulas, e.g., increased cardiac output and congestive heart failure, are seldom seen with this lesion (10).

Numerous aneurysms involving the splenic, hepatic, or other visceral arteries have been diagnosed since the advent of arteriography (7,8,10–14,30–36). Iatrogenic causes of hepatic artery aneurysm and arterioportal fistula include trauma induced during cholecystectomy, bile duct exploration, and percutaneous liver biopsy (14,35,36) (Fig. 9-8). The resultant lesion may cause hemobilia and be overlooked as the source of gastrointestinal bleeding until arteriography is performed (13,14,31) (Fig. 9-9).

Aortoenteric and paraprosthetic-enteric fistulas are communications between the gastrointestinal tract and the aorta following graft replace-

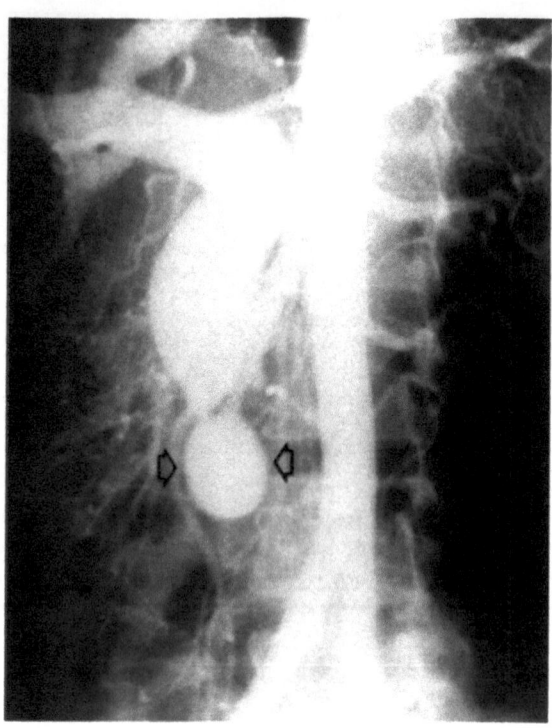

Fig. 9-7. Postsurgical arteriovenous fistula. The 56-year-old man had had partial gastrectomy and Billroth II procedure because of peptic ulcer disease. Three years later he had recurrent episodes of severe cramping pain suggestive of abdominal angina. Aortogram demonstrates a large aneurysm of gastroduodenal artery *(arrows)* with fistulous communication to a markedly distended portal vein.

ment for abdominal aortic aneurysms and occlusive vascular disease. Their incidence is about 1% (37,38). The fistulas have been reported to occur from 3 weeks to 10 years postoperatively, with an average of 6 months to 2 years (38,39). Clinical presentation consists of gastrointestinal hemorrhage, abdominal pain, and perhaps a pulsatile mass or signs of infection. The bleeding is seldom exsanguinating initially, and there are often quiescent periods varying from days to months. Signs of infection can occasionally be dominant (40). The mortality in graft-intestinal fistulas of 70% (37) is related to both the frequent delay in diagnosis and the technical difficulties of surgical repair. A high index of suspicion and an aggressive diagnostic evaluation are essential to reduce the mortality in this condition (38,41–43).

In aortoenteric fistula there is direct communication between the aortic lumen and the intestine, and in paraprosthetic-enteric fistula the

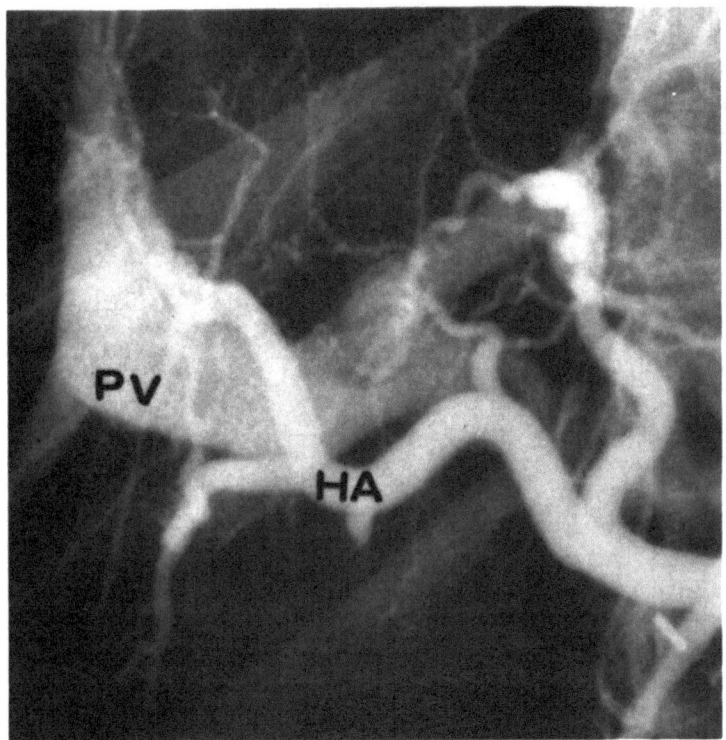

Fig. 9-8. Hepatic arteriportal fistula secondary to percutaneous liver biopsy. Four months after liver biopsy showing micronodular cirrhosis in a 52-year-old male alcoholic, he developed bleeding esophageal varices. Selective celiac arteriogram demonstrates fistula between a central hepatic artery (*HA*) and the portal vein (*PV.*) There is marked enlargement of the right branch of the portal vein. (Baer J: Hepatic arterioportal fistula related to a liver biopsy. Gastrointest Radiol 2:297–299, 1977.)

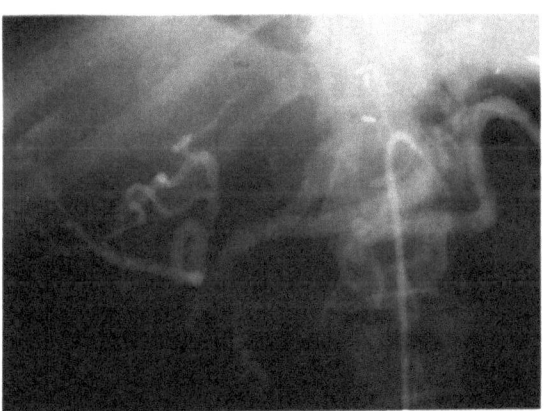

a

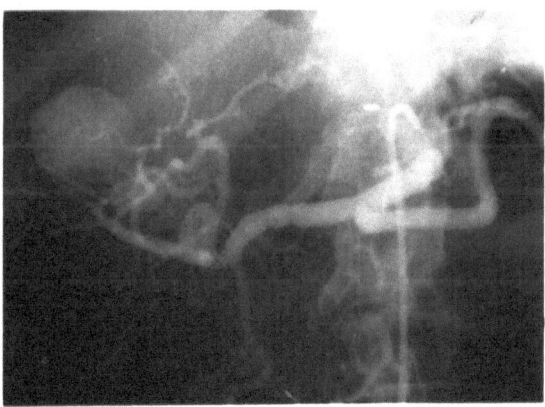

b

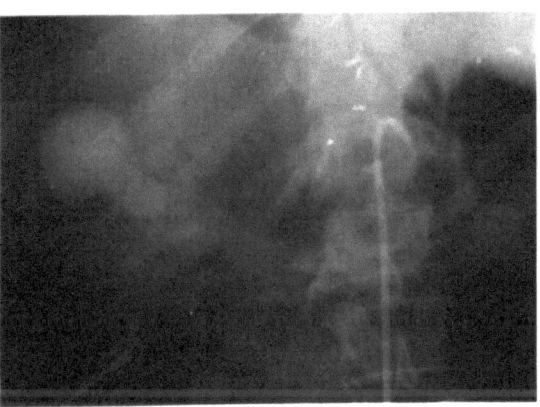

c

Fig. 9-9, a–c. Postoperative hemobilia due to mycotic intrahepatic aneurysm. The 60-year-old man with previous history of aortic valve replacement and gastrectomy developed intestinal bleeding and mild jaundice. **a** In the early phase celiac arteriogram appears unremarkable. **b** Few seconds later a large cavity is opacified within the right lobe of the liver. **c** Late venous phase shows retention of contrast material in the pearshaped pseudoaneurysm. (Ranniger K et al: Angiographic diagnosis of an intrahepatic aneurysm as a cause of unexplained bleeding. Radiology: 90:507–509, 1968)

communication is between the graft bed and intestine. Fistulization after grafting usually occurs at the proximal aortic anastomosis, and in 80% of cases there is communication with the duodenum, most frequently the adjacent third portion (37,44) (Fig. 9-10).

The mechanism of development of the fistula is either pseudoaneurysm formation and erosion into the adherent duodenum or dehiscence of the suture line secondary to infection caused by leak of intestinal content through a duodenum whose blood supply has been compromised at surgery (37–39).

Other sites of fistulization include the remainder of the duodenum, the stomach, jejunum, ileum, colon, and appendix (38,39,42). The fistula involves the distal suture line in about 20% of the cases. Two cases of fistula between a renal artery bypass graft and the jejunum have been reported (42). Modern surgical techniques to reduce the complications of fistulization include replacement of homografts and Teflon grafts

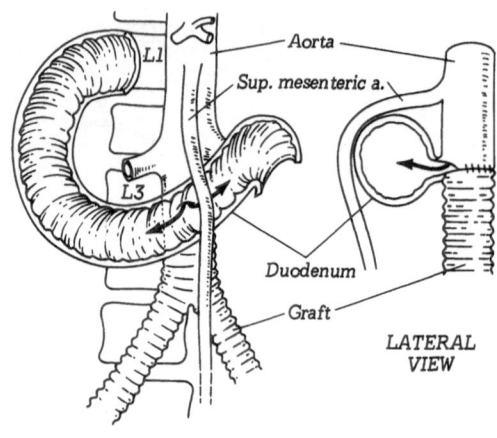

Fig. 9-10. Aortoduodenal fistula. This developed at the proximal anastomosis of abdominal aortic graft.

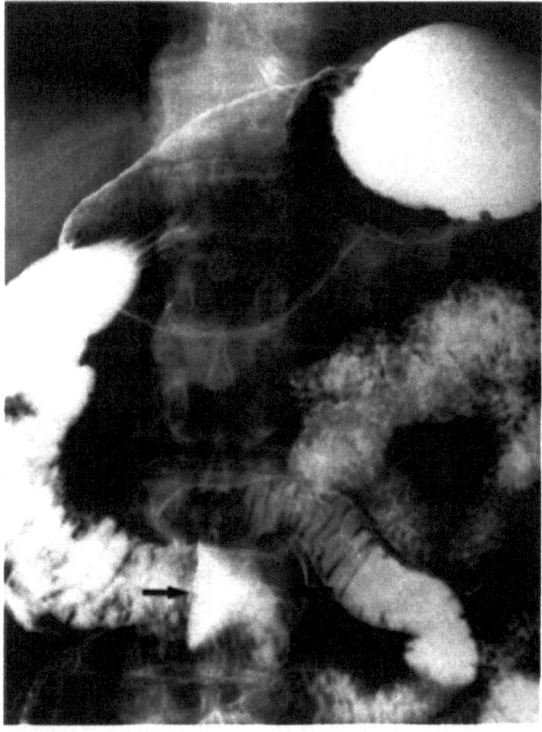

a

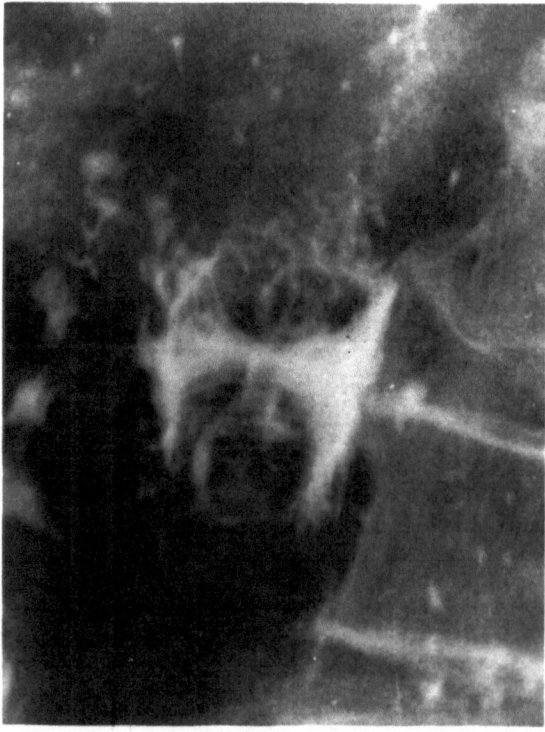

b

Fig. 9-11, a and b. Aortoduodenal (paraprosthetic-enteric) fistula. a Upper gastrointestinal series 1 year after Dacron graft replacement of abdominal aortic aneurysm shows localized extravasation of contrast material from the third portion of the duodenum (arrows). b Lateral spot film demonstrates extraluminal barium outlining the rings of the Dacron graft. (Hall DA, Jones B: Telepaque—The ubiquitous contrast. Gastrointest Radiol 4:405–406, 1979)

with more suitable Dacron grafting material, use of nonabsorbable synthetic suture material, and interposition of tissues between the patient's intestine and the graft suture lines (37).

Radiologic evaluation is critical for precise diagnosis. Plain films are usually unrewarding but may show a mass secondary to false aneurysm, retroperitoneal hematoma, or abscess. These conditions may also be revealed by abdominal ultrasonography (45). An upper gastrointestinal series may demonstrate evidence of extrinsic pressure or submucosal mass with or without erosion with extravasation of barium into the paraprosthetic space (37,38,40,46) (Figs. 9-11,9-12). Intraperitoneal extravasation (Fig. 9-12) is very uncommon and indicates gross erosion at the fistula site (40). A small-bowel study should be included since the loops may be displaced by a false aneurysm or hematoma. Bar-

ium enema study in patients with lower-intestinal bleeding may demonstrate a mass or area of ulceration and possible extravasation along the limb of the graft (38,46). Aortograms can be normal if the fistula is due to a defect in the proximal suture line without any signs of pseudoaneurysm formation, but in one series findings were abnormal in six of seven cases (38). In a patient with gastrointestinal bleeding, angiographic finding of a false aneurysm with no evidence of extravasation should indicate the need for surgical exploration of the graft (38). Definitive diagnosis rests on demonstration of extravasation of contrast material with enteric opacification. Since the bleeding point is on the anterior aortic wall (Fig. 9-10), the fistula may be evident in the lateral or prone rather than the frontal projection (38).

The diagnosis of aortoenteric fistula can be made endoscopically if the bleeding prosthesis

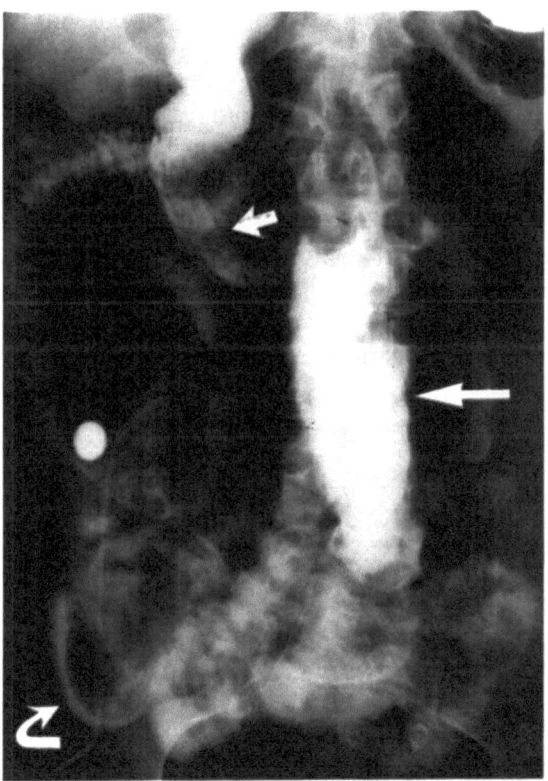

a

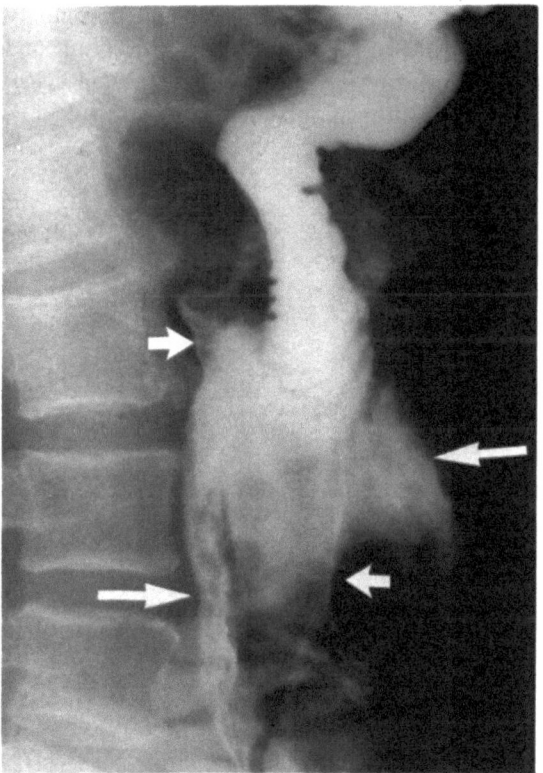

b

Fig. 9-12. Aortoduodenal (paraprosthetic-enteric) fistula. This developed within weeks after Dacron graft replacement of a large leaking abdominal aortic aneurysm with perforations of the posterior wall of the duodenum. **a** Gastrografin swallow demonstrates extrinsic pressure on the duodenum *(small arrow)* and contrast material in the paraprosthetic space *(large arrow)* and free in the peritoneal cavity *(curved arrow)*. **b** Lateral film from the same study shows contrast material outlining the graft *(small arrows)* and in the paraprosthetic space *(large arrows)*. (Lautin EM, Friedman AC: A complicated case of aortoduodenal fistula. Gastrointest Radiol 4:401–404, 1979)

or aneurysm is seen (47). It should be considered if a pulsatile structure is seen in a visceral wall or lumen, if arterial bleeding is noted in the third or fourth portion of the duodenum, or if a suture line or ulceration is seen in a patient who has had vascular reconstructive surgery.

Intramural Hemorrhage

Hematoma can develop within the wall of the gastrointestinal tract after blunt abdominal trauma or in patients with hemophilia (48–53). Iatrogenic factors include anticoagulant therapy and trauma during gastrointestinal endoscopy or surgery (15,16,54,55).

In contrast to postoperative intraluminal bleeding, bowel-wall hematoma complicating surgery is infrequently diagnosed. Submucosal or subserosal hemorrhage and edema commonly occur after procedures involving resection and anastomosis of the gastrointestinal tract (1,4,16). Bleeding is often minimal and confined, subsides spontaneously, and resolves without sequelae.

Only when the hematoma is large enough to obstruct the lumen or manifest other recognizable symptoms are contrast studies or endoscopy performed (2,3,55). In several cases illustrated in this chapter the diagnosis of postoperative hematoma was made possible primarily because upper gastrointestinal series were obtained within the first 2 weeks after surgery.

Intramural hematoma of the esophagus has been reported as a complication of vagotomy (15). Rabiah and Elliott described a patient who developed chest pain and almost complete obstruction of the distal esophagus within a few days after transabdominal bilateral vagotomy (15). Reexploration disclosed a large organized intramural hematoma surrounding the esophagogastric junction. The authors noted that the clinical and radiographic findings of esophageal hematoma can simulate transient postvagotomy achalasia and thus be erroneously diagnosed. In one of our patients the esophagogram obtained 8 days after surgical repair of a hiatus hernia showed submucosal hematoma in the distal esophagus (Fig. 9-13).

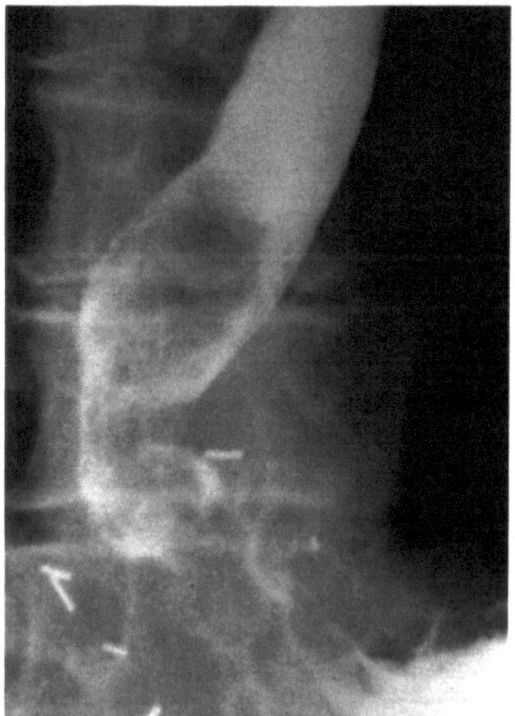 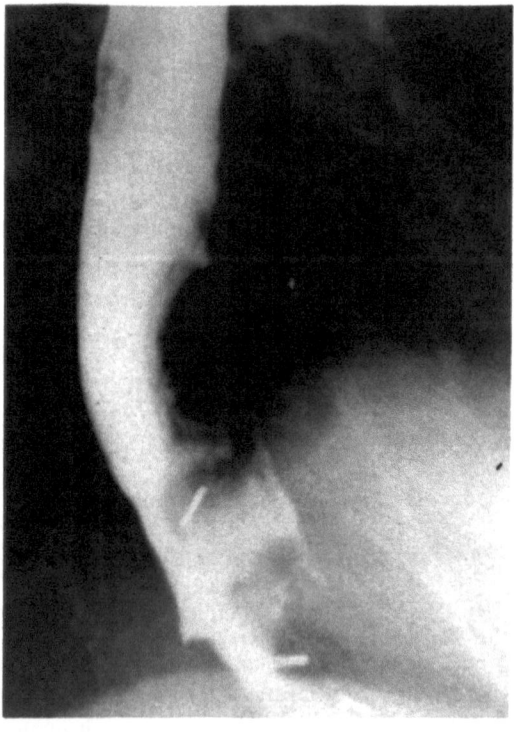

a   b

Fig. 9-13, a and b. Submucosal hematomas of distal esophagus. These are demonstrated in this study performed 8 days after surgical repair of a hiatus hernia.

Intramural hematoma of the esophagus can occur in patients with hemophilia (48) or uremia (56) and as a complication of trauma induced by ingestion of a foreign body or by endoscopy (49,55). Submucosal dissection of a hematoma and its communication with the lumen of the esophagus can present radiographic findings strikingly similar to those of a dissecting aortic aneurysm as seen angiographically (49,57,58). In the esophagus, subsequent leakage of material from the lumen into the space created by a hematoma can lead to formation of an intramural abscess (57). Paraesophageal hematoma may develop as the result of esophageal surgery or trauma, causing extrinsic compression and displacement of the esophagus (15) (Fig. 9-14).

Intramural gastric hematoma may develop as a result of hemocoagulation disorders, penetrating peptic ulcers, and trauma induced during gastroscopy (50,51,54,55). In patients who have recently undergone gastric surgery a mass-like deformity due to associated hematoma and inflammatory edema may be seen about the suture line or stoma (1,3,4). Radiographically larger hematomas closely resemble benign gastric tumors such as leiomyomas (50,51). In the two cases illustrated here (Figs. 9-15,9-16), submucosal hematoma presented as a pseudotumor of the gastric pouch on postoperative upper gastrointestinal series. Endoscopy further verified the diagnosis. In another patient, gradual resorption of multiple hematomas occurred with conservative management (Fig. 9-17).

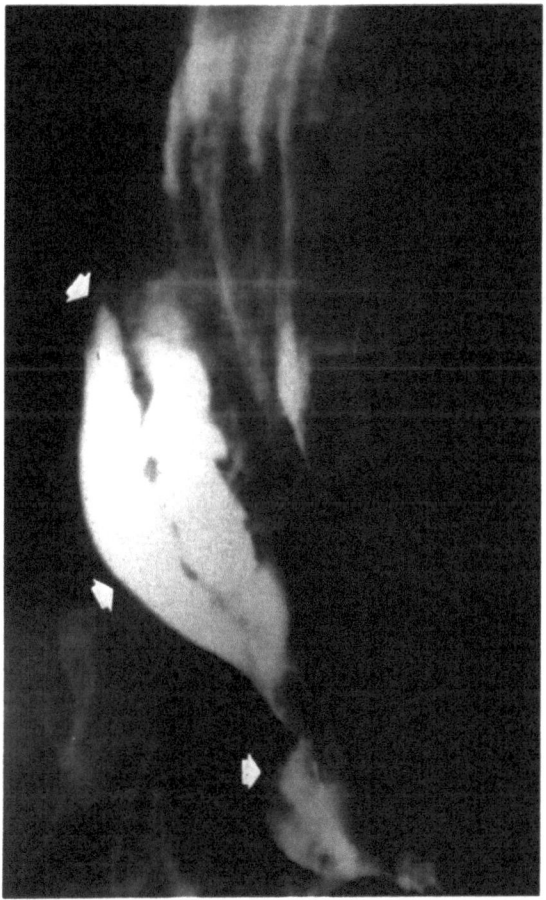 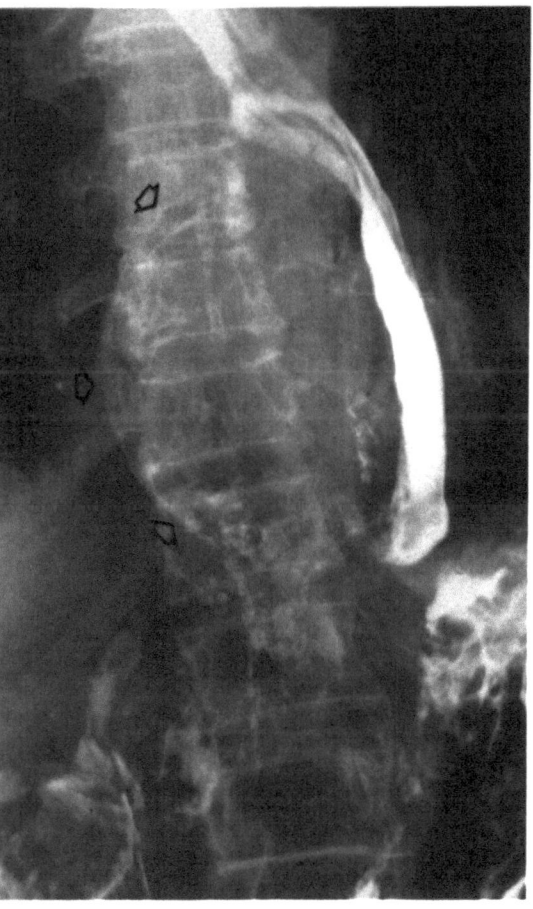

a   b

Fig. 9-14, a and **b. Iatrogenic posterior mediastinal hematoma. a** Esophagogram obtained immediately after pneumatic dilatation for achalasia in a 77-year-old female demonstrates a large tear of the distal esophagus *(arrows)* and inferior extension of extraluminal barium into the lesser sac. **b** A repeat study 5 days after surgical closure of the esophageal rupture and the performance of Heller's myotomy indicates development of a paraesophageal hematoma, outlined by residual barium *(arrows)* and displacing the distal esophagus to the left.

G. G. Ghahremani, M. A. Meyers, S. -O. Hietala, and W. H. Brewer

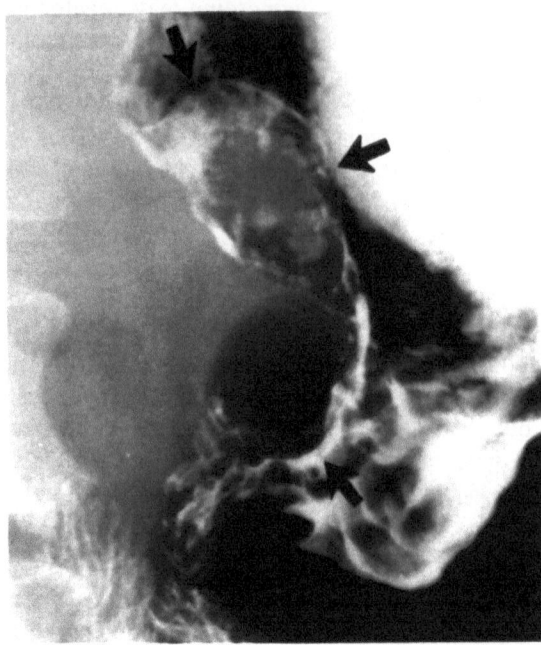

Fig. 9-15. Intramural hematoma of the stomach *(arrows).* This occurred as a complication of partial gastrectomy and Billroth I anastomosis. This localized hematoma closely resembles a leiomyoma.

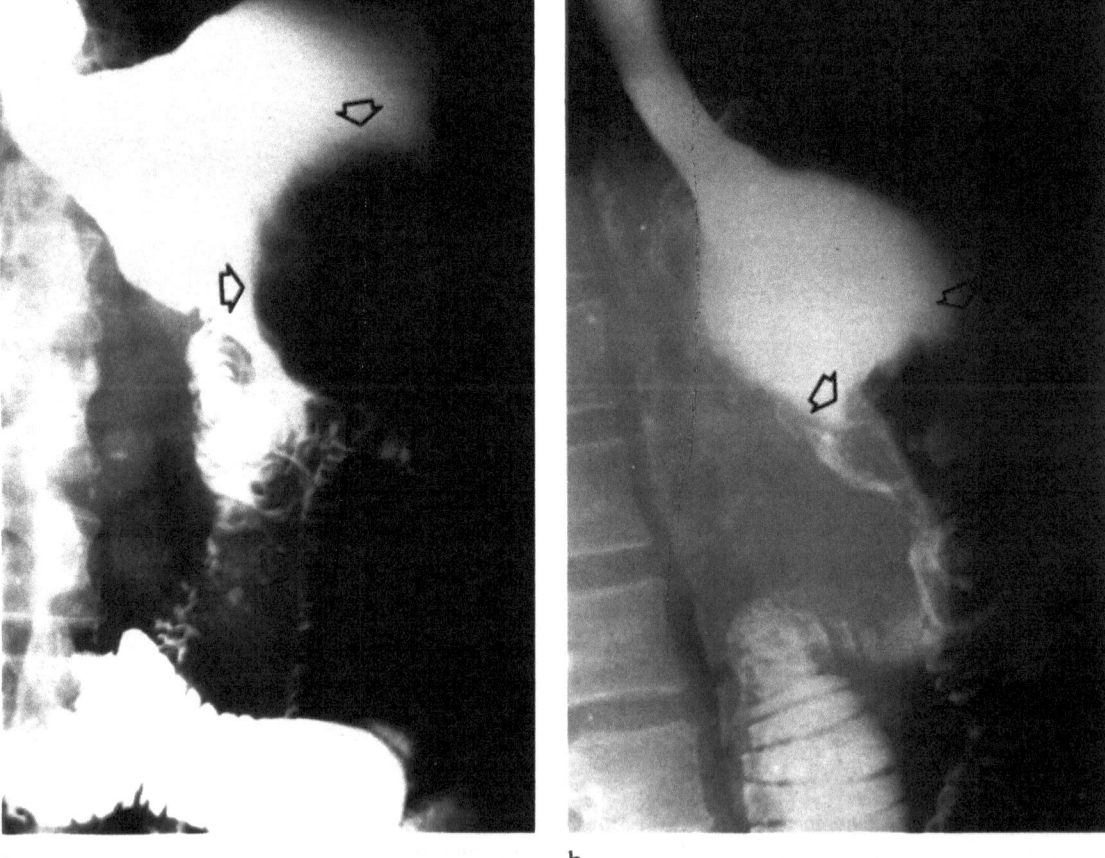

a   b

Fig. 9-16, a and b. Large intramural hematoma of the gastric pouch *(arrows).* The upper gastrointestinal series was done 10 days after partial gastrectomy and Billroth II gastrojejunostomy.

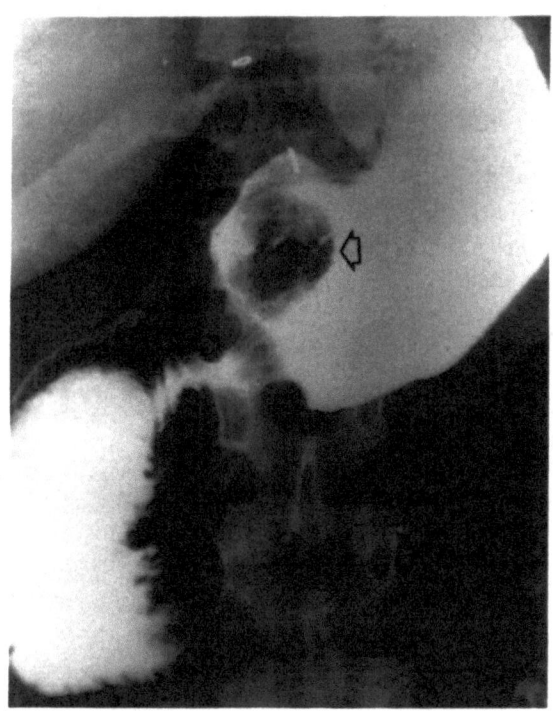

a

Fig. 9-17, a–c. Multiple localized hematomas. The 51-year-old woman previously had hiatus hernia repair. She later underwent antrectomy and Billroth I gastro-duodenostomy because of a bleeding ulcer. Postoperative hemorrhagic diathesis developed as a result of coagulation defects caused by repeated transfusions.

a Gastrografin study 1 week after surgery shows an intramural mass in the gastric pouch (arrow) and obstruction of third portion of the duodenum. b Two weeks later examination demonstrates partial resorption of the gastric (arrow) and duodenal (curved arrows) hematomas. c Upper gastrointestinal series 1 year after surgery is unremarkable. The persistent deformity of the fundus is due to fundoplication defect.

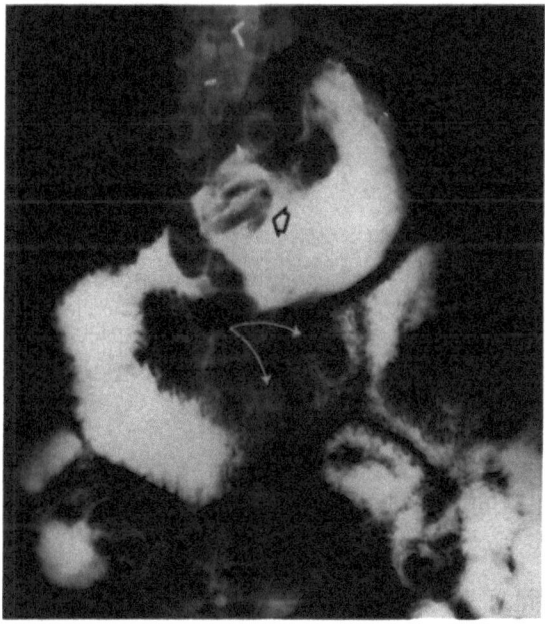

b

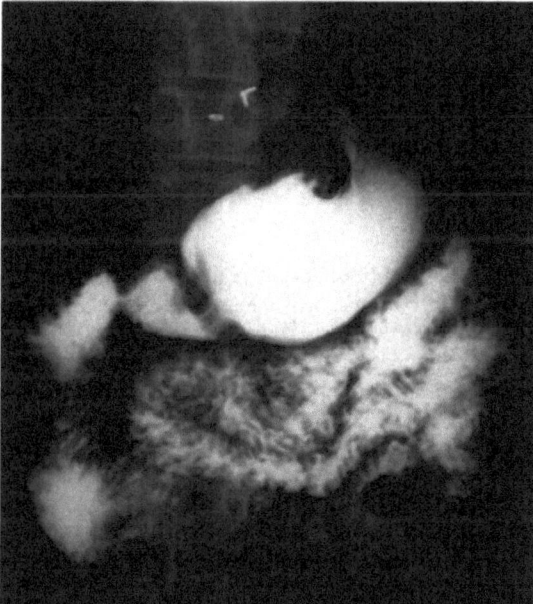

c

Intramural hematoma of the duodenum is most frequently a result of blunt abdominal trauma (52,54). It can also occur as a complication of gastroduodenal surgery and operation upon the gallbladder or bile ducts (2,4,16,52). Heidenblut and Holz reported two patients who developed localized intramural hematoma of the periampullary duodenal segment soon after cho-

lecystectomy and bile duct exploration (16). This type of iatrogenic mechanism was also responsible for production of duodenal hematomas in two of our patients (Figs. 9-18,9-19).

Intramural hematomas complicating gastrointestinal surgery resolve rather slowly over several weeks or months without leaving any significant permanent deformity (1,16). Conservative

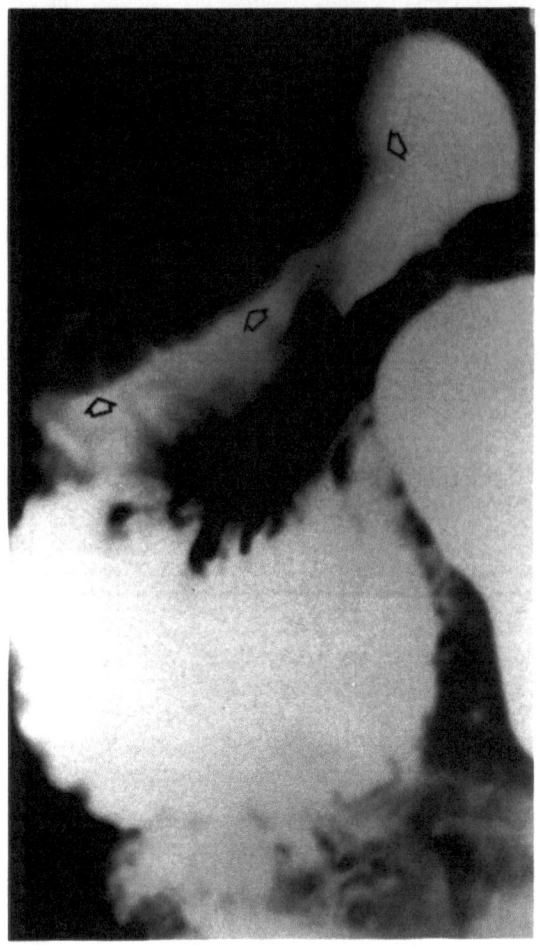

a

b

Fig. 9-18, a and b. Postoperative duodenal hematoma. A 19-year-old woman with a large choledochal cyst underwent cholecystectomy and Roux-en-Y choledochocystojejunostomy. **a** Upper gastrointestinal series 3 weeks after surgery shows a lobulated intramural mass *(arrows),* representing an organized hematoma of the duodenal wall. **b** Repeat study 5 months later demonstrates complete resorption of the hematoma. There is air within the choledochal cyst *(arrows).*

management is preferred, and operative evacuation is reserved for large obstructive or infected hematomas (15,52,53,55,57,59). Fiberoptic endoscopy, follow-up contrast studies, computed tomography, and ultrasound scanning can be most helpful in monitoring the size and evolution of intramural hematomas (55,60–62).

Other Sites of Postoperative Bleeding

Intraperitoneal hemorrhage is fortunately quite uncommon after abdominal surgery (3,4). When the operative field is adequately drained the sub-sequent appearance of blood is often the clue to this complication. Plain radiographs of the abdomen can show evidence for accumulation of fluid or blood within the peritoneal cavity. Arteriography, ultrasound, and computed tomography may further assist in evaluation prior to surgical intervention (5,8,13,26,28,60–62).

Rectus sheath hematoma can result from trauma to the epigastric vessels induced during abdominal operations (63). The usual symptoms are localized pain, palpable mass, and ecchymosis of the anterior abdominal wall (63–66). Fever, nausea, and vomiting may be associated findings, and shock can develop when blood loss has been excessive. Recent studies have clearly demonstrated ultrasound scanning as the method of choice for the diagnosis of this entity (63,64,-66). The procedure is easily performed, readily tolerated by acutely ill patients, and can be repeated to follow the course of evolution and resolution of the hematoma (64). The ultrasonographic appearance is characteristic: a sonolucent cyst-like mass corresponding to the anatomic location of the rectus sheath (Fig. 9-20). It is usually spindle shaped on the longitudinal sections and ovoid with slightly flattened base on transverse scans. The highest part of the hematoma is close to the anterior abdominal wall, but its inferior margin may extend toward the pelvis to impinge on the anterior wall of the urinary bladder and become palpable on pelvic or rectal examination (63,65).

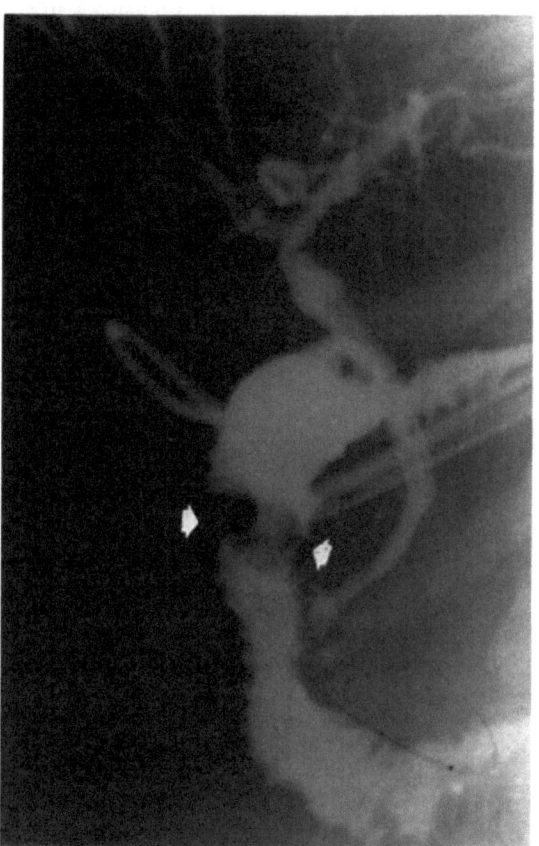

Fig. 9-19. Intramural duodenal hematoma. T-tube cholangiogram shows localized narrowing of the duodenum *(arrows)*, representing an intramural hematoma induced during cholecystectomy and bile duct exploration.

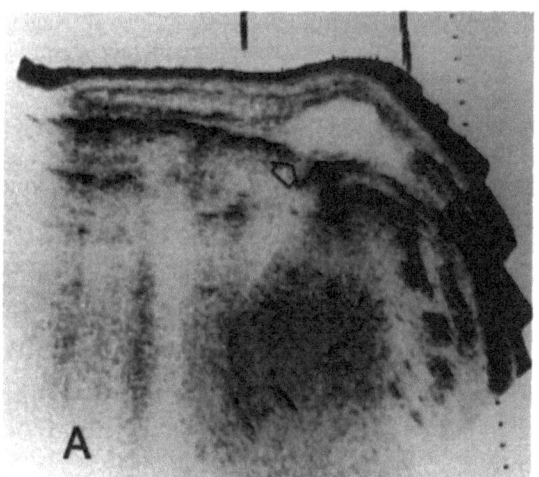 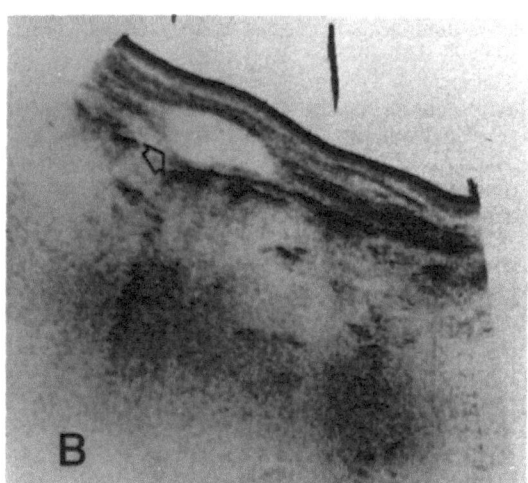

Fig. 9-20. Ultrasonographic appearance of a postoperative rectus sheath hematoma. Transverse (A) and longitudinal (B) sections of the left upper abdominal wall demonstrate an echo-free ovoid mass (arrow) representing a localized hematoma in the left rectus sheath.

References

1. Burhenne HJ: Postoperative defects of the stomach. Semin Roentgenol 6:182–192, 1971

2. Burhenne HJ: The postoperative stomach. In Margulis AR, Burhenne HJ (eds): Alimentary Tract Roentgenology, vol. 1, St. Louis: Mosby 1973, pp 740–783

3. Ochsner SF, Watson JD: Radiologic evaluation of early postoperative abdominal complaints. South Med J 58:1439–1446, 1965

4. Cen M, Dihlmann W: Roentgenbefunde am operierten Magen in Abhängigkeit vom postoperierten Intervall. Radiologe 9:187–195, 1969

5. Athanasoulis CA, Waltman AC, Ring EJ, et al: Angiographic management of postoperative bleeding. Radiology 113:37–42, 1974

6. Nusbaum H, Baum S, Blakemore WS: Clinical experience with the diagnosis and management of gastrointestinal hemorrhage by selective mesenteric catheterization. Ann Surg 170:506–514, 1969

7. Silverberg PW: The arteriographic demonstration of bleeding in the duodenal stump. Radiology 100:315–317, 1971

8. Walter JF, Bookstein JJ, Kramer RA, et al: Therapeutic angiography: Its value to the surgical patient. Arch Surg 113:432–439, 1978

9. LeVeen HH, Falk G, Diaz C, et al: Control of gastrointestinal bleeding. Am J Surg 123:154–159, 1972

10. Korobkin M, Kantor I, Pollard JJ, et al: Arteriovenous fistula between systemic and portal circulations following partial gastrectomy. Radiology 109:311–314, 1973

11. Casarella WJ, Galloway SJ, Taxin RN, et al: Lower gastrointestinal tract hemorrhage: New concepts based on arteriography. Am J Roentgenol 121:357–368, 1974

12. Blackwell TL, Whelan TJ: Arteriovenous fistula as a complication of gastrectomy. Am J Surg 109:197–200, 1965

13. Koehler PR, Nelson JA, Berenson MM: Massive extra-enteric gastrointestinal bleeding: Angiographic diagnosis. Radiology 119:41–44, 1976

14. Anderson PT: Traumatic false aneurysm of the right hepatic artery: An unusual complication of cholecystectomy. Aust NZ J Surg 40:273–277, 1971

15. Rabiah FA, Elliott HB: Intramural hematoma of the esophagus—An unusual complication of vagotomy. Am J Dig Dis 13:925–928, 1968

16. Heidenblut A, Holz K: Intramural hematoma of the duodenum after operation on gallbladder and bile ducts. Fortschr Geb Roentgenstr Nuklearmed 112:609–614, 1970

17. Bushkin FL, Wickbom G, DeFord GW, et al: Postoperative alkaline reflux gastritis. Surg Gynecol Obstet 138:933–939, 1974

18. Delaney JP, Broadie TA, Robbins PL: Pyloric reflux gastritis: The offending agent. Surgery 77:764–772, 1975

19. Herrington JL Jr, Sawyers JL, Whitehead WA: Surgical management of reflux gastritis. Ann Surg 180:526–539, 1974

20. Rosenkrantz JG, Bartlett MK: Hemorrhage from gastritis: An analysis of 44 proven cases. Ann Surg 153:617–624, 1961

21. Lulu DJ, Dragstedt LR: Massive bleeding due to acute hemorrhagic gastritis. Arch Surg 101:550–554,1970

22. Rösch J, Dotter CT, Rose RW: Selective arterial infusion of vasoconstrictors in acute gastrointestinal bleeding. Radiology 99:27–36, 1971

23. Ghahremani GG, Hietala SO: Arteriography of a bleeding duodenal diverticulum. Am J Dig Dis 22:445–448, 1977

24. Walters W: Six to ten-year follow-up of the surgical treatment of duodenal, gastric, and gastrojejunal ulcers. Gastroenterologia 93:15–25, 1960

25. Walters W, Priestley JT, Belding HH: Vagotomy in treatment of gastrojejunal ulceration: Postoperative clinical and laboratory study. JAMA 148:803–808, 1952

26. Alavi A, Dann RW, Baum S, et al: Scintigraphic detection of acute gastrointestinal bleeding. Radiology 124:753–756, 1977

27. Baum S, Ward S, Nusbaum M: Stress bleeding from the mid-duodenum. An often unrecognized source of gastrointestinal hemorrhage. Radiology 95:595–602, 1970

28. Goodman AA, Frey CF: Massive upper gastrointestinal hemorrhage following surgical operations. Ann Surg 167:180–184, 1968

29. Fogelman MJ, Garvey JM: Acute gastroduodenal ulceration incident to surgery and disease. Analysis and review of eighty-eight cases. Am J Surg 112:651–656, 1966

30. Boijsen E., Göthlin J, Hallböök T, et al: Preoperative angiographic diagnosis of bleeding aneurysms of abdominal visceral arteries. Radiology 93:781–791, 1969

31. Ranniger K, Menguy R, Kittle CF, et al: Angiographic diagnosis of an intrahepatic aneurysm as a cause of unexplained bleeding. Radiology 90:507–509, 1968

32. Metzger DG, Hamilton RF, Stephenson DV Jr: Mesenteric arteriovenous fistula. Unusual cause of distal gastrointestinal bleeding. Am J Surg 124:767–769, 1972

33. Grafe WR, Steinberg I: Superior mesenteric arteriovenous fistula following small bowel resection. Gastroenterology 51:231–235, 1966

34. Van Way CW, Crane JM, Riddell DH, et al: Arteriovenous fistula in the portal circulation. Surgery 70:876–889, 1971

35. Baer JW: Hepatic arterioportal fistula related to a liver biopsy. Gastrointest Radiol 2:297–299, 1977

36. Wallace S, Medellin H, Nelson RS: Angiographic changes due to needle biopsy of the liver. Radiology 105:13–18, 1972

37. Elliott JP Jr, Smith RF, Szilagyi DE: Aortoenteric and paraprosthetic-enteric fistulas. Arch Surg 108:479–488, 1974

38. Thompson WM, Jackson DC, Johnsrude IS: Aortoenteric and paraprosthetic-enteric fistulas: Radiologic Findings. Am J Roentgenol 127:235–242, 1976

39. Wyatt GM, Rauchway MI, Spitz HB: Roentgen findings in aortoenteric fistulae. Am J Roentgenol 126:714–722, 1976

40. Lautin EM, Friedman AC: A complicated case of aortoduodenal fistula. Gastrointest Radiol 4:401–404, 1979

41. Reckless JPD, McColl I, Taylor GW: Aortoenteric fistulae: An uncommon complication of abdominal aortic aneurysms. Br J Surg 59:458–460, 1972

42. Shaigany A, Gillespie L, Mock JP, et al: Aortoenteric fistula. Arch Intern Med 136:930–932, 1976

43. Ray FS, McAfee RE, Hiebert CA, et al: Aortoduodenal fistula: primary repair with saphenous vein patch graft. JAMA 236:2423–2425, 1975

44. Schramek A, Weisz GM, Erlik D: Gastro-intestinal bleeding due to arterioenteric fistula. Digestion 4:103–108, 1971

45. Wolson AH, Kaupp HA, McDonald K: Ultrasound of arterial graft surgery complications. Am J Roentgenol 133:869–875, 1979

46. Ng E, Cooperman LR: Erosion of the small intestine with hemorrhage following aortic resection: Roentgen findings. Clin Radiol 21:87–89, 1970

47. Baker MS, Fisher JF, vander Reis L, et al: The endoscopic diagnosis of an aortoduodenal fistula. Arch Surg 111:304, 1976

48. Oldenburger D, Gundlach WJ: Intramural esophageal hematoma in a hemophiliac. An unusual cause of gastrointestinal bleeding. JAMA 237:800, 1977

49. Benjamin B, Hanks TJ: Submucosal dissection of the esophagus due to hemorrhage. A new radiographic finding. J Laryngol Otol 79:1032–1038, 1965

50. Wright FW, Matthews JM: Hemophilic pseudotumor of the stomach. Radiology 98:547–549, 1971

51. Rothstein JD, Sandusky WR, Keats TE: Hematoma as a cause of radiographic deformity of stomach. Radiology 90:116–117, 1968

52. Felson B, Levin EJ: Intramural hematoma of the duodenum. A diagnostic roentgen sign. Radiology 63:823–831, 1954

53. Altner PC: Constrictive lesions of the colon due to blunt trauma to the abdomen. Surg Gynecol Obstet 118:1257–1263, 1964

54. Hyson EA, Burrell M, Toffler R: Drug-induced gastrointestinal disease. Gastrointest Radiol 2:183–212, 1977

55. Meyers MA, Ghahremani GG: Complications of gastrointestinal fiberoptic endoscopy. Gastrointest Radiol 2:273–280, 1977

56. Chen P, Lebowitz R, Lewicki AM: Spontaneous hematoma of the esophagus. A complication of uremia. Radiology 100:281–282, 1971

57. Lichter I, Borrie J: Intramural esophageal abscess. Br J Surg 52:185–188, 1965

58. Lowman RM, Goldman R, Stern H: Roentgen aspects of intramural dissection of the esophagus. The mucosal stripe sign. Radiology 93:1329–1331, 1969

59. Lampert EG, Goodfellow JD, Wachowski TJ: Traumatic subserosal hemorrhage causing small bowel obstruction. Ann Surg 140:768–770, 1954

60. Schaner EG, Balow JE, Doppman JL: Computed tomography in the diagnosis of subcapsular and perirenal hematoma. Am J Roentgenol 129:83–88, 1977

61. Korobkin M, Moss AA, Callen PW, et al: Computed tomography of subcapsular splenic hematoma. Clinical and experimental studies. Radiology 129:441–445, 1978

62. Lee TG, Brickman FE, Avecilla LS: Ultrasound diagnosis of intramural intestinal hematoma. JCU 5:423–424, 1977

63. Wyatt GM, Spitz HB: Ultrasound in the diagnosis of rectus sheath hematoma. JAMA 241:1499–1500, 1979

64. Kaplan GN, Sanders RC: B-scan ultrasound in the management of patients with occult abdominal hematomas. JCU 1:5–13, 1973

65. Adams AT: Rectus sheath hematoma. In Schwartz SI (ed): Principles of Surgery, 2nd edn. New York: McGraw-Hill 1974, pp 1313–1315

66. Kaftori JK, Rosenberger A, Pollack S, et al: Rectus sheath hematoma: Ultrasonographic diagnosis. Am J Roentgenol 128:283–285, 1977

10 Postoperative Abdominal Abscesses

Morton A. Meyers, Gary G. Ghahremani,
and Burton M. Gold

Intraperitoneal abscesses are now seen most commonly as a postoperative complication and are particularly frequent following cholecystectomy and gastric operations. In Wetterfor's series of subphrenic abscesses, biliary tract diseases and peptic ulceration were responsible for the great majority, with acute appendicitis accounting for only 10% (1); in 60% of the total cases, however, the abscess occurred as a complication of surgery. *Escherichia coli* and other gram-negative bacteria are the dominant organisms cultured, but streptococci and staphylococci still play an important role. Many postoperative abscesses are secondary to anastomotic leaks (2).

Wound abscesses are usually quite apparent, but true intraabdominal abscesses are often clinically insidious, presenting with mild abdominal pain, malaise, and a slight fever. Early radiologic identification and localization are of extreme importance, since morbidity and mortality increase with delay in treatment.

Radiologic Signs and Accuracy in Intraabdominal Abscess

Intraabdominal abscesses may be indicated by conventional radiologic techniques by the demonstration of (a) a soft-tissue mass, (b) a collection or pattern of extraluminal gas, (c) visceral displacement, (d) loss of normally visualized structures, (e) fixation of a normally mobile organ, or (f) opacification of a communicating sinus or fistulous tract (3). Secondary signs include scoliosis, elevation or splinting of the diaphragm, localized or generalized ileus, and pulmonary basilar changes.

Ultrasonography has a sensitivity of almost 95% and a specificity approaching 100% in the diagnosis and localization of intraabdominal abscesses (4). These present generally as irregular fluid collections with indistinct margins.

Computed tomography (CT) may reveal an abscess as a mass with low attenuation value displacing surrounding structures, occasionally with a peripheral rim of higher density that may show contrast enhancement; there may be thickening or obliteration of neighboring fascial planes, and the presence of gas bubbles or air-fluid levels usually allows definitive diagnosis. CT may diagnose and accurately define the extent of involvement in at least 90% of cases, depending upon the size of the abscess (5). The characteristic signs on ultrasonography and CT usually permit clear distinction from other postoperative fluid collections such as seroma and lymphocyst.

The overall accuracy for gallium-67 citrate examination is highly dependent on the type of patient studied; the presence of a surgical incision, as well as nonspecific uptake in inflammatory but nonsupporative lesions, bowel, and tumors, may be confused with an abscess cavity (4).

Dynamic Anatomic Considerations and Localizing Features

Anatomic-radiologic correlations by Meyers have established the preferential pathways by

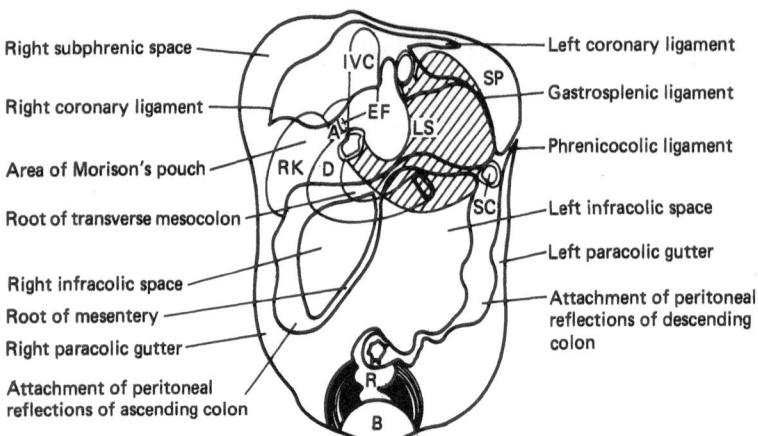

Fig. 10-1. Posterior peritoneal reflections and recesses. *Sp*, spleen; *LS*, lesser sac; *IVC*, inferior vena cava; *EF*, epiploic foramen of Winslow; *RK*, right kidney; *D*, duodenum; *A*, adrenal gland; *SC*, splenic flexure of colon; *R*, rectum; *B*, urinary bladder. (Meyers MA: Dynamic Radiology of the Abdomen: Normal and Pathologic Anatomy. New York: Springer-Verlag 1976)

which a remote abscess develops from a primary site of infection (3,6–9). The posterior peritoneal attachments and associated recesses serve as watersheds directing the spread and compartmentalization of contaminated material (Fig. 10-1.) Following is a radiologic-anatomic classification of intraperitoneal abscesses most commonly encountered as postoperative complications (3).

Supramesocolic
  Right subphrenic: anterior, posterior
  Right subhepatic: anterior, posterior (Morison's pouch)
  Left subphrenic
  Lesser sac
Inframesocolic
  Pelvic
  Paracolic, right, left
  Infracolic, right, left

The most common site for a localized intraperitoneal abscess is the pelvis, particularly its central cul-de-sac (pouch of Douglas) (Figs. 10-2 to 10-4). From the pelvis, contaminated fluid ascends the paracolic gutter, on the right preferentially, to the subhepatic spaces (Figs. 10-5 to 10-8), seeking especially the posterior subhepatic space (hepatorenal fossa); this site, lying in the paravertebral groove, is also known as Morison's pouch, and is the second most common intraperitoneal area for localized abscess formation (Figs. 10-9 to 10-11). The contamination, however, may not coalesce here, and the infection then may be contained in the right subphrenic space (Figs. 10-12 to 10-14). In generalized peritonitis the lesser sac as a rule remains sterile, presumably because the epiploic foramen of Winslow is promptly sealed off by inflammatory adhesions.

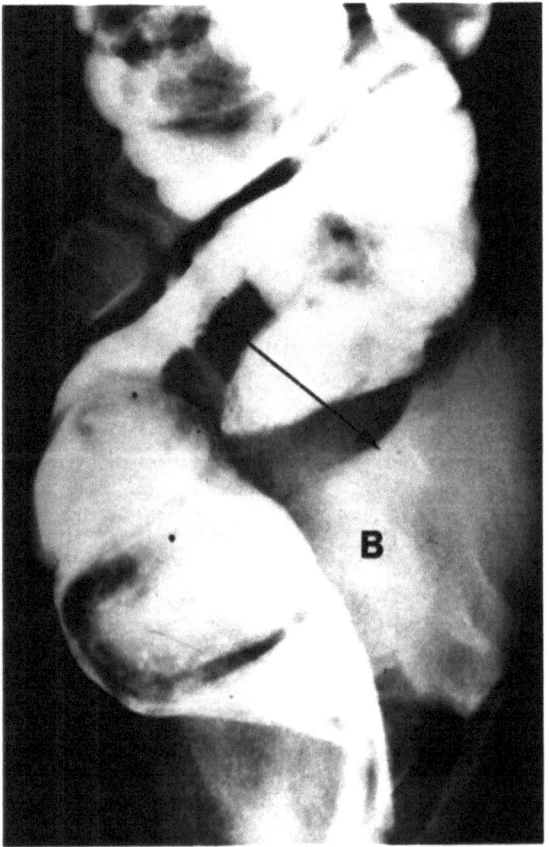

Fig. 10-2. Pelvic abscess. After appendectomy in a child a large soft-tissue mass compresses and separates the rectosigmoid junction and the urinary bladder (*B*). A redundant sigmoid loop seen in this lateral view projects in this area but is truly off the midline.

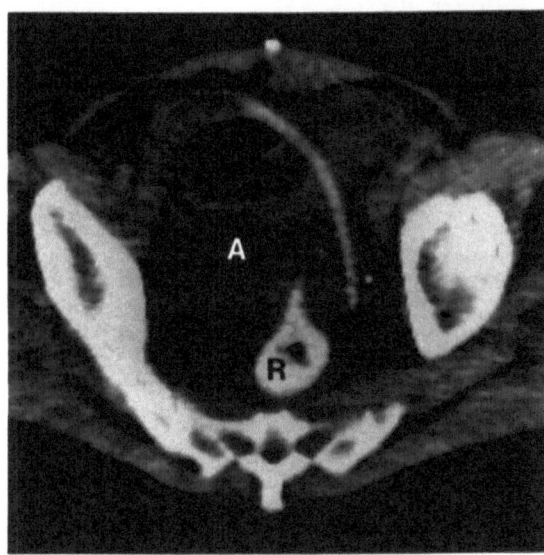

◀Fig. 10-3. Pelvic abscess. Ten days after sigmoid resection for carcinoma, CT demonstrates extensive pelvic abscess (A) with air-fluid levels displacing the contrast-filled rectum (R). A blindly introduced drainage catheter (arrowheads) is not in optimal position. (Courtesy of L. Love, MD, Maywood, Illinois)

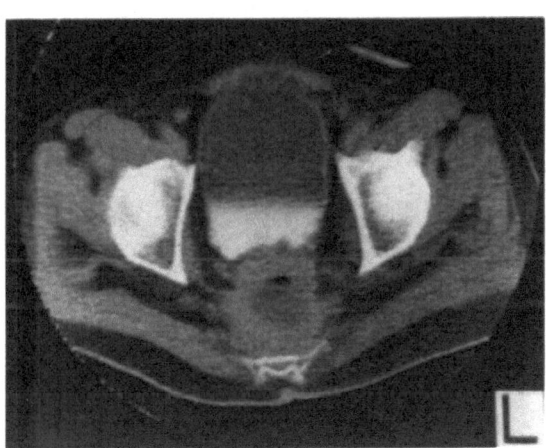

a

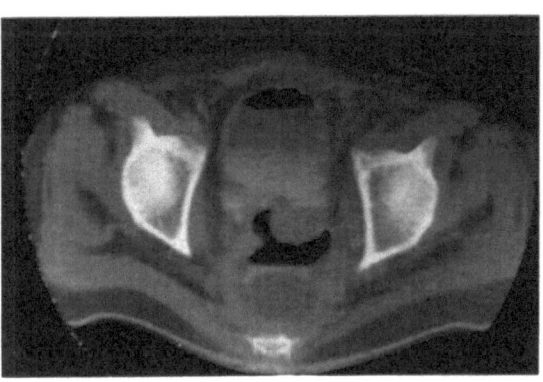

c

b

Fig. 10-4, a–c. Pelvic abscess. The abscess was demonstrated by CT after abdominoperineal resection for carcinoma of the rectosigmoid. a and b Supine and decubitus scans after intravenous injection of contrast medium were obtained 6 weeks postoperatively. The abscess is defined as a soft-tissue mass with a prominent gas collection, producing irregular indentations on the posterior wall of the urinary bladder. Colostomy device is anteriorly over the skin. c Follow-up study, several weeks after drainage of the pelvic abscess and recurrence, shows a large irregular abscess cavity communicating with the bladder (outlined by gas). The abscess had involved an adjacent ileal loop, producing a fistulous tract to soft tissues of the pelvis and bladder.

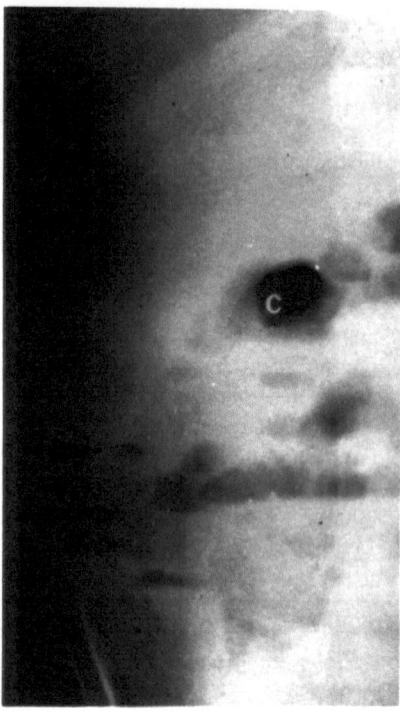

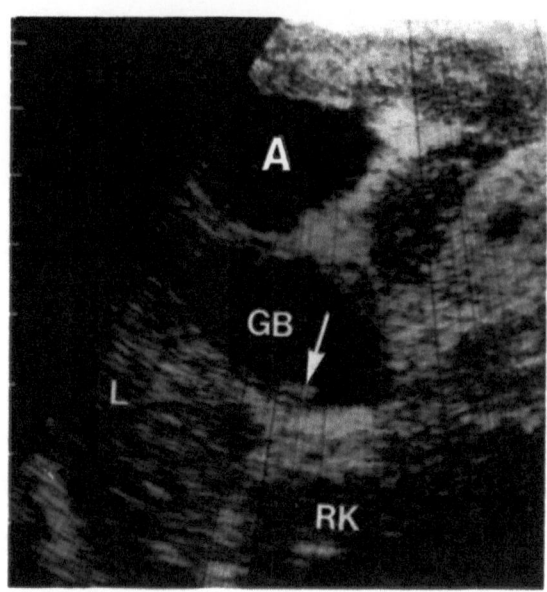

Fig. 10-5. **Right paracolic and anterior subhepatic abscesses after appendectomy.** Exudate containing a few gas bubbles *(arrows)* extends up the right paracolic gutter to a subhepatic abscess. This depresses the proximal transverse colon (*C*) and, by lifting the edge of the liver from its bed of extraperitoneal fat, results in loss of visualization of the hepatic angle. (Meyers MA: Dynamic Radiology of the Abdomen: Normal and Pathologic Anatomy. New York: Springer-Verlag 1976)

Fig. 10-6. **Right anterior subhepatic abscess.** Ultrasonography demonstrates a large abscess cavity (*A*) beneath the liver (*L*) anterior to distended gallbladder (*GB*), which, incidentally, contains a gallstone *(arrow)*. The right kidney (*RK*) is seen posteriorly. (Taylor KJW et al: Ultrasound and gallium for the diagnosis of abdominal and pelvic abscesses. Gastrointest Radiol 3:281–286, 1978)

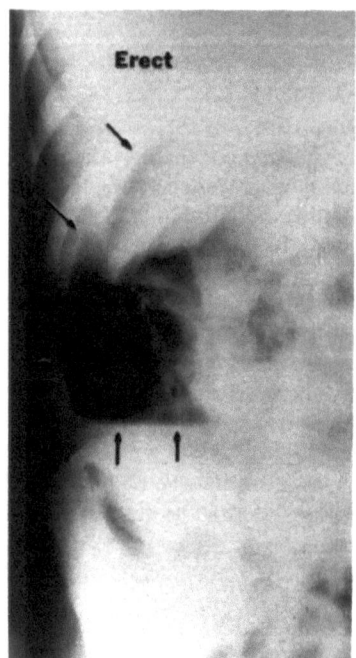

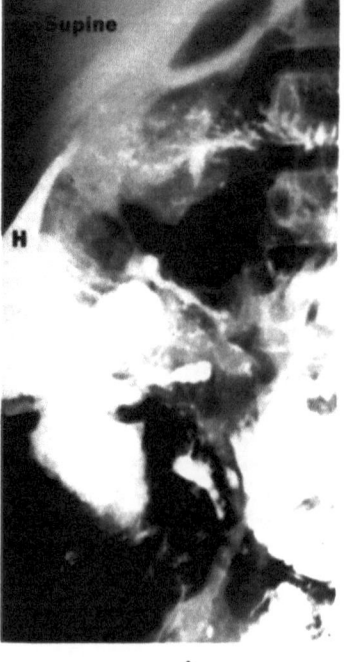

a   b

Fig. 10-7, a and b. **Sequential development of multiple abscesses after appendectomy. a** A large gas-containing abscess occupies the right paracolic gutter and extends along the right subhepatic space *(arrows)*. **b** Small-bowel series demonstrates extravasation in the area of an abscess along the hepatic angle (*H*), leading toward Morison's pouch. (Meyers MA: Dynamic Radiology of the Abdomen: Normal and Pathologic Anatomy. New York: Springer-Verlag 1976)

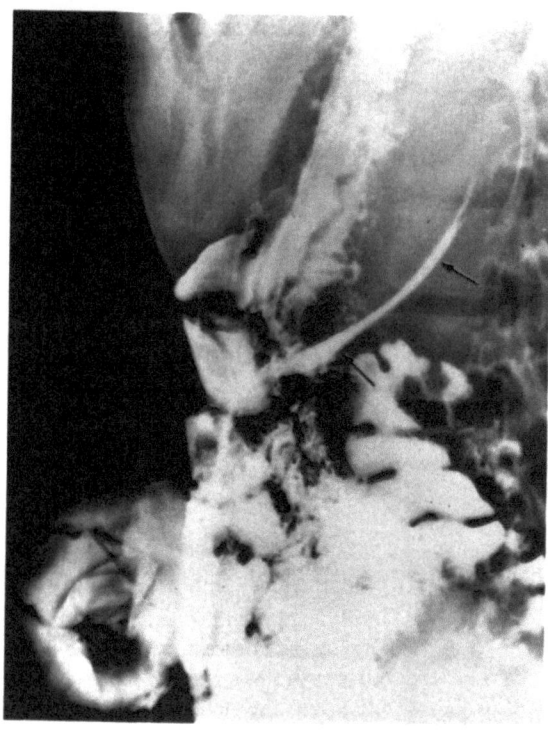

Fig. 10-8. Leak from anastomotic site following ileo-transverse colostomy. Extravasation seeks the right subhepatic space *(arrow)*. (Meyers MA: Dynamic Radiology of the Abdomen: Normal and Pathologic Anatomy. New York: Springer-Verlag 1976)

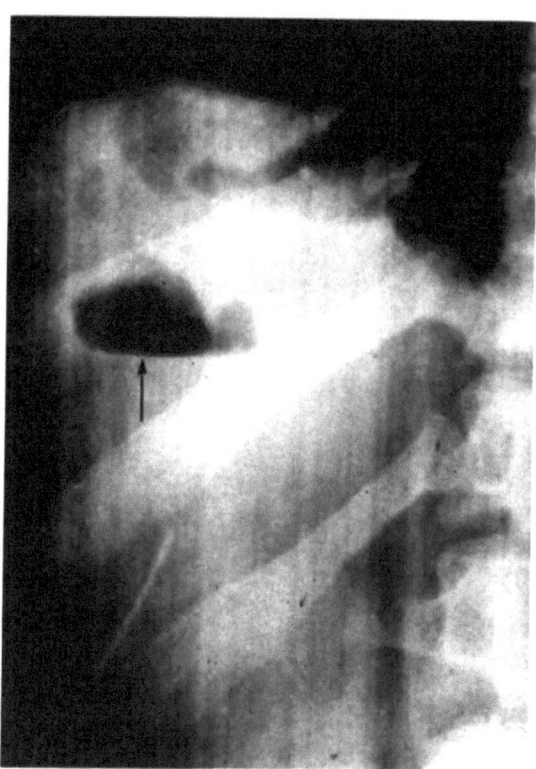

Fig. 10-9. Abscess of Morison's pouch. Erect view identifies a conspicuous air-fluid level *(arrow)* characteristically projecting anterior to the upper pole of the right kidney at the level of the 11th rib. (Meyers MA: Dynamic Radiology of the Abdomen: Normal and Pathologic Anatomy, New York: Springer-Verlag 1976)

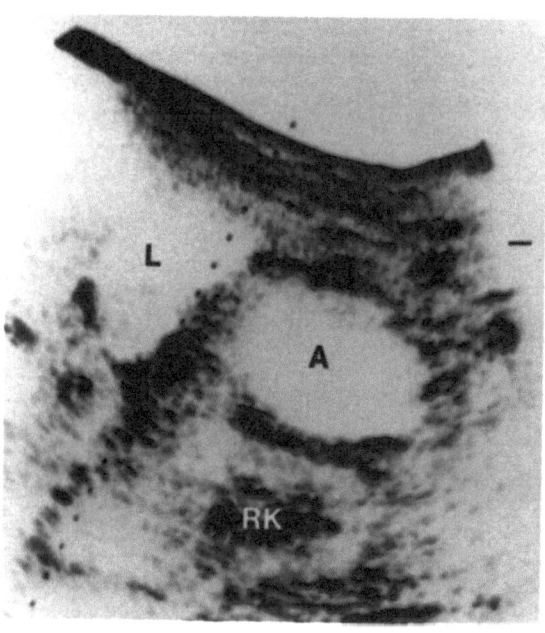

Fig. 10-10. Abscess of Morison's pouch. Ultrasonography demonstrates that a large abscess (A) has coalesced immediately anterior to the right kidney (RK), beneath the liver (L).

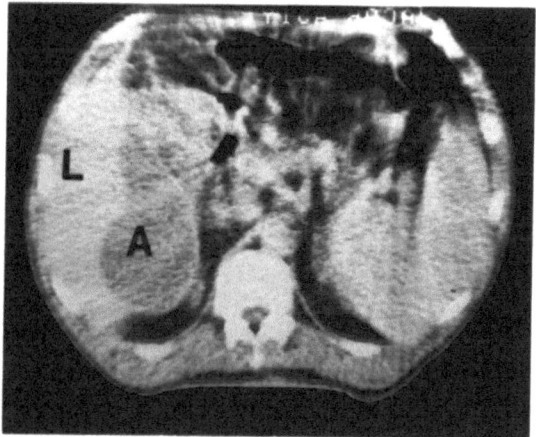

Fig. 10-11. Right posterior subhepatic abscess. This is demonstrated by CT 12 days after cholecystectomy. After contrast enhancement a clearly visible rind of peripheral enhancement outlines a 7 × 11-cm abscess (A) in Morison's pouch medial to the liver (L). (Gerzof SG et al: Computed tomography in the diagnosis and management of abdominal abscess. Gastrointest Radiol 3:287–294 1978)

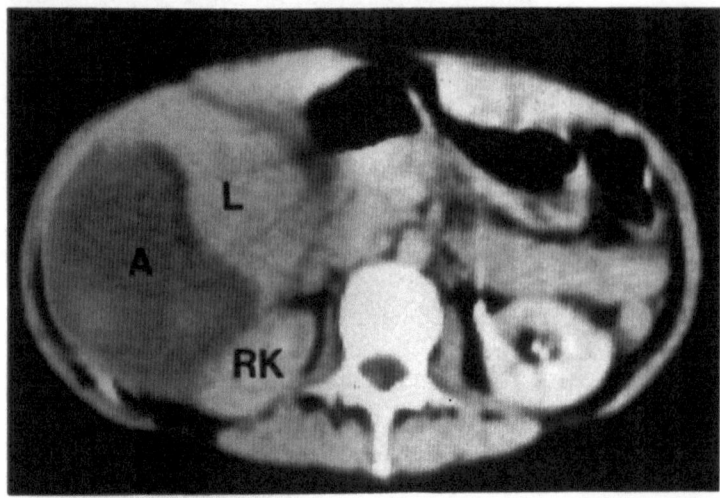

a

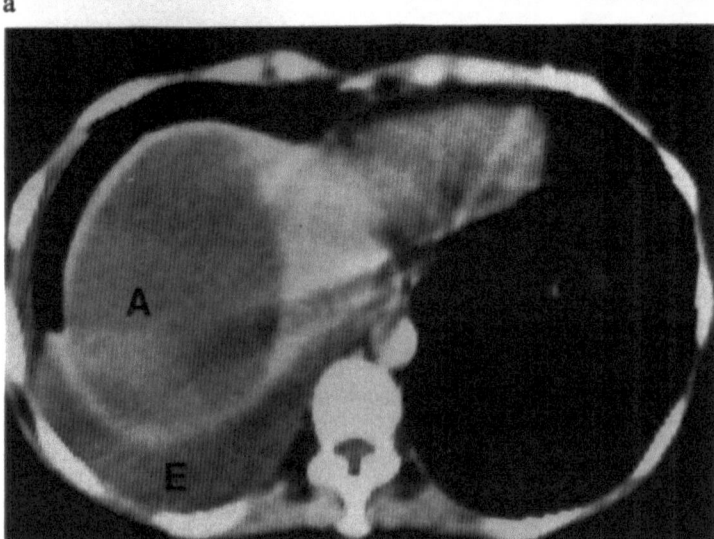

b

Fig. 10-12, a and b. Right subhepatic and right subphrenic abscesses. a Following contrast enhancement CT demonstrates a large abscess (A) that displaces the right kidney (RK) meidally, extending from Morison's pouch around the lateral margin of the liver (L) and markedly compressing and displacing that organ. b A more cephalad scan reveals its continuity with a large subphrenic collection (A) associated with reactive pleural effusion (E) in the dependent costophrenic sulcus. Note the rim of inflammatory enhancement in both subhepatic and subphrenic abscesses. (Courtesy of L. Love, MD, Maywood, Ill.)

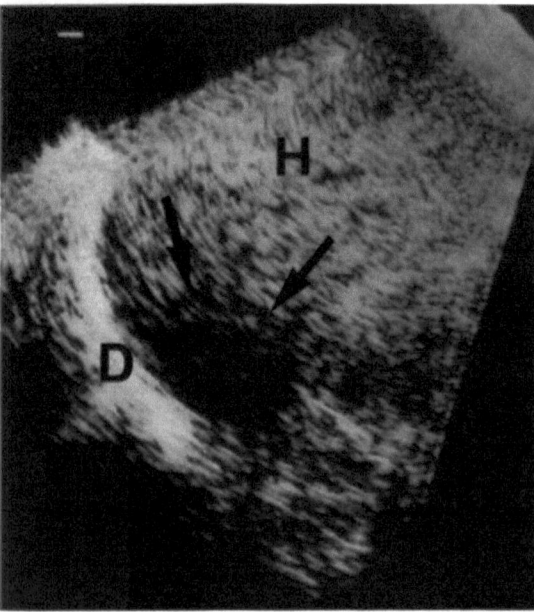

Fig. 10-13. Right subphrenic abscess. This is shown by ultrasonography. Vector scan of liver (H) demonstrates defect of abscess (arrows) beneath the right hemidiaphragm (D). (Taylor KJW et al: Ultrasound and gallium for the diagnosis of abdominal and pelvic abscesses. Gastrointest Radiol 3:281–286, 1978)

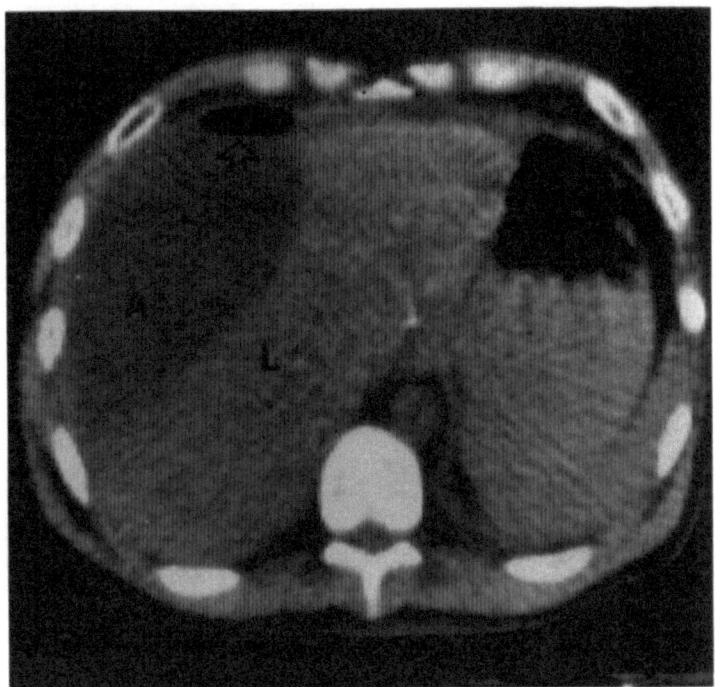

Fig. 10-14. Right subphrenic abscess. CT shows a large abscess (*A*) with an air-fluid level *(arrowhead)* compressing the lateral margin of the liver (*L*) near its dome. (Courtesy of L. Love, MD, Maywood, Illinois)

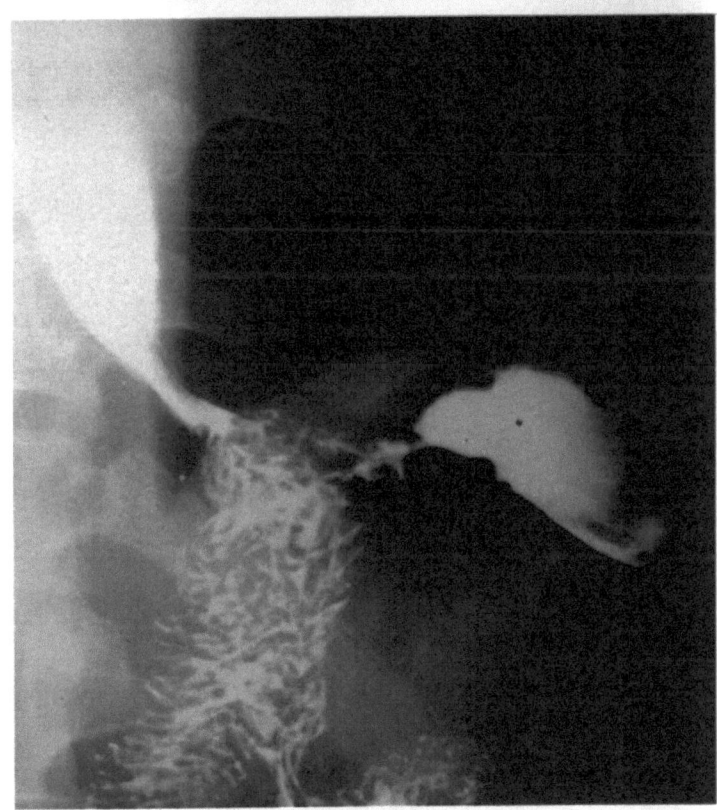

Fig. 10-15. Chronic loculated left subphrenic abscess. Secondary to anastomotic leak, the abscess developed following gastrectomy and esophagojejunostomy. (Meyers MA: Dynamic Radiology of the Abdomen: Normal and Pathologic Anatomy. New York: Springer-Verlag 1976)

Left subphrenic abscesses, in contrast, usually result from immediately contiguous sites and are seen following operations on the stomach, spleen, or splenic flexure of the colon (Figs. 10-15 to 10-19). The left paracolic gutter, being narrow and shallow, is generally not a significant avenue for the transmission of infections (Fig. 10-20); furthermore, the phrenicocolic ligament serves to disrupt continuity between this recess and the left subphrenic space.

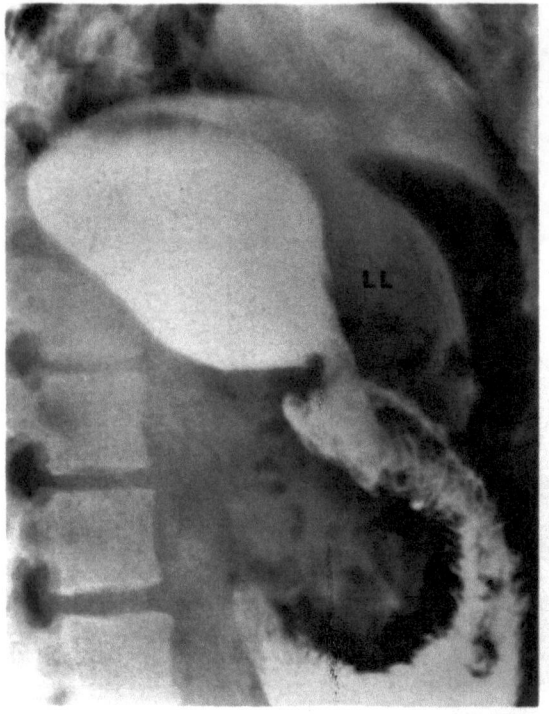

a

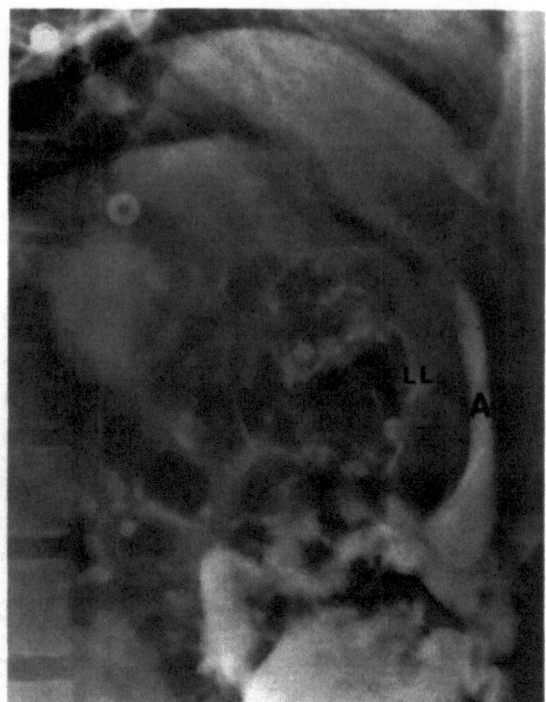

b

Fig. 10-16, a and **b. Left subphrenic abscess.** The abscess (*A*) is secondary to anastomotic leak after Billroth II procedure. The collection, first filled with gas and later opacified, seeks the subphrenic area anterior to the left lobe of the liver (*LL*). (Meyers MA: Dynamic Radiology of the Abdomen: Normal and Pathologic Anatomy. New York: Springer-Verlag 1976)

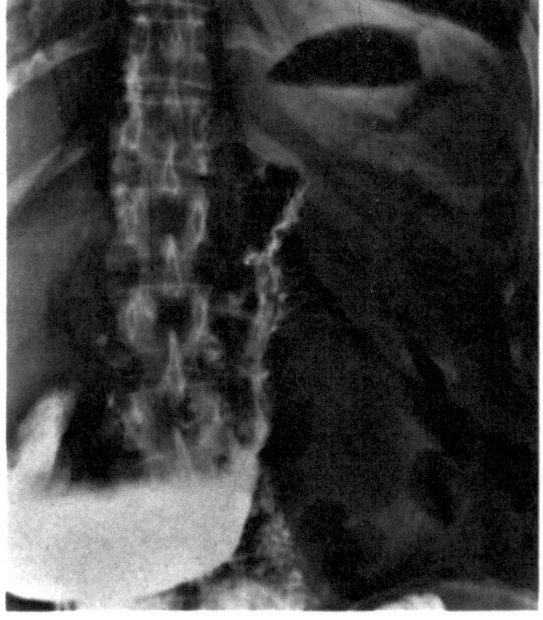

a

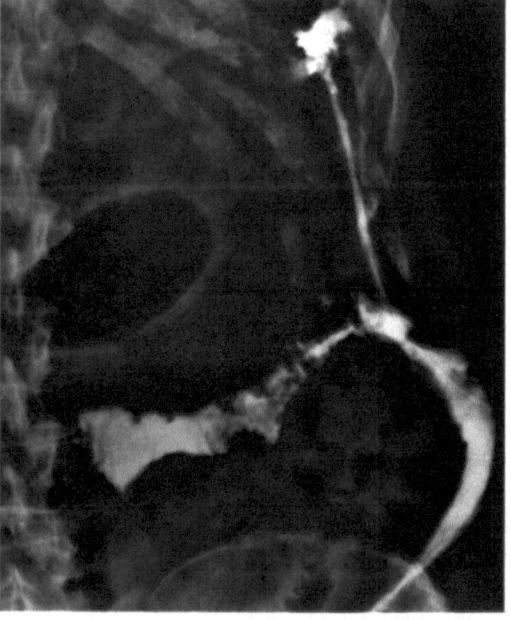

b

Fig. 10-17, a and **b. Left subphrenic abscess.** The abscess developed after splenectomy. **a** Erect frontal view demonstrates a large air-fluid collection extending lateral and superior to the stomach. **b** Barium enema study shows postsurgical perforation of the splenic flexure with a sinus tract leading to the subphrenic abscess. (Meyers MA: Dynamic Radiology of the Abdomen: Normal and Pathologic Anatomy. New York: Springer-Verlag 1976)

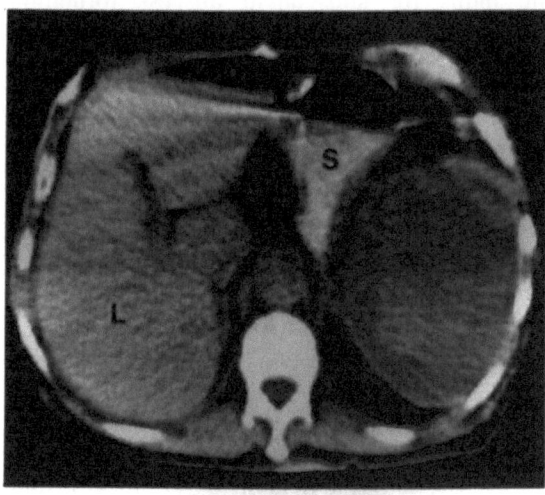

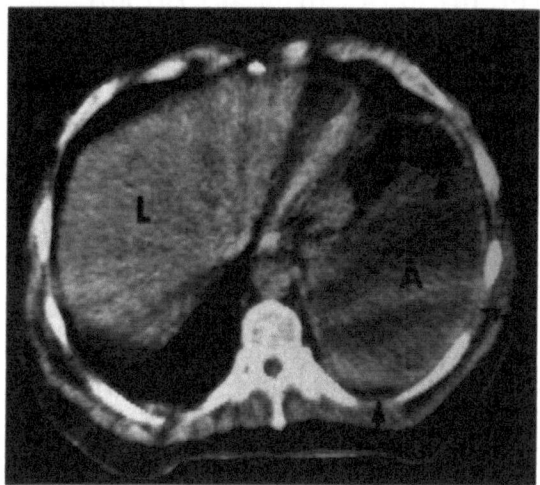

Fig. 10-18. Left subphrenic abscess. The abscess developed after splenectomy. CT demonstrates a huge abscess (A) with peripherally increased density displacing the contrast-filled stomach (S) medially. L, liver. (Courtesy of L. Love, MD, Maywood, Illinois)

Fig. 10-19. Left subphrenic abscess. Seven days after splenectomy, CT shows a 10 × 16-cm abscess (A) with an air-fluid level *(arrowhead)* elevating the left hemidiaphragm and obliterating the posterior costophrenic sulcus *(arrows)*. Note rind of peripheral enhancement. L, liver. (Gerzof SG et al: Computed tomography in the diagnosis and management of abdominal abscesses. Gastrointest Radiol 3:287–294, 1978)

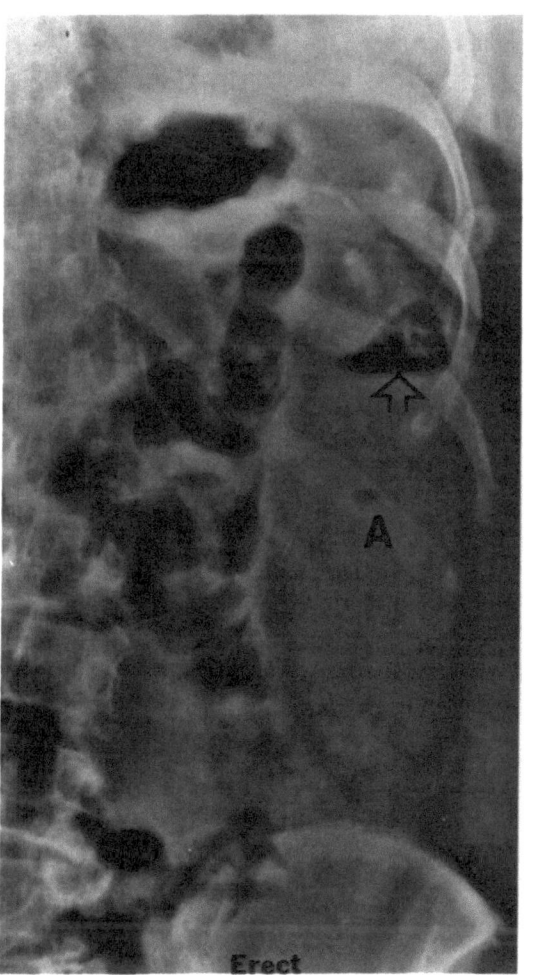

Fig. 10-20. Abscess of left paracolic gutter extending into perisplenic space. Following resection of the sigmoid colon with mobilization of the splenic flexure and excision of the phrenicocolic ligament, the large abscess (A) with an air-fluid level *(arrowhead)* within the gutter is not restrained from progressing into the perisplenic area. (Meyers MA: Dynamic Radiology of the Abdomen: Normal and Pathologic Anatomy. New York: Springer-Verlag 1976)

Retention of Surgical Foreign Bodies

An infrequent but alarming cause of postoperative abscesses is retention of surgical foreign bodies. The objects include various types of sponges, pads, drains, forceps (Fig. 10-21), needles, metallic irrigator tips, and tantalum mesh (10-12). A laparotomy sponge is the most commonly retained surgical foreign body because of the frequency of its use and the depth of the cavities into which it is placed (11).

Surgical sponges are usually made of inert cotton and do not undergo decomposition or biochemical reaction (11); however, in some cases they may become distorted by folding, twisting, and partial disintegration (13). Occasionally they may cause no apparent problem other than medicolegal liability. Retained sponges may stimulate an inflammatory reaction, with development of fibrosis, adhesions and foreign-body granuloma (14), which can result in bowel obstruction (11,13). The retained sponge may also serve as

the nidus for subsequent abscess formation (Figs. 10-22 to 10-24). In addition, a sinus tract and fistula into a hollow viscus may form in an attempt by the body to extrude the foreign material (10,15).

Tantalum mesh is an inert, although relatively rigid, material that has been increasingly used in hernia repairs. The rigidity can lead to fragmentation, extrusion through the skin, and erosion into the peritoneal cavity, with development of bowel fistulas, sinuses, and abscesses (12).

Because of past difficulty in recognizing retained surgical sponges, most institutions now routinely use only sponges that have been manufactured with radiopaque markers (11) (Fig. 10-25). Detection of the opaque marker may be hindered by its distortion and by overlying bony structures (13). In addition, retained sponges may even now be found in patients operated on before the use of radiopaque sponges. Other radiographic signs suggesting the presence of retained surgical sponges include a well-circumscribed mass, whorl-like gas patterns in the sponge's meshwork, abnormal gas collections due to abscess formation adjacent to the sponge, and rarely, development of calcification around

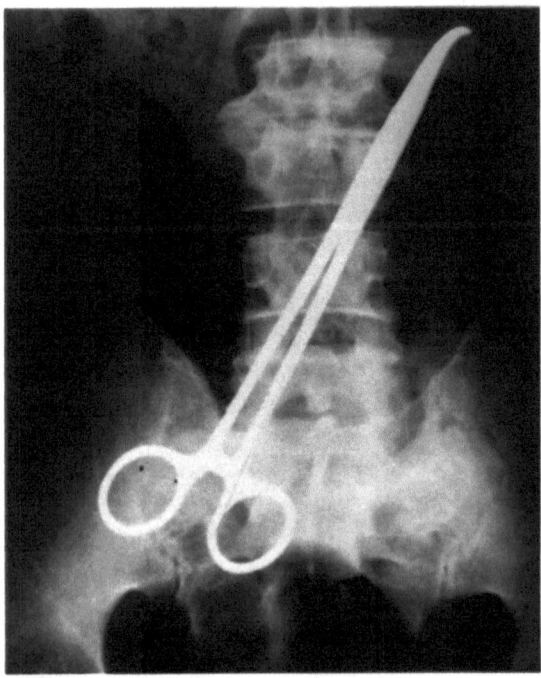

Fig. 10-21. Intraabdominally retained hemostat. This was revealed in an elderly male several years after the last of multiple abdominal operations.

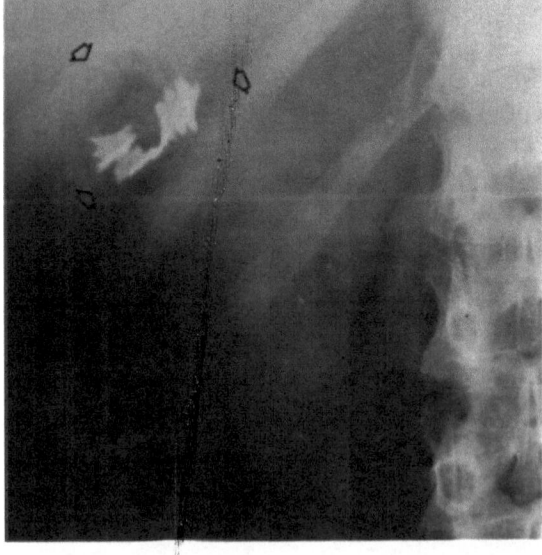

Fig. 10-22. Abscess surrounding retained sponge. Mottled gas bubbles *(arrows)* indicate the abscess; the sponge was identified by characteristic metallic densities in the gallbladder fossa. The sponge subsequently perforated into bowel and was passed per rectum. (Courtesy of M. Burrell, MD, New Haven, Connecticut)

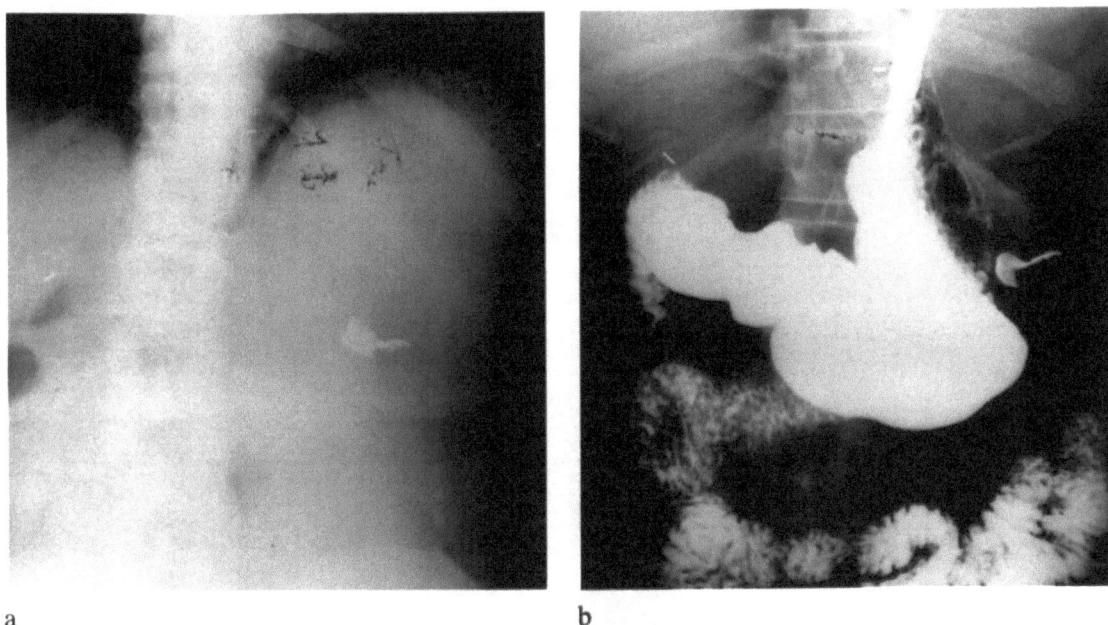

a   b

Fig. 10-23, a and **b. Large left upper-quadrant abscess surrounding retained sponge.** This occurred following splenectomy; it is distorting and displacing the stomach. (Courtesy of M. Burrell, MD, New Haven, Connecticut)

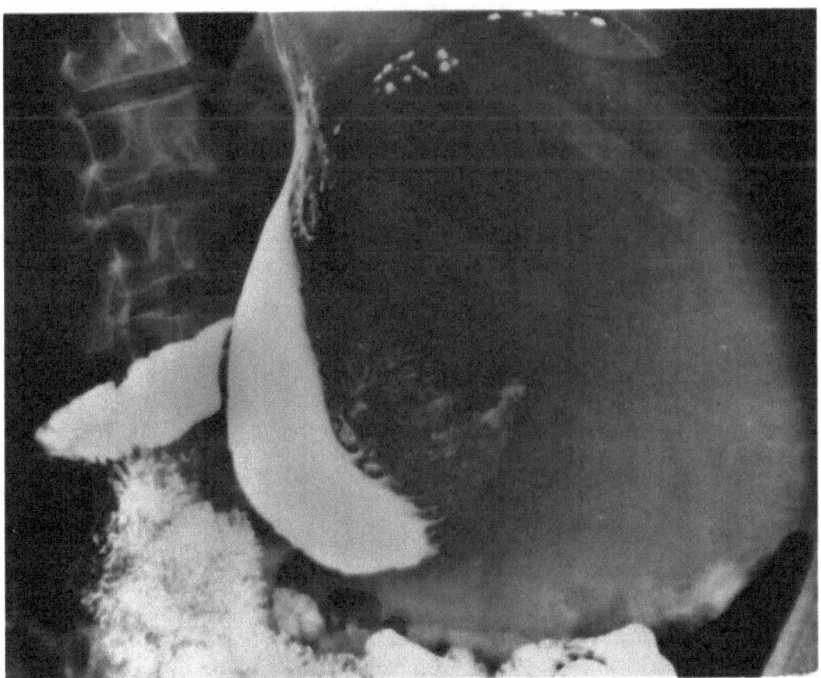

Fig. 10-24. Huge abscess secondary to retained laparotomy sponge. A 56-year-old female had had cholecystectomy 12 years earlier and hysterectomy 15 years earlier. Upper gastrointestinal series demonstrates a large soft-tissue mass in the left upper quadrant with some small oval metallic densities near the periphery of the mass. (Carsky EW, Haswell DM: Huge laparotomy pad granuloma simulating a gastric wall tumor. Am J Roentgenol 131: 909–910, 1978)

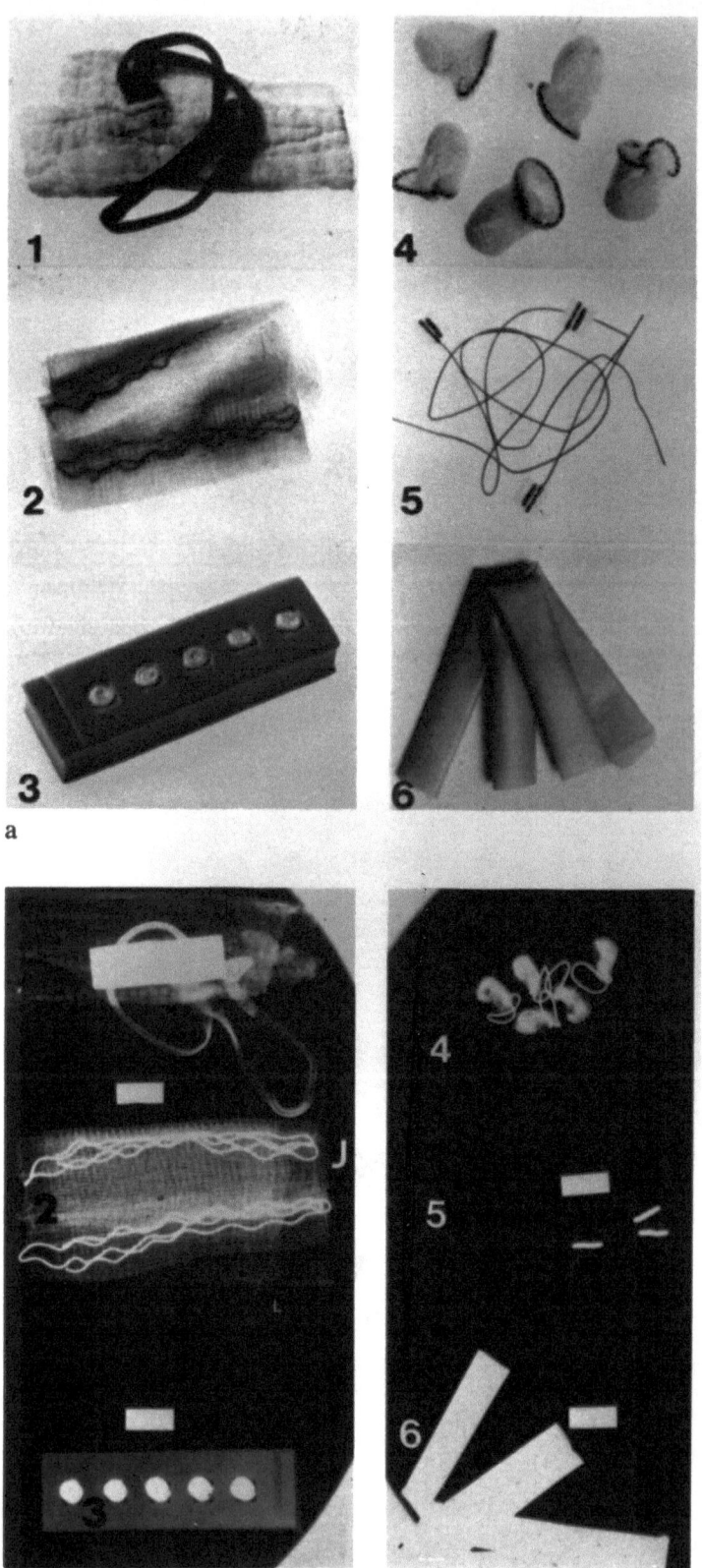

Fig. 10-25, a and b. Commonly used sponges and their radiopaque markers. Sponges (a) and radiographs (b) illustrating their opaque markers are shown with the same coding: *1*, Laparotomy sponge; *2*, 4 × 4 sponge; *3*, Kittner sponges; *4*, peanut sponges; *5*, surgical "patties" or neurosponges; *6*, Penrose drain. (Williams RG et al: Gossypiboma—The problem of the retained surgical sponge. Radiology 129:323–326, 1978)

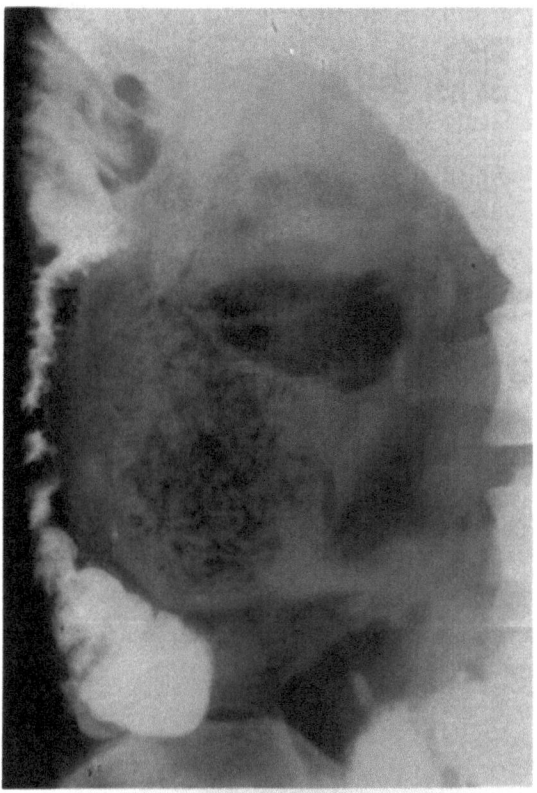

Fig. 10-26. Abscess secondary to retained laparotomy pad. The abscess is shown by swirled pattern of gas loculations, and the pad demonstrates localized opacities. The abscess distorts and compresses the ascending colon.

a retained sponge (11,13) (Fig. 10-26). In patients with a sinus tract, injection of contrast material usually identifies the meshwork of the retained sponge, and a bizarre filling defect in the intestinal lumen may be found on contrast examination in patients with sponges that erode into the intestine.

Management

The presence of an intraabdominal abscess and its precise site, as determined radiologically, dictate the most appropriate route of surgical drainage (9) (Fig. 10-27). Although antibiotics play an important role, operative drainage remains the cornerstone of therapy. A transperitoneal approach is generally employed for drainage of anterior subphrenic and subhepatic, left subphrenic, lesser sac, and multiple abscesses. An

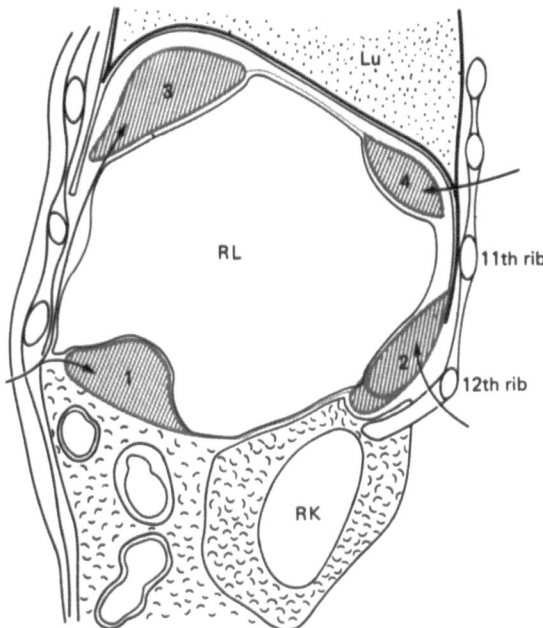

Fig. 10-27. The four sites of localized abscesses around right lobe of liver (*RL*) and surgical approaches. The site of the abscess determines the route of surgical drainage. RK, right kidney; LU, lung. (Meyers MA: Dynamic Radiology of the Abdomen: Normal and Pathologic Anatomy. New York: Springer-Verlag 1976)

abscess compartmentalized to the right posterior subhepatic space is best drained by means of Ochsner's extrapleural approach through the bed of the resected 12th rib. The right posterior subphrenic space is drained via Trendelenburg's transpleural route. Drainage of postsplenectomy abscesses is usually done posteriorly through the bed of the 12th rib to prevent contamination of the peritoneal cavity and provide the most dependent drainage (16). Ultrasound- and CT-guided aspiration and drainage of intraabdominal abscesses represent recent advances in management (17,18).

References

1. Wetterfors J: Subphrenic abscess: A clinical study of 101 cases. Acta Chir Scand 117:388–408, 1959
2. Samuel E, Duncan JG, Philip T, et al: Radiology of the postoperative abdomen. Clin Radiol 14:133–148, 1963
3. Meyers MA, Whalen JP: Radiologic aspects of intraabdominal abscesses. In Ariel I, Kazarian K: The Diagnosis and Treatment of Intraabdominal Abscesses. Baltimore: Williams & Wilkins 1971

4. Taylor KJW, Sullivan DC, Wasson JF, et al: AT: Ultrasound and gallium for the diagnosis of abdominal and pelvic abscesses. Gastrointest Radiol 3:281–286 1978

5. Aronberg DJ, Stanley RJ, Levitt RG, et al: Evaluation of abdominal abscess with computed tomography. J Comput Assist Tomogr 2:384–387, 1978

6. Meyers MA: Roentgen significance of the phrenicocolic ligament. Radiology 95:539–545, 1970

7. Meyers MA: The spread and localization of acute intraperitoneal effusions. Radiology 95:547–554, 1970

8. Meyers MA, Peritoneography: Normal and pathologic anatomy. Am J Roentgenol 117:353–365, 1973

9. Meyers MA: Dynamic Radiology of the Abdomen: Normal and Pathologic Anatomy. New York: Springer 1976

10. Crossen HS, Crossen DF: Foreign Bodies Left in the Abdomen. St. Louis: Mosby 1940

11. Williams RG, Bragg DG, Nelson JA: Gossypiboma—The problem of the retained surgical sponge. Radiology 129:323–326, 1978

12. Bothra R: Late onset small bowel fistula due to tantalum mesh. Am J Surg 125:649–650, 1973

13. Olnick HM, Weens HS, Rogers JV Jr: Radiological diagnosis of retained surgical sponges. JAMA 159:1525–1527, 1955

14. Sturdy JH, Baird RM, Gerein AN: Surgical sponges: A cause of granuloma and adhesion formation Ann Surg 165:128–134, 1967

15. Robinson KB, Levin EJ: Erosion of retained surgical sponges into the intestine. Am J Roentgenol 96:339–343, 1966

16. Jordan, GL Jr.: Complications of pancreatic and splenic surgery. In Artz CP, Hardy JD (eds): Management of Surgical Complications, 3rd edn. Philadelphia: Saunders 1975, pp 534–572

17. Haaga JR, Alfidi RJ, Havrilla TR, et al: CT detection and aspiration of abdominal abscesses. Am J Roentgenol 128:465–474, 1977

18. Gerzof SG, Robbins, AH, Birkett DH: Computed tomography in the diagnosis and management of abdominal abscesses. Gastrointest Radiol 3:287–294, 1978

11 Iatrogenic Abdominal Hernias

Gary G. Ghahremani and Morton A. Meyers

Abdominal hernias occur in 1.5% of the population, usually as a congenital or acquired primary condition, and account for over half a million operations per year in the United States (1). The increased frequency of surgical intervention has resulted in a significant incidence of iatrogenic hernias. These may be divided into three major categories: (a) incisional hernias (b) recurrences after previous hernial repair, and (c) internal herniation through surgically created mesenteric or peritoneal defects. An abdominal hernia may also occur as a complication of certain diagnostic or therapeutic procedures such as laparoscopy (2) and ventriculoperitoneal shunt placement (3,4).

Clinical diagnosis of incisional and recurrent groin hernias is usually by inspection and palpation. Radiologic studies may be used for preoperative delineation of the hernial content or evaluation of intestinal obstruction and other associated complications and, most importantly, in the diagnosis of postoperative hernias involving the diaphragm or various compartments within the abdominal cavity (5).

Incisional Hernias

Protrusion of abdominal viscera at the site of a previous surgical incision accounts for nearly 2% of all hernias. Depending upon the type of operation, the incidence of this complication may be 0.5%–13.9% (6), and about half of all cases are encountered following appendectomy or hysterectomy. In a comprehensive study of 500 inci-

sional hernias by Akman, one-half had developed within 6 months and two-thirds within 1 year of the operation. Contributing factors include:

1) *Wound infection,* particularly by anaerobic bacteria, which tend to destroy the fascial structures, is followed by incisional hernia in 5%–20% of the cases (6).

2) *Wound dehiscence* complicating infection, faulty healing, or loosening of the sutures is probably the single most important factor. Among 103 instances of wound dehiscence studied by Grace and Cox, 45% resulted in an incisional hernia despite resuturing (8).

3) *Type of incision* is significant because of its documented influence on wound healing. Both transverse and midline incisions markedly decrease the possibility of a complicating hernia. Paramedian incisions, which transect the fascial aponeurotic fibers, are more prone to disrupt the suture line when the abdominal pressure is increased by coughing, straining, or postoperative intestinal distention.

4) *Advanced age of the patient and preexisting diseases* (e.g., obesity, collagen vascular disorders, cancer, and uremia) adversely affect the process of wound healing and increase the potential for an incisional hernia (6).

The symptoms depend upon the diameter and rigidity of the hernia's aperture, the extent of visceral protrusion, and the existence of adhesions between the hernial sac and its content. The properitoneal fat or edge of the greater omentum are often the initial content of a small incisional hernia, and may cause vague abdominal discomfort and tenderness in the area of the

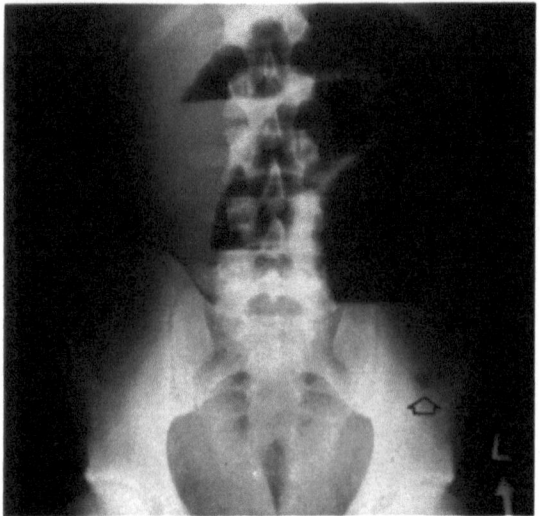

a

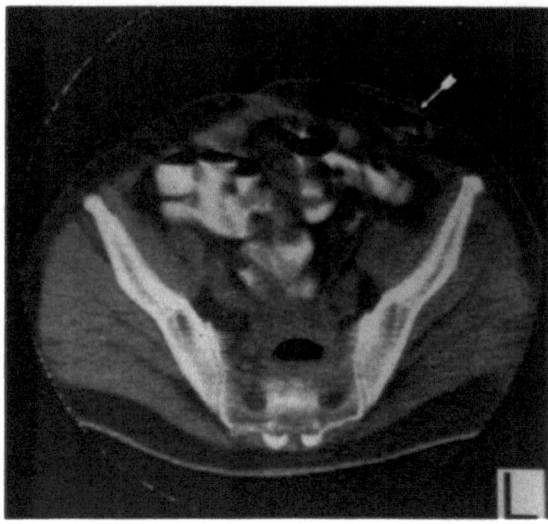

b

Fig. 11-1, a and **b. Incarcerated incisional hernia.** The patient developed intermittent small-bowel obstruction 8 months after laparotomy for stab wounds in his lower abdomen. **a** Upright film shows marked distention of the jejunal loops. A separate gas collection is noted in the left lower quadrant *(arrow)* in the area of healed incision. **b** CT section at that level clearly demonstrates a herniated intestinal loop within the anterior abdominal wall *(arrow)*.

healed scar. Diagnosis by physical examination alone, particularly in obese patients, may be difficult or even misleading. Ultrasonography is extremely useful for visualization of the defect in deeper layers of the abdominal wall and the associated interparietal hernial content (9–11). Computed tomography can also document the existence of an incisional hernia before the lesion has become large enough to be detectable by physical examination (Fig. 11-1).

Even the initially small incisional hernias progressively enlarge, and successful surgical repair becomes more difficult. A localized tender mass is produced when the greater omentum and intraperitoneally mobile segments of the small or large intestine become incarcerated. This complication occurs in about one-third of incisional hernias, but strangulation is noted in only 5% (1,12). Radiographs of the abdomen may show evidence of intestinal obstruction and a tumor-like density of the protruded viscera (Fig. 11-2).

Significant additional information is often provided by coned-down tangential views of the involved abdominal wall, utilizing soft-tissue technique. The herniated omentum presents as radiating stripes of soft tissue and fat density projecting through the abdominal-wall defect (Fig. 11-3). In the presence of gas-containing

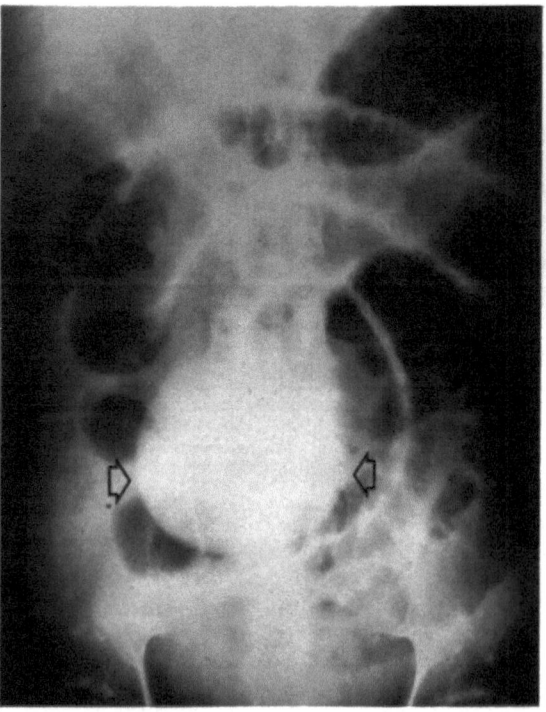

Fig. 11-2. Strangulated midline incisional hernia. Supine film of the abdomen demonstrates the well-defined soft-tissue density of the herniated viscera *(arrows)* and the associated small-bowel obstruction.

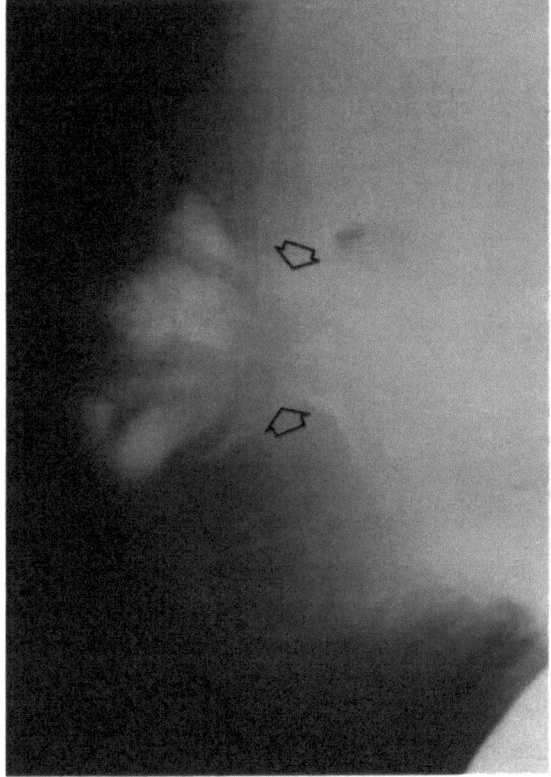

Fig. 11-3. Strangulated umbilical hernia. Coned-down lateral view of the anterior abdominal wall shows the soft-tissue and fat densities of the small bowel and omentum within the abdominal wall as they emerge from a small hernial orifice *(arrows).*

loops within the hernial sac and associated air-fluid levels in the distended proximal intestine, strangulation should be suspected. Contrast studies of the gastrointestinal tract prior to onset of intestinal obstruction (Figs. 11-4, 11-5) are helpful for clear demonstration of the herniated viscera and detection of their possible involvement by ischemic, inflammatory, or neoplastic processes (12).

Therapeutic pneumoperitoneum has recently gained popularity in the management of large incisional or other ventral hernias. Since the protruded viscera gradually "lose the right of domicile", pneumoperitoneum is utilized to expand the volume of the abdominal cavity and provide the necessary space for return of the herniated intestine (6).

Although the majority of incisional hernias involve the ventral wall of the abdomen, other potential sites should also be considered. An

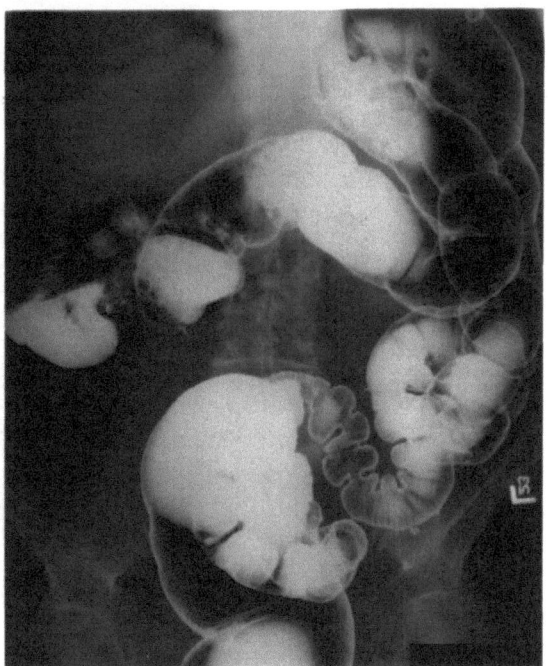

a

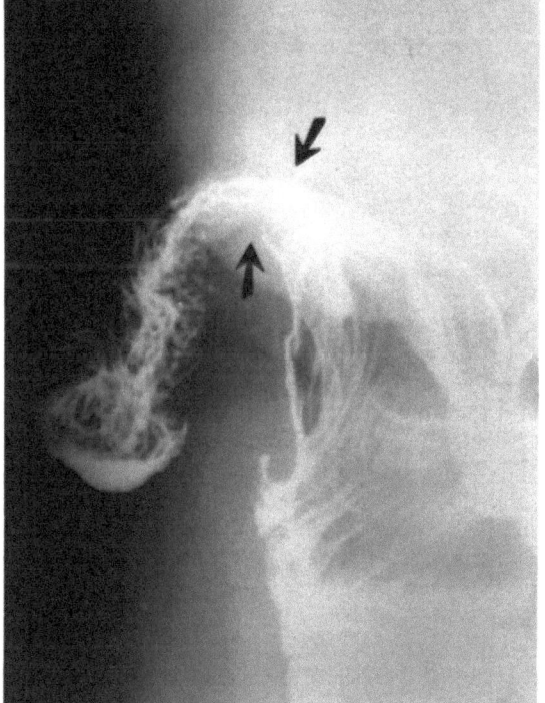

b

Fig. 11-4, a and **b. Incisional hernia complicating cholecystectomy. a** Barium enema examination reveals a deformed and partially obstructed hepatic flexure of the colon. **b** Spot film shows herniation of the colon through the right subcostal incision *(arrows).*

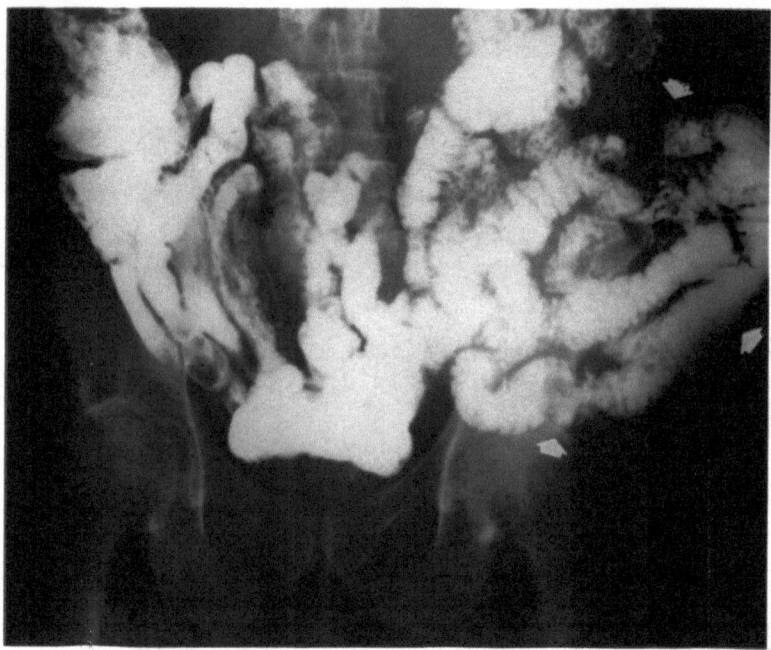

a

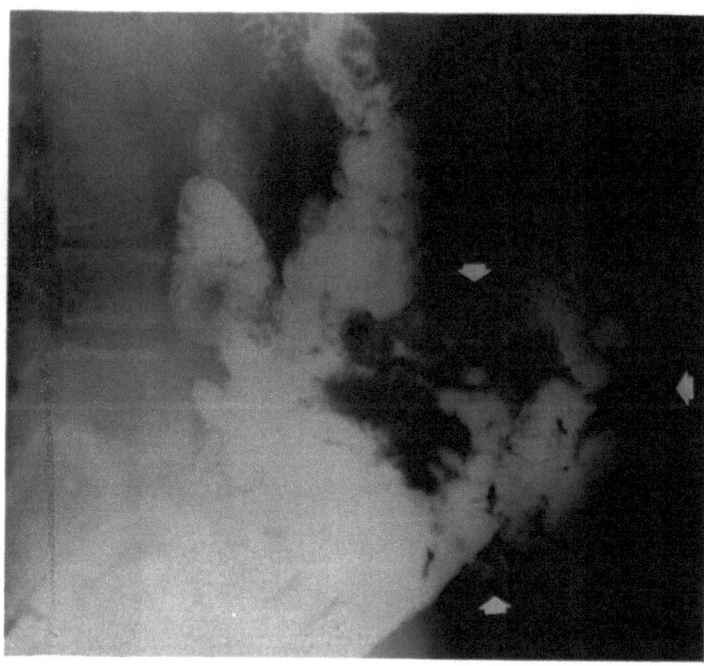

Fig. 11-5, a and b. Large incisional hernia. Supine (a) and left lateral (b) films during small-bowel series show herniation of multiple jejunal loops *(arrows)* involving a left lower-abdominal incision. Previous recto-sigmoid resection for carcinoma had been complicated by wound infection and dehiscence.

b

acquired lumbar hernia may develop in the region of a previous flank incision, particularly after nephrectomy (13). An incisional perineal hernia may occasionally complicate abdomino-perineal resection or other operations involving the pelvic floor (14). A parastomal herniation of the omentum or small intestine may occur where the distal bowel loop has been tunneled through the abdominal wall to form a permanent stoma (6,15).

Recurrent Hernias

Recurrence of a hernia following surgical repair is a formidable problem. It often indicates inadequacy of operative technique or failure in carrying out the correct procedure. This complication is particularly significant due to the enormous number of inguinal and esophageal hiatus hernias that are treated with a variety of operative methods each year. Obviously, the risk of recurrence cannot be completely eliminated because the inherent weakness of muscular and supportive tissues in the regions prone to herniation persists after the primary repair and advances further with age (1,12).

Depending upon the type of operation and follow-up period, inguinal hernias recur in 0.5%–21%, the average rate being about 8% (16–18). Postlewait studied 300 cases, including 176 indirect recurrences mainly due to low ligation or missed hernial sacs, 106 direct inguinal, and 11 femoral hernias (19). Some of these recurrences actually represent a second hernia, particularly in the femoral canal, which coexisted but was overlooked at the time of initial surgery (Fig. 11-6). Approximately half of all recurrences are

manifest within 5 years, and more than 75% by the end of 10 postoperative years. The radiographic features and associated complications of primary and recurrent hernias are quite similar. Barium studies of the gastrointestinal tract, with upright views while the patient is straining, often help in early detection of recurrence (Fig. 11-7). Positive-contrast peritoneography has also proven to be an excellent means of diagnosis (20,21). Even after a second operation the rate of recurrence may be as high as 33%. In a series of 1874 inguinal hernias reoperated on by Glassow, 1449 had recurred once, 360 had recurred twice, and 65 had undergone 3 to 5 unsuccessful repairs (17).

The recurrence rate of epigastric hernias in several series has been 10%. About half may represent new herniations involving other defects in the linea alba that were not initially recognized and corrected (22).

Despite the development of sophisticated techniques for repair of esophageal hiatus hernias, 6%–14% recur postoperatively (23,24). A major cause is the improper placement or subsequent failure of fixation sutures necessary to anchor the stomach in its infradiaphragmatic position. The radiographic features of this com-

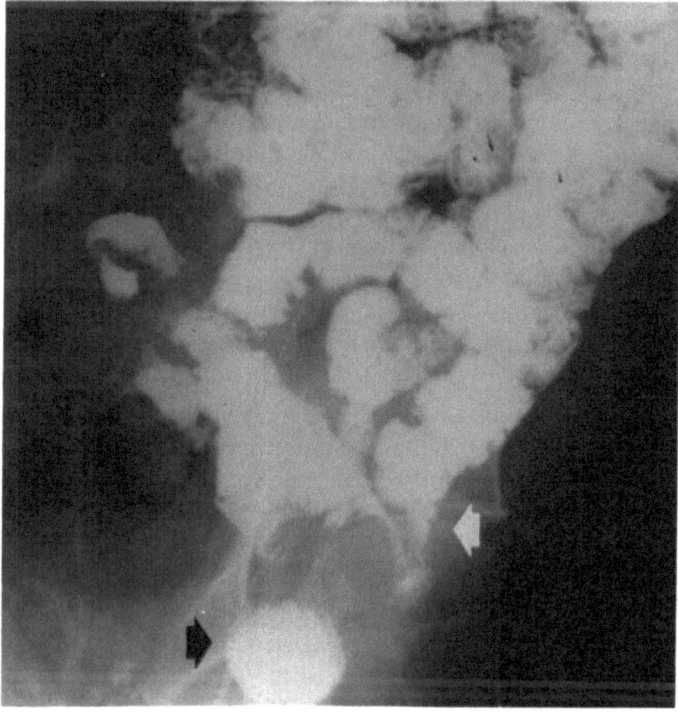

Fig. 11-6. Coexisting groin hernias. Small-bowel examination demonstrates an indirect inguinal hernia *(black arrow)* associated with a small femoral hernia *(white arrow)* on the same side. Lesions like the latter may be thought to be a recurrence if not recognized and treated at the time of inguinal hernia repair.

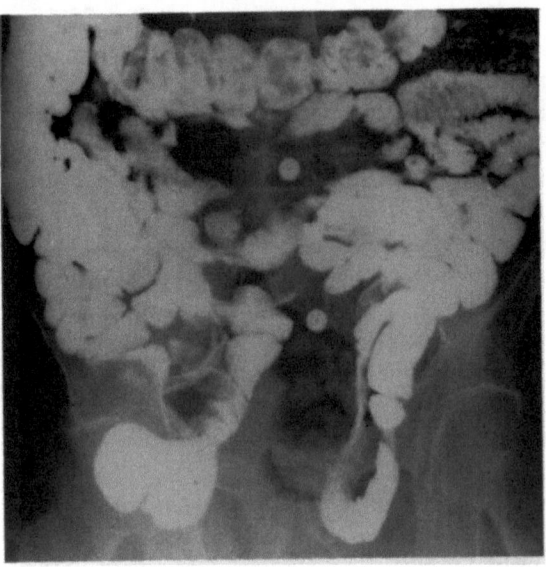

Fig. 11-7. Recurrent inguinal hernia. A 57-year-old man had previously undergone right inguinal herniorrhaphy. Small-bowel examination reveals recurrence on the same side, with adhesions deforming the adjacent ileal loops. A reducible left inguinal hernia is also demonstrated.

plication are presented in Chapters 5 and 6. A rare type of iatrogenic diaphragmatic hernia may develop after the transthoracic approach (25–27). This procedure requires an incision in the left hemidiaphragm through which the abdominal cavity is entered for placing the gastropexy and fundoplication. Occasionally the sutures closing the incision are too widely spaced or become disrupted after surgery. A "disparaesophageal" hernia can result when the gastric fundus protrudes through the defect, separated from the esophageal hiatus by an intervening segment of the diaphragm (26). In four cases reported by Balison et al., there were volvulus and incarceration of the herniated supradiaphragmatic portion of the stomach (25). In another patient the splenic flexure protruded through the diaphragmatic incision and became obstructed.

Postoperative Internal Hernias

Internal hernia represents the protrusion of a viscus through a defect in the mesentery or peritoneum, leading to encapsulation of the bowel in another compartment within the confines of the abdominal cavity. These hernias are found in 0.2%–0.9% of autopsies (5). Many small and easily reducible hernias remain clinically silent or produce intermittent and vague symptoms. However, incarcerated internal hernias still account for 2%–4% of all intestinal obstructions (28). Mortality due to bowel strangulation and gangrene exceeds 50% (5). Most internal hernias develop as a result of congenital anomalies of intestinal rotation and peritoneal attachment. Acquired defects of the mesentery and peritoneum may also serve as a hernial ring. Among 39 cases of internal hernia reported by Mayo et al., 20 were secondary to previous surgery (29). This iatrogenic complication has gained importance because of the increase in number of abdominal operations in the past few decades.

A typical example is the retroanastomotic hernia that may occur following partial gastrectomy and gastrojejunostomy in 0.5%–3% of the cases (30–34). The original Billroth II operation is now being performed in a variety of modifications. The anastomosis may be antecolic, retrocolic, isoperistaltic, or antiperistaltic. In each instance a potential hernial sac is created by the surgeon immediately behind the gastrojejunal anastomosis (31). Thus the efferent jejunal limb and, less commonly, an exceedingly long afferent loop can protrude into the retroanastomotic space. The herniation frequently occurs in a right-to-left direction. The involved small intestine becomes entrapped and may be palpable as a tender mass in the left upper quadrant of the abdomen. About half of these hernias are manifest within 1 month and another 25% within 1 year after surgery (30). The usual presenting symptoms are cramping abdominal pain, vomiting, and other signs of proximal small bowel obstruction. The findings may be mistaken for postoperative stomal edema, gastric outlet obstruction, or pancreatitis. Delay in diagnosis with eventual strangulation of the herniated loops is the principal cause for mortality in 32% of surgically treated patients (31). An upper gastrointestinal series provides crucial information when retroanastomotic hernia is suspected. It reveals that the obstruction is not at the gastric stoma but more distally in either of the anastomotic limbs. The commonly herniated efferent loop may be visualized posterior and lateral to the gastrojejunostomy (Fig. 11-8), forming a localized mass of distended loops retaining the contrast material.

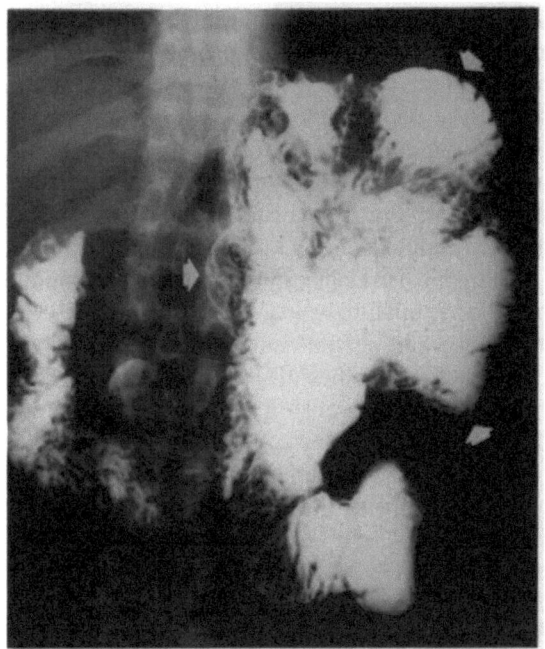

Fig. 11-8. Retroanastomotic hernia. The patient experienced recurrent epigastric pain and vomiting after subtotal gastrectomy and retrocolic gastrojejunostomy. Upper gastrointestinal series shows the herniated efferent loop encapsulated in the left upper abdomen *(arrows)*. The afferent loop with a duodenal diverticulum is also opacified with barium.

The diagnosis of afferent loop herniation is more difficult because it may not be opacified or may be delayed despite the patency of the anastomosis and efferent limb. The findings include epigastric pain and tenderness, nonbilious vomiting, and elevation of serum amylase levels (30–32).

While the retroanastomotic space is the most common, it is not the only location for iatrogenic internal hernias. In patients with retrocolic gastrojejunostomy, for example, both anastomotic limbs occasionally protrude upward through the surgically created opening in the transverse mesocolon (5,33,35). This complication is likely to occur as a result of absence or subsequent disruption of sutures between the mesocolon and the gastrojejunal segment. Upper gastrointestinal series may disclose a localized constriction of afferent and efferent loops a short distance below the anastomosis (5).

The lesser sac is another potential site. Post-

surgical defects in the transverse mesocolon, which constitutes its floor, can serve as an orifice for internal herniation of the bowel loops (35,36). Similarly a large opening is created in the anterior wall of the lesser sac by removing the gastrohepatic ligament during partial or total gastrectomy (37). As a result, the small intestine or transverse colon can protrude upward within the confines of the lesser sac (Fig. 11-9). In one case, incarceration of small intestine occurred within the remnant of the omental bursa (36). A variety of other mesenteric and omental defects produced during abdominal operations can also lead to internal herniation. However, it often cannot be differentiated from obstructive adhesions on the basis of clinical and radiographic features (5,28–37).

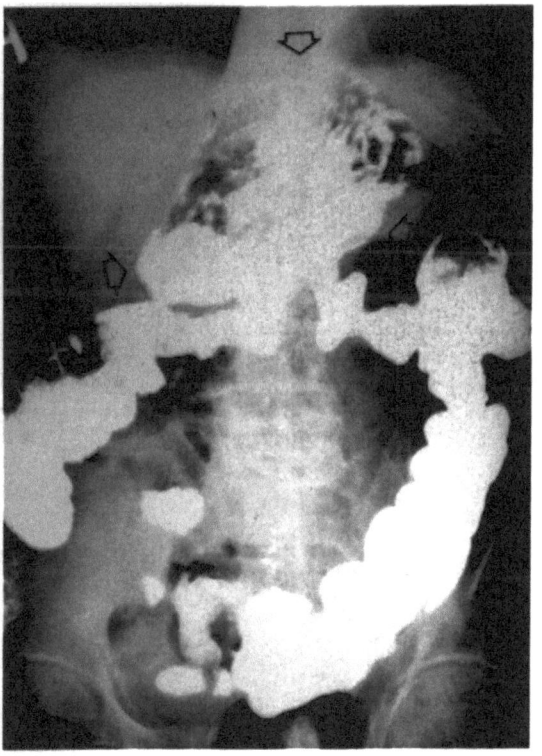

Fig. 11-9. Postoperative herniation of the colon into the lesser sac. Previous resection of the stomach and the gastrohepatic ligament in the patient had created a large defect in the anterior wall of the lesser sac. Barium enema examination shows upward herniation of the transverse colon within the confines of the lesser sac *(arrows)*.

Other Iatrogenic Hernias

Diagnostic and therapeutic procedures are occasionally the causal or contributory factors in the development of abdominal hernias. A prime example is the inguinal hernia complicating ventriculoperitoneal shunt for treatment of hydrocephalus (3,4). The underlying mechanism is increased intraabdominal pressure caused when the volume of diverted cerebrospinal fluid exceeds the rate of its peritoneal absorption. A hernia is likely to develop particularly if the processus vaginalis is patent. In one study 31 of 185 pediatric patients (16.8%) developed inguinal hernia after shunt surgery (4). The mean postoperative interval was 6.8 months. Bilateral inguinal hernias occurred in 75% of the cases, and incarceration was noted in 25%.

Diagnostic laparoscopy is another procedure that may result in a ventral hernia at the site of insertion of the instrument (2,6).

The use of a full-thickness iliac bone graft has become popular in orthopedic surgery. The peritoneum and viscera may subsequently protrude through the created bony defect and become incarcerated (38,39). The components often include the cecum, terminal ileum, and appendix on the right side, and the descending colon, sigmoid, or jejunal loops on the left. Operative reduction of the hernia and repair of the bony defect with a prosthesis are recommended.

Following surgical removal of an abdominal organ the remaining viscera may occupy the created space and become entrapped there by peritoneal folds and adhesions (5,29). After nephrectomy, intestinal loops or the opposite kidney may herniate into the vacant renal fossa (40) (Fig. 11-10). After splenectomy, small bowel loops can protrude into the left subphrenic space (Fig. 11-11). Guba et al. (41) described an unusual iatrogenic hernia developing after radical retroperitoneal lymphadenectomy (41). In their patient most of the small intestine had herniated beneath the skeletonized iliac artery, causing strangulation and perforation of the bowel.

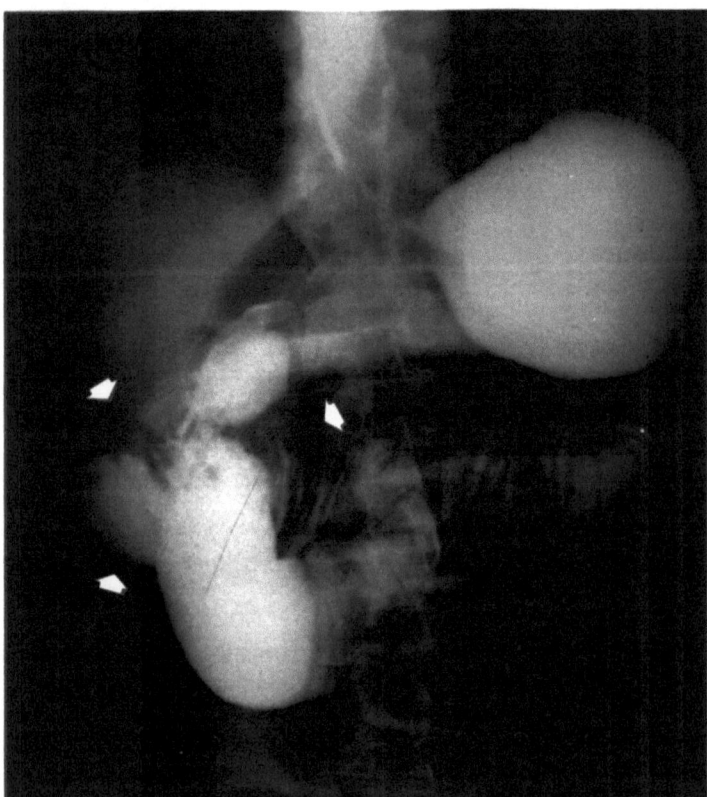

Fig. 11-10. Herniation of the small bowel after nephrectomy. Upper gastrointestinal examination reveals dilation of the duodenum and proximal jejunum, partly protruding into the right renal fossa (arrows). At surgery, multiple small-bowel loops were found entrapped by adhesion within the space vacated by the right kidney.

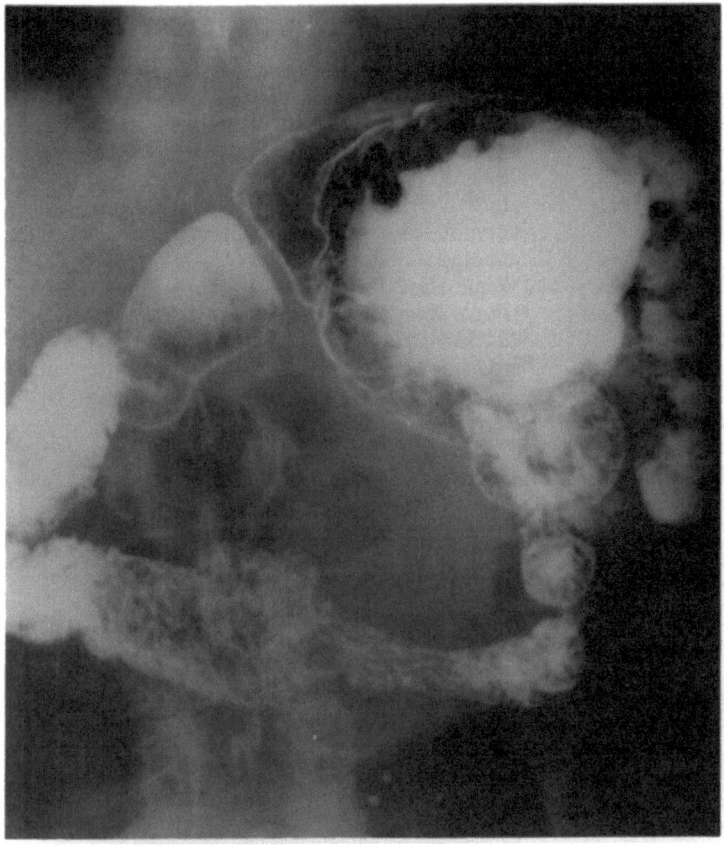

Fig. 11-11. Subphrenic migration of jejunal loops following splenectomy. Upper gastrointestinal series shows the proximal jejunum and the stomach occupying the vacant left subphrenic space.

References

1. Nyhus LM, Bombeck CT: Hernias. In Sabiston DC Jr. (ed): Davis-Christopher Textbook of Surgery, 11th edn. Philadelphia: Saunders 1977, pp 1335–1360

2. Bourke JB: Small-intestinal obstruction from a Richter's hernia at the site of insertion of a laparoscope. Br Med J 2:1393–1394, 1977

3. Grosfeld JL, Cooney DR: Inguinal hernia after ventriculoperitoneal shunt for hydrocephalus. J Pediatr Surg 9:311–315, 1974

4. Grosfeld JL, Cooney DR, Smith J, et al: Intra-abdominal complications following ventriculoperitoneal shunt procedure. Pediatrics 54:791–796, 1974

5. Ghahremani GG, Meyers MA: Internal abdominal hernias. Curr Probl Radiol 5(6):1–30, 1975

6. Baker RJ: Incisional hernia. In Nyhus LM, Condon RE (eds): Hernia, 2nd edn. Philadelphia: Lippincott 1978, pp.329–341

7. Akman PC: A study of five hundred incisional hernias. J Int Coll Surg 37:125–142, 1962

8. Grace RH, Cox SJ: Incidence of incisional hernia following dehiscence of the abdominal wound. Proc R Soc Med 66:1091–1092, 1973

9. Thomas JL, Cunningham JJ: Ultrasonic evaluation of ventral hernias disguised as intra-abdominal neoplasms. Arch Surg 113:589–590, 1978

10. Spangen L: Ultrasound as a diagnostic aid in ventral abdominal hernia. JCU 3:211–213, 1975

11. Fried AM, Meeker WR: Incarcerated spigelian hernia: Ultrasonic differential diagnosis. Am J Roentgenol 133:107–110, 1979

12. Zimmerman LM, Anson BJ: Anatomy and Surgery of Hernia. Baltimore: Williams & Wilkins 1967

13. Koontz AR: An operation for massive incisional lumbar hernia. Surg Gynecol Obstet 101:119–121, 1955

14. Koontz AR: Perineal hernia. In Nyhus LM, Condon RE (eds): Hernia, 2nd edn. Philadelphia: Lippincott 1978, pp.453–462

15. Thorlakson RH: Technique of repair of herniations associated with colonic stomas. Surg Gynecol Obstet 120:347–350, 1965

16. Welch CE: Abdominal surgery. N Engl J Med 288:661–672, 1973

17. Glassow F: The Shouldice repair for inguinal hernia. In Nyhus LM, Condon RE (eds): Hernia, 2nd edn. Philadelphia: Lippincott 1978, pp.163–174

18. Thieme ET: Recurrent inguinal hernia. Arch Surg 103:238 241, 1971

19. Postlewait RW: Causes of recurrence after inguinal herniorrhaphy. Surgery 69:772–775, 1971

20. Oh KS, Dorst JP, White JJ, et al: Positive-contrast peritoneography and herniography. Radiology 108:647–654, 1973

21. Oh KS, Condon VR, Dorst JP, et al: Peritoneographic demonstration of femoral hernia. Radiology 127:209–211, 1978

22. McCaughan JJ: Epigastric hernia. In Nyhus LM, Condon RE (eds): Hernia, 2nd edn. Philadelphia: Lippincott 1978, pp.369–374

23. Orringer MB, Skinner DB, Belsey RHR: Long-term results of the mark IV operation for hiatal hernia and analyses of recurrences and their treatment. J Thorac Cardiovasc Surg 63:25–33, 1972

24. Hill LD, Ilves R, Stevenson JK, et al: Reoperation for disruption and recurrence after Nissen fundoplication. Arch Surg 114:542–548, 1979

25. Balison JR, Macgregor AMC, Woodward ER: Postoperative diaphragmatic herniation following transthoracic fundoplication. A note of warning. Arch Surg 106:164–166, 1973

26. Hoyt T, Kyaw MM: Acquired paraesophageal and disparaeosphageal hernias. Complications of hiatal hernia repair. Am J Roentgenol 121:248–251, 1974

27. Effler DB: Allison's repair of hiatal hernia: Late complication of diaphragmatic counter incision and technique to avoid it. J Thorac Cardiovasc Surg 49:669–676, 1965

28. Sufian S, Matsumoto T: Intestinal obstruction. Am J Surg 130:9–14, 1975

29. Mayo CW, Stalker LK, Miller JM: Intra-abdominal hernia. Review of 39 cases in which treatment was surgical. Ann Surg 114:875–882, 1941

30. Bastable JRG, Huddy PE: Retro-anastomotic hernia. Eight cases of internal hernia following gastrojejunal anastomosis, with a review of the literature. Br J Surg 48:183–189, 1960

31. Markowitz AM: Internal hernia after gastrojejunostomy. Surgery 49:185–194, 1961

32. Rutledge RH: Retroanastomotic hernia after gastrojejunal anastomoses. Ann Surg 177:547–553, 1973

33. Hardy JD: Problems associated with gastric surgery. A review of 604 consecutive patients with annotation. Am J Surg 108:699–716, 1964

34. Wang HH: Internal herniation of the efferent jejunal loop after gastroenterostomy. Am J Surg 124:587–590, 1972

35. Addison NV: Herniation through the transverse mesocolon following partial gastrectomy. Br J Surg 47:381–387, 1960

36. Sorensen T: Intra-abdominal herniation of the bowel. A late complication of gastric resection. Acta Chir Scand 139:108–109, 1973

37. Boras J, Sparberg M, Poticha SM: Internal hernia with gastric outlet obstruction. Arch Surg 113:756–757, 1978

38. Pyrtek LJ, Kelly CC: Management of herniation through large iliac bone defects. Ann Surg 152:998–1003, 1960

39. Reid RL: Hernia through an iliac bone-graft donor site. A case report. J Bone Joint Surg 50:757–760, 1968

40. Cho KJ, Walter JF, Konnak JW: Contralateral renal herniation after nephrectomy: A cause of pseudo-crossed renal ectopia. Am J Roentgenol 129:1099–1100, 1977

41. Guba AM Jr, Lough F, Collins GJ, et al: Iatrogenic internal hernia involving the iliac artery. Ann Surg 188:49–52, 1978

12 Radiation Injury of the Gastrointestinal Tract

Lee F. Rogers

The physician is made constantly aware of the delicate therapeutic balance between cure and complication—the risk of treatment against the gain of control of disease. To achieve the maximum cure rate in the treatment of malignant disease it is necessary to accept a certain number of complications. To realize the optimum therapeutic balance it is necessary to attempt full eradication of the tumor while simultaneously maintaining the rate of complication at an acceptable minimum. Even under the best of circumstances some injury to normal surrounding tissues is inevitable (1).

Previously radiotherapists were limited by the nature of their equipment. Kilovoltage machines were not capable of delivering adequate central tumor doses without exceeding the tolerance of the skin. With megavoltage equipment, skin tolerance is no longer a significant problem, and high tumor doses can be administered. Unfortunately the administration of doses at sufficient depth substantially increases the likelihood of radiation injury to the normal gastrointestinal tract within the treatment field.

Radiation injuries of the alimentary tract have proven particularly vexing to all physicians involved in their diagnosis and management. Despite the presence of severe clinical symptoms, the radiologic changes may be subtle and easily overlooked. Moreover, extensive changes may be easily confused with those created by recurrent malignant disease or postoperative adhesions (2–4). However, diagnostic radiologists are in a position to suggest inadvertent radiation injury as an explanation for clinical symptoms in a patient treated for neoplastic dis-

ease. Awareness of the radiation tolerance of the bowel and the general principles of radiation treatment of various malignant diseases and knowledge of the radiologic features of radiation injury are necessary. The intention of this chapter is to provide some understanding of the factors involved in radiation injury of the gastrointestinal tract, present the spectrum of radiologic findings, and correlate them with the pathologic features.

There are two principal factors involved in radiation injury to the gastrointestinal tract (5,6). The first is related to the treatment method, and the second consists of factors inherent in the patient. The higher the radiation dose, the shorter the time over which it is administered, and the larger the treatment volume, the greater the likelihood of injury. As a general rule, radiation injuries of the gastrointestinal tract are seldom encountered with tumor doses below 4200–4500 rads delivered to the pelvis, utilizing treatment fields of approximately 15 by 15 cm (Fig. 12-1) over a period of 4–4.5 weeks (2,6). The frequency of injury increases steadily between 4500 and 6000 rads given over 4.5–6 weeks and increases sharply beyond these limits (6–8). In general, gynecologic cancer requires treatment of larger ports to a higher dose than utilized for other forms of malignant disease. Lymphomas account for a large proportion of the remaining malignant neoplasms that require treatment of the abdomen. A dose of 3500–4500 rads ordinarily is utilized, and treatment commonly is protracted by administering a tumor dose of less than 1000 rads/week. Thus one can anticipate an appreciably lower incidence of bowel injury in

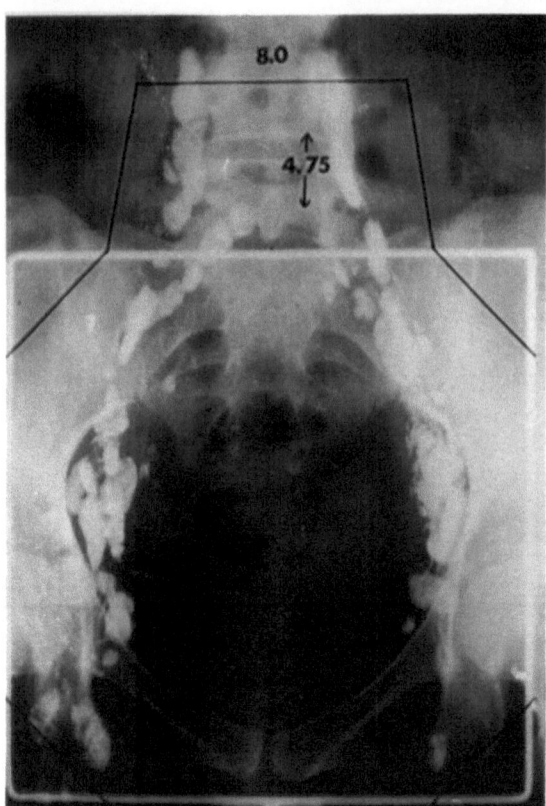

Fig. 12-1. Pelvic treatment field. The *white frame* outlines a typical 15 × 15 cm-pelvic irradiation portal. The *black line* outlines a modification of the standard pelvic treatment portal. It has been extended upward to include the lowest paraaortic lymph nodes.

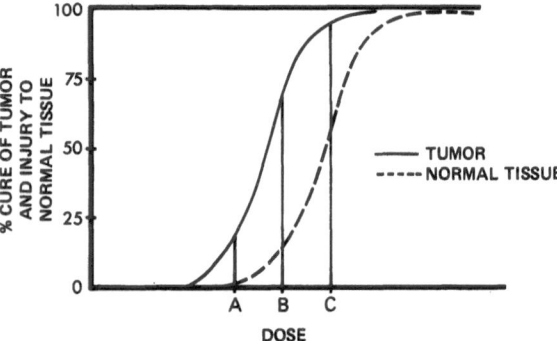

Fig. 12-2. Theoretical cure versus complication curve. Selection of dose *A* results in relatively few cures and no complications. By increasing the dose to *B* the cure rate rises appreciably at the expense of a small percentage of complications. An attempt to increase the cure rate by increasing the dose to *C* results in a small increase in cures but an unacceptable increase in the rate of complications. Dose *B* is the most acceptable compromise between cure and complication. After Fletcher (1)

the treatment of lymphomatous diseases. Most radiation injuries of the esophagus are secondary to treatment for bronchogenic carcinoma (9,10). The dose required for the treatment of bronchogenic carcinoma is in the range of 4500–6000 rads in 4–6 weeks. Radiation injury is to be anticipated at this dose level. The fact that the survival rate is low probably reduces the incidence of clinically significant radiation injury.

The rate of complications is likely to be increased in proportion to any increase in total dose, fractional dose, or dose per treatment; to volume of tissue irradiated; and to utilization of certain concurrent chemotherapeutic regimens (1). With a particular treatment regimen there may be no or minor complications, but with a small increase in one of the treatment factors, complications may appear. The balance between cure and complications can be graphically demonstrated (1). Note that the curve is sigmoid with a steep slope for both the tumor response and complications (Fig. 12-2). Therefore an attempt to increase the cure rate may simultaneously result in a significant increase in the complication rate. This may prove unacceptable. Therefore the dose and volume selected must take into account the radiosensitivity of the tumor and the potential for complications.

The two principal tissue sites involved in the genesis of radiation injury of the bowel are the mucosa and the vasculoconnective tissue within the bowel wall. The effect of radiation on the mucosa is potentially reversible, whereas the effect on the vascular tissue is prolonged and gradually progressive. Radiation injury to the vascular tissue consists of obliterative endarteritis, which results in tissue hypoxia and is the critical factor in the pathogenesis of bowel injury. The ultimate outcome is dependent upon the degree of vascular injury.

Advanced age and previous history of abdominal surgery, pelvic inflammatory disease, concomitant arteriosclerosis, diabetes, or hypertension increase the likelihood of injury (11–14). Adhesions limit motion of the small bowel and fix loops within the treatment field. Normally the small bowel is free to move, and, therefore, in the absence of adhesions it is less likely that the same segment of bowel will lie within the field during each treatment. Arteriosclerosis, diabetes, and hypertension diminish the vascularity of the bowel. Since radiation affects the small vessels, tissues that are already compromised by preexisting vascular disease are more susceptible to injury (5,15,16).

An important and unpredictable factor is individual sensitivity. For unexplained reasons, within any given dose range some individuals undergo treatment without any ill effects, whereas others who are treated similarly develop radiation injury. For the most part it is not possible to predict which individual will sustain radiation injury.

Pathologic Features

Gross inspection reveals dense peritoneal adhesions in the abdomen. The affected bowel is shortened and the mesentery thickened and contracted (12,17,18). The external surface of the bowel is gray and opaque, and telangiectasia is evident (15). The bowel wall is thickened and the lumen stenotic. The mucosa is edematous, atrophic, and frequently ulcerated.

Microscopically the bowel thickening is found predominantly in the submucosa (Fig. 12-3). It consists of edema and hyalinized fibroblastic proliferation with or without nodule formation. The small vessels demonstrate obliterative

endarteritis, consisting of endothelial proliferation, hyaline rings, and subendothelial foam cells (14,16,19).

The most prominent histologic feature of chronic radiation esophagitis is marked thickening of the submucosal and muscular layers due to edema and fibrosis (9,20). Disruption of the muscle layer is demonstrated (3,20). Vascular changes appear to be less important in the esophagus than the direct effect of radiation upon the connective and muscular tissue. This is in contradistinction to the importance of vascular changes in the development of radiation injury in the remainder of the gastrointestinal tract.

Occurrence

Radiation injury to the gastrointestinal tract has been variously reported to occur in 0.6%–17% of all individuals receiving radiation therapy for abdominal or pelvic cancer or both (12,13,21,22). The mean rate of reported occurrence is approximately 6%. The incidence of injury of the upper gastrointestinal tract is said to be less than that of the colon or small bowel. This is probably more a function of the relative infrequency of

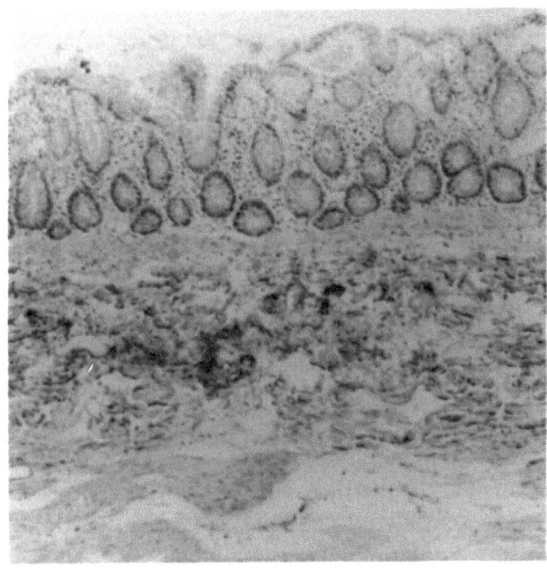 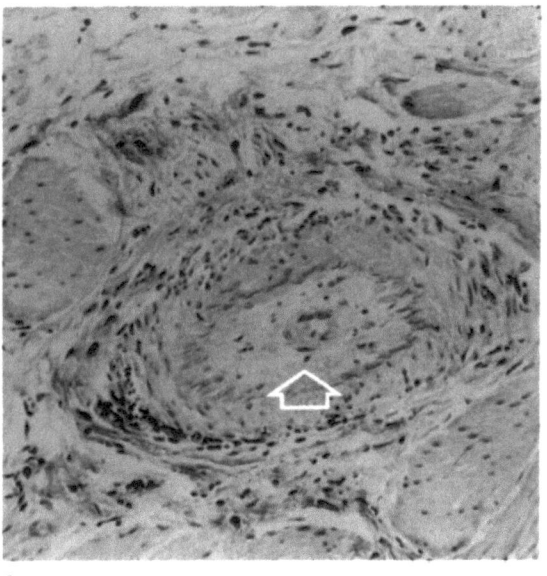

a   b

Fig. 12-3, a and b. Radiation injury of the intestine. a Injury to the rectum resulted in muscosal atrophy and thickening of the submucosal tissue. **b** Radiation injury of the vasculoconnective tissue, submucosa of colon. Endothelial proliferation is present, and the lumen of this small artery is markedly narrowed *(arrow)*.

treatment to the epigastrium, as opposed to the pelvis, than an index of the radiosensitivity of the respective organs involved.

In most series, treatment for carcinoma of the cervix accounts for approximately 75% of radiation-induced gastrointestinal disease (5,15,23). This is a reflection of the frequency of carcinoma of the cervix and of the higher doses required to eradicate the disease. Intracavitary radiation sources are utilized, which, depending upon pelvic anatomy, may result in high doses to the rectum and sigmoid. With advanced neoplasm, the anatomy is significantly distorted, space is limited, and the potential for injury is increased. Treatment of carcinoma of the ovary, bladder, and endometrium accounts for most of the remaining radiation injuries to the gastrointestinal tract. A small percentage occurs as a result of treatment of carcinoma of the prostate, testis, kidney, and adrenal and treatment of lymphoma. Radiation enteritis and colitis therefore appear predominantly in females, with a ratio of approximately 9:1.

The uncommon occurrence of radiation injury to the stomach and duodenum is more likely due to the relative infrequency of high-dose irradiation treatment to the epigastrium in comparison with the lower abdomen and pelvis (9). When the paracaval and paraaortic nodes are treated with doses in the range of 4500–6000 rads, there is an appreciable incidence of radiation damage to the stomach and duodenum (9,24–26). This was demonstrated in the Walter Reed Army Hospital series of patients who received supervoltage radiation for testicular carcinoma in the 1940s (26) and more recently in a series from M.D. Anderson Hospital where these nodes were treated as an extension of the pelvic portals for carcinoma of the cervix. The minimum incidence of gastric injury in the latter series was over 8% (9).

The incidence of radiation injury of the esophagus is not precisely determined (27). As would be anticipated, most of the patients who sustain injury have undergone high-dose treatment for carcinoma of the lung. A smaller number have received treatment for metastatic disease of the breast or testis. Although the mediastinum is commonly treated for lymphomatous disease, the dose required is lower, and the occurrence of clinically apparent radiation injury to the esophagus is infrequent.

Clinical Features

Symptoms frequently occur during actual treatment. Depending upon the area treated, some degree of dysphagia, anorexia, nausea, and diarrhea is quite common. Usually these are satisfactorily managed with conservative measures and resolve following cessation of treatment. At times the acute symptoms are of sufficient magnitude to require some reduction in the daily dose and protraction of the treatment.

The symptoms of chronic radiation injury usually occur within 6 months to 2 years of completion of therapy (6,15). Occasionally symptoms may appear somewhat earlier, or they may not appear for 10 or more years. Rarely the acute symptoms continue unabated, becoming chronic. The appearance of chronic injury cannot be predicted on the basis of the acute symptoms.

Radiologic Features

Distinct sequential, acute, and chronic stages of radiation injury are not often seen. Considerable overlap occurs, and combinations of both subacute inflammatory and chronic fibrotic changes are to be expected. The radiographic findings of radiation injury to the gastrointestinal tract are largely the manifestations of an ischemic process (7,17,23,28). In many cases of pelvic irradiation both the small intestine and colon are affected (15,27), and therefore a complete radiologic examination must include both a small-bowel series and barium enema study (16,27). However, if either examination is normal, it does not exclude the possibility of injury in the other portion of the bowel.

Esophagus

Patients who undergo mediastinal irradiation commonly experience dysphagia or substernal burning during treatment. This is presumed to represent inflammation within the esophagus and is transient. Commonly only those who complain of persistent symptoms following radiation therapy are studied roentgenographically (9,10).

Most patients do not demonstrate any evidence of morphologic abnormalities. An alteration in motility is by far the most frequent roentgenologic manifestation of radiation injury to the esophagus (9,20) (Fig. 12-4a). The disordered motility often is characterized by interruption of primary peristaltic waves at the proximal level of the mediastinal irradiation. Distal to this point there are nonperistaltic tertiary contractions, and occasionally the inferior esophageal sphincter fails to relax. Although delayed emptying of the esophagus is commonly encountered, neither esophageal dilatation nor complete absence of peristalsis is a feature of this disorder.

A smaller percentage of patients develop an esophageal stricture within the field of previous irradiation (Fig. 12-4b). These strictures have a benign appearance with tapered margins and relatively smooth mucosal surfaces. This narrowing may be due in part to radiation changes involving surrounding mediastinal structures. On occasion, angulation of the esophagus is encountered at or near the level of the stricture, suggesting adherence to adjacent structures.

Frank ulceration at the site of radiation is the least common morphologic finding (9) (Fig. 12-4c). When ulceration does occur, healing is poor, and subsequent development of an esophageal fistula is likely.

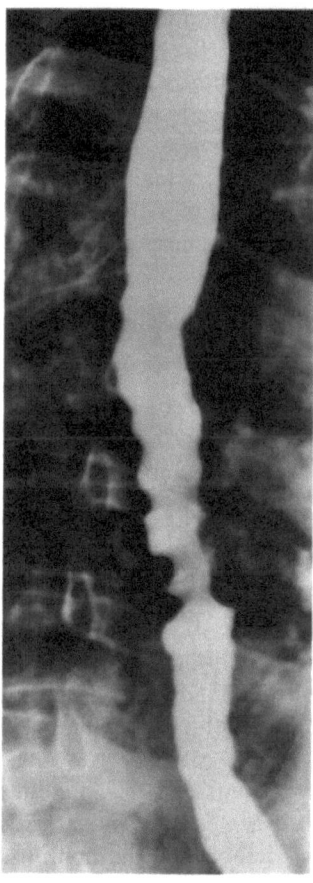
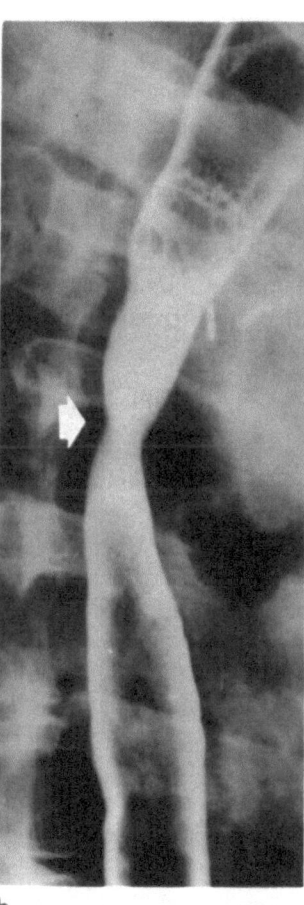
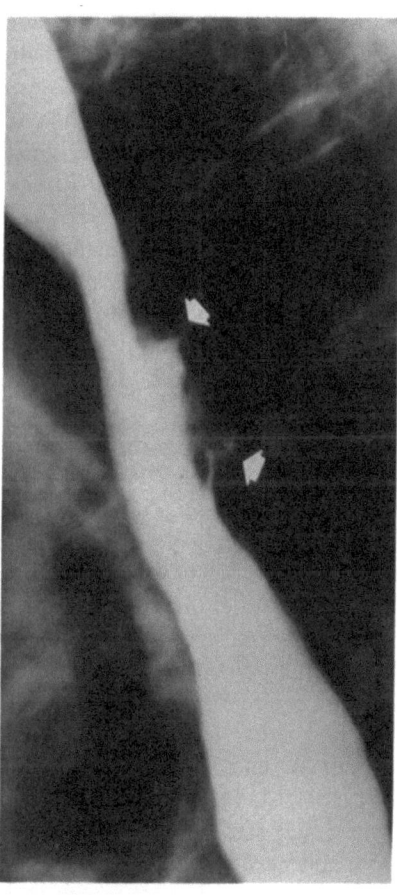

a   b   c

Fig. 12-4, a–c. Radiation injury of the esophagus. a In motility disturbance of the esophagus, note the tertiary contractions beginning at the upper margin of the port utilized in treatment of carcinoma of the lung. **b** The patient had received irradiation treatment 7 months previously for bronchogenic carcinoma and now complains of dysphagia. A smooth tapered stricture of the esophagus is identified *(arrow)*. **c** A 59-year-old man received 5818 rads to the mediastinum for bronchogenic carcinoma. The esophagogram 5 months later reveals an irregular ulceration along the posterior esophageal wall at the level irradiated *(arrows)*. (Goldstein HM, et al: Radiological manifestations of radiation-induced injury to the normal upper gastrointestinal tract. Radiology 117:135–140, 1975)

The most common complication of radiation esophagitis is obstruction of the esophageal lumen at the proximal margin of the stenotic segment.

An esophageal stricture at the site of previous irradiation must be differentiated from persistent or recurrent mediastinal neoplastic disease. The smooth appearance of the stricture and the absence of an identifiable surrounding mass are the principal features that allow this important distinction to be made with confidence.

Stomach and Duodenum

The chief symptom of radiation injury of the stomach and duodenum is epigastric pain. In contradistinction to pain associated with peptic ulceration, pain associated with radiation-induced ulcer or injury is often unrelenting and has no relation to meals. A high incidence of perforation and hemorrhage of radiation-induced ulcers has been reported (9,10,17). Healing of these ulcerations is characteristically negligible despite intense medical management. This is most likely due to underlying vascular damage rather than to failure of regeneration of the epithelium. Because of the persistence of the ulcer and its attendant symptoms, surgery is frequently required.

There are two common radiologic patterns of injury of the stomach (9). The first consists of a prepyloric ulcer and associated deformity indistinguishable from benign peptic ulceration (6,29–31) (Fig. 12-5a). Usually these are not associated with gastric outlet obstruction. Corresponding to the lack of clinical improvement with treatment, only a small percentage of these ulcers heal with conservative management (9,32,33). The second pattern consists of narrowing and deformity of the antrum and pylorus without demonstrable ulcer craters (Fig. 12-5b to d). This portion of the stomach appears rigid when palpated at fluoroscopy, and peristalsis is frequently diminished or absent. Its mucosal contour may be irregular and serrated, indicating multiple superficial ulcerations (Fig. 12-5b,d). The mucosal folds may be quite prominent and nodular or entirely effaced (Fig. 12-5c).

In the duodenum the most prominent manifestations of radiation injury are found in the second portion and vary from ulcerations (Fig 12-6a) to smooth strictures (9,10,17) (Fig. 12-6b,c). Diffuse thickening and coarsening of the mucosal pattern may be encountered (Fig. 12-6d). Often there is an associated gastric injury.

Radiation injury of the stomach and duodenum is characterized by lack of healing, and therefore acute or chronic hemorrhage may appear as a result of erosion of vessels within the bowel wall. Perforation is possible either into the peritoneal cavity, associated with peritonitis, or posteriorly into the pancreas, associated with pancreatitis. Progressive stenosis may lead to gastric outlet or duodenal obstruction.

The radiologic features of radiation-induced ulceration of the upper gastrointestinal tract are indistinguishable from those of peptic ulcer disease (9). Ulcers associated with radiation injury, however, are characterized by the history of previous irradiation and the relentless nature of the associated symptoms despite adequate medical therapy. Mucosal irregularity may be of sufficient degree to suggest a primary malignant neoplasm (34). The fixed narrowing of the stomach must be differentiated from primary gastric carcinoma or encasement of the gastric antrum by serosal implants of metastatic disease (9,10,17)

Small Bowel

Since the ileum is located within the pelvis it is irradiated routinely in the treatment of carcinoma of the cervix and other pelvic malignant disease. Injuries of the small bowel are clinically manifest by nausea, anorexia, or diarrhea, alone or in combination. Crampy abdominal pain associated with vomiting suggests obstruction (27).

The radiographic manifestations are due to a combination of pathologic changes within the bowel wall and mesentery, chiefly edematous, fibrotic, or both within the submucosa. This results in the typical appearance of straightening and thickening of the valvulae conniventes (Fig. 12-7a,b). Nodular filling defects and thumbprinting are also the result of edema, fibrous nodule formation, or both within the submucosa (Fig. 12-8). Thickening of the bowel wall causes separation of loops (Figs. 12-7a,b,12-9a,b,12-10a). With progressive damage, considerable luminal narrowing may occur over short (Fig. 12-9b) or long (Figs. 12-9a,b,12-11) segments of small bowel (19). It is unusual to demonstrate mucosal

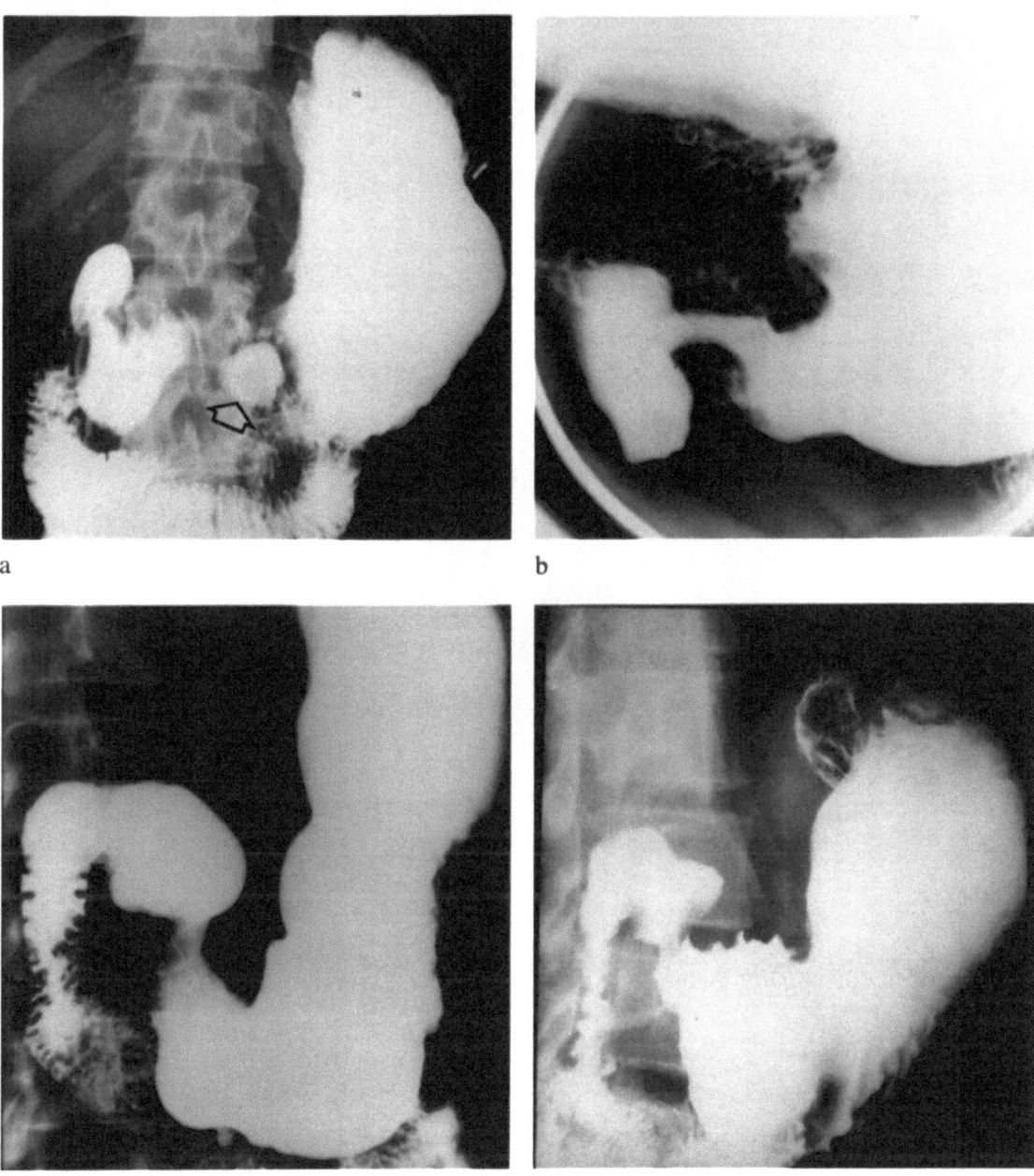

a

b

c

d

Fig. 12-5, a–d. Radiation injury of the stomach.

a A large ulcer is present in the gastric antrum *(arrow)*. Six months previously this patient had received 5000 rads to the epigastrium.

b There is a stricture in the gastric antrum. Note the irregular mucosal surface along lesser curvature. The patient had received approximately 5000 rads to the epigastrium 1 year prior to this examination.

c A 39-year-old woman received 4250 rads to the paraaortic region. One month later rigidity and fine serrations of the prepyloric and pyloric regions of the stomach are evident. The mucosal pattern is effaced.

d A 29-year-old woman received 5441 rads for metastatic cervical carcinoma. Six months later the upper gastrointestinal series showed rigidity and an irregularly serrated mucosal contour distal to the incisura angularis. (Goldstein HM, et al: Radiological manifestations of radiation-induced injury to the normal upper gastrointestinal tract. Radiology 117:135–140, 1975)

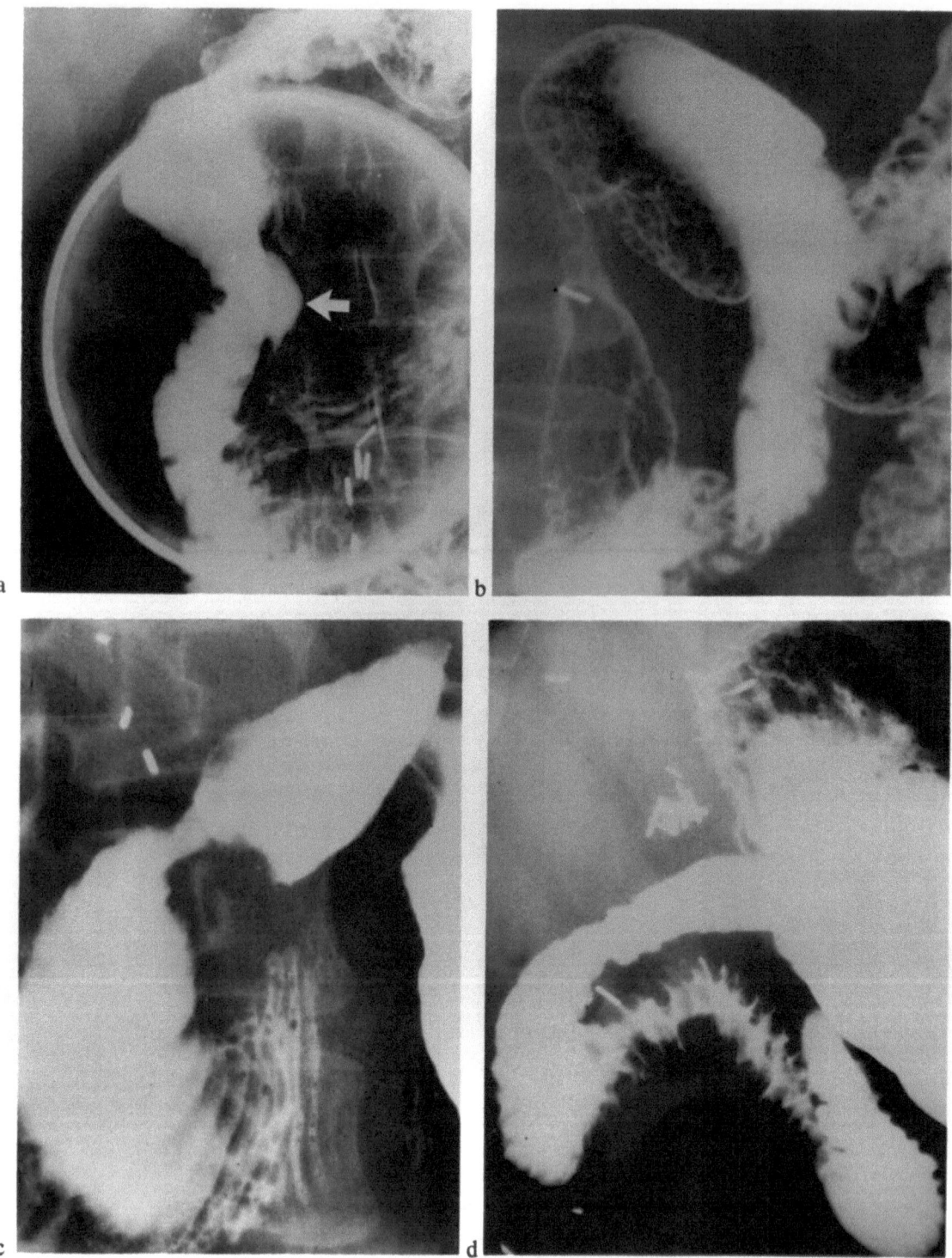

Fig. 12-6, a–d. Radiation injury of the duodenum. a
Radiation duodenitis with frank ulceration in a 63-year-old woman who received 5440 rads to the paraaortic area. Upper gastrointestinal series demonstrates a large postbulbar ulcer *(arrow)* with associated deformity. (Goldstein HM, et al: Radiological manifestations of radiation-induced injury to the normal upper gastrointestinal tract. Radiology 117:135–140, 1975) **b** Postbulbar stricture of the duodenum 13 months after irradiation for angiosarcoma of right kidney. The mucosal pattern is irregular. **c** In a young patient who was treated for an adrenal tumor the mucosal folds are thickened and a postbulbar stricture is present. **d** A 10-year-old boy received abdominal irradiation for neuroblastoma. Upper gastrointestinal series demonstrates marked thickening of the duodenal mucosal pattern.

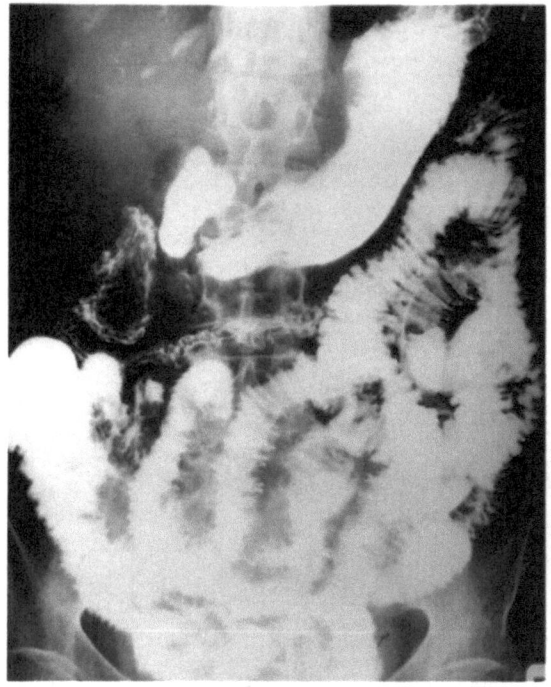

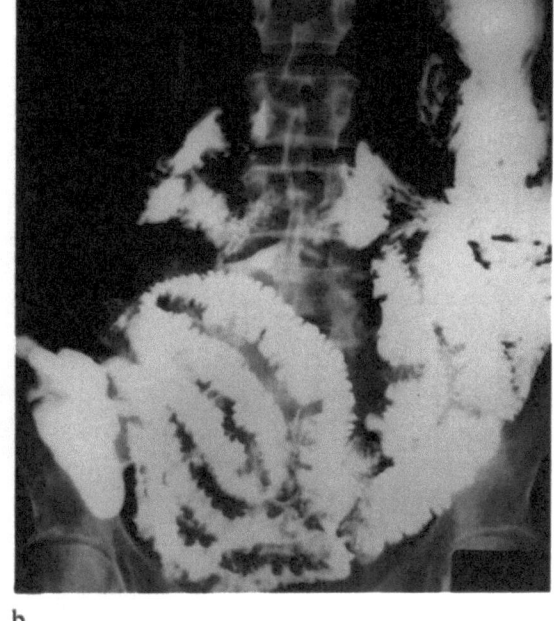

a

b

Fig. 12-7, a and b. Radiation injury of the small intestines. a In the first patient the bowel wall is thickened, and the bowel loops appear separated. The mucosal folds are prominent because of submucosal edema. **b**
Radiation changes are present in the ileum of the second patient. Nodular filling defects are present in the submucosa. The bowel wall is thickened, and mucosal edema is noted in more proximal loops.

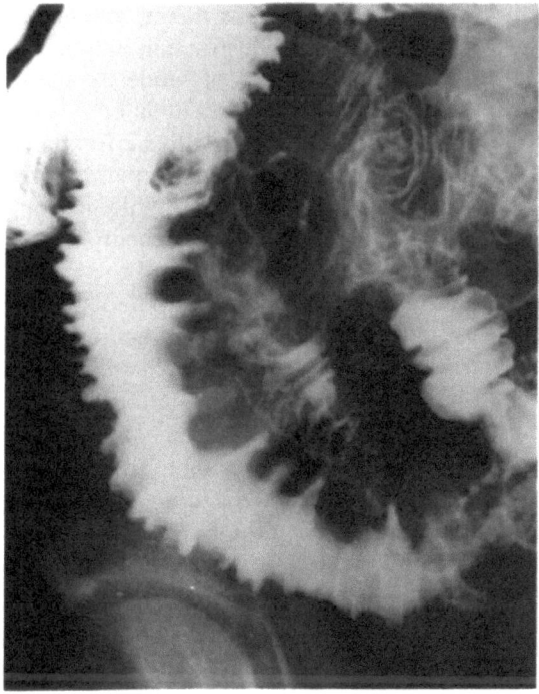

Fig. 12-8. Marked radiation ileitis. Demonstrated are thickening of the mucosal fold and actual nodular filling defects secondary to submucosal inflammation. (Reproduced with permission from Rogers LF, Goldstein HM: Roentgen diagnosis of radiation injury of the gastrointestinal tract. In M.D. Anderson Hospital and Tumor Institute, Houston: Radiologic and Other Biophysical Methods in Tumor Diagnosis. Copyright © 1975 by Year Book Medical Publishers, Inc., Chicago)

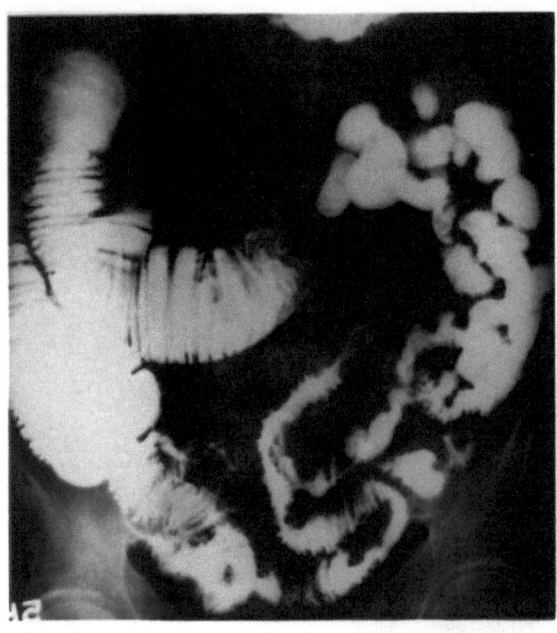
a

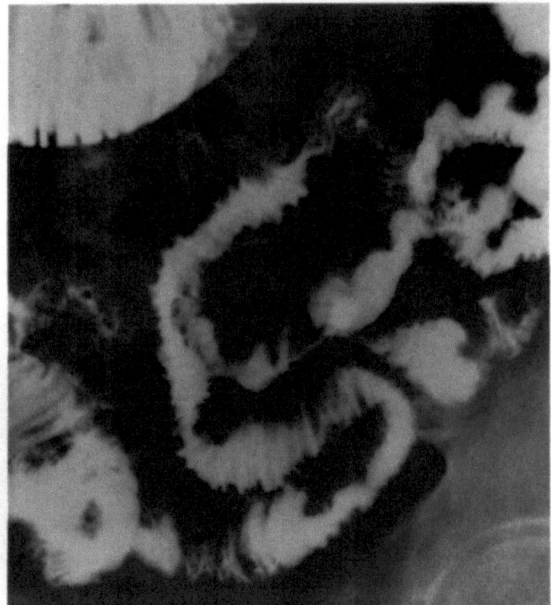
b

Fig. 12-9, a and b. Radiation enteritis with proximal small-bowel obstruction. a No focal point of narrowing was identified, but rather several long segments of rigid loops were present. **b** Close-up demonstrates notable thickening and straightening of the mucosal folds with compression of the intervening barium-filled troughs. The affected loops were rigid, with little peristaltic activity. (Reproduced with permission from Rogers LF, Goldstein HM: Roentgen diagnosis of radiation injury of the gastrointestinal tract. In M.D. Anderson Hospital and Tumor Institute, Houston: Radiologic and Other Biophysical Methods in Tumor Diagnosis. Copyright © 1975 by Year Book Medical Publishers, Inc., Chicago)

ulcerations roentgenographically because of their superficial nature and small size; however, on occasion small ulcers similar to those seen in granulomatous enteritis may be identified.

In addition to the changes of the bowel wall, there are associated changes within the mesentery, consisting of adhesions, thickening, and contraction (16,27). These are reflected in the radiographic appearance of the small bowel. The bowel loops are fixed, matted together, and may be displaced by palpation only enmasse (Fig. 12-10a). Adhesions cause abrupt angulation of the bowel. The foreshortening of the mesentery causes a mass impression on the bowel and creates a traction or pulling effect on the adjacent bowel wall (Fig. 12-12b). This appearance is accentuated with any peristaltic activity. The mesenteric changes may be confused with recurrent neoplastic disease.

The most common complication is bowel obstruction (6,15,17,22,35). This usually occurs in the mid or distal ileum (Figs. 12-9a,b,12-11,12-12a,b). The obstruction may be due to focal intrinsic stenosis or adhesions at one or more points, but equally severe obstruction may also occur from longer segments of modestly narrowed or rigid bowel loops (Figs. 12-9a,b,12-11).

Necrosis of the bowel wall with perforation into the peritoneal cavity results in peritonitis (17,27,35). This is usually a catastrophic occurrence. More commonly the necrosis leads to fistula formation between the bowel and the adjacent structures (Figs. 12-13,12-14). The fistulas may occur between the small bowel and colon, bladder, vagina, or skin in any combination.

Recurrent neoplasm must be differentiated when there is mesenteric involvement and fistula formation. The distinction cannot always be made with absolute certainty. During the acute and subacute phases when the bowel mucosa is fixed and thickened, regional enteritis, lymphoma, and other infiltrative enteropathies should be considered in the radiologic differential diagnosis (16,27).

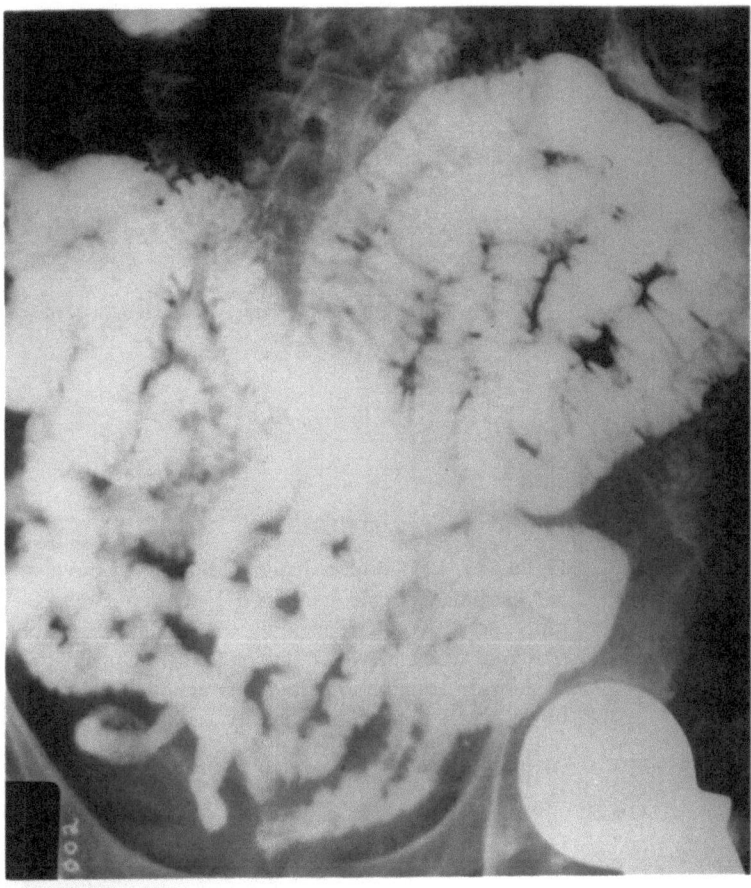

Fig. 12-10, a–c. Radiation enteritis. a Small-bowel examination demonstrates narrowing of multiple ileal loops within the pelvis. The bowel wall is thickened and edematous. b Midarterial phase of superior mesenteric angiogram demonstrates crowding, angular distortion, and tortuosity of the small arteries in the affected loops of ileum *(arrows)*. c Late arterial phase of superior mesenteric angiogram demonstrates a blush in the bowel wall *(open arrows)* and early draining veins in the involved area *(closed arrows)*.

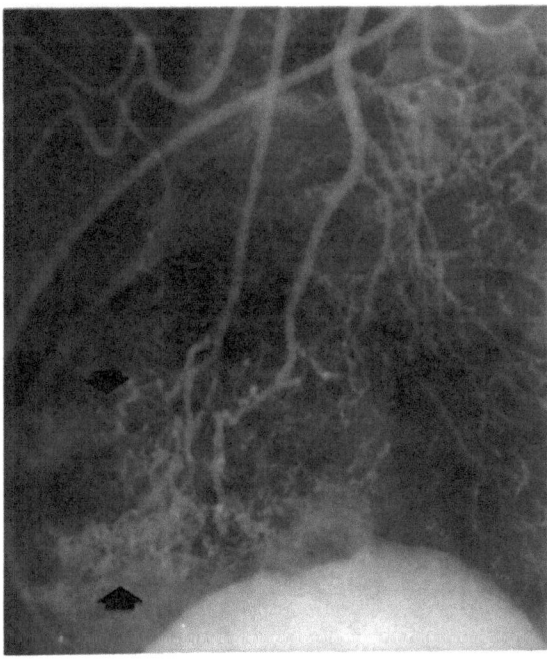

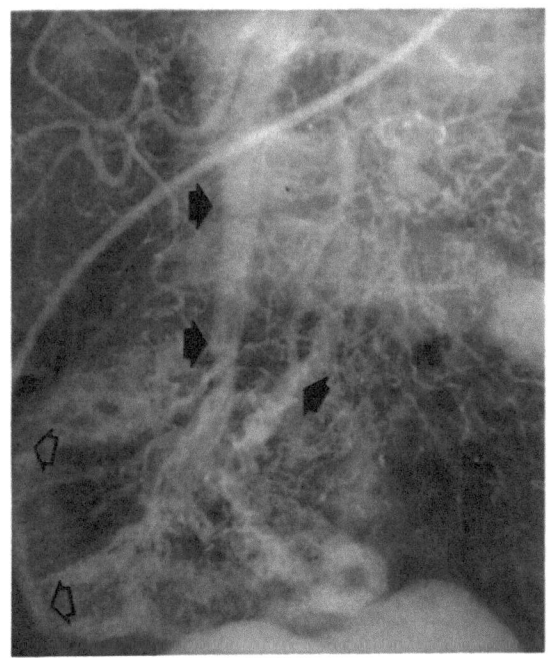

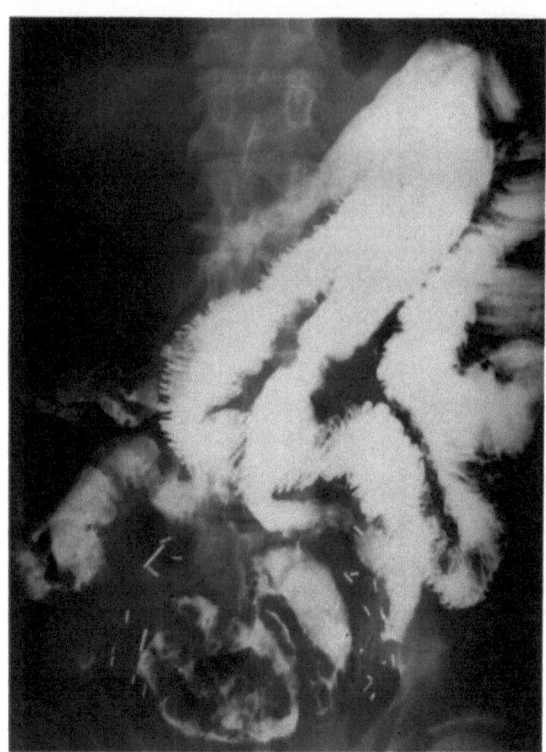

Fig. 12-11. Partial obstruction of the small bowel. A 58-year-old male was examined 1 year after cystectomy, pelvic lymphadenectomy, and administration of 6000 rads whole pelvic irradiation for carcinoma of the bladder. In addition to partial obstruction of the small bowel, gross mucosal irregularity and a long stenosis of the distal ileum are evident.

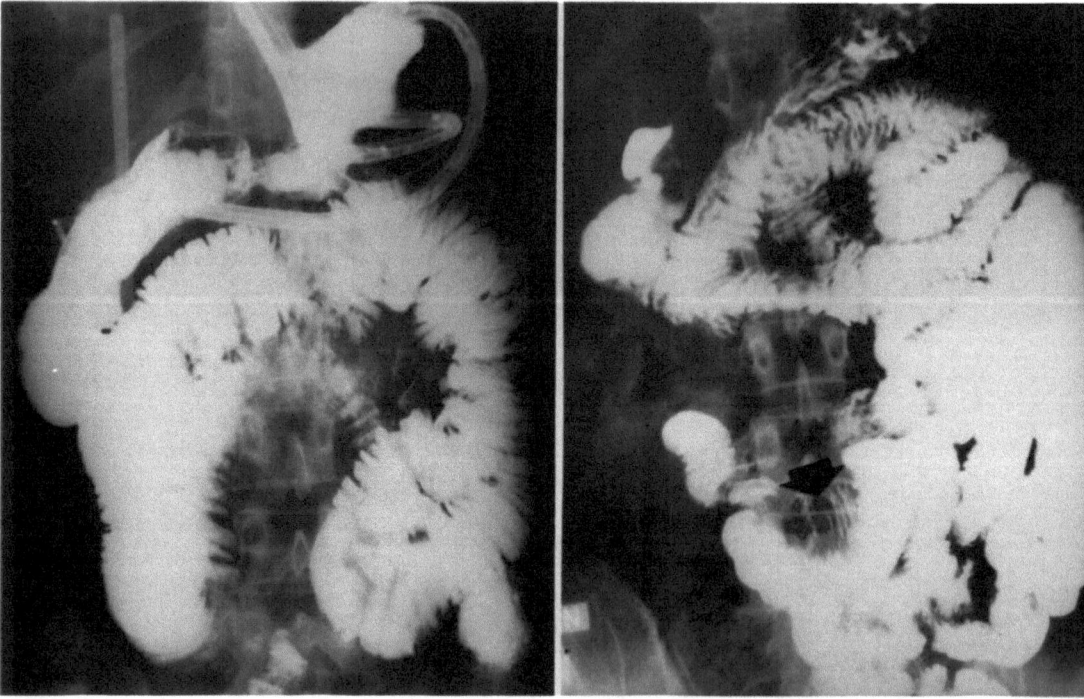

a

b

Fig. 12-12, a and b. Radiation enteritis with mesenteric involvement and obstruction. a The proximal bowel loops are markedly dilated in the first study. b In the second, thickening of the mesentery causes angular distortion of the bowel lumen. Note the traction changes on one side of the stretched loops of small intestine (arrow). This mimics the appearance of metastatic neoplasms in the mesentery.

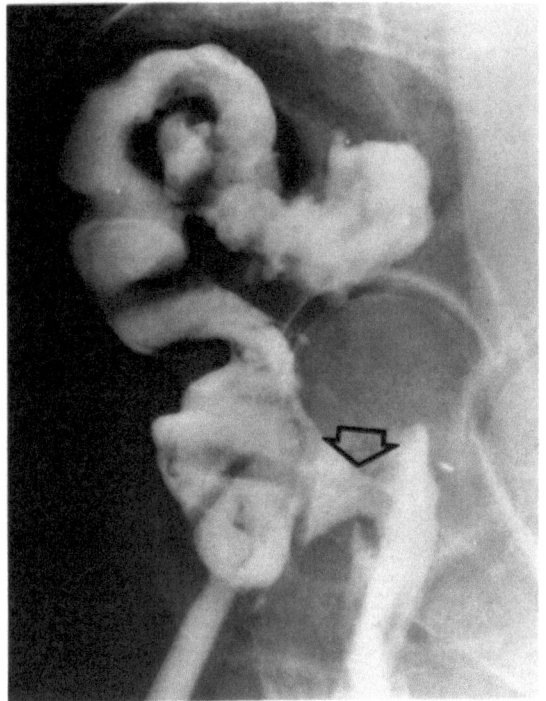

a

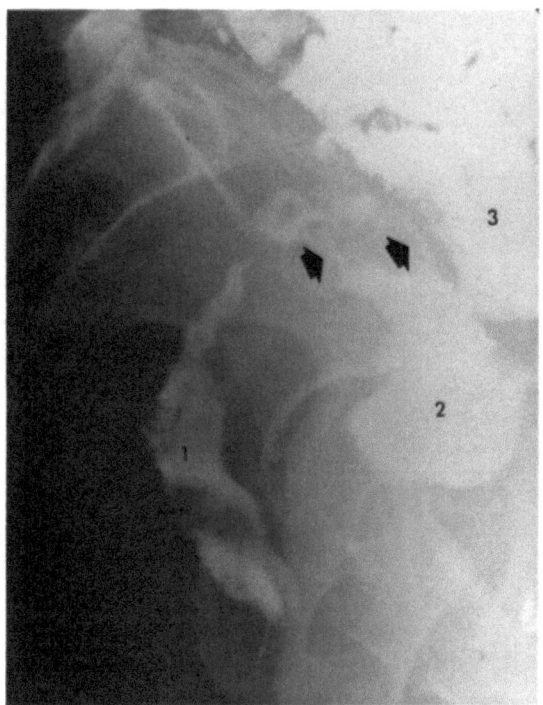

b

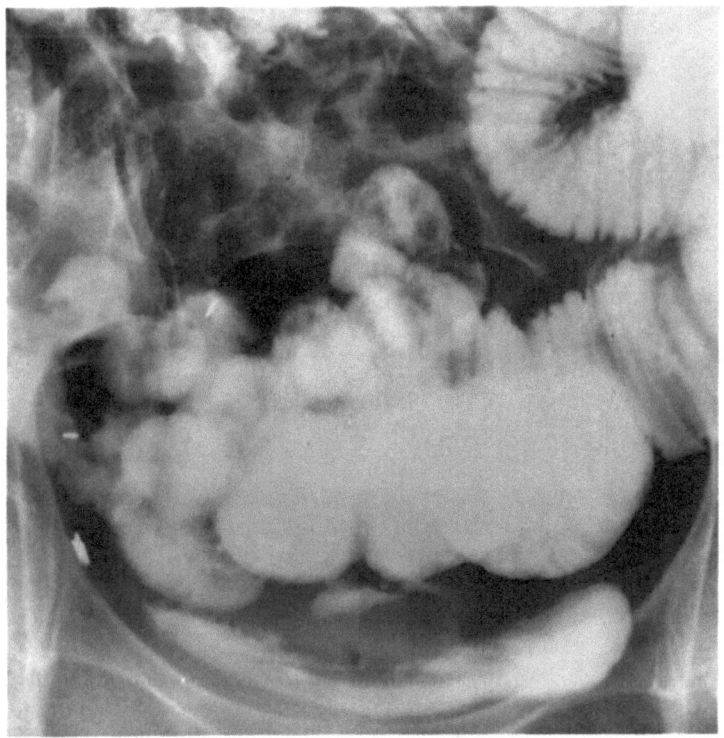

c

Fig. 12-13, a–c. Fistula formation complicating radiation enteritis after treatment for carcinoma of the cervix. a Lateral view in barium enema study demonstrates a large rectovaginal fistula (arrow). b Lateral view in small-bowel examination of second patient demonstrates enterorectovesical fistulas (arrows) (1, rectum; 2, bladder; 3, small bowel). c In the third patient there is an enterovesical fistula arising from the distal ileum. (Reproduced with permission from Rogers LF, Goldstein HM: Roentgen diagnosis of radiation injury of the gastrointestinal tract. In M.D. Anderson Hospital and Tumor Institute, Houston: Radiologic and Other Biophysical Methods in Tumor Diagnosis. Copyright © 1975 by Year Book Medical Publishers, Inc., Chicago)

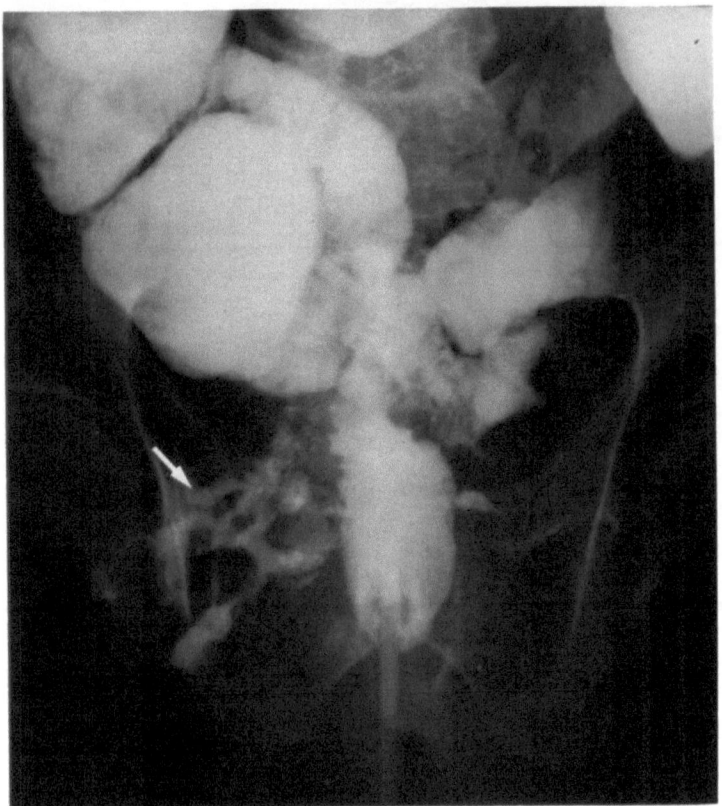

a

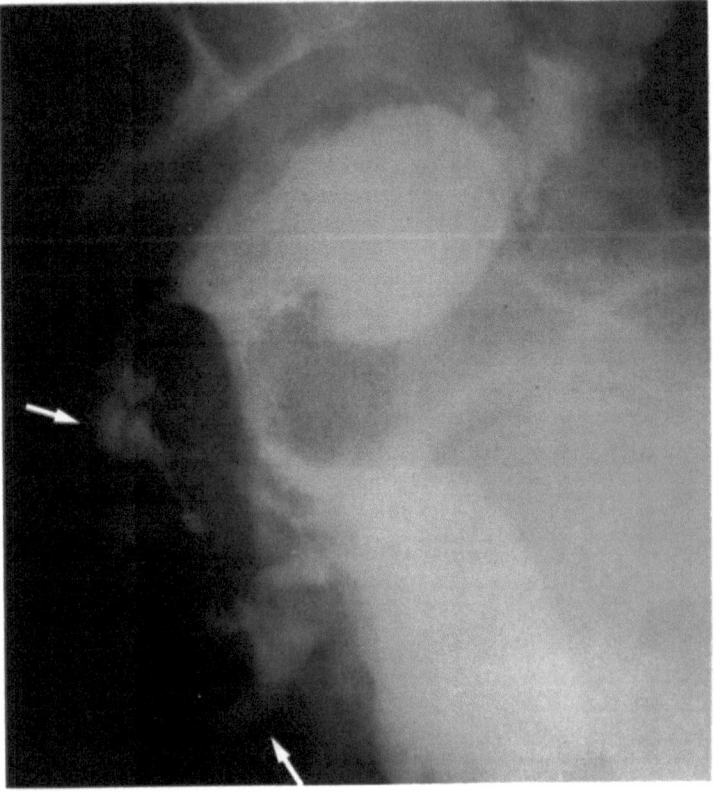

b

Fig. 12-14, a and b. Radiation colitis
with fistula formation. The 74-year-
old male was previously treated for
carcinoma of the bladder. a Barium
enema study reveals narrowing of
rectosigmoid colon with extensive
fistula formation (arrow). b Lateral
projection shows that most of the fistulas extend into the posterior peri-
rectal space (arrows).

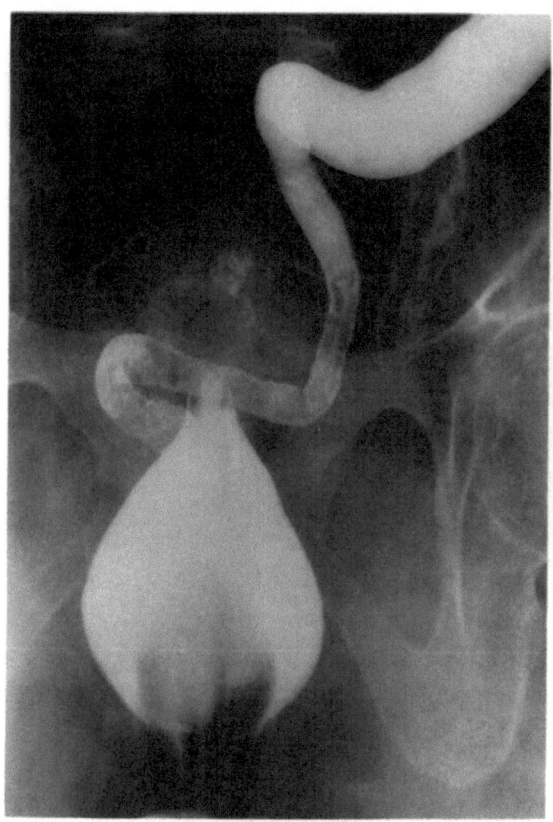

a

Colon

The rectum and sigmoid are the most common sites of radiation injury of the large bowel, although any portion of the colon may be affected. Clinical manifestations are abdominal pain, diarrhea, tenesmus, and bright red rectal bleeding. The clinical management is difficult since the disease is progressive. Surgical resection may be necessary, and postoperative complications are frequent because of the compromised vascularity of the bowel.

The most common radiographic manifestation is a smooth, elongated narrowing of the rectum and sigmoid colon (23,25) (Figs. 12-15a,b). The affected segment is frequently straightened and often elevated out of the pelvis because of combined thickening of the bowel wall and the surrounding pelvic tissues. When a radiation-induced colonic stricture is relatively short and has rather abrupt transition margins, it may closely resemble primary carcinoma (4). Ulceration of the mucosa is frequent; it may be superficial (Fig. 12-15c) or penetrating (Figs. 12-16a,b). Sinus tracts are encountered that may at times appear similar to diverticulitis. Submu-

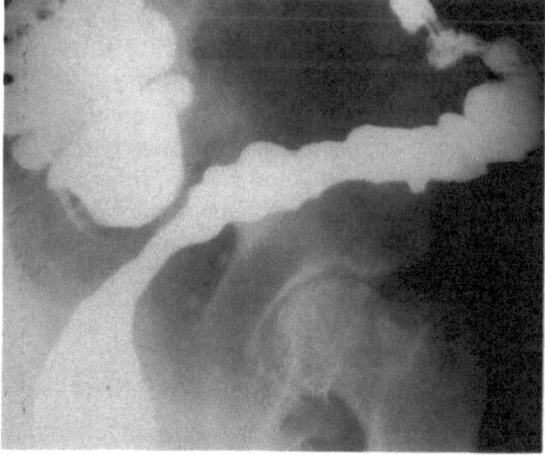

b

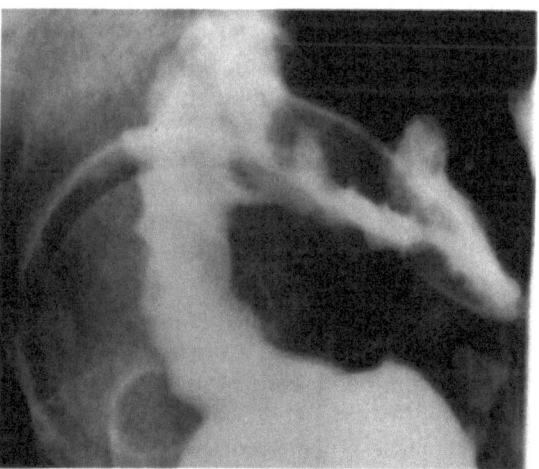

c

Fig. 12-15, a–c. Radiation injury of the colon. a In this patient barium enema study demonstrates the characteristic finding of radiation colitis: a smooth stricture of the rectosigmoid and distal sigmoid colon. **b** In a patient who received treatment for carcinoma of the prostate a slightly undulating, elongated stricture of the rectosigmoid colon is identified. **c** There is a long, irregular stricture of the rectosigmoid. When this type of stricture is shorter it mimics primary carcinoma.

The patient was previously treated for carcinoma of cervix.

(Fig. 12-15 a reproduced with permission from Rogers LF, Goldstein HM: Roentgen diagnosis of radiation injury of the gastrointestinal tract. In M.D. Anderson Hospital and Tumor Institute, Houston: Radiologic and Other Biophysical Methods in Tumor Diagnosis. Copyright © 1975 by Year Book Medical Publishers, Inc., Chicago.)

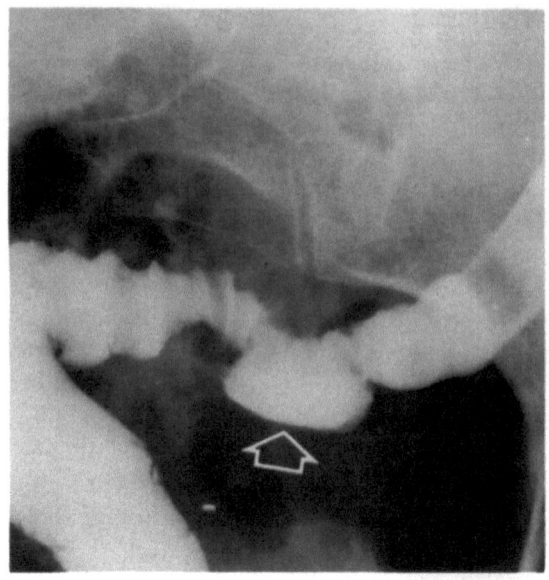

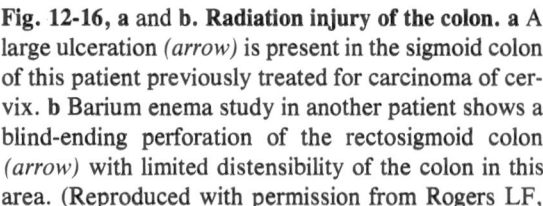

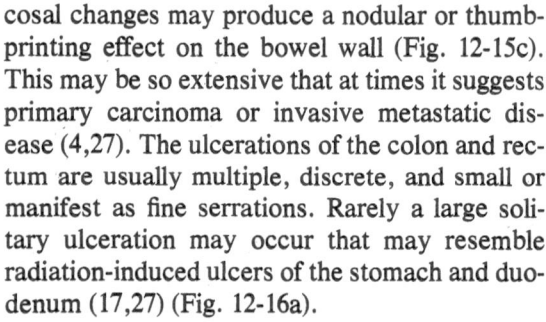

a

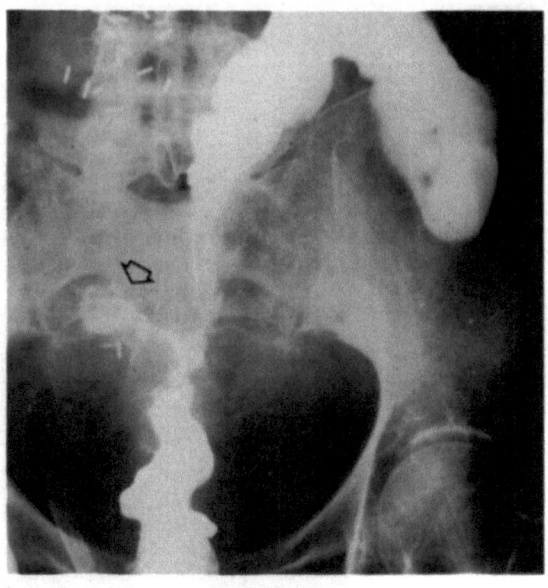

b

Fig. 12-16, a and **b. Radiation injury of the colon. a** A large ulceration *(arrow)* is present in the sigmoid colon of this patient previously treated for carcinoma of cervix. **b** Barium enema study in another patient shows a blind-ending perforation of the rectosigmoid colon *(arrow)* with limited distensibility of the colon in this area. (Reproduced with permission from Rogers LF, Goldstein HM: Roentgen diagnosis of radiation injury of the gastrointestinal tract. In M.D. Anderson Hospital and Tumor Institute, Houston: Radiologic and Other Biophysical Methods in Tumor Diagnosis. Copyright © 1975 by Year Book Medical Publishers, Inc., Chicago)

cosal changes may produce a nodular or thumbprinting effect on the bowel wall (Fig. 12-15c). This may be so extensive that at times it suggests primary carcinoma or invasive metastatic disease (4,27). The ulcerations of the colon and rectum are usually multiple, discrete, and small or manifest as fine serrations. Rarely a large solitary ulceration may occur that may resemble radiation-induced ulcers of the stomach and duodenum (17,27) (Fig. 12-16a).

Rectal bleeding is a most common complication of radiation injury to the colon. Bleeding may occur in the absence of identifiable ulceration. Clinically significant obstruction may occur but is much less common than small-intestinal obstruction. Fistula formation is frequent, particularly rectovaginal (Fig. 12-13a).

Carcinoma of the rectum or sigmoid has been reported to arise within areas of chronic radiation injury (14,36,37), within an area of stenosis and demonstrating irregular and abrupt margination with mucosal destruction. This usually occurred a long time after the initial radiation. I am unaware of such a case in my clinical experience. The incidence of this complication is certainly low. In fact, there is some dispute whether this is a sequela of radiation injury or a coincidental de-novo carcinoma.

The differential diagnosis of radiation injury of the colon includes inflammatory colitis, from which it can be readily distinguished by the clinical history, and, in some cases, primary carcinoma or secondary involvement from recurrent neoplasm. In primary or recurrent neoplasm, distinction may not be made with certainty, and biopsy may be necessary.

Complications: Diagnosis and Management

Obstruction is the most common complication of gastrointestinal radiation injury (6,15,22,35). Usually occurring in the small bowel, it may occasionally occur in the sigmoid colon (Fig. 12-17a). The obstruction may result from significant narrowing due to intrinsic stenosis or adhesions at one or more points, but obstruction of equal severity may also occur from longer segments of less narrow but rigid bowel (Figs. 12-9a,b;12-11).

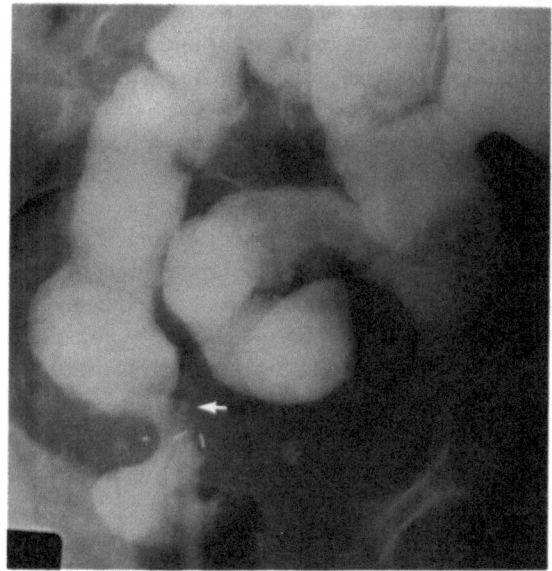

a

Rectal bleeding is a common complication of radiation injury. It is usually chronic from single or multiple ulcerations in the small or large bowel. Bleeding may be present without radiologic demonstration of ulceration, particularly in the small bowel. Mesenteric angiography has been utilized to evaluate and localize bleeding sites in radiation enteritis (Fig. 12-10) and colitis (38–40) (Fig. 12-17). Arterial stenosis and occlusions are identified; the vasa recta are tortuous, distorted, and crowded, indicating bowel shortening. The bowel wall may be avascular, or a capillary blush may be demonstrated. The draining veins are occasionally stenotic with irregular lumina; at times, arteriovenous shunting is demonstrated. Transcatheter embolization has been utilized in the treatment of bleeding from radiation injury in the rectum and sigmoid colon (Fig. 12-17).

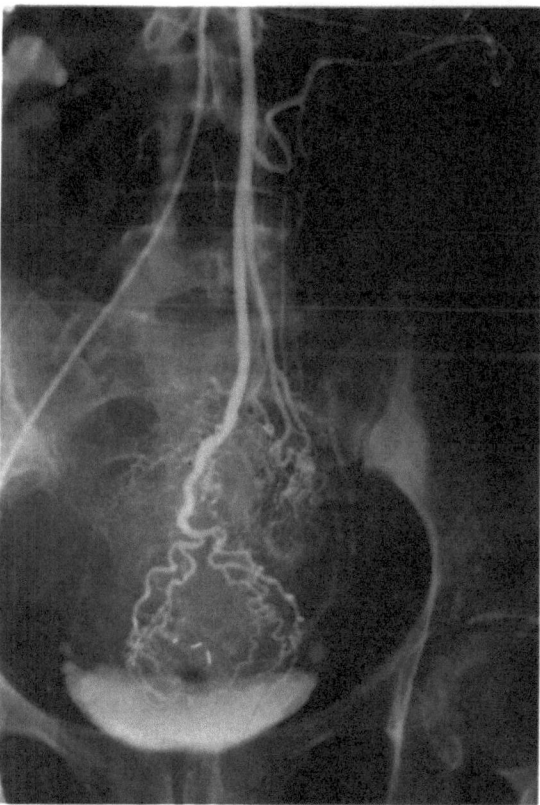

b

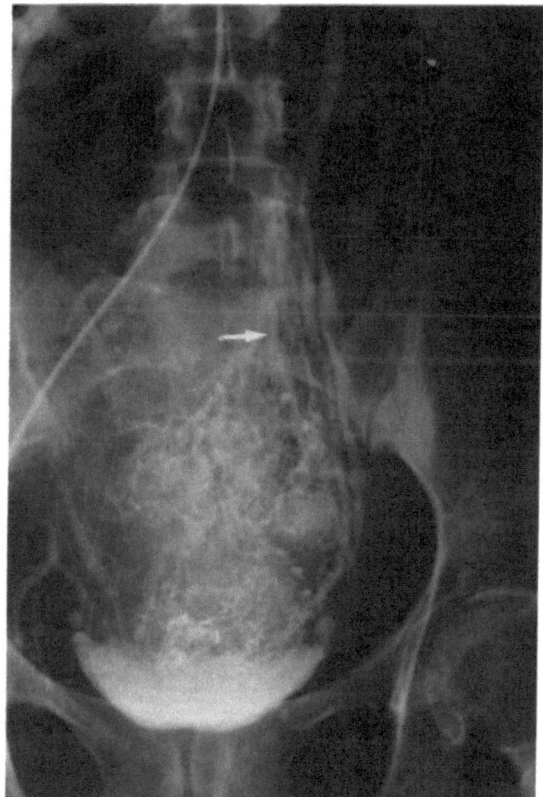

c

Fig. 12-17, a–c. Radiation colitis. A 42-year-old female treated 10 months previously for stage IIb carcinoma of the cervix now has profuse bleeding from the rectosigmoid colon. a Barium enema examination demonstrates stenosis of rectosigmoid colon with ulceration *(arrow)*. b Inferior mesenteric angiogram shows angular distortion and tortuosity of the smaller arterial branches supplying the rectosigmoid. c In the late arterial phase early draining veins are demonstrated *(arrow)*. The bleeding was successfully treated by gel foam embolization of the inferior mesenteric artery. The patient died 7 months later of disseminated disease without recurrence of colonic bleeding.

Fistula formation is a frequent consequence of radiation enteritis and colitis and may occur between any adjacent hollow viscera—small bowel, distal colon, bladder, vagina, and skin in any combination. Rectovaginal, enterovaginal, and enterovesical fistulas are particularly common (Fig. 12-13). Radiologic demonstration of a fistula is important to the clinical management of the patient. Overlapping of the vagina, bladder, small bowel, and rectum makes demonstration of a fistula between these structures very difficult on the frontal projection. Steep oblique and lateral views of the pelvis and lower abdomen are particularly important since the fistulas are frequently best demonstrated in these projections (17,18,27) (Fig. 12-13). Examination in the upright position may also be helpful. Sinus tract formation is frequent (Figs. 12-14, 12-16).

Free perforation of necrotic bowel into the peritoneal cavity may also occur and result in an acute surgical emergency.

Thickened, nodular, fixed, and possibly ulcerated bowel may be easily confused with regional enteritis, lymphoma, and especially recurrent metastatic disease. The various colonic changes might be confused with acute or chronic inflammatory colitis, ischemic colitis, and primary carcinoma. If any question exists the diagnosis should be proved by biopsy before the patient is consigned to treatment for recurrent or metastatic disease.

A small number of individuals receiving pelvic irradiation will sustain injuries to the ureters and bladder. Therefore, full evaluation of pelvic radiation injury requires intravenous pyelography and possibly cystography in search of ure-

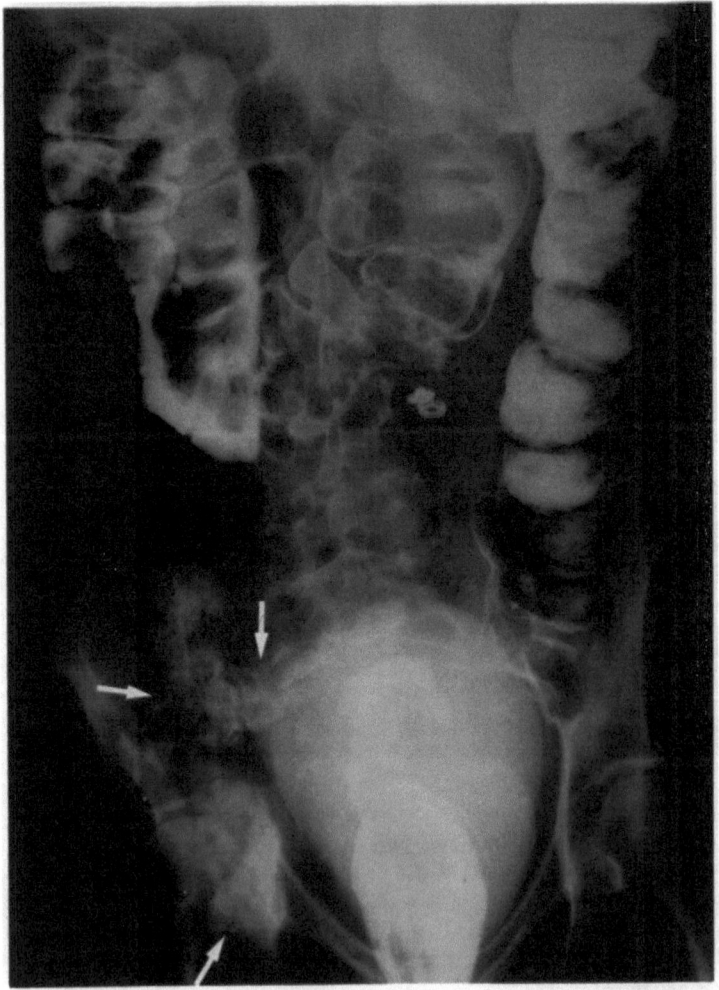

Fig. 12-18. Radiation colitis associated with radiation osteitis complicated by osteosarcomatous degeneration. The 51-year-old female had received two full courses of pelvic irradiation for carcinoma of the cervix, 15 and 16 years prior to this examination. She now complains of pain in the right hip. Radiation colitis is present with partial obstruction due to a sigmoid stricture. An irregular lytic and blastic destructive lesion of the right hemipelvis is demonstrated (arrows), which proved to be osteosarcoma.

teral stenosis and bladder contraction. In an even smaller number roentgenographic evidence of radiation osteitis will be manifest by irregular sclerosis in portions of the pelvic bones, particularly the ilium and sacrum. This is ordinarily not clinically significant, but it can serve as a clue to the etiology of associated abnormalities of the bowel. Rarely, radiation-induced sarcoma of bone occurs (Fig. 12-18).

Although most chronic radiation injury of the bowel becomes apparent 6–24 months following completion of therapy, at times there may be a delay of 10 years or more before the injury is manifest. It may then become evident because supervening atherosclerotic changes frequently associated with hypertension, diabetes, or aging accentuate preexisting radiation vascular injury of the bowel. Similarly the vascular compromise may be increased and symptoms precipitated by abdominal surgery, such as elective cholecystectomy, for circumstances unrelated to either the primary cancer or irradiation injury.

The *prognosis* associated with radiation injury to the bowel is guarded. The mortality is reported to be 15%–37% (35). Many of the deaths occur in the absence of identifiable malignant disease. Surgical resection is frequently required and carries with it an appreciable risk of complications. In any event the problem is difficult to control, and those afflicted rarely become symptom free despite the best pharmacologic and surgical management.

References

1. Fletcher GH: Parameters in radiotherapy complications. In Libshitz HI (ed): Diagnostic Roentgenology of Radiotherapy Change. Baltimore: Williams & Wilkins pp1–2, 1979
2. Localio SA, Stone A, Friedman M: Surgical aspects of radiation enteritis. Surg, Gynecol Obstet 129:1163–1172, 1969
3. Phillips TL, Margolis L: Radiation pathology and the clinical rsponse of lung and esophagus. In Vaeth JM (ed): Radiation Effect and Tolerance, Normal Tissue. Basic concepts in radiation pathology. Proc. Sixth Annual SanFrancisco Cancer Symposium, October 1970. Front Radiat Ther Oncol 6:254–273, 1972 Baltimore: University Park Press
4. Todd TF: Rectal ulceration following irradiation treatment of carcinoma of the cervix uteri, pseudo-carcinoma of the rectum. Surg Gynecol Obstet 67:617–631, 1938
5. Rubin P, Casarett G: Alimentary tract: Small and large intestines and rectum. In Rubin P, Casarett G: Clinical Radiation Pathology. Philadelphia: Saunders 1968, pp.193–240
6. Strockbine MF, Hancok JE, Fletcher GH: Complications in 831 patients with squamous cell carcinoma of the intact uterine cervix treated with 3,000 rads or more whole pelvis irradiation. Am J Roentgenol 108:292–304, 1970
7. Roswit B, Malsky SJ, Reid CB: Severe radiation injuries of the stomach, small intestine, colon and rectum. Am J Roentgenol 114:460–475, 1972
8. Roswit B: Complications of radiation therapy: The alimentary tract. Semin Roentgenol 9:51–63, 1974
9. Goldstein HM, Rogers LF, Fletcher GH, et al: Radiological manifestations of radiation-induced injury to the normal upper gastrointestinal tract. Radiology 117:135–140, 1975
10. Goldstein HM: Esophagus, stomach and duodenum. In Libshitz HI (ed): Diagnostic Roentgenology of Radiotherapy Change. Baltimore: Williams & Wilkins 1979, pp. 69–84
11. Jampolis S, Martin P, Schroder P, et al: Treatment tolerance and early complications with extended field irradiation in gynecological cancer. Br J Radiol 50:195–199, 1977
12. Joelsson I, Raf L, Soderberg G: Stenosis of the small bowel as a complication in radiation therapy of carcinoma of the uterine cervix. Acta Radiol 10:593–604, 1971
13. Maruyama Y, Van Nagell JR, Jr., Utley J, et al: Radiation and small bowel complications in cervical carcinoma therapy. Radiology 112:699–703, 1974
14. Kaplan AL, Hudgins PT, Wall JA: Injury of the small intestine following irradiation for gynecologic cancer. South Med Journal 58:1109–1114, 1965
15. DeCosse JJ, Rhodes RS, Wentz WB, et al: The natural history and management of radiation induced injury of the gastrointestinal tract. Ann Surg 170:369–384, 1969
16. Rubin P, Casarett GW: Clinical Radiation Pathology. Philadelphia: Saunders 1968, pp. 153–192
17. Rogers LF, Goldstein HM: Roentgen diagnosis of radiation injury of the gastrointestinal tract. In MD Anderson Hospital and Tumor Institute: Radiologic and Other Biophysical Methods in Tumor Diagnosis. Chicago: Year Book 1975, pp. 345–357
18. Goldstein HM: Small bowel and colon. In Libshitz HI (ed): Diagnostic Roentgenology of Radiotherapy Change. Baltimore: William & Wilkins 1979, pp. 85–100
19. Perkins DE, Spjut HJ: Intestinal stenosis following radiation therapy, a roentgenologic-pathologic study. Am J Roentgenol 88:953–966, 1962
20. Seaman WB, Ackerman LV: The effect of radiation on the esophagus. A clinical and histologic study of the effects produced by the betatron. Radiology 68:534–540, 1957

21. Kottmeier HL: Complications following radiation therapy in carcinoma of the cervix and their treatment. Am J Obstet Gynecol 88:854–866, 1964

22. Smith AN, Douglas M, McLean N, et al: Intestinal complications of pelvic irradiation for gynecologic cancer. Surg Gynecol Obstet 127:721–728, 1968

23. Mason GR, Dietrich P, Friedland GW, et al: The radiological findings in radiation-induced enteritis and colitis, a review of 30 cases. Clin Radiol 21:232–247, 1970

24. Brick IB: Effects of million volt irradiation on the gastrointestinal tract. Arch Intern Med 96:26–31, 1955

25. Fletcher GH, Rutledge FN: Extended field technique in the management of the cancers of the uterine cervix. Am J Roentgenol 114:116–122, 1972

26. Friedman M: Calculated risks of radiation injury of normal tissue in the treatment of cancer of the testis. Proc Second National Cancer Conference. New York: American Cancer Society 1954, pp. 390–400

27. Rogers LF, Goldstein HM: Roentgen manifestations of radiation injury to the gastrointestinal tract. Gastrointest Radiol 2:281–291, 1977

28. Chau PM, Fletcher GH, Rutledge FN, et al: Complications in high dose whole pelvis irradiation in female pelvic cancer. Am J Roentgenol 87:22–40, 1962

29. Hamilton FE: Gastric ulcer following radiation. Arch Surg 55:394–399, 1947

30. Sell A, Skov Jensen T: Acute gastric ulcers induced by radiation. Acta Radiol 4:289–297, 1966

31. Sylven B, Vikterlof KH, Schnurer LB: Gastric ulceration following cobalt teletherapy, estimation of the tolerance dose. Acta Radiol 8:183–188, 1969

32. Bowers RF, Brick IB: Surgery in radiation injury of the stomach. Surgery 22:20–40, 1947

33. Feiring W, Jampol ML: Perforation of a gastric ulcer following intensive radiation therapy. N Engl J Med 242:751–753, 1950

34. Lane D: Irradiation gastritis simulating carcinoma. Med J Aust 2:576–577, 1970

35. Wellwood JM, Jackson BT: The intestinal complications of radiotherapy. Br J Surg 60:814–818, 1973

36. Black WC, Acker LV: Carcinoma of the large intestine as a late complication of pelvic radiotherapy. Clin Radiol 16:278–281, 1965

37. McMahon CE, Rowe JW: Rectal reaction following radiation therapy of cervical carcinoma: Particular reference to subsequent occurrence of rectal carcinoma. Ann Surg 173:264–269, 1971

38. Bosniak MA, Hardy MA, Quint J, et al: Demonstration of the effect of irradiation on canine bowel using in vivo photographic magnification angiography. Radiology 93:1361–1368, 1969

39. Dencker H, Holmdahl KH, Lunderquist A, et al: Mesenteric angiography in patients with radiation injury of the bowel after pelvis irradiation. Am J Roentgenol 114:476–481, 1972

40. Sprayregen S, Glotzer P: Angiographic demonstration of radiation colitis. Am J Roentgenol 113:335–337, 1971

Index